# Contents

HEINEMANN
AVCE

ADVANCED

# Health and Social Care

Editor: Neil Moonie
Richard Chaloner
Kip Chan Pensley
Beryl Stretch
David Webb

FOR THE 2000 STANDARDS



ELIZABETH MUSADZIRUMA

LONDON BRITTANNIA College

46 Peartree Way, Stevenage

Heinemann Educational Publishers,
Halley Court, Jordan Hill, Oxford OX2 8EJ
Part of Harcourt Education

Heinemann is the registered trademark of Harcourt Education Limited



First published 1996

Third edition published 2000

2004
10 9

A catalogue record for this book is available from the British Library on request.

ISBN 0 435 45589 3



Edited by Linda Claris Mellor

Picture research by Jennifer Johnson

Typeset by TechType, Abingdon, Oxfordshire

Printed and bound in Great Britain by Scotprint

Tel: 01865 888058 www.heinemann.co.uk

# Introduction to the 2000 edition

This book has been written to support students who are studying for a Vocational A-level in Health and Social Care. The book is designed in six units or chapters, which cover the Compulsory units of the new Curriculum 2000 National Standards.

The six compulsory units will form the core of the different Vocational A-level awards that will be offered by all awarding bodies.

These six units are:

Unit 1: Equal Opportunities and Client's Rights

Unit 2: Communicating in Health and Social Care

Unit 3: Physical Aspects of Health

Unit 4: Factors Affecting Human Growth and Development

Unit 5: Health, Social Care and Early Years Services

Unit 6: Research Perspectives in Health and Social Care

Each chapter unit of this book has been organised to follow the content specified for the corresponding unit of national standards. Headings are designed to make it easy to follow the content of each unit and to find all the knowledge and other details needed in order to achieve a high grade.

## Assessment

Units will be assessed either by an assignment or by an external test, which will be set and marked by the awarding body. At the time of writing this book the authors expected Unit 1 and Unit 4 to be externally tested. Units 2, 3, 5 and 6 are likely to be assessed through project work marked internally within the school or college delivering the A-level.

External tests are expected to require short written answers to questions. These questions may often be based on case studies or brief descriptions of situations. All the chapter units in this book have a brief test at the end. This is not because all units will be tested. The tests are intended to offer a revision check for students who wish to test their understanding of the chapter unit. The tests may also provide some outline guidance to help preparation for the external tests.

## Special features of the book

Throughout the text there are a number of features which are designed to encourage reflection and discussion and to help relate theory to practice in Health and Social Care. Many activities may also help to develop **key skills** by practising numeracy, communication and ICT. The features are:

**Think it over** — thought provoking questions or dilemmas, which can be used for individual reflection or possibly for group discussion

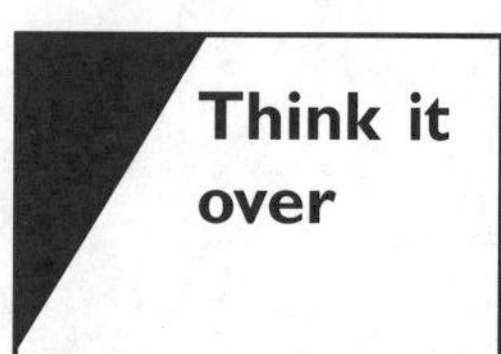


**Did you know?** — interesting facts or snippets of information about Health and Social Care issues

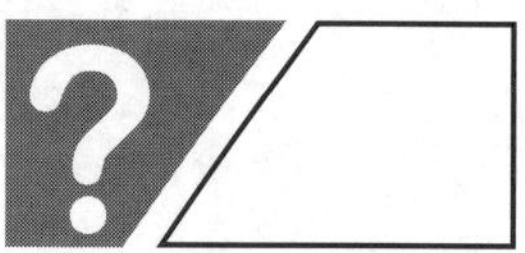

**Try it out** activities to encourage the application of theory in practice

| **Try it out** | |
|---|---|

**Case studies** brief stories or situations which help to explain the relevance of key issues and how theory relates to practise.

**Assessment guidance** each chapter unit offers some ideas to help prepare for the standards expected at an E grade level, C grade level and A grade level. This assessment guidance has been developed from the assessment grid provided for each unit within national standards.

There are further useful features at the end of each chapter unit:

**Fast facts** a glossary of key terms

**References** a list of references, recommended further reading and useful web sites.

At the end of the book is a comprehensive index.


## Acknowledgements

The authors and publishers would like to thank the following individuals and organisations for permission to reproduce tables, photographs and other material.

The Controller of HMSO – Crown copyright material reproduced with permission
Gareth Boden
Camera Press/William Conran
Format/Roshini Kempadoo
Format/Sally Lancaster
Format/Maggie Murray
Format/Joanne O'Brien
Format/Ulrike Preuss
Sally & Richard Greenhill
Health Promotion England
Kate Makepeace for her contribution to Unit 1
Sheila Mulvenney for contributing sections to the book on Early Years organisations
The National Centre for Social Research
School for Urban Studies, University of Bristol
Gerald Sutherland
Popperfoto
The Winged Fellowship Trust.

Tel: 01865 888058 www.heinemann.co.uk

# Equal opportunities and clients' rights

Unit 1

**Anyone who works in the health and social care sector needs to know about equal opportunities and how to promote equality and challenge discrimination. Equal opportunities is both a legal and a moral issue. On the legal side there is legislation and policies in place that have to be implemented in practice in the working environment. On the moral side, it is the responsibility of every individual to promote equality and work within the framework of care values.**

**The unit is organised in five sections. You will learn about:**

- **promoting equality in care practice**
- **the legislation, policies and codes of practice for promoting equality**
- **how care organisations promote equality**
- **the effects of discriminatory practices on individuals**
- **the role and functions of organisations that challenge discrimination.**

**The unit concludes with advice on meeting the test requirements for unit 1.**

## 1.1 Promoting equality in care practice

All human societies, and large-scale social groupings, need to have rules or principles which establish how people are expected to behave in relation to other people. One of the oldest and most well known set of principles for regulating society is the 'Law of Moses', known as the Ten Commandments in the Old Testament of the Bible. These principles have established a foundation for Jewish, Christian and Islamic societies. They include rules about the importance of human life, 'Thou shalt not kill', laws about property, 'Thou shalt not steal', and laws about family life, 'Thou shalt honour thy father and mother' and 'Thou shalt not commit adultery'.

### Principles which underpin equality of opportunity

Foundational principles such as these provide a structure for the organisation of a society. However, whilst all effective societies must have principles, not all societies share the same principles. Even the importance of human life has not been accepted or seen in the same way by all human societies. There have been societies which have made a virtue of male aggression and where the social status of a man, including his right to marry and have children, has depended on the number of people he has killed. The philosophy behind this was that a high level of aggression would increase the military power of the society and enable it to conquer and exploit other societies. However, the lesson of history appears to be that a society which develops this way tends to become completely disorganised as individuals compete with each other. Far from achieving military dominance, such societies may collapse and be taken over by more socially cohesive and organised cultures.

Some societies have avoided the idea of property rights. Tools, clothes and equipment are 'owned' communally, i.e. people use things as they wish and as they need them – they do not belong to any individual. Such a principle might work, and it is possible to find examples of successful communities which share everything. The problem lies in organising very large-scale societies, with millions of people, so that everyone is fed, housed and has their basic needs met. Without the 'institution' or social belief in property rights there may be difficulties in organising a society.

The principles of equality and individual rights and choice are not merely simple ideas about being nice to others or about being 'good'. Like principles about the importance of life, or rules about property, equality and individuality are foundational values which will influence how a society functions.

Modern western societies describe themselves as *democracies.* The democratic theory is that political power and economic control depend on the wishes of a majority of the population. The majority voice their wishes by electing a 'party' to power. The party then makes day-to-day decisions about the operation and regulation of society.

As a generalisation, a democracy depends on the principle of individuals having the freedom to voice differing political opinions. Democracy balances a wide range of individual freedoms with the general wishes of a *majority* (or 'greater number of people'). Respect for individual rights, and having individual rights to make choices, are an essential part of the principles which underlie a society organised as a 'democracy'.

By contrast, centralised Communist societies do not organise themselves around principles of individual rights. In some recent Communist societies it was essential that people understood themselves not as individuals but solely as members of a large group. Conformity to group belief systems and behaviour patterns was seen as a foundational principle of some Communist societies. Sometimes the Communist system has been confused with personality cults.

## Democracy and competition

Western democracies adopt the notion of competition as an organisational principle of society. Individuals must compete with one another to make money and achieve economic success. Part of this competitive ethic, or principle, is that no group should be discriminated against or prevented from the opportunity to compete. Equality of opportunity legislation is aimed at ensuring that factors like gender, race and disability do not exclude certain groups of people from the chance to compete. This principle

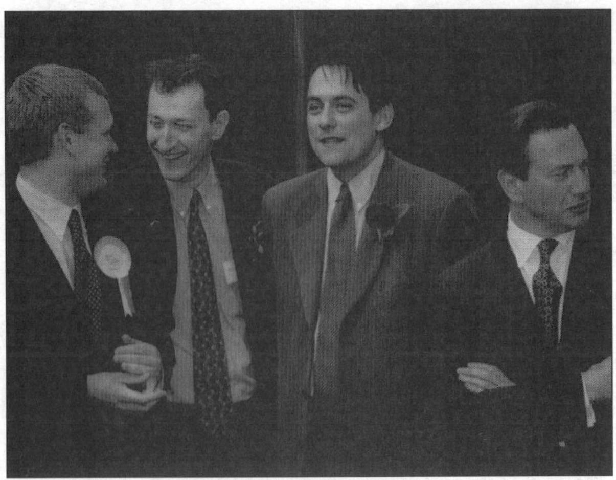

**Figure 1.1 In democracy people are allowed to express different political opinions**

of equality does not necessarily mean that every person has the same chance in the 'competition'. It is a principle of not excluding people because of their group membership or origins.

Another reason for equal opportunity principles relates to the multicultural nature of western societies. Britain has been a society with a variety of religions, including people of different racial origins and different customs and practices, for many centuries. There is an argument that Britain has a long history of being multicultural (meaning, many customs, cultures and beliefs). For a multicultural society to function smoothly it may be important that the equality between different cultures, as well as individual rights, are respected.

These principles of democracy, individual rights and choice, and equality have resulted in laws aimed at promoting equality of opportunity. These principles and laws will influence how our society functions.

## The care value base

Health and care work in a democratic society takes place in the context of beliefs about individual rights, choice and freedom. David Seedhouse (1988) argues that health and care work should not simply be about meeting physical needs or curing disease and illness. Seedhouse quotes the World Health Organisation's definition that: 'Health is a state of complete physical, social and mental well-being, not merely the absence of disease, illness and infirmity'. Seedhouse goes on to argue that, 'Curing disease and illness and increasing the length of life remain important, but not as important as creating and increasing the autonomy of people who request, or need health care . . . [and] respecting people's choices even if they conflict with given advice' (page 9). The central purpose of health and care work is to improve quality of life and this means enabling people to take control of their own life or to be 'autonomous'. If care workers are to improve the quality of life for clients then they must meet people's emotional and social needs and not just focus on physical needs.

Abraham Maslow (1908–1970) established a way of understanding human need which has become very well known (see Chapter 4 for details of this theory). In outline, Maslow believed that people have a range of different types of need. Adults can only live a fulfilled and worthwhile life when their physical, safety, belonging and self-esteem needs are met. (See Figure 4.60 on page 322.)

Authors such as David Seedhouse argue that health and social care workers have a moral obligation to work in ways which go beyond meeting basic physical needs. Workers must also create psychological safety and help people to maintain or establish links with family, friends and society. Care workers must be sensitive to and try to meet the self-esteem needs of clients.

Most professions have ethical codes, codes of conduct or value statements which guide the behaviour of members of that profession. Values are particularly important in care work. People who receive health or social care services are usually vulnerable. Clients might be afraid, in pain, unhappy or just simply young and easy to influence. National Vocational Qualifications in Care include a Unit which defines the values which should guide care practice.

Figure 1.2 provides an outline of the main principles of the Care Value Base, which has three main elements. If carers work within the guidance of these values they may foster

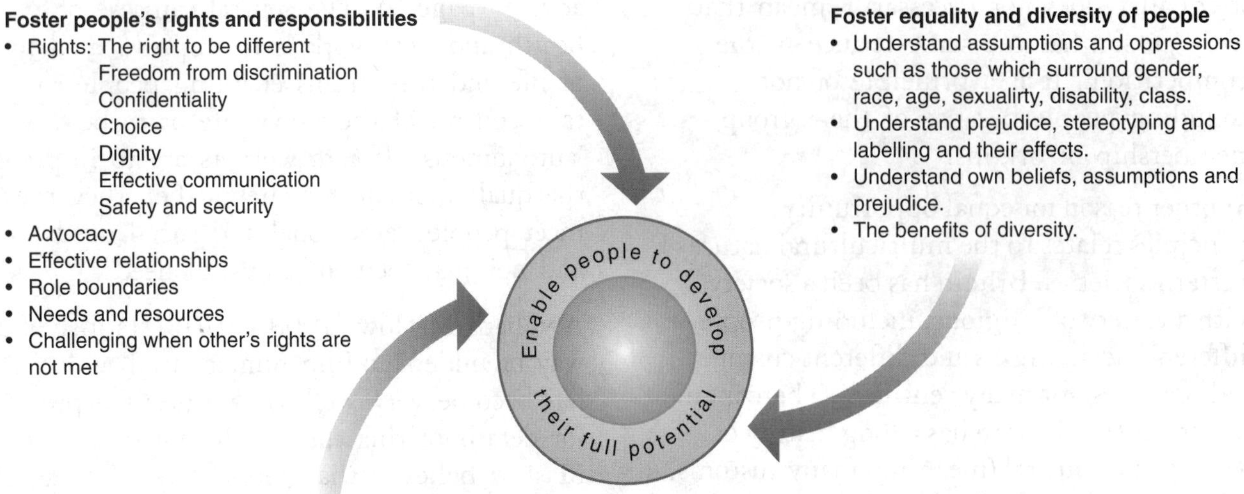


**Maintain the confidentiality of information**

The legal framework: Data Protection Acts, 1984 and 1998,Access to Personal Files Act 1987

- The security of recording systems
- The need and right 'to know'
- Confidentiality can value and protect a client
- Policies, procedures and guidelines
- Boundaries and tensions in maintaining confidentiality.

**Figure 1.2 The care value base: foster people's equality, diversity and rights**

Care Value Base

- **Foster equality and diversity of people**

Carers need to value the ways in which people are different. Carers also need to understand that there are prejudices, stereotypes and assumptions which can discriminate against people from different gender, race, age, sexual orientation, disability or class groups. Carers need to be able to prevent prejudices and assumptions from damaging the quality of care provided to clients.

- **Foster people's rights and responsibilities**

People have a right to their own beliefs and lifestyle, but no one has a right to damage the quality of other people's lives. This means that rights often come with responsibilities toward other people.

The easiest way of understanding this idea is to think about smoking. Adults have a right to choose to smoke, even though smoking usually damages health and often shortens a person's life. Smokers have a responsibility to make sure their smoke is not breathed in by other people. This means that smoking is only allowed in special places nowadays.

- **Maintain the confidentiality of information**

Confidentiality is an important right for all clients. It is important because:

- clients may not trust a carer if the carer does not keep information confidential
- clients may not feel valued or able to keep their self-esteem if their private details are shared with others
- clients' safety may be put at risk if details of their property or their habits are widely known
- a professional service that maintains respect for individuals must keep private information confidential
- there are legal requirements to keep personal records confidential.

**Trust** is important. If you know that your carer will not pass things on, you may feel able to tell him or her what you really think and feel.

**Self-esteem** is involved, because if your carer promises to keep things confidential, it shows that he or she respects and values you; it shows that you matter.

**Safety** is an issue, because you may have to leave your home empty at times. If other people know where you keep your money and when you are out, someone could be tempted to break in. Carers need to keep personal details confidential to protect clients' property and personal safety.

Medical practitioners and lawyers have always strictly observed confidentiality as part of their professional role. If clients are to receive a professional service, care workers must copy this example.

people's equality, diversity and rights. They may also meet human needs in a way which will enable people to develop to their full potential.

## Valuing diversity

People are all different. Because people are different it can be easy to think that some people are better than others, or that some views are right while other views are wrong.

Our own socialisation, culture and life experience may lead us to make assumptions as to what is right or normal. When we meet people who are different, it can be easy to see them as 'not right' or 'not normal'. Different people see the world in different ways. Our own way of thinking may seem unusual to others.

Because people are different there is always the danger of discrimination. Some ways in which people are different from one another are listed below.

- **Age** People may think of others mainly in terms of their age, i.e. as being children, teenagers, young adults, middle aged or old. Discrimination can creep into our thinking if we see some age groups as being 'the best' or if we make assumptions about the abilities of different groups.
- **Gender** People are classified as male or female. In the past, men often had more rights and were seen as more important than women. Assumptions about gender can still create discrimination.
- **Race** People may understand themselves as being Black or White, as European, African or Asian. Many people have specific national identities such as Polish, Nigerian, English or Welsh. Assumptions about racial characteristics lead to discrimination.
- **Class** People differ in their upbringing, the kind of work they do and the money they earn. People also differ in the lifestyles they lead and the views and values that go with levels of income and spending habits. Discrimination against others can be based on their class or lifestyle.
- **Religion** People grow up in different traditions of religion. For some people, spiritual beliefs are at the centre of their understanding of life. For others, religion influences the cultural traditions that they celebrate; for example, many Europeans celebrate Christmas even though they might not see themselves as practising Christians. Discrimination can take place when people assume that their customs or beliefs should apply to everyone else.
- **Sexual orientation** Many people see their sexual orientation as very important to understanding who they are. Gay and lesbian relationships are often discriminated against. Heterosexual people sometimes judge other relationships as 'wrong' or abnormal.
- **Ability** People may make assumptions about what is 'normal'. People with physical disabilities or learning difficulties may be labelled or stereotyped.
- **Health** People who develop illnesses or mental health problems may feel that they are valued less by other people and discriminated against.
- **Relationships** People choose many different lifestyles and emotional commitments, such as: marriage, having children, living in a large family, living a single lifestyle but having sexual partners, being single and not being

sexually active. People live within different family and friendship groups. Discrimination can happen if people think that one lifestyle is 'right' or best.

- **Presentation and dress** People express their individuality, lifestyle and social role through the clothes, hairstyle, make-up and jewellery they wear. While it may be important to conform to social expectations at work, it is also important not to stereotype individuals.

## Learning about diversity

In order to learn about other people's culture and beliefs, it is necessary to listen and watch what other people say and do. Learning about diversity can be interesting and exciting, but some people feel that finding out about different lifestyles can be stressful. We may feel that our own culture and beliefs are being challenged when we realise the different possibilities that exist. Our emotions may block our abilities to learn.

Skilled carers have to get to know the people they work with in order to avoid making false assumptions. In getting to know an individual, carers will also need to understand the ways that class, race, age, gender and other social categories influence the person. A person's culture may include all the social groups they belong to.

There are many different ethnic groups in the world, many different religions, many different cultural values, variations in gender role, and so on. Individuals may belong to the same ethnic group yet belong to different religions or class groups. Knowing someone's religion will not necessarily tell you all of that person's beliefs, or general culture.

You can pick up background knowledge on different ethnic and religious customs, but it is impossible to study all the differences that might exist for individual clients. The best way to learn about diversity is to listen and communicate with people who lead different lives from ourselves.

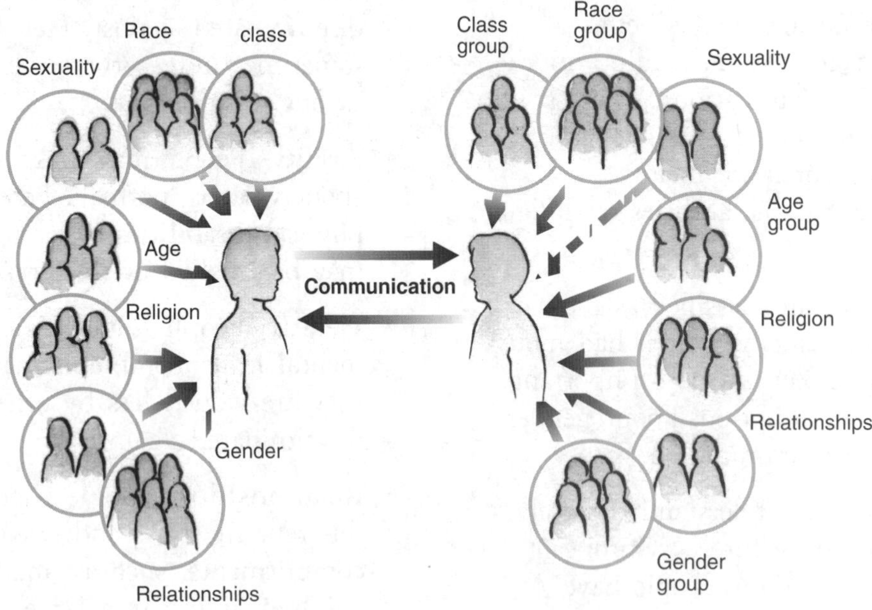


**Figure 1.3 Learning about diversity**

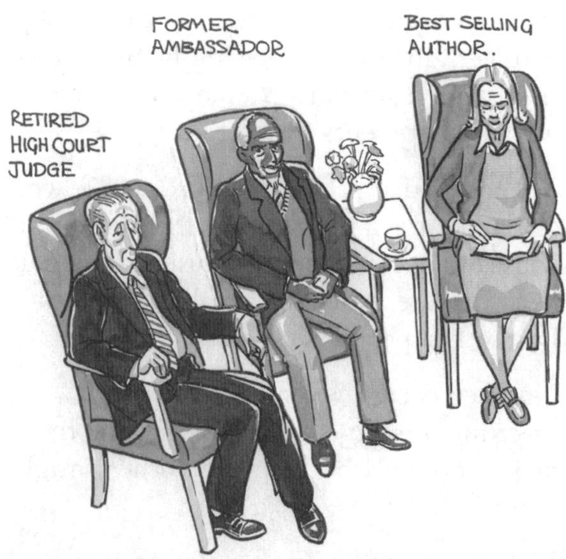


Figure 1.4 Valuing diversity means not assuming everyone is the same

Valuing diversity will enrich your own life. If you are open to understanding other people's life experiences and differences you may be able to become more flexible and creative, because you can imagine how other people see things. You may develop a wider range of social skills because you have met different people, and learning about other cultures may provide you with new experiences – such as new foods to try and new places to visit. Understanding other people's lives may also help you to adapt your own lifestyle when you have to cope with change. For instance, if you talk to people who get married or who have children, you may be more prepared for the changes involved if you choose these roles.

Employers are likely to want to employ people who value diversity because:

- effective non-discriminatory care depends on staff valuing diversity
- people who value diversity are likely to be flexible and creative
- people who value diversity may make good relationships with one another and with clients
- diverse teams often work together effectively. If everyone has the same skills and interests, then team members may compete. If people have different interests there is more chance that the team will cover all the work and enjoy working together.

Within a care setting, everyone should receive service of an equal quality which meets with their own personal needs. This is not the same as everyone receiving the same service. Treating people as individuals with different beliefs, abilities, likes and dislikes is at the heart of caring for others.

If you come across a situation where services are not of equal quality for different groups of people, the best way to start to change this is to raise the subject with management. In care settings there should be policies to help to protect individuals against any discrimination they might meet. Policies on equal opportunities will help to stop discrimination (see section on codes of practice in this chapter, page 39). Equal opportunity policies will help both clients and staff in a care setting by providing standards to which people have to keep.

### Think it over

We live in the 'Communication Age'. It is possible to e-mail around the world and to communicate and trade with a vast range of different people. Prejuidice and stereotyping will limit the possibility of communication and also trade between people.

What problems might exist for people who were prejuidiced in the modern world? Would a prejuidiced person be likely to have restricted job opportunities, leisure opportunities and even a restricted range of friends?

## Rights and responsibilities

The law, codes of practice, employers' policies and national standards outline rights for clients of health and social care services. These rights include:

- freedom from discrimination
- a right to independence and choice
- respect and dignity
- safety and security
- confidentiality.

Table 1.1 provides some examples of rights and responsibilities.

- **Freedom from discrimination**

In care work, discrimination means treating some groups of people less well than others. People are often discriminated against because of their class, race, gender, religion, sexuality or age.

Discrimination may take the following forms:

- **Physical abuse** means hitting, pushing, kicking or otherwise assaulting a person. People may commit assault because they hate certain groups, or simply because they feel frustrated or annoyed by those who are different.
- **Verbal abuse** means insults, 'put downs' or damaging language. Like physical abuse, it may happen because individuals feel they are more powerful if they can hurt other people.
- **Neglect** occurs when people are discriminated against by being ignored or not offered the help that others might receive.
- **Exclusion** is a more subtle form of discrimination, and may be hard to prove. Exclusion means stopping people from getting services or jobs because they belong to a certain class, race or other group. Disabled people may still be excluded from certain services because access is difficult – some buildings do not have full disabled access. Some jobs may not be advertised in all local areas, therefore excluding certain communities.

| People receiving care have a right to: | People receiving care have a responsibility to: |
|---|---|
| • not be discriminated against | • not discriminate against others |
| • have control and independence in their own lives | • help others to be independent and not try to control other people |
| • make choices and take risks | • not interfere with others, or put others or themselves at risk |
| • maintain their own beliefs and lifestyle | • respect the different beliefs and lifestyles of others |
| • be valued and respected | • value and respect others |
| • a safe environment | • to keep things safe for others |
| • confidentiality in personal matters. | • respect confidentiality for others. |

Table 1.1 Rights and responsibilities of clients of health and social services

- **Avoidance** is where people try to avoid sitting next to people or working with people who are different from them. Those who discriminate against others may try to avoid contact – perhaps so that they do not need to learn or re-think any of their prejudices.
- **Devaluing** involves seeing some types of people as less valuable than others. Some people are helped to build self-esteem because they receive praise and their ideas are valued, but people who are 'different' may be criticised and find their ideas ignored. People who are subjected to constant discrimination and prejudice may develop a low sense of self-esteem.

- **Independence and choice**

Although most people think of themselves as being independent, there are times in everybody's life when they need help from others. Independence in care settings can be increased by giving the client control and choice over aspects of their care. It is important to recognise the difference between doing things to/for clients, and doing things *with* clients.

> **Think it over**
>
> Discuss the difference between working *with* clients and working to do things *for* clients. What might be the effects on clients of constantly having things done *for* them?

Wherever possible, clients should be helped to take control over their own care. When people cannot do things for themselves, they can still be asked for their opinion on how they would like the care to be given. This is **empowering** the client. Feeling independent may increase a client's self-esteem and personal satisfaction. Feeling dependent may cause the opposite effect and make the client feel vulnerable.

- **Dignity and respect**

In some care situations it might be difficult to feel dignified. Suppose that tomorrow you were in an accident which put you into hospital. You used to be in control, but now you need help with washing and going to the toilet. How would you feel about another person helping you to use the toilet? If a carer showed respect for your feelings and treated you with dignity, you might not feel so bad.

It is important for clients to feel that they are treated with respect. When working with clients who need help with washing, dressing, using the toilet or eating, it is vital to help them to keep their sense of self-worth and dignity. This means showing respect in the way you give support to clients, not showing negative attitudes and providing privacy.

- **Safety and security**

All clients have the right to feel that they are safe and secure while they are receiving care. They should not have to worry about themselves or their property, but remain free from concern.

The Health and Safety at Work Act (1974) made it a duty of employers to ensure 'the health, safety and welfare at work of employees'. Equally, 'Employees have a duty to take reasonable care for the health and safety of themselves and others'.

When working in a care role it should become part of the daily routine to assess the safety of any situation. If you are working with clients who have impaired movement or poor sensory perception, it is doubly important to ensure that the setting is free from hazards.

### Confidentiality

Confidentiality is a right, but it is so important that it has become a specific area of the NVQ care value base.

The Data Protection Acts 1984 and 1998, Access to Personal Files Act 1987 and Access to Health Records Act 1990, create a legal duty for health and social care agencies to keep clients' details confidential. Further details of these laws can be found later in this chapter.

Often you will be told personal information about the individuals you are caring for. This information needs to be kept confidential and not used freely. Personal information which is passed to the wrong people might lead to the client being discriminated against, or could put them in a position of danger. For example, an old person living alone could be in danger if people found out that she kept her life savings under the mattress.

Clients could lose control over their lives if relatives or neighbours know details of their medical condition and make assumptions. Suppose that you had been ill and then your next-door neighbour started to treat you as though you had a terminal illness, when you thought you were getting better?

## Ethical issues

Ethics are the principles an individual uses, in order to make decisions in life and when applying the values of a given profession. The value base informs the decision-making process for the individual, but ethical principles also have to be used.

> **Think it over**
>
> Imagine professional ethics as a bunch of specially made keys. These keys have been carefully prepared to uphold the value base of health and social care staff.
>
> When faced with a problem a decision has to be reached. The keys enable the worker to open the appropriate door, thereby making a sound professional judgement. Ethics are the essential tools of the trade to uphold professional standards of care.

### Ethical dilemmas

There are different schools of thought regarding the function of professional ethics. Each school of thought will tackle situations in different ways.

**Utilitarianism**, or **consequentialism**, was developed by Jeremy Bentham (1748–1832) and John Stuart Mill (1806–1873). A utilitarian will believe that a morally right act has to bring about the greatest happiness for the greatest number of people. Utilitarians equate happiness with good, so a morally right act (from this viewpoint) is one which creates the greatest good for the greatest number of people.

Utilitarian philosophy holds that all knowledge comes from experience (*empiricism*). The situation or social context is a major factor, as is the effect or consequences of any action; i.e. whether a doctor tells a patient that they are terminally ill will depend on the doctor's knowledge and experience of that individual and on the effect the news is expected to have on the person. It can be seen that utilitarian philosophy, like most ethics, involves making personal judgements, rather than following strict rules in a given situation.

Ethical systems of thought always encounter problems. It is difficult sometimes to define what is good. How can you guarantee that all possible consequences have been considered prior to action being taken? The concept of the greatest good for the greatest number of people is not straightforward. At face value this idea seems an admirable concept but does it always work in practice? For example, keeping an ailing business going to prevent redundancy may in time bring down the whole business. If some staff had been made redundant in the beginning then the jobs of the majority might have survived.

### Think it over

If every decision was made simply on the basis of the greatest happiness of the greatest number of people then all sorts of injustice and abuses could be justified. If the people in a particular neighbourhood wanted to prevent a care home being built, they could argue that there were more of them and that more happiness would result from their ability to exercise their prejudice than would result from providing care for people with learning disability. Tax payers could argue that more happiness for more people would result from not paying tax rather than meeting the needs of people with disability and so on. It was for this reason that John Stuart Mill argued that utilitarianism had to be just a principle of decision-making: a principle that could only be used after the more important principle of justice had been checked through.

The idea of creating the greatest happiness for the greatest number of people has to be used as a principle to *guide* the construction of codes of professional conduct, or for designing laws and systems of social regulation. Utilitarianism does not work very well when it is applied to day-to-day decisions, or day-to-day actions. The first reason for this is that very few people can predict the future and manage to work out what will create future happiness.

The second reason that utilitarian principles don't work well when applied to acts of behaviour is that most people are very biased in their judgement of happiness.

OH WOW, A TEN POUND NOTE.
SHOULD I TRY TO FIND OUT WHO THIS MONEY BELONG TO - OR SHOULD I KEEP IT? WHAT DOES UTILITARIAN PHILOSOPHY SAY?
YES KEEP IT! THE HAPPINESS THIS MONEY BRINGS ME IS SO GREAT THAT IT MUST CREATE MORE HAPPINESS FOR ME TO KEEP THE MONEY THAN TO DO ANYTHING ELSE.

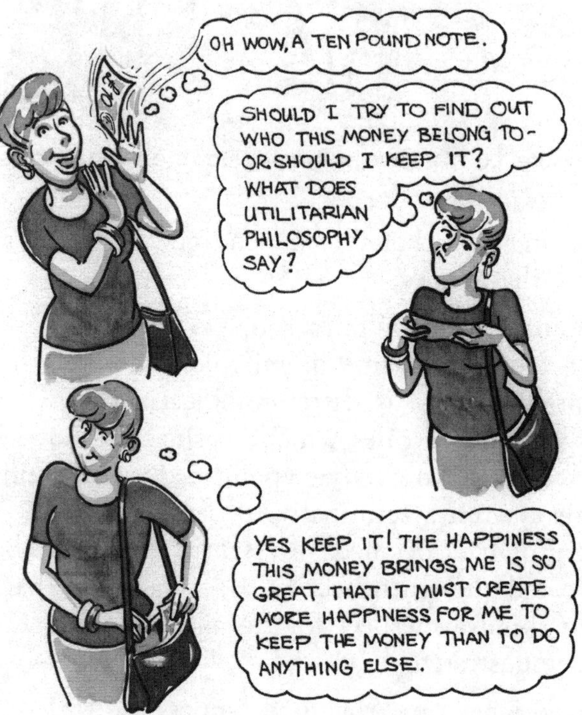

**Figure 1.5 Utilitarian principles applied to a day-to-day decision**

So the idea of greatest happiness may be a helpful principle of social justice, but not a useful way to make moment-by-moment decisions in care work.

Immanuel **Kant** (1742–1804) argued that the same rules should apply to all people and that knowledge comes from a process of reasoning. Whether an action is right or

DOROTHY IS WATCHING HER FAVOURITE T.V. PROGRAMME BUT WE NEED TO GET THE BATH ROTA DONE. OK, ACT UTILITARIANISM- LET'S SEE, TWO OF US WOULD BE VERY HAPPY IF WE DRAGGED HER OFF- SHE WOULDN'T BE HAPPY. OK, TWO AGAINST ONE, WE WIN- SHE GETS A BATH!
BUT THE CARE VALUE BASE SAYS I HAVE A RIGHT TO DIGNITY, RESPECT AND CHOICE-THESE RIGHTS ARE JUSTIFIED IN TERMS OF SOCIETY'S VALUE AND QUALITY CARE - THIS IS WHERE THE PRINCIPLE OF UTILITARIAN DECISION-MAKING COMES IN- NOT IN JUSTIFYING INDIVIDUAL ACTIONS.
VALUES
OK, DOROTHY WINS, WE HAVE TO ACT IN TERMS OF THE VALUE BASE - THE VALUE BASE MIGHT BE JUSTIFIED IN TERMS OF THE GREATEST HAPPINESS FOR PEOPLE IN SOCIETY.

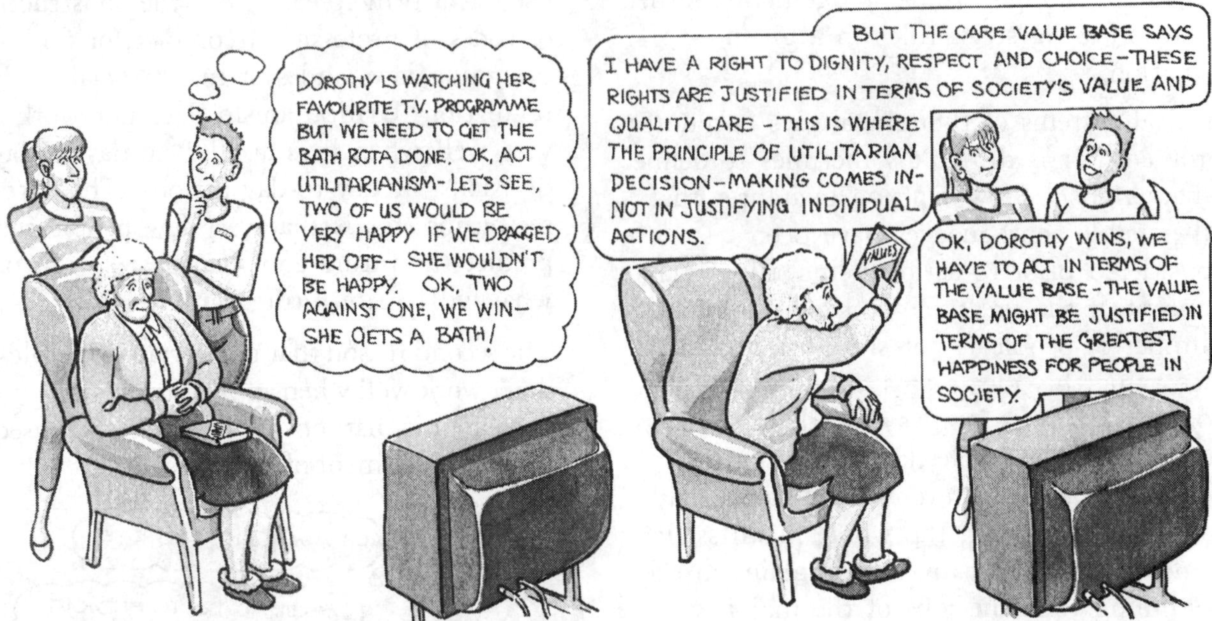

**Figure 1.6 An alternative logical theory of ethics**

wrong will therefore depend on the motives for the action.

Kant's theory is universal, i.e. everyone has to follow the same moral rules whatever the situation, and is therefore objective, i.e. there are set rules which all should follow. According to this viewpoint a doctor would always tell a terminally-ill patient the truth. It is deemed an essential duty always to tell the truth because Kant believed that in this way respect for the individual is demonstrated.

Kantians argue that it is impossible to have a meaningful relationship unless it is based on truth. In this example, the patient has free will and, if he asks for a diagnosis, the truth must be told. In this way the doctor has done the right thing by telling the truth to the patient and has therefore demonstrated respect for that individual.

Critics of Kantianism state that the definition of duty can be interpreted in different ways by different people. The essential dictate (rule) always to tell the truth may place an individual in an impossible situation; for example, being told something in confidence by one person then instructed to tell the truth about the confidence by another. Kant would expect both!

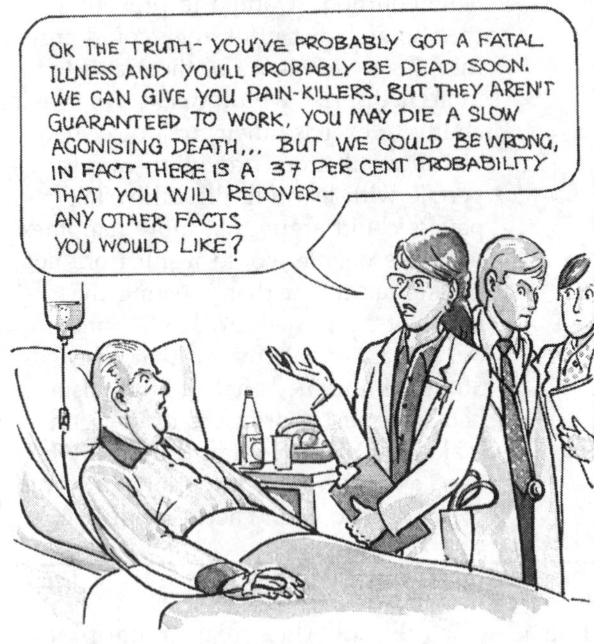


**Figure 1.7 The truth isn't always best**

Pure logic and absolute truth seem a good idea at first, but when used as a basis for day-to-day decision-making the idea does not lead to acceptable practice on its own. It is not enough simply to be logical or truthful. Communication has to show respect for individual beliefs and identity. The care value base does not suggest that it might be acceptable to lie or mislead clients, but it does suggest that truth and logic are not the sole issues in care work.

Decision-making in health and social care cannot depend on simple principles like utilitarianism or logic: but nor can decision-making be left to the beliefs that individuals have been brought up with, or socialised into. Professional value bases or codes of practice are needed to help workers make decisions. The problem is that decision-making is still a difficult task, even when staff understand value bases and codes of practice. Many situations require professional levels of judgement.

David Seedhouse (1988) combines the theories of utilitarianism and Kant's notion of consistency into one theory. Seedhouse argues that when an ethical decision needs to be taken care workers should weigh up:

1 The facts of the situation. Decisions depend on workers collecting all relevant details about client need, legal rights and so on.

2 The extent to which a decision may create a good outcome for everyone. This principle is the same as the idea of utilitarianism, proposed by John Stuart Mill.

3 Fairness and consistency in any decision that is taken. People have a right to an equal quality of service or treatment. People must not be discriminated against. This principle is similar in some ways to Kant's ideas about consistency.

4 The degree to which the decision empowers vulnerable clients and increases their control over their own life (autonomy). Decisions should not result in 'control' of others unless this is definitely in the greater interests of the majority of people.

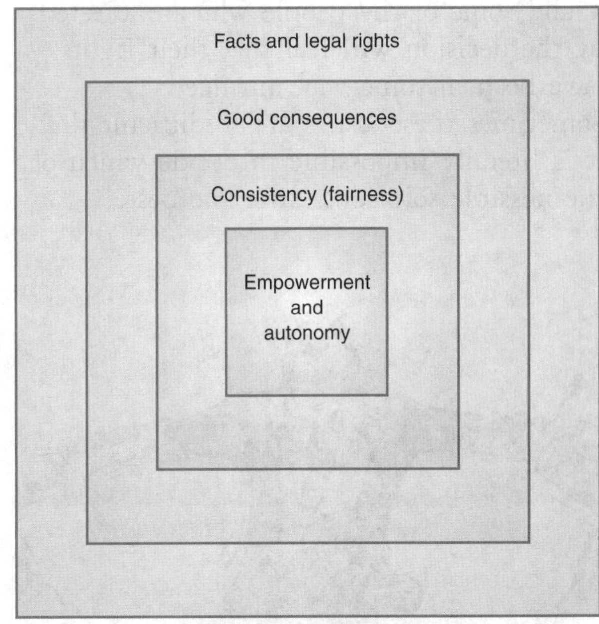


**Figure 1.8** Four levels of principles which should influence ethical decisions, based on Seedhouse's theory

## Rights and responsibilities

Individuals have rights; and for every right, there are corresponding duties and responsibilities on others to uphold it. There are, however, no guarantees that rights and duties will never conflict, and because of this care workers in all situations encounter ethical issues. An ethical issue is a particular type of problem: one that has two sides to it, both of which have a moral dimension. A simple straightforward choice between right and wrong is not an ethical issue, nor is a practical problem; although as will become clear, some practical problems do have a moral dimension. An ethical issue is to do with conflicting rights, obligations, duties or responsibilities. There are arguments on both sides and there is no clear-cut correct answer.

Whatever decision is made, the person doing it will feel bad about some aspect of it and some of the people who are affected by the decision will feel that their rights have been in some way infringed. Sometimes these issues are so difficult that it is literally impossible to decide which of the possible solutions is for the best.

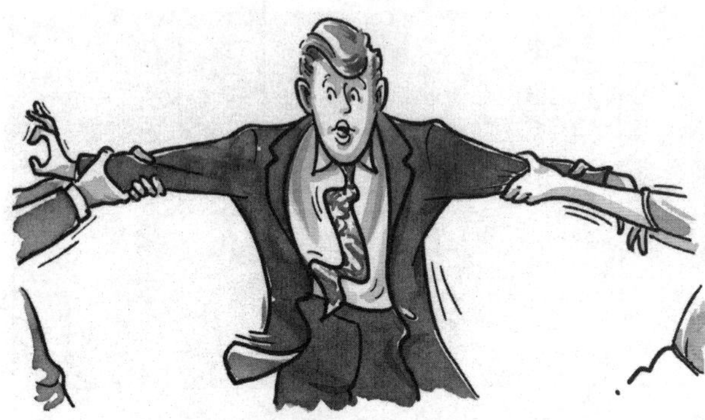

**Figure 1.9** An ethical issue always involves conflict

> An ethical issue:
> - has at least two sides
> - involves a conflict of rights, responsibilities, duties or obligations
> - has no clear-cut right or wrong answer.

Ethical issues may arise for a number of reasons:

- **The rights of one person may clash with the rights of others.** For instance, an older person becomes confused and wanders at night, repeatedly waking the neighbours with claims that they have been burgled. The neighbours demand something is done but when a social worker offers the older person residential care, they refuse it. The right of the person to choose is conflicting with the right of the neighbours to lead an undisturbed life. Whose rights should take precedence?
- **Two different rights which a person has may conflict.** For instance, a child reveals to a care worker that they are being abused, and asks the care worker to keep it secret. The right of the child to confidentiality is conflicting with the right to be protected from harm. Which right is more important?
- **Two obligations of a care worker may conflict.** A home care assistant has a good relationship with a client who is severely disabled with a degenerative disease. The worker calls one day to discover that the client has taken a large overdose of medication, and has left a note saying that they wish to be left to die in peace. The care assistant has an obligation to the client, but also has responsibilities as an employee of a social services department. What is the first responsibility of the worker?
- **Cultural or religious values may conflict.** Parents who are Jehovah's Witnesses may refuse permission for their child to have a blood transfusion, requiring the doctors to overrule the parents if they are to treat the child. Would it ever be right to agree with the parent's wishes? Might a degree of risk to the child be acceptable in order to do so?
- **Practical decisions such as resource allocation may have an ethical**

**dimension.** For instance, a health authority has a limited budget, and cannot meet all the health needs of its population. Suppose a critically ill child needs a very expensive experimental operation with a low chance of success to have any chance of survival? We may think that life is precious, and no expense should be spared in preserving it. But for the cost of that operation (which after all may not be successful), the health authority could carry out hundreds of hip operations that would reliably improve the mobility and quality of life of large numbers of people. Which is the most important?

### Think it over

Think about the principles outlined by David Seedhouse. How far can these ideas help you to solve the problems above?

It is clear that some ethical issues are easier to handle than others. An ethical issue may be seen as something like a pair of scales, and we do talk about weighing up choices or options. Some rights and some responsibilities are much more important than others, and by altering some facts we can change the balance of the scales. The case of the abused child is quite straightforward. If the abuse is serious, it is obviously more important that it be stopped than that the child's confidentiality be respected; but even after making the decision, you would probably feel that you had some explaining to do to the child. Now suppose that it is an adult who is being abused, does that alter the balance of the scales? And if it is an older person or someone with severe disabilities being abused by someone they are dependent upon, is that different again?

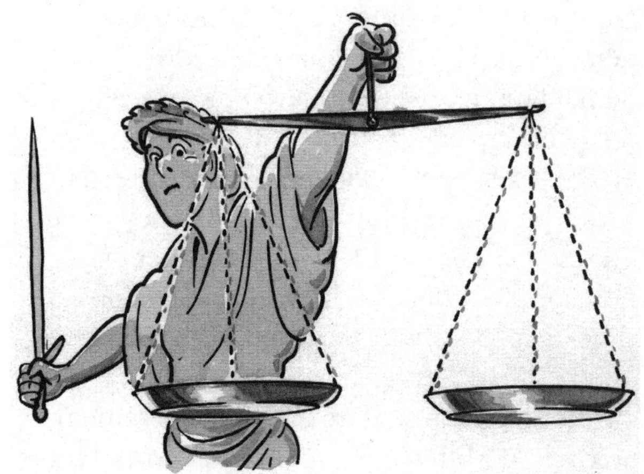

**Figure 1.10 Ethical issues involve weighing up choices or options. There are often no 'right' answers**

There are a number of factors that might go into the scales to balance the decision one way or another. Care workers may find themselves in the position where they have to decide what are the best interests of the client. A number of considerations will go into this decision.

### 1 Competence

Is the client able to make their own decisions? This is known as competence. Several factors might affect this:

- age – is a child too young to fully understand the consequences of the decision?
- mental state – might a person with dementia be too confused or forgetful to make their own decision?
- learning difficulties – these may have a bearing on a client's ability to make some decisions
- mental disorders – this might distort a client's viewpoint and impair their ability to make some decisions
- unconsciousness – this obviously prevents someone from making decisions for themselves.

If someone is unable to make decisions for themselves, then someone must do so for them. This may be a relative, a professional care worker, or a court. If a relative, is it certain that they always have the interests of the person at heart, or might they have interests of their own which conflict with those of the client? These considerations come into play when people with parental responsibility are either giving or withholding consent to medical treatment for their children. The case of parents who are Jehovah's Witnesses refusing a blood transfusion for their child is one side of this, but there are also instances where parents insist on treatment being undertaken when doctors are convinced that it is not in the best interests of the child.

**2 Risk**

If we are considering overriding the choices of a client on the grounds of risk to themselves or others, what is the level of risk to which the client is exposed, and does this justify overriding their personal preferences? We need to assess the level of risk to make the decision. How serious must a risk be to justify overriding a client's right to choose? If someone is competent to make their own decisions, should they be allowed to put their lives at risk if they choose? We might be reluctant to leave an older person at home where they might have an accident when we would not consider stopping a younger person from taking part in a dangerous sport, for instance rock climbing.

### Think it over

Think about Seedhouse's principles, can they guide action in these situations? Which criteria would be ethical using his system?

Risk to others is a different matter, but again it is necessary to assess the degree of risk. The older person who wanders at night and disturbs the neighbours is causing inconvenience and irritation. Is this enough to justify overriding their wishes? Supposing she started turning on the gas fire and not lighting it, and there was a real risk of explosion? And supposing she lived in a flat, rather than a detached house, so that the danger to neighbours was increased? How would this tilt the scales in favour of one decision or another?

**3 Resources**

How do we balance the need of one individual against another? There will never be enough resources to meet all needs, and offering a service to one person often means it is not available to someone else. Somebody has to decide whose needs are most important. This has to be done in a way that is as fair as possible to everyone. Doctors often have to decide where treatment will be most efficient and a whole range of criteria may be applied:

- people's ability to contribute to their own care – some types of operation may not be offered to smokers or people who are very overweight
- some operations might be refused to people over a certain age
- preference to people in employment or with family responsibilities might be considered

**4 Cultural values**

Where there is a clash of values, which is the more important? Even within a single culture, there may be widespread differences of view on very contentious matters. Think of abortion, for instance, and the divergence of views between those who support a woman's right to choose and those who agree with the pro-life lobby. The variation of belief between different cultures may be even greater. People have a right to respect for their cultural values, but if they are widely at variance with the predominant culture – let's say arranged marriages – which should take precedence?

### 5 Safety and protection

Very serious issues arise when there are questions of protecting vulnerable people. Suppose it is suspected that a child is being maltreated. Two systems of values clash: the right to protection of family life and the right to protection from inhuman treatment. Both are guaranteed by the European Convention on Human Rights, and social workers have been criticised on both counts for misjudging the point at which they should intervene. These arguments are currently being played out in the controversy over whether corporal punishment of children should be banned.

> **Think it over**
>
> Would a government ban on smacking children be a child protection measure, or an unacceptable infringement of parents' rights to discipline their children? What are the arguments on both sides? Use Seedhouse's four principles to help guide your decisions.

## Ethical dilemmas: applying the Care Value Base

What is common to all the cases shown below is that although a decision must be made, usually someone will feel that it was the wrong decision, or that their rights have been violated. The other important thing about them is that they all contain issues of principle and we go to court for them to be decided because they have important implications for others. For instance, we may be tempted to think in the case of the pregnant woman, that of course she should be made to have a caesarean section to preserve the life of her child. But if we concede the principle that an individual can be forced to have an operation for the benefit of another, would it also be right for a child to be forced to donate a kidney to save the life of a sick parent? Think about Seedhouse's principles and how they might assist in this situation.

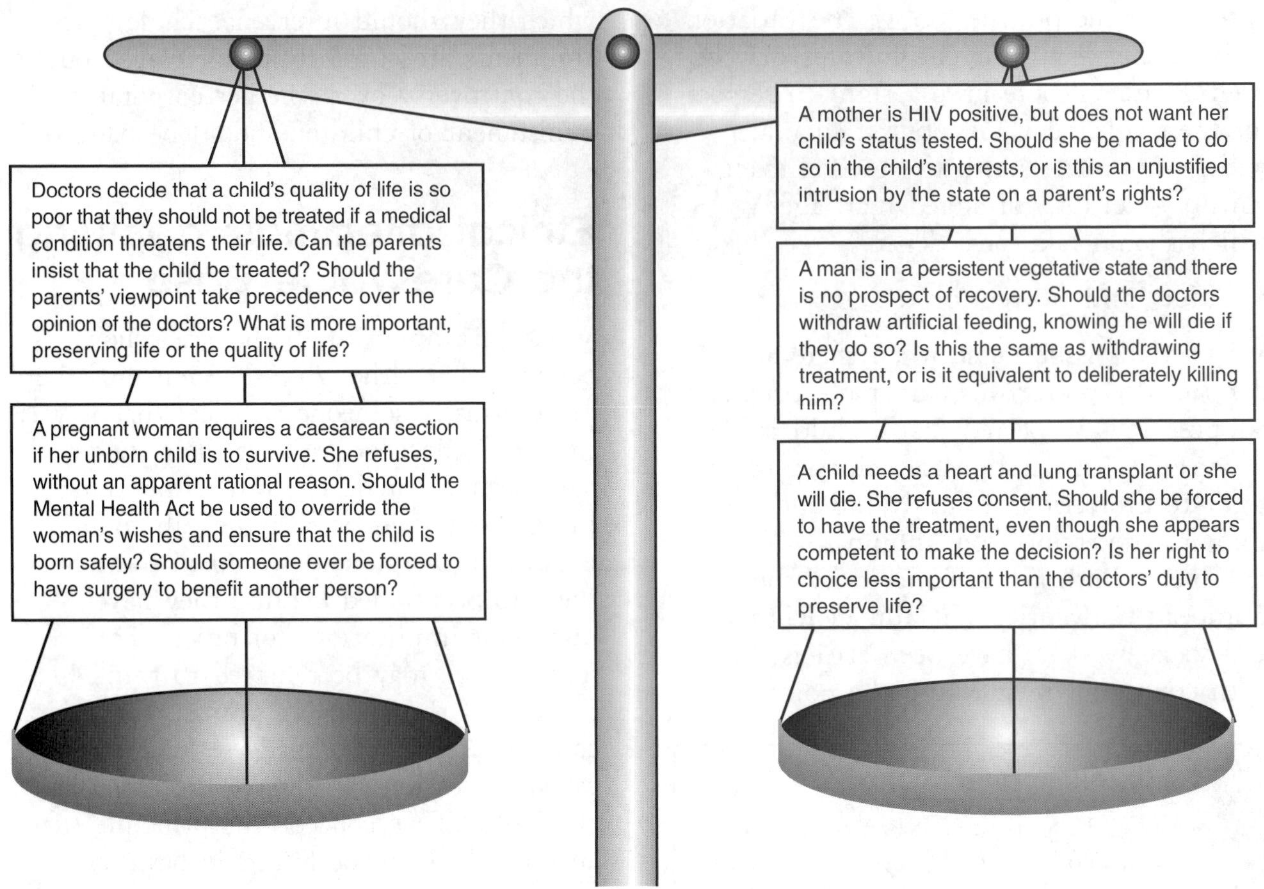


**Figure 1.11** Ethical dilemmas

## 1.2 Legislation, policies and codes of practice for promoting equality

A number of Acts of Parliament make discrimination on the basis of gender, race and disability illegal. There are no laws against discrimination on the basis of age or sexual orientation. The current legislation is:

- The Equal Pay Act 1970
- The Sex Discrimination Acts 1975 and 1986
- The Race Relations Act 1976
- The Disability Discrimination Act 1995.

Northern Ireland has its own legislation. The Race Relations Act was extended to Northern Ireland in 1977. The Fair Employment Acts 1976 and 1989 deal with religious and political discrimination there, which are not matters covered by the laws of the United Kingdom.

### The historical background of equal opportunities legislation

In 1942, the **Beveridge Report** looked at the state of the nation. The Second World War continued until 1945 and the role of women had changed dramatically in order to take over work in the factories and on the land while the men (and some women) were in the forces. A radically new concept emerged from the Beveridge Report, which aimed to rid the country of what was termed the 'five giants' of *want, disease, ignorance, squalor* and *idleness.* The idea of the Welfare State had been conceived.

The Welfare State was set up to provide for the welfare of every citizen 'from the cradle to the grave'. The Education Act 1944 provided education for all from the age of 5 to 15 years. The National Health Service was created in 1948 to provide medical care and advice for all ages. This system included Social Services, dentists, general practitioners and pharmacists: no longer would poorer people suffer because of their inability to pay for medical help. Mothers would receive care and advice before, during and after the birth of their children. Children would be monitored by health visitors, and seen by doctors and dentists, to ensure their appropriate physical and mental development. Housing and social security benefits meant that those who were on low incomes, or were unemployed, had somewhere to go for advice and assistance. In all, the aim was to rebuild a nation following two devastating world wars: a nation where provisions and services were more widely available to all.

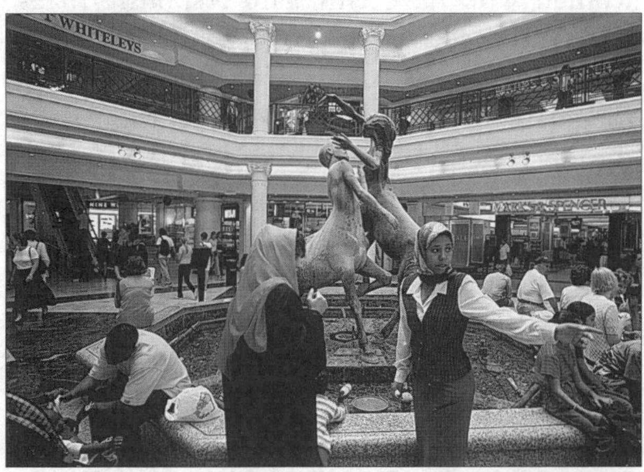


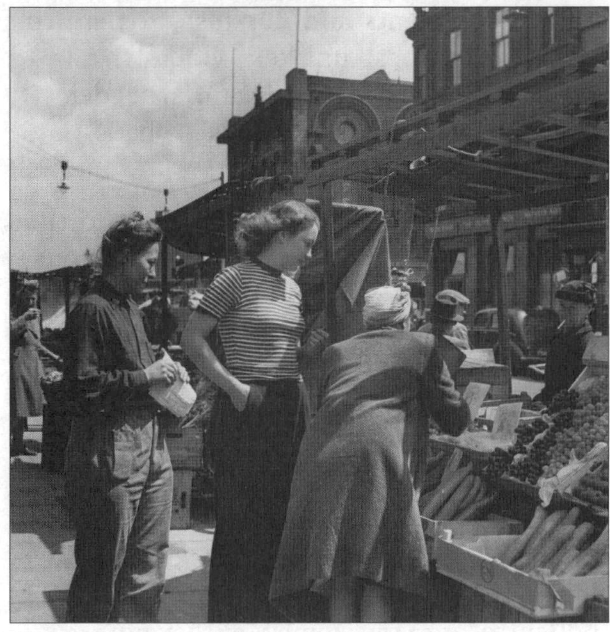

Britain now and Britain in the 1940s

Many changes have taken place in the years since the introduction of the Welfare State, not least in the rise in population and the change in the population in terms of the ethnic mix. Britain is a multicultural society; industry has become more complex and competition from around the world is greater. The demands on the Welfare State are very great compared to those of the 1940s; social values and roles have changed as society evolves to keep pace with events.

In order to ensure that all members of society have equal opportunities in the workplace, several pieces of legislation have been implemented over the last thirty years in particular.

## Equal Pay Act (1970)

The rising number of women in the workforce, in the late 1960s and early 1970s, saw the introduction of the **Equal Pay Act 1970.** This made it unlawful for firms to discriminate between men and women in terms of their pay and conditions in the workplace. This Act came about as a direct result of the Treaty of Rome (1957), Article 119, which stated that,

*Each Member State shall during the first stage ensure and subsequently maintain the application of principle that men and women should receive equal pay for equal work.*

Later, **the Equal Pay Act** 1975 and the Equal Pay (Amendment) Regulations (1983) made it possible to claim equal pay for work which was considered to be of 'equal value' to that done by a member of the opposite sex. This, too, came about following proceedings by the European Commission against the British Government. This amendment to the original Act brought Britain further into line with mainland Europe.

## Sex Discrimination Acts (1975 and 1986)

The **Sex Discrimination Act** 1975 built on the Equal Pay Act of 1970 by further ensuring that women were not discriminated against in education or employment on the grounds of their gender or marital status. It is interesting to note that the provisions of this Act apply equally to discrimination against both sexes. Women are the major beneficiaries, however, as they are more likely to face inequality on the grounds of their gender in the workplace.

The Sex Discrimination Act is concerned with the recruitment, training and promotion of employees, as well as other aspects of employment. In all these aspects it is essential that an employer does not discriminate against a person on the grounds of gender.

The Act established two forms of discrimination – direct and indirect – both of which are unlawful. *Direct discrimination* arises when a person of one sex is treated less favourably than another purely on the grounds of their gender. So it is unlawful to refuse to employ a woman because a position is a 'man's job'; for example, the position of school caretaker has in the past been seen as a man's job. If a woman applied for such a post and fulfilled all the relevant criteria, then she should be given equal consideration for the job; failure to do so could lead to a case being brought before a tribunal if the evidence is clear that the woman was not appointed solely because she was a woman.

Discrimination is illegal on the grounds of marital status for either sex. In the past, women who have childcare responsibilities were often seen as a potential liability to a firm or business. Under the Act it is illegal to take this into consideration to the detriment of the individual; for example, no questions should be asked at an interview regarding domestic or childcare arrangements. It has to be assumed that the person would not have applied for the job without considering the implications for their personal and family life. If an employer considers such a question to be important then they must ask all applicants and not just women; this is, however, most unlikely. Equally it is good practice to try and gain a gender balance on an interview panel where possible.

*Indirect discrimination* arises when conditions are applied which favour a person on one sex rather than another. If these conditions cannot be justified, then the employer is deemed to be acting illegally. For example, in 'Hurley v. Mustoe', the applicant for a waiter/waitress job was a woman with four young children. The manager decided to give her a trial but on the first night the proprietor of the restaurant asked her to leave. He said that it was against his policy to employ women with young children as he thought they were unreliable. The woman took her case to a tribunal, who ruled that she had been directly discriminated against on the grounds of sex contrary to Section 1(1)(a) and indirectly discriminated against on grounds of marital status contrary to Section 3(1) (b).

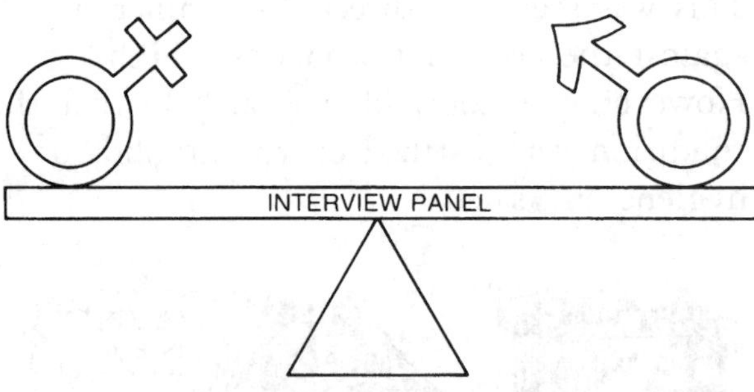


**Figure 1.12 Achieving a gender balance on the interview panel is one of the principles of good recruitment practice**

Following the EEC Equal Treatment Directive (76/207/EEC), major amendments were made to the Sex Discrimination Act 1975. These amendments affected discrimination in collective agreements, employment for the purpose of private households, employment in firms with five or fewer employees and retirement age. All were brought together to widen the scope of the original Act and to bring Britain in line with mainland Europe through the **Sex Discrimination Act 1986.** The EEC Directive also means that decisions made by the British courts and tribunals are subject to the overriding views of the European Court of Justice applying Article 119 of the Treaty, and the Equal Pay Directive. In the event of any disputed interpretation of these issues, it is European Law which will apply.

In 'Worringham v. Lloyd's Bank', female clerical officers under the age of 25 were not required to contribute to a pension scheme. However, male clerical officers under the age of 25 were required to contribute 5 per cent of their salary to the scheme. To compensate for this, male staff were paid 5 per cent more than female staff. The Equal Pay Act (Section 6) (1A) (b) excluded terms relating to death or retirement, or any provision made in relation to death or retirement. Contributions to a pension scheme are therefore outside the scope of the Equal Pay Act.

The female clerical officers took their case to the European Court of Justice as they considered that they were not being afforded equal pay and conditions. The European Court of Justice ruled that, under Article 119, there was an enforceable Community right on all individuals within the EEC. The right to equality of pay meant that the Bank was in violation of Article 119 which took precedence over the Equal Pay Act: the female staff won their case!

## Race Relations Act (1976)

In the same way that Europe influenced British social policy in terms of discrimination on the grounds of sex, so it did with race. The treaty of Rome 1957 made it unlawful to discriminate against EEC workers on grounds of nationality and citizenship.

The British government introduced the **Race Relations Act 1965** which made it unlawful to discriminate on the grounds of colour, race, ethnic or national origins in places of public resort. The Act also made it an offence to incite racial hatred. The Race Relations Board was set up to enforce the law, acting as a 'watch-dog'. A Local Government Act 1966 made money available to local authorities for work with 'immigrants' from the New Commonwealth. Some of this money was used to create 'section eleven' posts to meet specific need, for example to pay for staff to support learning in schools and colleges.

The 1965 Act was replaced by the **Race Relations Act 1968.** The provisions under the Act were widened to include areas of employment, education, and the provision of housing and services.

This law was repealed by the introduction of the **Race Relations Act 1976.** This law, currently in force, seeks to close several loopholes left by previous legislation. Modelled closely on the Sex Discrimination Act, the Race Relations Act 1976 identifies direct and indirect discrimination in the area of race.

*Direct discrimination* occurs when a person treats another person less favourably because of their 'group membership'. In the case of racial discrimination, the actual race of the person discriminated against is immaterial. It is possible, for example, for Jonathan to discriminate against Stuart on the grounds of Jamal's colour: i.e. Jonathan may dismiss Stuart in order to give Jamal a job because Jamal is black. Stuart would win his case for unfair dismissal at a tribunal under Section 1 (1)(a) of this Act.

Equally, it is unlawful to segregate people on racial grounds, as this constitutes less favourable treatment. Providing separate facilities for black and white staff is unlawful. However, if a group of black care staff negotiate to work together on a particular shift that is acceptable – unless the manager states that all black staff should work a specific shift. The former is negotiated by choice, the latter imposed by reason of race.

*Indirect discrimination* occurs when a condition(s) is applied which places people from one race in a more advantageous position than people of another race. Any criteria for a job which an applicant 'must' have is deemed discriminatory if it disadvantages a person of one race in favour of another. If a firm can demonstrate that the requirements or conditions are justified, then the complaint will not succeed. For example, in 'Panesaar v. Nestle & Co Ltd.' a factory rule prohibited beards and long hair. This was seen as indirect discrimination against the applicant who was a Sikh. However, the Court of Appeal held that the condition was justified on the grounds of hygiene and safety.

VACANCY FOR SCOTS COOK
MY SPECIALITY IS EGG AND CHIPS!

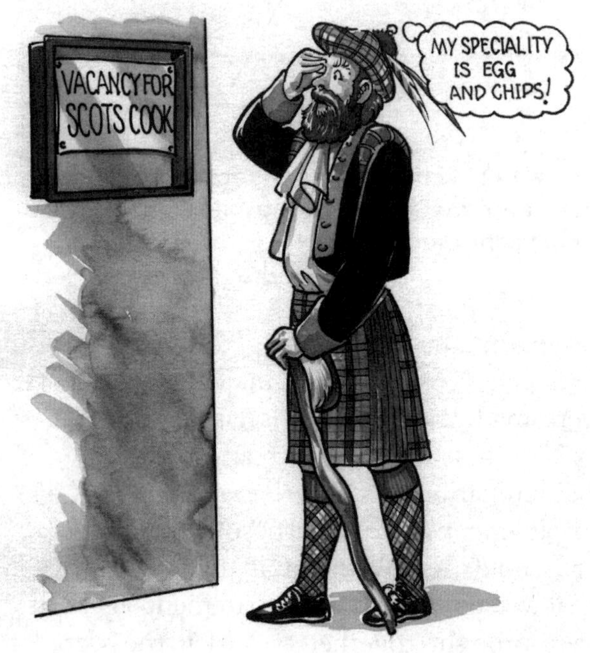

**Figure 1.13 Should the advert ask for 'a person skilled in Scottish cooking'?**

The Race Relations Act makes it unlawful to discriminate on *racial grounds*. The Act defines racial grounds as being colour, race, nationality or ethnic or national origins. A House of Lords ruling in 'Ealing Borough Council v. Race Relations Board', held that the term 'national origins' meant race rather than citizenship. This is now overruled, being replaced by the term 'nationality' to cover both meanings.

This is a complex issue, as was demonstrated by a much publicised debate about an advert for a 'Scots cook'! It was ruled that it was unlawful to advertise in this way and it was suggested that the advert should read, 'a person skilled in Scottish cooking'!

The debate centred on whether Scotland is a separate nation, or an ethnic or racial group. This is a matter of concern for several groups. The Act does not appear to cover religion as such, which can cause confusion. Are all Muslims deemed to be of the same racial, ethnic or national origins? What about Hindus, Christians or Jews? The law as it stands is not very clear.

In 'Mandla v. Dowell Lee', the House of Lords held that the term 'ethnic' was appreciably wider than 'race'. What constitutes an ethnic group? Under the Act, such a group must be able to demonstrate particular characteristics:

a they must have a long history shared and kept alive by all its members
b a cultural tradition with shared social traditions and customs.

Other factors which may be relevant include:

- a common geographical origin or common ancestors
- common language (this may not necessarily be peculiar to the group)
- common literature
- common religion different from their neighbouring groups
- being either a minority or a dominant group within a large community.

An example of an ethnic group fulfilling these criteria would be Sikhs. They share common religious beliefs, have social customs and traditions which are shared by all.

The 1976 Act denotes important exemptions, such as 'positive action'; for example, a social service department wishing to recruit a social worker to have responsibility for meeting the needs of a particular ethnic group. It is perfectly acceptable within the law for positive action to be taken to advertise the post by stating that the post is for someone from that particular ethnic group. The rationale for this is that a person from the same ethnic group will have a better understanding of the needs of the group. The person will therefore be in a more favourable position to identify and meet those needs. This is covered by Section 5, 'genuine occupational qualifications'.

| **Try it out** | Look at the websites for the Commission for Racial Equality and the Equal Opportunities Commission for more information about their roles, responsibilities and current activities. |
|---|---|

The Race Relations Act and the Sex Discrimination Act are similar in many ways. Both cover three main areas of discrimination:

- employment
- education
- the provision of goods and services.

Both the Race Relations and Sex Discrimination Acts make two forms of discrimination illegal: *direct* and *indirect discrimination*. They also make *victimisation* and *harassment* illegal.

**Direct discrimination** is where an individual is discriminated against because of their race or sex; for instance if someone was not given an interview or turned down for a job or refused a service on the basis of their race or sex.

**Example** Ian is black, and has a Scottish accent. He phones about a job vacancy and is asked to attend for an interview. When he arrives, he is told that someone has just been appointed to the job. He suspects that this is not true, and that he has been refused the job on racial grounds and would never have been asked to attend for the interview if the employer had known he was black. The next day he asks a white friend to phone about the job, and they are told that it is still available. Ian takes advice from a solicitor at a law centre, and decides to take the employer to an Employment Tribunal.

There does not need to be any intention to discriminate, it is enough that someone suffers discrimination.

**Example** Maria, a black woman, applies for a job in a private care home for older people. The owner refuses her the job because two of the residents have very racist views. They had been very offensive to a black care assistant who worked there before, and made it difficult for the manager to organise work rotas because they refused to allow the care assistant to do anything for them. Maria suffered discrimination, although this was not the motivation of the home owner.

**Indirect discrimination** is rather more complicated. It may occur even when people are apparently treated alike. It covers situations where a condition is made which is harder for one group to meet than another, and where there is no good reason for it. Suppose an employer, for instance, gives preferential treatment to applicants who are related to existing employees, all of whom are white. The effect would be to discriminate against other applicants who were not white. Similarly, an employer who did not accept job applications from certain postcode areas could be indirectly discriminating if that area contained a higher proportion of black residents. An example of indirect discrimination on the basis of gender would be an employer giving less favourable access to a pension scheme to part-time workers, or being reluctant to employ people on a part-time basis for no good reason. Since women make up the greater proportion of part-time workers, this would have the effect of indirectly discriminating on the basis of gender.

**Example** Jane is a single parent with two school-aged children. She has worked for some years as an ambulance driver. Her employers decide to change the shift patterns of the job. Jane tells them that the new shift patterns will make it very difficult for her to do her job, as they do not fit in with childcare arrangements. Her employer refuses to reconsider the decision to change the shift and Jane has to give up her job. She takes her case to an Employment Tribunal on the grounds that the new shift patterns will affect female employees more than males because more female employees have childcare responsibilities.

Both Acts also make **victimisation** illegal. This means that an employer should not treat someone unfavourably because they have made a claim under this legislation, or helped someone else to do so. The person does not have to be in the group which is discriminated against: for instance, a white person can take action for victimisation against an employer if they think they have been victimised as a result of supporting a black colleague.

**Example** A black care assistant in a residential home fails to get promotion on a number of occasions. Peter, a white colleague, gives evidence on her behalf to an Employment Tribunal, and she wins her case. Peter then applies for promotion himself, but fails to get it. Instead, a less qualified colleague is promoted over his head. He is advised by his Trade Union to make a claim under the Race Relations Act against his employer on the grounds of victimisation.

Sexual and racial **harassment** are also unlawful under the legislation. This means, for example, subjecting someone to racial abuse or unwanted sexual attentions. Other illegal activities would be verbal or physical bullying, jokes, or excluding people because of race or sex.

**Example** The male manager of a female member of staff continually brushes up against her, makes unwanted remarks about her physical appearance and, despite her refusals, often asks her to go out for a drink with him.

**Example** Sean, an Irish worker, is subjected to a constant stream of derogatory jokes about the Irish by his colleagues. He complains to his manager who does nothing about it, telling him that he has no sense of humour. Sean becomes depressed and takes time off work. When he returns, he is sacked on the grounds that he doesn't fit in. He goes to the Citizens Advice Bureau where he is advised to take the company to an Employment Tribunal on the grounds of racial harassment.

Although there are laws against discrimination on the basis of race and sex, job advertisements such as the ones below do appear.

### Think it over

These advertisements are legal because the Race Relations Act and the Sex Discrimination Act allow exceptions in some circumstances. Why do you think these advertisements are allowed?

**AFRICAN CARIBBEAN SOCIAL WORKER – ADOPTIONS PROJECT DEVELOPMENT**

Qualified social worker to recruit, train, assess and support black adopters and support the adoption needs of black children.

**We are an equal opportunities employer. This post is advertised under Section 5(2) of the Race Relations Act 1976**

ASIAN SENIOR CHILD PROTECTION TELEPHONE COUNSELLOR

We are planning an Asian languages service. To help us create this we are looking for two qualified and experienced Asian social workers.

**These posts are advertised under S5(2) of the Race Relations Act 1976 and are only open to applicants who are Asian and who are fluent in at least one of the following languages: Bengali, Gujarati, Hindi, Punjabi or Urdu.**

**Female Social Worker**

**Abuse Survivors Counselling Service**

Counsellor required to provide individual counselling to young women aged 12 to 21 and to mothers who are survivors of sexual abuse.

**Section 7(2) of the Sex Discrimination Act 1975 applies**

> **Male Senior Practitioner**
>
> **Young Abusers Counselling Project**
>
> Your role will involve risk assessment and counselling of young sexual abusers, provision of therapeutic help to young people and their carers, and giving advice and consultation to other professionals.
>
> **This post is advertised under Section 7(2) of the Sex Discrimination Act 1975**

The Sex Discrimination Act allows an employer to recruit someone of a particular gender if:

- there is a good reason why a job needs to be done by someone of a particular sex – for instance, an actor playing a part in a play
- there are reasons of decency, for instance a toilet attendant
- accommodation is provided and it is not practical to supply separate sleeping accommodation for both sexes
- the job is in a single sex institution
- it is a personal service best performed by one sex, for instance a care assistant performing intimate tasks for clients, or intimate counselling of people of one sex or the other
- the job is in a country where laws require it to be performed by a member of one sex.

The Race Relations Act allows similar exemptions in the case of:

- entertainers, actors, artists' and photographers' models where the use of someone of a particular race is necessary for reasons of authenticity
- waiters and waitresses if it is a requirement of a particular type of restaurant e.g. Chinese or Indian
- personal welfare services that could be administered best by members of a particular racial group.

These exceptions are called **genuine occupational qualifications**.

| **Try it out** | Monitor job advertisements in the general and specialist press. Collect those that claim exemption under the Race Relations and Sex Discrimination Acts. On what grounds do employers claim exemption? |
|---|---|

It is important to note that these Acts do *not* make discrimination generally illegal, only in the contexts in which they operate, that is in employment, education and the provision of goods and services. There is protection against discrimination in other contexts, but it is provided by other laws. Inciting racial hatred, for instance, is an offence under the Public Order Act 1986, and racial and sexual harassment are offences under the Criminal Justice and Public Order Act 1994.

## Disability Discrimination Act (1995)

The Disability Discrimination Act is different from the Sex Discrimination and Race Relations Acts in a number of ways. Discrimination only occurs if someone is treated less favourably on the basis on their disability, and this treatment cannot be justified under the Act. This means that there is not as strong a requirement for equality of treatment as in the other anti-discriminatory legislation, and there is no reference in the law to indirect discrimination against people with disabilities.

The Disability Discrimination Act changed the law relating to people with disabilities in a number of ways. It is important to know that it repealed those parts of the Disabled Persons (Employment) Act 1944 that dealt with the registration of people with disabilities and employment quotas. In their place, the new law makes discrimination illegal in the areas of:

- obtaining goods, services or facilities
- buying or renting land or property
- employment.

Under the law, discrimination takes place when:

- a disabled person is treated less favourably than someone else
- the treatment is for a reason related to the person's disability and
- the treatment cannot be justified

or:

- there is a failure to make a reasonable adjustment for a disabled person and
- the failure cannot be justified.

People who provide services must not refuse a service, or provide services of a worse standard or in a worse manner, and must not provide service on less favourable terms to people with disabilities. From October 1999 service providers must take reasonable steps to change practices, policies or procedures which make it impossible or unreasonably difficult for disabled people to use a service. From 2004 service providers will have to take reasonable steps to remove, alter or provide reasonable means of avoiding physical features that make it impossible or unreasonably difficult for disabled people to use a service.

The Act does not guarantee people with disabilities the same services as others under all circumstances, and in particular no one is required to do anything that would endanger the health and safety of any person, including the disabled person. For instance, a person with certain physical disabilities may not be able to safely use a ski lift, and it would not be unlawful to refuse to allow them to do so. Neither is anyone obliged to enter into a contract with a disabled person if the person cannot understand the contract because of their disability. A person with disabilities cannot be refused a service without good reason. For instance, if a shopkeeper refused to serve people with learning difficulties from a nearby hostel because she thinks their appearance would put off other customers, she would be acting illegally. However, if a cinema manager refused entry to someone whose disability caused them to shout frequently, he might be justified under the law on the grounds that this would disrupt the enjoyment of other customers.

The Act does introduce the concept of what adjustments it is reasonable for an employee to make to enable a person with disabilities to perform a job. Generally speaking, this will depend on how much the adjustment would cost, compared to the resources of the organisation (firms employing fewer than 20 people are excluded from the legislation altogether), whether outside funding is available and how effective the adjustment would be. Reasonable adjustments might include:

- transferring minor duties that are not an essential part of the job to another person if they are difficult for the person with disabilities to perform
- finding suitable alternative employment within the organisation for a worker who develops a disability
- moving a work station to a more accessible location
- providing additional training, for instance for someone who is visually impaired to use speech recognition software on a computer
- providing specialised equipment to enable someone with a disability to perform their job.

### Stop press!

Watch out for the Disability Rights Commission Act which is currently going through Parliament. This will establish the Disability Rights Commission which will have powers to:

- work towards the elimination of discrimination against disabled people
- promote equal opportunities for disabled people
- provide information and advice to disabled people, employers and service providers
- prepare codes of practice and encourage good practice
- keep the workings of the Disability Discrimination Act under review
- investigate discrimination and ensure compliance with the law, and
- arrange for a conciliation service between service providers and disabled people to help resolve disputes in regard to access to goods and services.

## Systems of redress

Because these Acts convey statutory rights, there are corresponding formal means of redress for people who think that their rights have been infringed. These will differ according to whether the discrimination has taken place in employment or one of the other protected areas.

For employment matters relating to sex and race discrimination, the aggrieved person can obtain advice from the relevant Commission. Because of the currently more limited powers of the National Disability Council, a disabled person with an employment problem could approach the Advisory, Conciliation and Arbitration Service (Labour Relations Agency in Northern Ireland) who can make the services of a conciliation officer available. In all cases of discrimination in employment, if informal means fail to resolve the problem, then the aggrieved person may complain to an Employment (previously Industrial) Tribunal. Details of how to do this can be obtained from Job Centres or a Citizens Advice Bureau.

For complaints to do with matters other than employment, advice is available from the Commissions, Citizens Advice Bureau and local advice centres and voluntary organisations. Redress is obtained from the County Court, and the person who thinks they have been discriminated against would normally approach a solicitor to assist. Free advice from a solicitor is often available from law centres or advice agencies.

## European Convention on Human Rights

It may not seem immediately obvious why it is necessary to know about the European Convention on Human Rights and its associated bodies, the European Commission of Human Rights and the European Court of Human Rights. However, newspaper stories like the ones illustrated below will give an idea of the impact that European law has had on the law and practice in Britain.

## UK guilty of child neglect

Five children were subjected to 'torture or inhuman or degrading treatment' when a Social Services department failed for more than four years to remove them from 'horrific' parental neglect, the European Commission for Human Rights has ruled.

If the European Court of Human Rights follows the ruling next year, it will have implications for local councils and other public bodies. A child law expert said, 'Children will be able to claim damages as a result of local authority negligence in investigating child abuse'.

## Armed forces ban on gays is lifted

The ban on homosexuals in the armed forces has been lifted in a move forced on the government by the European Court of Human Rights. The Defence Secretary told the House of Commons that the ban was no longer legally justifiable following the Court's judgement that sexual orientation was a private matter.

Rights are given by society, but they can also be taken away. We accept, for example, that people can be detained against their will if they commit criminal offences or they are a danger to themselves and others as a result of a mental disorder. However, most people would also agree that there should be limits to how far people's rights should be removed and under what circumstances.

There was widespread horror at the extent of the violations of human rights which took place under Nazi Germany before and during the Second World War. People were persecuted on the basis of their race, health status, physical and mental disabilities and political beliefs. There was a determination that this should not be repeated, which gave rise to the European Convention on Human Rights. This was drawn up under the auspices of the Council of Europe, which is a separate organisation from the European Community. The Convention gives a number of protections against

**The European Convention on Human Rights**

| | |
|---|---|
| **Article 2:** | Protection of life |
| **Article 3:** | Freedom from inhuman treatment |
| **Article 4:** | Freedom from slavery, servitude or forced or compulsory labour |
| **Article 5:** | Right to liberty and security of person |
| **Article 6:** | Right to a fair and public hearing |
| **Article 7:** | Freedom from retrospective effects of penal legislation |
| **Article 8:** | Right to respect for privacy |
| **Article 9:** | Freedom of thought, conscience and religion |
| **Article 10:** | Freedom of expression |
| **Article 11:** | Freedom of association and assembly |
| **Article 12:** | Right to marry and found a family |
| **Article 13:** | Right to an effective remedy before a national authority |
| **Article 14:** | Prohibition of discrimination on the grounds of: |

sex, race, colour, language, religion, political or other opinion, national or social origin, association with a national minority, property, birth or other status.

discrimination. Article 14 prohibits discrimination in the application of all the other rights of the Convention.

This treaty has had a major effect on UK legislation. By becoming a signatory, the UK agreed to be bound by its provisions, and this has had two effects. First, British courts must take the Convention into account when making decisions. Secondly, the European Court of Human Rights set up by the Convention acts as a final court of appeal against the decisions of British courts, with the power to rule against the governments of member states.

The Convention can give protection against discrimination where there is no specific UK protection. As a result, being a signatory to the Convention has had dramatic effects on British government policy. For instance, a number of gay and lesbian people have brought the UK before the European Court of Human Rights because they were dismissed from the Armed Forces. Despite there being no statutory protection in Britain against discrimination on the basis of sexuality, the court found in their favour because their right to respect for private and family life (article 8) had been violated. UK policy about whether gay and lesbian people should be allowed to serve in the Armed Forces had to be reviewed as a result.

People who believe they have been discriminated against cannot approach the European Court of Human Rights directly. They have to try all the available national remedies first. Only when this has been done can the Court be approached through the European Human Rights Commission. Once the Commission has decided that there is a case to answer, the case can go forward to the Court.

The Convention has the potential to have far-reaching effects on care organisations in the UK. In November 1999, for instance, the European Commission of Human Rights found against the UK in a child care case. A local authority social services department failed to remove some children from a home in which they suffered extreme neglect. The UK was found to have violated article 3 by failing to protect the children. The UK was also found to have breached their rights under article 6 because the House of Lords (the final appeal court in the UK) refused the children permission to sue the council responsible because it was against public policy. If the Court agrees with the Commission's findings, this will change UK policy, and the authority concerned may have to pay compensation to the children in the case.

The European Convention has been important because it has given people rights that they would not have had under either UK or European Community law:

- it has given people protection against sexual discrimination in areas not covered by either UK or EU law – for instance, the equalisation of pension ages of men and women
- it has given protection against discrimination to groups that had no protection under existing UK law – for instance, the gay service people.
- it may give people new rights of redress that they did not have under UK law – for instance new rights for clients to sue social services departments which do not act properly to protect them.

### Stop press!

The European Convention on Human Rights will soon be fully incorporated into British law by the Human Rights Act 1998, which comes into force in October 2000. From that date, all new laws must meet the requirements of the Convention, and it will be unlawful for public bodies to act in a way that is incompatible with the Articles of the Convention. This might, for instance, mean that if a local authority has a child in its care involuntarily, and the child has no means of contesting this, it would be in breach of the legislation. Public bodies will also lose their immunity from claims for damages, and service users will be able to sue them.

### Pension ages of men and women to be equalised

The government has announced that state pension ages for men and women are to be equalised at the age of 65 by 2020. This action has been forced on the government by two recent judgements in the European Court of Human Rights. In the first decision, the court ruled that dismissal by an employer at the current state pension age (60 for women and 65 for men) was discriminatory on the basis of sex. The second judgement ruled that occupational pension schemes could not discriminate on the basis of sex by offering different terms to men and women. The government has decided that because of these decisions, it is not possible to have a different pension age for men and women in the state system when occupational pension schemes are obliged to provide pensions on the same terms to men and women.

## The European Community

The laws concerning discriminatory behaviour in employment have also been affected by Britain's membership of the European Community. The UK signed the Treaty of Rome in 1973 and as a result is bound by Article 119 of the Treaty that establishes the principle of equal pay for equal work. The Equal Pay Directive, the Equal Treatment Directive and the Pregnancy Directive make further requirements on equal pay and equal treatment between the sexes, and are binding on UK courts. National courts can refer questions of EC law to the European Court of Justice. The Court can deal with matters of discrimination on the basis of nationality (Article 6 of the EC Treaty) and Sex (Article 119). However, the Court has no jurisdiction in matters of race, as there are no provisions covering racial discrimination in the EC Treaty. Decisions of the European Court of justice have influenced British law in matters far beyond employment protection, as is illustrated below.

### Important

Do not confuse the European Court of Justice with the European Court of Human Rights. The European Court of Human Rights sits in Strasbourg and was set up under the Council of Europe to ensure the observance of the European Convention on Human Rights. The European Court of Justice sits in Luxembourg and deals with questions of EU law referred to them by national courts.

## Overriding clients' wishes

The law assumes that all adults are capable of making decisions about their lives unless it can be demonstrated otherwise. But the law does allow the liberty of individuals to be restricted under certain circumstances. **The Mental Health Act 1983** permits the detention of someone in hospital for the purpose of assessment or treatment if they fulfil the following requirements:

- they are suffering from a mental disorder
- detention is necessary for the patient's own health or safety, or for the protection of others.

Two doctors and a social worker (or the patient's nearest relative) must agree it is necessary, although in an emergency, one doctor and a social worker may do so. The police also have powers to detain someone in a public place if they have reason to suspect that they are suffering from a mental disorder.

**Example** Mrs Greene has become very agitated. She has not slept for three nights and is not eating or drinking. She is talking continuously and is constantly active with pointless tasks such as moving the furniture around. Her husband calls the GP. She is in danger of becoming exhausted and dehydrated, but refuses to take medication or go to hospital, as she does not believe she is ill. The GP calls the social worker and the consultant psychiatrist. Together they decide that Mrs Greene should be admitted to hospital for a period of assessment.

People who are detained in hospital have the right to appeal to a Mental Health Review Tribunal that has the power to discharge them from hospital, if they believe that there is no need for them to be detained any longer.

## Children

The position of children is different, and they are not automatically regarded as being competent to make decisions in their own interests. The other side of this is that they are not necessarily considered to be fully responsible for their actions. The law has always recognised this by setting ages at which children are allowed to do certain things. Children under 10 years old cannot be charged with criminal offences: this is known as the age of criminal responsibility. At 13 years old, a child can get a part-time job, and at 16 years old a child can leave school and get a full-time job. At 16 years, a child can leave home with parental consent and even without it is unlikely to be forced to return. A girl can consent to sexual intercourse, and people can marry with parental consent. At 17 a young person can drive a car, and be interviewed by the police about criminal offences without an 'appropriate adult' being present. The age of majority is held to be 18 years, when it is generally held that people become adult. At 18 people can vote. Young people of 18 can leave home and marry without parental consent, serve on a jury, buy alcohol and bet.

Some important rights of children are based on their understanding rather than their age. Consent to medical treatment is probably the most important area. Children of any age can give consent to medical treatment, providing that they understand fully what is proposed. This principle was established by the Gillick case, in which a mother tried to obtain a court judgement preventing her underage daughter from getting contraceptive advice from her GP without parental consent. She failed, and as a result children can consent to a range of medical procedures if they have sufficient understanding. In practice, this means that the more serious and hazardous the treatment, the older the child would have to be to consent to it. Refusing consent is slightly different. A child can refuse consent to treatment on the same basis, but the refusal can be overridden by anybody with parental responsibility giving consent.

## Children Act 1989

Children have rights within the law. The Children Act 1989 followed several well-publicised cases of child abuse and seeks to simplify the great complexity of child care law. The law applies to all statutory and voluntary organisations providing care for children and their families. It is essentially a balancing act between the rights of the child and the parents and the duty of the state to protect children deemed to be in need or at risk.

Children in need are defined as, '.... children whose health and welfare may suffer significantly without support from social services.' Any child with a disability is automatically deemed to be in need. The local authority must provide services to meet identified need, for example nurseries and family centres.

Race and culture were, for the first time, recognised as essential factors to be given consideration. Local authorities must carefully consider a child's race, religion, language and culture when deciding on fostering, day or residential care services. Department of Health guidelines state that day care services should promote the self-esteem and racial identity of the child. Any provider of child care services must be able to satisfy the local authority that they are able to meet the racial and cultural needs of the children in the area, in order to gain registration.

The Act requires local authorities to 'take preventive steps', to ensure that children may live as normal a life as possible. Care must be taken to ensure that children are safe from suffering and that disabilities are minimised. Care must also be taken to ensure that children do not commit offences, so avoiding the need for placing them in secure provision.

Other key features of the Act lie in a principle termed **paramountcy.** This term means that the child's welfare is paramount (the most important issue). Any decision made about the child has to be made in the child's best interest. Where a child is either mature enough or old enough, they have a right to be consulted about their wishes. These wishes must be given priority.

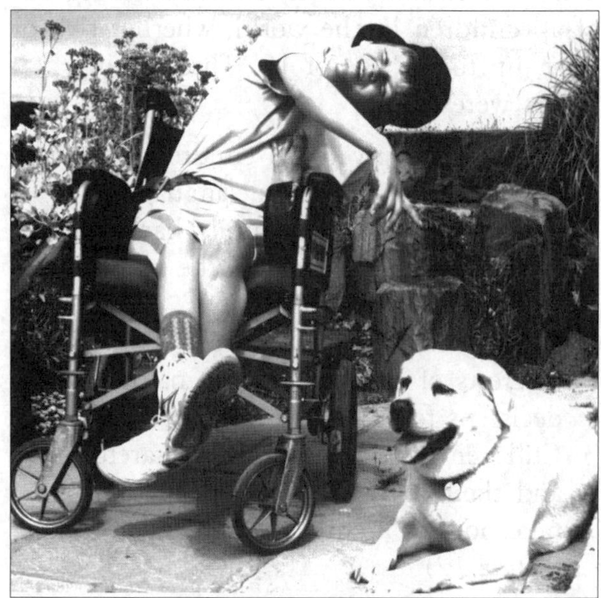

**Figure 1.14 A child's own wishes must be given priority**
**(Photo courtesy of Winged Fellowship Trust)**

The Act requires caring agencies and parents to work in partnership. Both work to plan and organise to meet the needs of the child at all stages. Parents are also still responsible for their child, even when that child is living in a local authority establishment. Any person may apply to be deemed responsible for the child, such as a friend or relative if it is appropriate; for example, the grandmother of a boy orphaned whilst his parents were on holiday in Eastern Europe.

Collaboration between parents, child care agencies and the child is essential to meet the needs of the individual child at all stages.

The UN Convention on the Rights of the Child was formalised by international agreement to protect the rights of children. This was in response to concerns raised across the world about the rights of children being ignored or forgotten.

The articles (statements) identify the rights of all children in the world, whether rich or poor, up to the age of 18. Three main rights were stated:

1 All rights apply to all children whatever their race, sex, religion, language, disability, opinion or family background. In other words, there will be no discrimination. (*article 2*)
2 Adults must always consider the best interests of the child when making decisions for them. (*article 3*)
3 Children must be listened to carefully and their opinions heard. Courts must take note of a child's wants and feelings. (*article 12*)

Other rights include civil and political rights, economic, social, cultural and protective rights. All are important issues which should be part of good child care practice. For example, Article 24 states that children have the right to live in a safe, healthy and unpolluted environment. Article 18 notes that children should have proper care from day to day with the family, but with government support if necessary. Article 20 looks at the day-to-day care with other families, or in a children's home if there is no family. Due respect must be taken of a child's race, religion, culture and language when a new home is sought.

The implications of the Children Act for those working in health and social care are great. Children must be provided with a safe environment where they may grow and develop to their full potential. That environment must acknowledge the child's race and culture, religion and language. This is essential for the child to develop a positive self-esteem, which will enable the child to grow into a confident adult, able to take his or her place in society.

**Think it over**

Does this sound familiar? You can clearly see how important this UN Convention was when looking again at the Children Act 1989!

You may wish to obtain a booklet, *The Rights of a Child – A Guide to the UN Convention* (CAG9), from the Department of Health, to further your understanding.

**STOP PRESS!**

The way young offenders are dealt with by the criminal justice system is being radically changed by the Crime and Disorder Act 1998. Before this Act, there was a presumption that children between the ages of 10 and 13 were incapable of telling the difference between serious wrong and simple naughtiness. They had to be proved capable of telling the difference before a prosecution could succeed. This is no longer the case, and children of 10 to 13 are now treated in the same way as 14 to 17 year olds.

Courts now have the power to impose Anti-Social Behaviour Orders on juveniles, banning them from specified areas if they create a nuisance. Local authorities have the power to impose local child curfew schemes, banning children from certain areas after a certain time, unless they are supervised by an adult. The police have the powers to pick up children they believe are truanting.

The courts have powers to impose secure training orders on:

- 10 to 11 years olds for persistent offending when custody is necessary to protect the public from further offending
- 12 to 14 year olds who are persistent offenders
- 15 to 17 year olds who commit imprisonable offences.

## Right to confidentiality

Apart from the Data Protection Acts, clients have no statutory right to confidentiality in UK law. Although Article 8 of the European Convention on Human Rights recognises the right of a person to respect for privacy, this is qualified by the need to prevent crime, protect health and protect the rights and freedom of others. These are the areas in which ethical issues are most likely to arise.

Under common law, an individual could go to court to ask for an injunction to make someone respect their confidentiality if:

- the information was confidential, such as medical or social work records
- the person with the information had a duty to keep it confidential, e.g. because of the nature of the relationship (doctor/patient or social worker/client)
- the way the information would be used would be incompatible with that duty, e.g. not covered by the European Convention qualifications.

In practice, this procedure would hardly ever be relevant in the vast majority of social care situations. However, the essence of the law is incorporated into the ethics of professional workers, charters, service standards of health and care organisations and contracts of employment of care workers. A breach of confidentiality would therefore constitute grounds for a complaint against a care organisation or an individual working for it, and grounds for disciplinary action by an employer against an employee.

There can be no such thing as complete confidentiality. Information about clients has to be shared between workers in care organisations to ensure good quality care, and it has to be shared with managers to ensure accountability and to enable standards to be monitored. Sometimes it will have to be passed to another agency to ensure continuity of service. Information is shared between social services and health care services because of overlapping responsibilities in community care. Social services departments contract out many services, such as home care services, so information about clients has to be passed to commercial organisations in order that they get a good service. Clients should understand what information is held about them, with whom it will be shared, and under what circumstances. Their permission should be sought before sensitive information is passed to others, and wherever possible they should be able to control disclosure about themselves. Care staff should only seek information about clients on a need-to-know basis.

There are circumstances where very sensitive information may have to be disclosed – even in the face of a refusal by the client. This arises where there is a likelihood of foreseeable harm if the information is not disclosed, and this consideration will override even the confidential nature of the doctor/patient relationship. Examples of where this may happen are:

- a GP has a patient suffering from a serious mental disorder, in need of hospital treatment but refusing it. The GP would have to provide information about the patient's condition to a social worker to enable the social worker to decide whether to make an application for compulsory admission to hospital
- a social worker suspects that a client is physically abusing their children. A Child Protection Case Conference is convened and the professionals concerned (paediatrician, GP, health visitor, teacher, nursery staff, police and social workers) meet to share information.

Clients have the right to know what information is held on them. The **Data Protection Act 1998** means that all records about clients which are filed will be seen as data, whether they are held electronically or on paper. The 1998 Act provides individuals with a range of rights including:

- the right to know what information is held about them and to see and correct the information if necessary
- the right to refuse to provide information
- the right that data should be accurate and up-to-date
- the right that information should not be kept for longer than necessary
- the right to confidentiality – that the information should not be accessible to **unauthorised people**.

The **Access to Personal Files Act 1987** and the **Access to Health Records Act 1990** gives social services clients and NHS patients access to their social work and health records. People who apply must be allowed to see their records, although certain types of information may be withheld from them. They can only see information about themselves, and information may be kept back if it would harm the applicant's or someone else's physical or mental health. Information may also be withheld if it is provided by another person other than a professional; this, for instance, would protect somebody who wished to tell the social services about a case of child abuse, but who wanted to preserve their anonymity.

## Charters

Other rights are conferred by various Citizen's Charters, such as the Community Care Charter that outlines people's rights to care in the community. One of the most important of these charters for workers in health and social care is the Patient's Charter (see next page).

In addition to these rights, the Patient's Charter also details a number of standards which patients should be able to expect from the NHS. These cover the following areas:

- respect for privacy, dignity, and religious and cultural beliefs
- the information to be made available to relatives and friends
- access to services for people with special needs
- waiting times for ambulances, in Accident and Emergency Departments, in outpatient clinics and for admission to hospital
- what should happen if an operation is cancelled
- quality of services from community nurses, midwives and health visitors
- quality of the hospital environment
- hospital discharge procedures
- changing your GP
- quality of services from optometrists, dentists and community pharmacists.

## Patient's Charter

Everyone has the right under the charter to:

- receive health care on the basis of clinical need
- be registered with a GP and change your GP easily and quickly if you want to
- get emergency medical treatment at any time
- be offered a health check when you join a GP's list
- ask your GP for a health check if you are aged 16 – 74 years and have not seen your GP for the past three years
- be offered a health check once a year in your GP surgery, or at your own home if you prefer, if you are 75 years or over
- receive information about the services your GP provides
- decide which pharmacy to use for your prescription and have the appropriate drugs and medicines prescribed
- get your medicines free if you are a pensioner, a child under 16, or under 19 in full-time education, pregnant or a nursing mother, suffering from one of a number of specified conditions, or on income support or family credit
- be referred to a consultant, acceptable to you, when your GP thinks it is necessary, and to be referred for a second opinion if you and your GP agree this is desirable
- have any proposed treatment, including any risks and any alternatives, clearly explained to you before you decide whether you agree to it
- receive dental advice in an emergency (if you are registered with a dentist) and treatment if your dentist thinks it is necessary
- receive a signed written prescription immediately after your eye test
- see your own health records, subject to any limitations in law, and know that everyone working in the NHS is under a legal duty to keep your records confidential
- choose whether or not you wish to take part in medical research or medical student training
- information about the standards of services you can expect, waiting times and local GP services
- have a complaint about NHS services investigated thoroughly and receive a full and prompt reply from the Chief Executive or General Manager
- be told before you go into hospital, except in an emergency, whether it is planned to care for you in a ward for men and women.

These rights differ in nature from the statutory rights that we looked at earlier, in that it is not possible to go to court to enforce them. However, as we have seen earlier, there may be instances where the way a service is provided, or not provided, may be in breach of the European Convention on Human Rights. There are means of redress available. If rights under the Patient's Charter are breached, someone can complain to the Chief Executive of the Hospital Trust or the Health Authority. The local Community Health Council can assist with making a complaint, and represent the person throughout the complaints procedure. If they are not satisfied with the way the complaint is dealt with, then they can ask the Health Service Commissioner (Ombudsman) to consider investigating the case.

### Think it over

A pregnant woman decides she would like to have her third baby at home. She phones the local midwifery service and is told that there are not enough midwives available so she will have to have her baby in hospital.

1. Find out what the woman's rights are in this situation.
2. Does the local health service have the right to refuse a home birth?
3. What are the legal implications if the woman decides to 'go it alone' with the help of her partner?

| Try it out | Monitor the broadsheet press for a month. Collect reports of court decisions relating to ethical issues. What decisions are made? How are they made? Do the decisions have implications for workers in health and social care?<br>Also read back copies of a magazine aimed at health and social care professionals. *Community Care* has a feature most weeks explaining an ethical issue which has arisen for a professional and describing how it was resolved. |
|---|---|

## 1.3 How care organisations promote equality

Some ethical issues are very finely balanced indeed – so much so that it is impossible to make a clear-cut decision about what is the right thing to do. As the range of difficulty varies, so there are a number of things that help the people concerned to deal with them.

### Training

Education and training will help a worker to recognise when a situation contains an ethical issue, and how to begin to deal with it. Ethical issues cannot be recognised without a sound knowledge of client rights and the care value base. It is as this knowledge is applied to real-life situations that it becomes obvious that life is not always straightforward, and that rights, duties and obligations may be incompatible with each other.

Workers who go on to further professional training will be equipped by their training to make decisions in a way that respects clients' rights. Professions have codes of conduct to guide their members in how to carry out their work, and there may be a controlling body with disciplinary procedures to deal with workers who do not meet acceptable standards.

### Organisational policies and procedures

Employing organisations may incorporate expectations of standards of behaviour in their contracts of employment. They will have guidelines and procedures about how to deal with certain situations. For instance, most employers will have equal opportunities policies. Most childcare settings will have 'abuse procedures' that would help in the case of the child disclosing abuse. Similarly, settings that care for older people are likely to have an elder abuse procedure. Most employers will also have general guidelines for staff to help them make day-to-day decisions about their relations with clients; for instance, whether it is permissible to accept a gift from a client, under what circumstances a worker should divulge information to another agency, and so on.

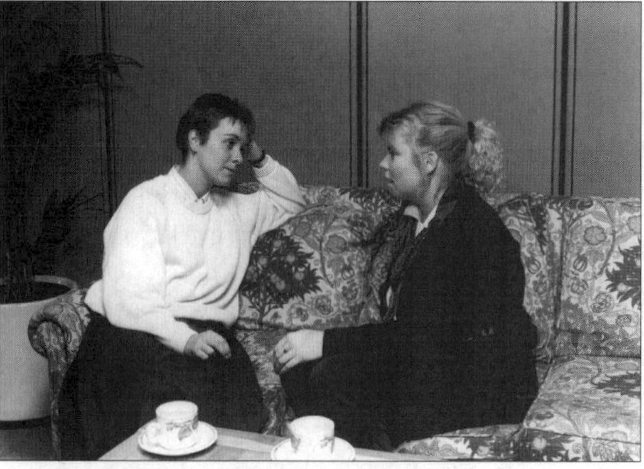

**Figure 1.15** It can be helpful to share problems with colleagues

Workers will have colleagues with whom they can discuss difficult decisions. Sometimes a more experienced colleague can be of help in resolving everyday problems. Some issues will be more complex and cannot be solved by talking them through with colleagues, or by referring to employer's guidelines. In such cases, one of the tasks of a manager is to supervise the work of their subordinates and offer advice and guidance in difficult situations. All organisations have *management structures*, and all workers within an organisation should be clear about the limits of their own responsibilities, and where they should go for assistance in resolving problems.

## External support

There may be some very difficult decisions where the ethical issue arises from something that an employer asks a worker to do, which the worker thinks conflicts with the rights of the client – perhaps a situation where resource shortage is leading to a client being deprived of their rights. If this cannot be resolved by consulting with a manager, it may be necessary to look outside the organisation for a solution. A worker may find their responsibility to their employer in conflict with their duty towards the client. Some groups of workers – for instance doctors, nurses and social workers – have professional associations that provide Codes of Practice for their members, and will also provide advice and guidance on particular circumstances. Professionals may have a particular need of such support systems and advice of this kind because they may have to accept personal responsibility for their actions in very difficult circumstances.

## Codes of practice and charters

Codes of practice and charters help to define the quality of care clients can expect if they receive care services and they can be used as a basis for measuring the quality of care provided.

### Codes of practice

What constitutes good care is not a matter of individual debate. Codes of practice are needed to define what quality means. These codes can then be used to measure whether or not a particular service is providing good quality. For example, *Home Life: a Code of Practice for Residential Care*, first published in

**STAFF**

**148** Staff qualities should include responsiveness to and respect for the needs of the individuals.

**149** Staff skills should match the residents' needs as identified in the objectives of the home.

**150** Staff should have the ability to give competent and tactful care, whilst enabling residents to retain dignity and self-determination.

**151** In the selection of staff at least two references should be taken up, where possible from previous employers.

**152** Applicants' curriculum vitae should be checked and for this purpose employers should give warning that convictions otherwise spent should be disclosed.

**153** Proprietors should consider residents' needs in relation to all categories of staff when drawing up staffing proposals.

**154** Job descriptions will be required for all posts and staff should be provided with relevant job descriptions on appointment.

**155** In small homes where staff carry a range of responsibilities, these must be clearly understood by staff.

**156** Any change of role or duty should be made clear to the member of staff in writing.

**157** Minimum staff cover should be designed to cope with residents' anticipated problems at any time.

**Figure 1.16 Home Life recommendations about staff quality**

1984, has a checklist of 218 recommendations for monitoring the quality of social care. Many of these recommendations have now been built into regulations which inspectors check before a residential home can be registered or for a home to remain registered. The first ten recommendations, which concern staff qualities, are listed in Figure 1.16.

Codes of practice often advise workers on how to behave. For example the Equal Opportunities Commission has published a code to help eliminate sexual discrimination, and the Commission for Racial Equality has issued a code that gives guidance on the elimination of racial discrimination. Similarly, the Department of Health has published a guide to the professional behaviour expected of social workers, doctors and the police when working with people who are mentally ill. These codes do not provide checklists to help in the assessment of qualities. Rather they provide guidelines for service managers when they are devising policies and procedures staff must follow.

Most professional bodies have a code of conduct or code of practice which explains the values that guide people who work in that profession. The British Association for Social Work (BASW) has published 12 principles for social work that are contained within its code of ethics (see Figure 1.17).

1. Social workers will contribute to the formulation and implementation of policies for human welfare, and they will not permit their knowledge, skills or experience to be used to further dehumanising or discriminatory policies and will positively promote the use of their knowledge, skills and experience for the benefit of all sections of the community and individuals.
2. They will respect their clients as individuals and seek to ensure that their dignity, individuality, rights and responsibility shall be safeguarded.
3. They will not discriminate against clients, on the grounds of their origin, race, status, sex, sexual orientation, age, disability, beliefs, or contribution to society, they will not tolerate actions of colleagues or others which may be racist, sexist or otherwise discriminatory, nor will they deny those differences which will shape the nature of clients' needs and will ensure any personal help is offered within an acceptable personal and cultural context. They will draw to the attention of the Association any activity which is professionally unacceptable.
4. They will help their clients both individually and collectively to increase the range of choices open to them and their powers to make decisions, securing the participation, wherever possible, of clients in defining and obtaining services appropriate to their needs
5. They will not reject their clients or lose concern for their suffering, even if obliged to protect themselves or others against them or obliged to acknowledge an inability to help them.
6. They will give precedence to their professional responsibility over their own personal interests.
7. They accept that continuing professional education and training are basic to the practice of social work, and they hold themselves responsible for the standard of service they give.
8. They recognise the need to collaborate with others in the interest of their clients.
9. They will make clear in making any public statements or undertaking any public activities, whether they are acting in a personal capacity or on behalf of an organisation.
10. They will acknowledge a responsibility to help clients to obtain all those services and rights to which they are entitled; and will seek to ensure that these services are provided within a framework which will be both ethnically and culturally appropriate for all members of the community; and that an appropriate diversity will be promoted both in their own agency and other organisations in which they have influence.
11. They will recognise that information clearly entrusted for one purpose should not be used for another purpose without sanction. They will respect the privacy of clients and others with whom they come into contact and confidential information gained in their relationships with them. They will divulge such information only with the consent of the client (or informant) except where there is clear evidence of serious danger to the client, worker, other persons or the community or in other circumstances, judged exceptional, on the basis of professional consideration and consultation.
12. They will work for the creation and maintenance in employing agencies of conditions which will support and facilitate social workers' acceptance of the obligations of the Code.

**Figure 1.17 The BASW principles for social work (taken from BASW Code of Ethics 1996)**

### Think it over

Compare *Home Life*, the BASW code, and the UKCC code. There are similarities among all three 'codes', but there are also differences because social workers have slightly different responsibilities from nurses.

Pick out three points that are similar in all codes of practice. Why do you think they are there?

The UK Central Council for Nursing, Midwifery and Health Visiting (UKCC) has similarly published a 16-point code of professional conduct (see Figure 1.18).

**As a registered nurse, midwife or health visitor, you are personally accountable for your practice and, in the exercise of your professional accountability, must:**

1 Act always in such a manner as to promote and safeguard the interest and well-being of patients and clients.
2 Ensure that no action or omission on your part, or within your sphere of responsibility, is detrimental to the interests, condition or safety of patients and clients.
3 Maintain and improve your professional knowledge and competence.
4 Acknowledge any limitations in your knowledge and competence and decline any duties or responsibilities unless able to perform them in safe and skilled manner.
5 Work in an open and co-operative manner with patients, clients and their families, foster their independence and recognise and respect their involvement in the planning and delivery of care.
6 Work in a collaborative and co-operative manner with health care professionals and others involved in providing care, and recognise and respect their particular contributions within the care team.
7 Recognise and respect the uniqueness and dignity of each patient and client, and respond to their need for care, irrespective of their ethnic origin, religious beliefs, personal attributes, the nature of their health problems or any other factor.
8 Report to an appropriate person or authority, at least the earliest possible time, any conscientious objection which may be relevant to your professional practice.
9 Avoid any abuse of your privileged relationships with patients and clients and of the privileged access allowed to their person, property, residence or workplace.
10 Protect all confidential information concerning patients and clients obtained in the course of professional practice and make disclosures only with consent, where required by the order of a court or where you can justify disclosure in the wider public interest.
11 Report to an appropriate person or authority, having regard to the physical, psychological and social effects on patients and clients, any circumstances in the environment of care which could jeopardise standards of practice.
12 Report to an appropriate person or authority any circumstances in which safe and appropriate care for patients and clients cannot be provided.
13 Report to an appropriate person or authority where it appears that the health or safety of colleagues is at risk, as such circumstances may compromise standards of practice in care.
14 Assist professional colleagues, in the context of your own knowledge, experience and sphere of responsibility, to develop their professional competence and assist others in the care team, including informal carers, to contribute safely and to a degree appropriate to their roles.
15 Refuse any gift, favour or hospitality from patients or clients currently in your care which might be interpreted as seeking to expert influence to obtain preferential consideration and
16 Ensure that your registration status is not used in the promotion of commercial products or services, declare any financial or other interests in relevant organisations providing such goods or services and ensure that your professional judgement is not influenced by any commercial considerations.

**Figure 1.18** The UKCC code of professional conduct

## Codes of practice: summary

- All codes of practice enable both members of the public and professionals to measure whether quality care is being delivered or not.
- *Home Life* includes a checklist to help people assess the quality of care. Other codes are perhaps more abstract but they still help people to decide whether a service is good or not.
- Some codes provide professionals with advice and guidelines; others define the detailed values relevant to a specific service.

## Charters

Recent governments have produced a series of charters that outline the standards people can expect from a wide range of services. These charters are like codes of practice but they are designed by government. The Citizen's Charter, in particular, sets out the quality people can expect from public services. The charter contains information about the services and gives advice about how to seek redress (follow up our rights) if a service does not fulfil all the stipulated standards. An important section of the Citizen's Charter is the **Patient's Charter**. A new NHS Charter is expected which provides a statement of national standards and offers a localised approach to the services patients can expect.

The existing charter (which was produced in January 1995) set out the rights and standards people could expect of the services (for example, waiting times for out-patient appointments and for operations).

Many GPs are now producing practice charters that give information about the standards of service provided by their particular health centres. These cover such information as opening times, test results collection, how to get a repeat prescription, facilities for people with disabilities and out-of-hours treatment.

The Department of Health requires all Local Authority social services departments to publish **Community Care Charters**. These charters explain what users and carers can expect from the community care services provided in that area and they also set out their services' commitments and standards.

### Think it over

Watch out for the implementation of the Care Standards Bill. It will probably initially apply to field social workers and residential staff working with children, but may eventually affect all care workers, including all residential staff, day care workers and domiciliary carers. The Act will set up the General Social Care Council (GSCC), which will:

- publish codes of conduct and standards of practice
- regulate standards of education and training
- maintain a register of staff who are appropriately trained and fit to practise
- investigate allegations of serious misconduct
- be responsible for registration, discipline and removal from the register.

Registration will be made a requirement for the employment of all staff in social care, and it is intended that the GSCC will both promote good practice and provide additional protection for clients.

Workers who do not have a professional association may be able to get advice from a trade union. In residential situations, the Inspection Unit of the local authority may be able to help. Other sources of help and advice are specialist charities dealing with specific client groups, e.g. MIND for people suffering from mental disorders. There are also government agencies, part of whose role is to give advice about the rights of groups that have protection under the law, e.g. the Equal Opportunities Commission, the Commission for Racial Equality, and the Disability Act Commission.

The law may help, although not all ethical problems are necessarily legal problems, and there is no guarantee that even if someone works strictly within the law that they might not feel badly about something they have to do. Some legislation, especially mental health and children's legislation, lays down the conditions under which people's liberty may be curtailed in order to protect themselves and others, and requires that people who undertake tasks concerning the liberty of clients have special training. Some pieces of legislation have Codes of Practice associated with them to guide practitioners in their role under the legislation.

Large employers, such as social services departments and Health Authorities, will have legal departments that will be able to advise workers about their legal responsibilities and powers in more complex situations.

However, sometimes even these measures are insufficient to help in the most complex situations. Many of the most difficult problems arise in the area of medicine, and in the most difficult cases health and care organisations, or the people themselves, take the case to court so that a judge can decide on the rights and wrongs of the situation.

# 1.4 The effects of discriminatory practices on individuals

### Think it over

Imagine you went into a shop and when you tried to pay for your goods other people were constantly served before you. Imagine that the shop assistants were friendly and pleasant to other people but that they were cold and very formal toward you. How would this make you feel?

You would probably feel 'excluded' by the staff in the shop and this would make you angry – you would decide not to use that shop again. But now imagine that every day you get the same treatment – not only when you shop, but while you are at work, while you travel, when you are out in the street. How would this influence you?

A single experience of discrimination may not make a large difference to the overall quality of a person's life, but general systematic discrimination may completely destroy the quality of someone's life.

Discrimination may occur in a variety of ways. These are summarised in Figure 1.19.

Discrimination can be understood as damaging the individual quality of life in relation to Maslow's analysis of human needs as set out in Figure 1.20. Discriminatory practice can affect clients' well-being in a number of different ways and we will look at some of these in turn.

DISCRIMINATORY PRACTICES
Physical assault of people who are different
Verbal abuse towards people who are different
Excluding people from activities
Excluding people from opportunities
Avoiding people because they are different
Negative non-verbal communication
Making assumptions Perhaps that everyone should be given the same experience or responded to in the same way
Devaluing people Treating their needs and interest as of less value than others

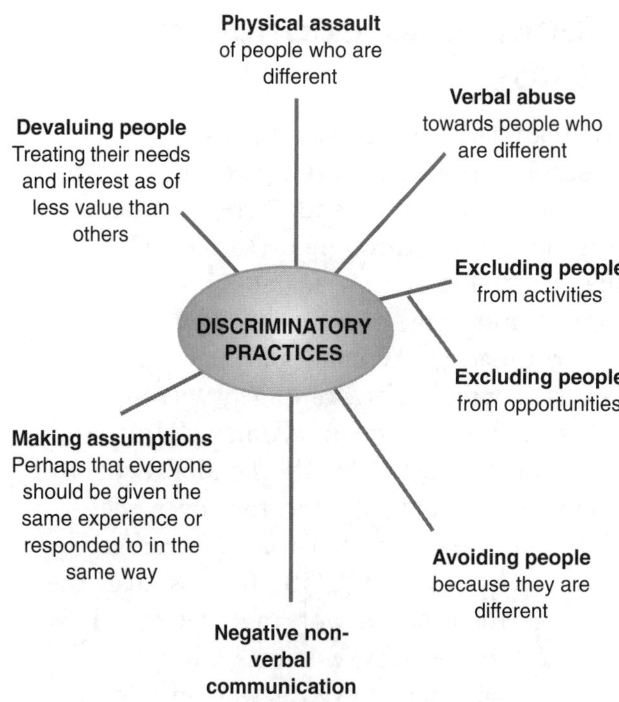

Figure 1.19 Types of discrimination and abuse

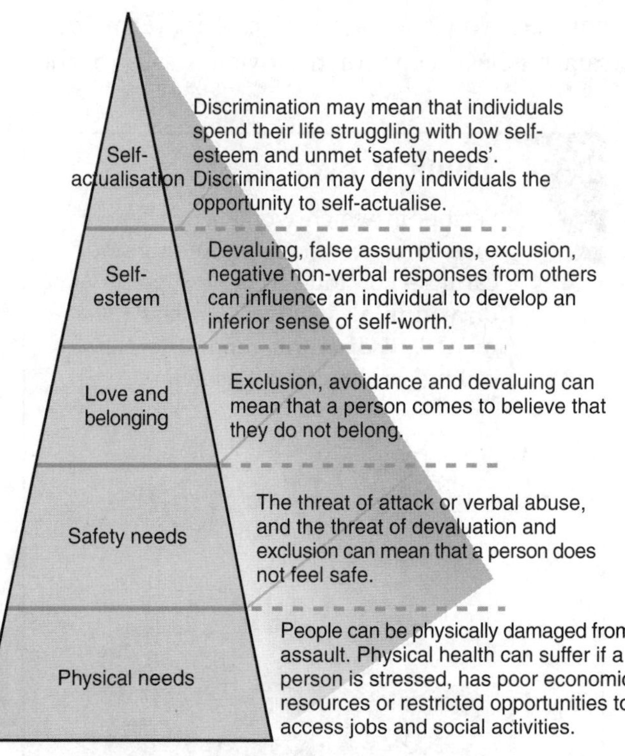


Figure 1.20 How discrimination may block human needs and change people

## Social and economic status

Although there are laws against discrimination, they are not enough on their own to eliminate it and there is structural discrimination throughout society. The law has had more success in reducing (though not eliminating) overt rather than covert discrimination. Women and black people are still widely disadvantaged within society. A government Women's Unit study published in 2000 by the London School of Economics (Women's Incomes over the Lifetime) demonstrated that an average woman would earn £250,000 less than the average man over a working lifetime. This is not explained by women taking time off to raise children – even a woman with no children earns on average £100,000 less. Women have made advances in education – the proportion of female undergraduates has risen from 25 per cent in the 1960s to 52 per cent today – but progress in terms of salaries has been much slower. In 1975 the top 10 per cent of women earners were paid 59.6 per cent of the earnings of comparable men. By 1999 this had increased, but only to 62.7 per cent.

### Think it over

Sectors in which women workers predominate – such as nursing and caring – continue to be low paid. Why do you think women earn less than men? Is it discrimination, 'the glass ceiling' or for other reasons?

The government report 'Opportunity for All' (1999) shows that people from some ethnic minorities are more likely to experience disadvantage than white people. 'Seven out of ten households with a Pakistani or Bangladeshi head were in the poorest fifth of the income distribution in 1996/97, and this was also true for three out of ten households with a black or Indian head' (page 26).

*Social Trends 2000* reports that between 1996-98, 17 per cent of white households fell into the category of low income (below 60 per cent medium income). But this compares with 28 per cent of black households, 27 per cent of Indian and 64 per cent of Pakistani households. There are clear relationships between income and ethnicity and discrimination undoubtedly plays a part in explaining these figures.

Women and people with a disability are also more likely to experience lower social and economic status than others. 'Opportunity for All' (1999) states: 'Women are particularly likely to live on low incomes at key stages of their life cycle: both lone mothers and single women pensioners are more likely to have persistently low incomes. People with disabilities are around six times more likely than those without a disability to be out of work and claiming benefits. Their chance of being in employment is only about half that of the general population. They are also more likely to experience greater problems with accessing goods, services and facilities' (page 26).

**Employees: by gender and occupation, 1991 and 1999**

United Kingdon — Percentages

| | Males | | Females | |
|---|---|---|---|---|
| | 1991 | 1999 | 1991 | 1999 |
| Managers and administrators | 16 | 19 | 8 | 11 |
| Professional | 10 | 11 | 8 | 10 |
| Associate professional and technical | 8 | 9 | 10 | 11 |
| Clerical and secretarial | 8 | 8 | 29 | 26 |
| Craft and related | 21 | 17 | 4 | 2 |
| Personal and protective services | 7 | 8 | 14 | 17 |
| Selling | 6 | 6 | 12 | 12 |
| Plant and machine operatives | 15 | 15 | 5 | 4 |
| Other occupations | 8 | 8 | 10 | 8 |
| All employees[2] (= 100%) (millions) | 11.8 | 12.4 | 10.1 | 10.8 |

[1]At Spring each year. Males aged 16 to 64, females aged 16 to 58.

[2]Includes a few people who did not state their occupation. Percentages are based on totals which exclude this group.

**Source: Labour Force Survey, Office for National Statistics**

*Social Trends 2000* notes that more women are becoming managers and professionals than in the past. But the figures still suggest that gender role stereotypes have a major effect on the type of employment that men and women achieve. The table (4.13) demonstrates how the largest male categories of employment in 1999 were management, craft and machine operatives, while for women, secretarial, personal (caring), and 'selling' formed the key sources of employment.

**Think it over**

Looking at the changes in male and female employment between 1991 and 1999, do you see evidence for changing gender role expectations or not? Do you think men and women have an equal opportunity to achieve well-paid jobs nowadays?

## Health

There is evidence of institutional racism within the National Health Service. A number of studies have suggested that non-white patients are treated differently to white patients within mental health services. This has been supported by a recent Mental Health Act Commission report which found that non-white patients, and particularly people of Afro Caribbean ethnicity, were far more likely to be compulsorily detained ('sectioned') under the Mental Health Act 1983. They are far more likely to have been admitted to hospital by the police under their powers of detention. Once in hospital they were more likely to be diagnosed as having a serious mental disorder, such as schizophrenia. They were also more likely to be treated in secure facilities, more likely to be treated with harsher forms of medication and more likely to be given physical forms of treatment such as electro-convulsive therapy (ECT). The Mental Health Act Commission report raised particular concerns that patients who did not have English as a first language, and some who spoke no English, were being forcibly treated in psychiatric units without the use of interpreters. Many ethnic minority patients in these units suffered racial harassment, and very few of the units had any policy for dealing with this.

Social services departments have also been accused of institutional racism. It is suggested that in some cases they have made unfounded assumptions about their ethnic minority populations. One assumption is that ethnic minority populations are made up of stable, multi-generational families who care for their own elderly people through community organisations or the extended family. This has led to failures to make appropriate provision for older people from ethnic minorities, particularly in preventative services. As a result, people from ethnic minorities are over-represented in areas of service provision which involve institutionalisation and social control, where their needs are not appropriately met. This over-representation applies also to the young, and children of Afro-Caribbean and mixed parentage are over-represented in the care system. This is compounded by frequent failure to recruit sufficient foster parents and prospective adopters form appropriate ethnic backgrounds.

The result of institutional racism is a frequent, although not universal, failure to provide appropriate services to ethnic minority communities, and a failure to provide information about services in appropriate languages. The Acheson report (1998) gathered extensive data on the nature of inequality in the area of health. The report found major differences between the health of people on low incomes compared with people who were financially better off. The report also found some evidence of inequalities between ethnic groups and gender. Further details can be found in Chapter 4.

## Self-esteem and empowerment

Have you ever experienced the situation when two members of your class at school were told to choose a team? Can you recall the feeling of unease as members of your group were gradually called to join one team or another? Do you remember the feeling of relief when you were chosen? Perhaps even a sense of smugness as you looked at the discomfort of the few remaining children left until last? Were they last because they were considered to be no good at the game to be played and therefore a liability? What effect do you think it had on the child who was always the one to be left until last? Why did you feel smug when chosen early on? People can be fickle and self-centred, even cruel, particularly (but not exclusively) in childhood.

You might have never had the experience of waiting to be picked for a team. Think then of a time when you had been 'put down' by an adult; remember how it felt, particularly if you believed their actions were unjust in some way. Can you remember the anger and frustration, the feeling of powerlessness? As a child you were expected to do what the adult said. Adults had power to control situations, whereas you as a child did not.

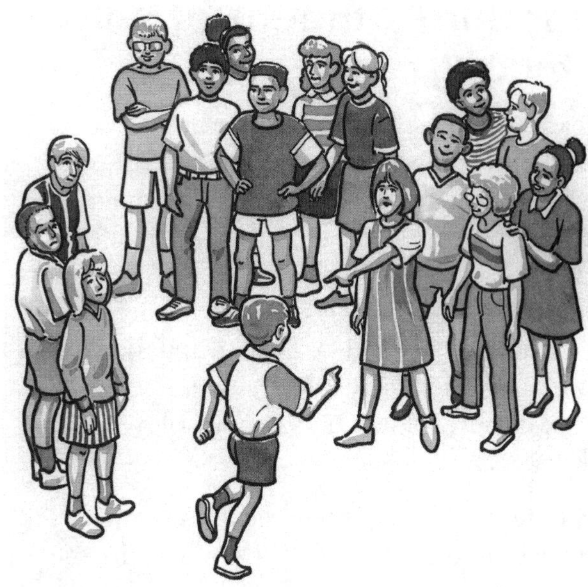

**Figure 1.21** It can be hard if you're always the last chosen

> **Think it over**
>
> Imagine now some adult experiences: the worker made redundant, the individual made homeless, the couple going through a divorce process, the ending of a relationship you felt would last forever. All these would have a profound effect on the way the individuals perceive themselves and the value they place on themselves. It takes time and support from others to rebuild a bruised and battered self-esteem.

Imagine that all your life people have put you down by the way they have spoken to you or behaved towards you. Perhaps at school there was a subject you found particularly difficult. However hard you tried you could not get it right. If the teacher at school – and also perhaps your family at home – were less than sympathetic to your efforts, and kept making comments about your low marks, you might begin to believe that you would never be any good at that subject. So in the end you stop trying – and then you never do succeed at that subject! Motivation to succeed when things are difficult comes from determination on the part of the individual – but also from the understanding and support of others.

Continuous episodes of discrimination are likely to have a major impact on a person's emotional development. People who experience devaluation or are 'put down' on a regular basis may develop a low sense of self-esteem. Some individuals may feel 'like a stranger' or 'estranged' from the broader society in which they live. Many people may develop a lack of self-confidence in their own abilities. This may result from the many subtle messages they receive while interacting with services such as health, care, education and law enforcement, where discrimination may be 'institutionalised'. Institutionalised discrimination means that exclusion, devaluing and inappropriate assumptions are built into the way systems, procedures and people work.

## Bandura's theory of self-efficacy

Learning to develop a low level of expectation about your own abilities (low self-confidence) is sometimes explained using the theory of self-efficacy. Bandura's theory of self-efficacy is explained in Unit 4 of this book (see page 274). Prolonged exposure to general or institutionalised discrimination may cause low self-efficacy in areas such as education and employability skills.

Where people experience extreme and persistent discrimination they may in the end simply give up and withdraw from attempting to control their lives. This might, for instance, result in withdrawing from looking for employment because people have learned not to bother in a system which seems to work against them. Giving up involves learning to become 'helpless'. The theory of learned helplessness is explained in more detail in Unit 2 (see page 101).

When people come to understand that they are not expected to succeed or achieve at school or in work they may 'fulfil the prophecies' of others. This means that people who develop low self-efficacy may find it easier to act in the way that teachers or employers expect. Some people come to accept or believe in the labels and stereotypes that others impose on them.

A summary of some of the outcomes of discrimination on self-esteem and empowerment is provided in Figure 1.22.

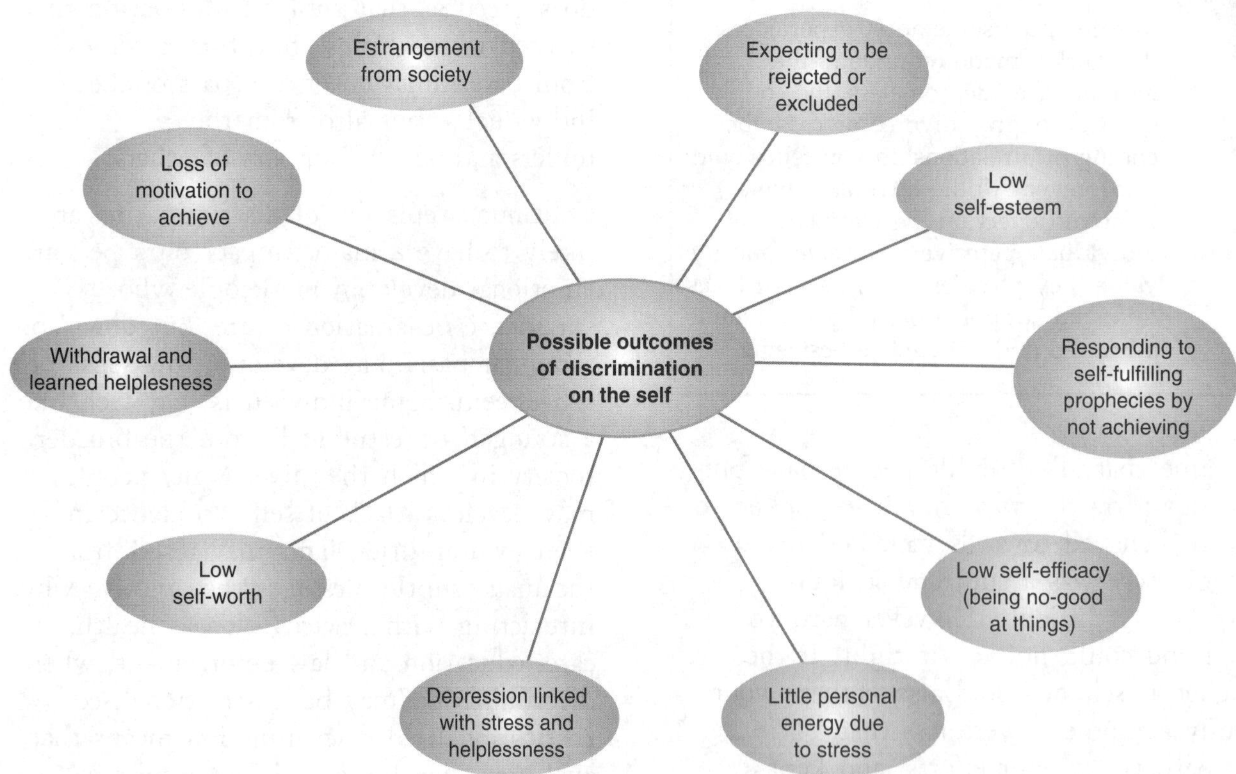


**Figure 1.22 Outcomes of discrimination on self-esteem and empowerment**

## Personal development and relationships

Children will be aware of differences between people from an early age, but they have to learn value judgements about those differences. Children will notice skin colour, but will not have a concept that one skin colour is 'better' than another unless they learn this. They will be aware of disability, but will not automatically generalise a disability in one area to all aspects of the person's life. This too is a learned attitude. This is what makes the attitudes of carers so important. Children not only learn what adults intend to teach them, but also learn from observing the world around them.

Children may hear their parents or other carers express prejudiced attitudes, and grow to accept them. They may learn about gender roles from an early age by experiencing how their own parents behave and allocate household and caring tasks. Through the way they are treated children may encounter stereotypes and prejudice from an early age, especially on the basis of gender. If they are given 'boys' and 'girls' toys to play with, or given messages such as 'girls don't fight' or 'boys don't cry', they will assimilate from an early age the kinds of behaviours and attitudes that are expected of them. They will also absorb messages from the media and, for instance, if people from some groups are not represented, or represented in a negative way, this will be damaging for children. Those in the favoured group may be confirmed in ethnocentric or prejudiced attitudes, the others will experience negative effects on their self-esteem. They may get the message that they are not valued because of their race or sex, or as a result of physical characteristic or disability. They may develop the belief that some opportunities are not available to them so there is no point in trying, which will limit their opportunities. They may be made to feel unattractive about physical characteristics they can do nothing about. If children are constantly bombarded with role models who are white and thin, people who do not have these characteristics may feel undervalued.

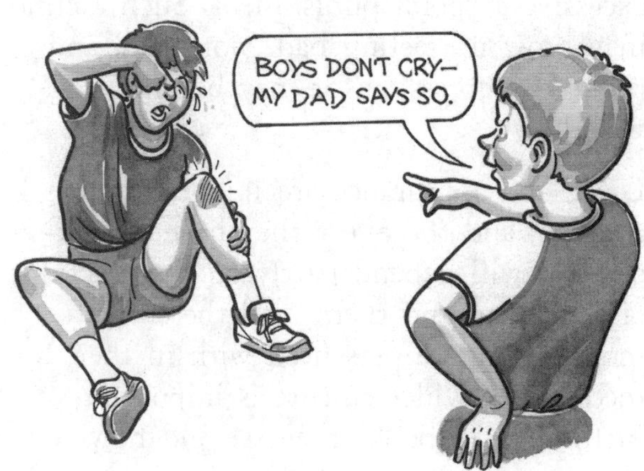


**Figure 1.23 Children assimilate attitudes from others from an early age**

As children get older, influences outside the home become more important. Children may be exposed to prejudiced attitudes that they had previously been protected from, especially concerning race and disability. Exposure to discrimination and prejudice is always likely to affect self-esteem adversely, although the extent to which it does may vary. It will depend partly on how the child has been prepared. This is one of the arguments advanced in favour of same race fostering and adoption.

Children's self-concept is initially strongly affected by the way they relate to other individuals, initially their close family and other carers, later with peers and other significant adults – teachers, etc. They will have a number of social roles – child, sibling, grandchild, then pupil, etc. – that will give them a sense of their place in the world. How these people react to them will be vital to their self-concept. For instance, a child who has loving and supportive parents who praise and encourage, and are consistent in the way they treat them, is more likely to grow up with a sense of their own worth than a child brought up by parents who criticise, belittle and use excessive corporal punishment. Such a child may grow up feeling bad, worthless, and prone to depression, or may become withdrawn.

Looks and appearance are important for self-concept, and the effect they have on self-concept will depend partly on the reactions of people around them, and the sort of models they are presented with in the media. The wider culture is important, including the books they see and how characters in them reflect their race or sex. The media and adverts which present ideals of beauty that are predominantly young, white, and thin affect how people view things, not only how they feel about skin colour and other racial characteristics, but also about body shape. Low self-esteem has consequences for eating disorders.

## Damaging self-esteem

The relationship between exposure to prejudice and discrimination and a person's self-esteem is a complex one. Although always damaging, if a person starts off with a strong sense of their own self-worth, they will be better able to face prejudice and discrimination without it severely affecting their self-esteem. The poem by Dorothy Law Nolte opposite gives a view of how the way a child is treated will affect his or her self-image and self-esteem.

The author of this poem is saying that a child who has loving and supportive parents, or other carers, who praise and encourage, and are consistent in the way they treat them is more likely to grow up with a sense of their own worth than a child brought up by people who criticise or devalue that person. Children treated in this way may grow up feeling worthless or may act their unhappiness out in the form of anti-social behaviour and find it difficult to form healthy relationships.

**Children Learn What They Live**

If children live with criticism<br>
They learn to condemn.<br>
If children live with hostility<br>
They learn to fight.<br>
If children live with ridicule<br>
They learn to be shy.<br>
If children live with shame<br>
They learn to feel guilty.

If children live with tolerance<br>
They learn to be patient.<br>
If children live with encouragement<br>
They learn to be confident.<br>
If children live with praise<br>
They learn to appreciate.<br>
If children live with fairness<br>
They learn justice.<br>
If children live with security<br>
They learn to have faith.<br>
If children live with approval<br>
They learn to like themselves.<br>
If children live with acceptance and friendship<br>
They learn to find love in the World.

As children grow older and move out into the world, the attitudes of others will become increasingly important. If they encounter widespread discrimination on the basis of their sex, the colour of their skin, or their culture, children will learn that some of their characteristics are not valued. How people react to this will depend on their self-concept, their self-esteem; whether they are able to deal with this with confidence may depend upon how they have been prepared.

### Think it over

Labelling becomes particularly important when a child enters education. If, for instance, a teacher really believes that boys are better at sciences and girls better at humanities then they may be guided this way in subtle ways, despite there being an official policy of equality. Similarly, a teacher who, perhaps unconsciously, has low expectations of black children may create an environment in which they underachieve. Disproportionate numbers of Afro-Caribbean children compared with white children are suspended and expelled from schools. How much is this self-fulfilling prophecy?

## Employability

Despite the legislation, people's life chances continue to be affected by prejudice and discrimination. Regular reports appearing in the press of Employment Tribunal findings and court judgements demonstrate this. People's prospects may be affected by overt or covert discrimination, but there may also be indirect effects resulting from exposure to discrimination affecting their self-esteem. People with low self-esteem may be discouraged from applying for jobs and, if they do apply, may not present themselves to the best advantage.

**Example** Sean and Daniel are both interviewed for a job, but neither gets it. Sean has high self-esteem. He is disappointed, but thinks that he was unlucky, or that he did not have the skills the employer was looking for. He asks the employer for some feedback on his performance in the interview and looks at ways in which he can acquire the skills he needs, and present the skills he has, for future applications. He is more confident the next time he applies for a job and is successful in his application.

Daniel has low self-esteem. He gets very depressed by being rejected and thinks he is useless and it must be all his fault. He goes along to his next interview feeling very low and expecting to be rejected again. He does not present himself very well, and does not get the job. He is even less confident when the next vacancy arises.

The way we react to circumstances as adults may be strongly affected by our early experiences, but experiencing discrimination as an adult is still a damaging experience. Everybody experiences rejection, whether in relationships or employment. If we have a positive self-image, we see it as a short-term set-back. If self-esteem has been eroded by constant exposure to prejudice, discrimination and abuse, then it may be much more difficult to handle rejection.

## Non-oppressive practice

Because of the importance of the effects that prejudice and discrimination may have on the social and emotional development of children, there is a particular responsibility for care workers in early years services to ensure that diversity is valued in those environments. The books, materials and toys provided should reflect ethnic diversity, and the activities undertaken should ensure that all children feel that their cultural backgrounds are valued equally. This is not only to promote the self-esteem of children of ethnic minority backgrounds, but also to promote tolerance and understanding in those from the ethnic majority group.

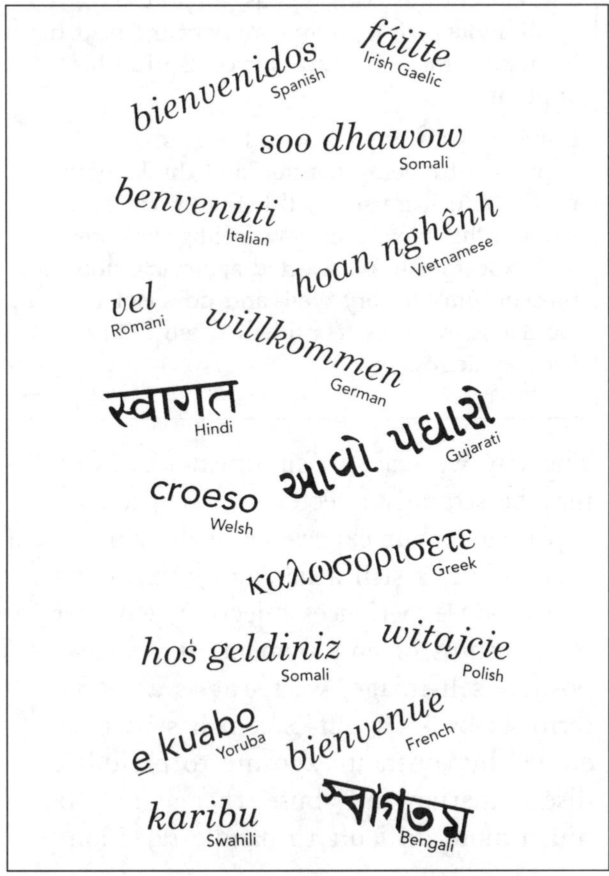


**Figure 1.24 All children should feel that their culture is valued**

It is also important not to stereotype children on the basis on their sex, and not to unconsciously steer boys into 'masculine' activities and girls into 'feminine' ones. This could happen either through the activities they are encouraged in or discouraged from, or by the examples they are offered in the books and materials which are provided for them. If children are not presented with choices during early years, then it may limit their options in later life.

It is important that carers avoid prejudice on any of the bases of discrimination, as this can result in clients being unreasonably deprived of services. The best way of avoiding prejudiced attitudes is to obtain knowledge. For instance, workers providing services to people with AIDS should understand how the infection is spread. Every worker has a duty under the legislation to safeguard their own health and safety, and should take sensible precautions in situations of risk. However, it is unacceptable for clients to be deprived of services, or to be treated in a discriminatory way, on the basis of mistaken and ill-informed beliefs about the risk of infection.

Similarly, there are widespread prejudiced views that people suffering from mental disorders are dangerous to others. It is undoubtedly true that a small number of people with certain mental disorders may, under some circumstances, be a danger to others. However, most people with a mental disorder do not present a threat to anybody, and those that do are more likely to harm themselves than other people. To talk as if all people with mental disorders are dangerous is prejudiced and labelling, and damaging to those people. Discrimination on the basis of health status may result in clients receiving inferior services, and prejudice results in fear which may also lead to clients being isolated and deprived of social contacts.

A lack of understanding of the needs of people with disabilities can easily lead to their being deprived of choice and a sense of empowerment and control over their lives. This is particularly true of people whose disabilities cause communication difficulties, for instance people with hearing problems or those who have had strokes. There is a responsibility to communicate effectively and sensitively to ensure that people are able to express preferences and choice. This may involve relatively simple techniques, such as taking time to listen carefully, speaking clearly and slowly, facing towards clients and not covering your mouth in order to facilitate lip-reading. It may require further measures, such as communicating in writing or developing skills such as signing, or obtaining the services of interpreters or advocates. People with disabilities frequently complain that prejudice often leads others to assume that they are unable to make decisions about wide areas of their lives. This results in exclusion and disempowerment.

Use of language is very important in avoiding prejudice and discrimination. Care should be taken to avoid using outdated terms which have acquired negative connotations. The Spastics Society, for instance, changed its name to SCOPE for precisely this reason.

Wherever possible, gender-specific language should be avoided as this may exclude or deter women, for example using terms like chairman, headmaster and foreman instead of chair, head teacher and supervisor.

Some language may reinforce stereotypes, such as using 'wheelchair bound' instead of 'wheelchair user'. The former term reinforces the discriminatory idea that people with disabilities are helpless. Similarly, people should be referred to as having illnesses, rather than suffering form them or being crippled by them. Worst of all is to refer to people in terms of their illnesses. Calling someone a schizophrenic, rather than someone with schizophrenia, or referring to 'the disabled' rather than 'people with disabilities' is discriminatory and the first stage in labelling. It is only a short step to seeing that label as the most important thing about the person and ceasing to respect their differences and individuality.

## Keys to good practice

Non-oppressive practice will involve:

- Ensuring that communication conveys a sense of value for all people. This may involve using the skills of understanding, warmth and sincerity. (Further details of these skills are covered in Chapter 2.)
- Using communication skills which demonstrate valuing diversity. This may include remembering personal details, perhaps learning to speak a few words of a client's language if their first language is different from yours.
- Being careful to avoid language terms which devalue others or which include stereotyped assumptions.
- Questioning assumptions which we might make as individuals. This involves checking for stereotypes which we might have to come to believe, and checking that we do not generalise our understanding of other groups to exclude individuality in others.
- Being prepared to apologise for mistakes if we do make assumptions which turn out to be incorrect.
- Understanding the rights and responsibilities of carers and clients being able to act in a way that promotes the dignity and autonomy of others.
- Maintaining confidentiality.

### Think it over

Look at the activities listed below. What problems might arise if these activities were presented in the same way to a diverse group of clients? Use the list of differences below to consider whether and how some of these activities could discriminate against certain people.

| Activities | Differences |
|---|---|
| Learn how to cook bacon | Religions |
| Take turns in washing up | Beliefs about what it is right to eat |
| Sing Christmas carols | Beliefs about alcohol |
| Play bingo | Countries of origin |
| Go to a sherry or drinks party | Ethnic groups |
| Play cards, gambling for pennies | Gender and gender roles |
| Learn to paint | Social class |
| Do old-time dancing | Levels of practical ability and disability |
| Talk about photographs of England in the 1920s | |

It is vital that health and care workers review their own practice to make sure that they do not discriminate and that they positively value diversity in other people. It is also important to remember that one of the key ways in which the damaging effects of discrimination can be prevented is for people who are discriminated against to support each other. If people build a positive self-concept, if people feel valued in their own community, they may be able to resist some of the damage that discrimination can create. Prejudice and discrimination may wreck a person's life if the result is learned helplessness or low self-efficacy. Helplessness and low self-efficacy may be prevented through group and community support, which builds an understanding of discrimination and its potential dangers. Positive action to empower people to develop and maintain their own self-esteem may be as important as the development of non-discriminatory practice in the struggle against oppression.

## 1.5 Organisations that challenge discrimination

There are a number of important organisations that act to challenge discrimination and work on the behalf of, and support, individuals. In this section we will look at the role and functions of these organisations.

### Equal Opportunities Commission (EOC)

At the same time as the Sex Discrimination Act was passed, the Equal Opportunities Commission (EOC) was set up to monitor, advise and provide information regarding the Sex Discrimination Act and its implementation. Individuals have the right to bring proceedings before an industrial tribunal should they face discrimination under this legislation. Help and advice is obtainable from the EOC should an individual feel that they have a case.

The EOC has issued a document, 'Guidance on Employment Advertising Practice'. This document helps employers to consider appropriate wording for advertising jobs. Appropriate wording is essential to remain within the law. It is unlawful to advertise a post in such a way as to discriminate against one sex in favour of another. The use of terms such as waitress, barman, steward and postmistress imply that applicant should be either male or female.

## Commission for Racial Equality (CRE)

The Race Relations Act 1976 abolished the Race Relations Board and set up the Commission for Racial Equality (CRE). This body monitors the Act, acts as an adviser and has extensive powers to investigate discrimination. Individuals have new rights to bring proceedings before an industrial tribunal should they be the victims of discrimination. The CRE may be asked to give information to an individual who wishes to take a case to a tribunal.

### The functions of the Commission for Racial Equality

The Commission for Racial Equality has three main duties, to:

- work towards the elimination of racial discrimination and promote equality of opportunity
- encourage good relations between people from different racial backgrounds
- monitor the way in which the Race Relations Act is working and recommend ways in which it can be improved.

It has the statutory powers to:

- directly advise or assist people who are complaining about racial discrimination, harassment or abuse
- conduct formal investigations of companies where there is evidence of possible discrimination, and make the organisation change the way it operates if discrimination is found
- take legal action against racially discriminatory advertisements and against organisations that attempt to pressurise or instruct others to discriminate.

To achieve this it:

- issues codes of practice
- advises employers, housing, health and education authorities, training bodies and other agencies
- advises government on race issues and the racial equality implications of legislation, policies and practice
- supports research into race issues
- runs public education campaigns.

## Sources of support and guidance

In terms of employment, workers who consider that they have been discriminated against have several avenues which they may explore. Information regarding the individual's rights may be obtained from the Commission for Racial Equality, if the issue is regarding race, or the Equal Opportunities Commission if the discrimination was on the grounds of gender – for either male or female employees.

A questionnaire has to be completed and returned within three months of the alleged incident. The next stage is then to go before an employment tribunal or county court. In the event of the discrimination being direct and intentional the employment tribunal or county court can award damages and make recommendations and a declaration of the law.

An incidence of discrimination on the grounds of race or gender which is outside employment may also be addressed by an employment tribunal or county court. If the discrimination was direct and intentional then, again, the employment tribunal or county court can award damages and make recommendations and a declaration of the law.

In either case, if the direct or indirect discrimination is proven to be unintentional, then the employment tribunal or county court can only make a declaration and/or recommendations; but no damages can be awarded.

Other routes to gain information regarding individual rights may be gained by visiting the local Law Centre or the Citizens' Advice Bureau. Trade unions will also be able to offer advice to their members.

It is possible to appeal against a decision made by an employment tribunal or county court. An appeal can only be made on a point of law to the Employment Appeal Tribunal. Any such appeal must be made within six weeks of the decision being given. In certain circumstances the case may be passed to the House of Lords and, finally, to the European Court in Luxembourg.

There is an Ombudsman for health and social care. The role is to consider any complaint about the service provision in this area. If an individual considers that his or her legal rights have been infringed, or that there has been unfair treatment or maladministration, then the Ombudsman may consider the case – unless it has already been to a court of law or employment tribunal.

The Ombudsman will require full details of the situation and will try to settle the dispute between the two parties. Failure to achieve this means that the Ombudsman will make a decision on the information received. Any decision made may be accepted or rejected; in the latter case the decision will lapse and the individual may take legal action against the organisation.

As stated earlier, organisations will have an equal opportunity statement or policy. Government Charters will have been interpreted by the organisation to form the basis for their own Charter or standards. These will include the method for making a complaint and the time element involved.

Most professional bodies have a code of practice for their staff; perhaps one of the best known is the Hippocratic Oath taken by doctors. The British Association of Social Workers, the United Kingdom Central Council and the British Psychological Society all provide such guidelines for staff, to name just a few.

Residential care, too, has seen a series of reports and codes of practice to ensure clients' rights and the quality of service are maintained. The **Wagner Report** stated that people moving into residential care should have real choices. These rights and choices include: the continued right as a citizen, for example, to vote in local and government elections etc; having access to community services and the right to complain if need be; the right to manage their own affairs, including their pensions; the right to make decisions and, where this is not possible, the right to a six-monthly review; and the right to have their cultural needs met.

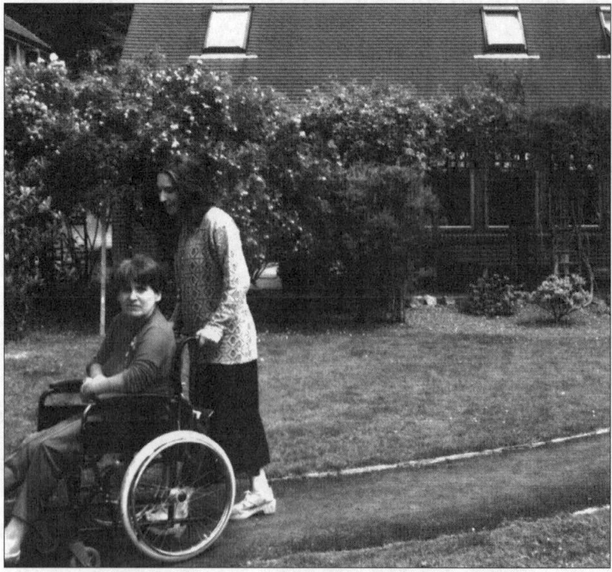

**Figure 1.25 People in residential care have rights and choices**
**(Photo courtesy of Winged Fellowship Trust)**

In 1984 **Home Life: A Code of Practice for Residential Care** was written. This stated that clients have the right to: individuality, dignity, esteem, fulfilment, autonomy, be able to take risks, have a quality of experience and have emotional needs met through personal/intimate relationships, if they wish.

**Community Life 1990** went a step further by saying that all care packages should reflect the informed choice of the client. Individuals should know their rights and responsibilities. They have the right to an advocate, and to make complaints if required. This placed responsibility on the providers of services to ensure that a complaints procedure was implemented and that provision for advocates was made. Providers have to ensure that all the service users are aware of possible choices and the potential outcomes of those choices. This also meant that clients could decide to take a calculated risk: for example, to make their own cup of tea despite some physical difficulty. The provider should take all necessary steps to minimise the risk but not prevent it.

Complaints procedures are made available to all service users; for example, a complaint regarding the service in a residential home would be made to the manager. Should the service user remain unsatisfied, the next step is to refer to the social services department or to the Registrar of Residential Establishments (the person who registers such establishments).

If it is a member of staff who has a complaint, this would be addressed to the immediate line manager. The staff member may wish to take the matter to the union for advice and guidance before taking the matter up with the employers. Should the case be one of discrimination on grounds of race or gender, then the matter may be referred to a tribunal as described earlier.

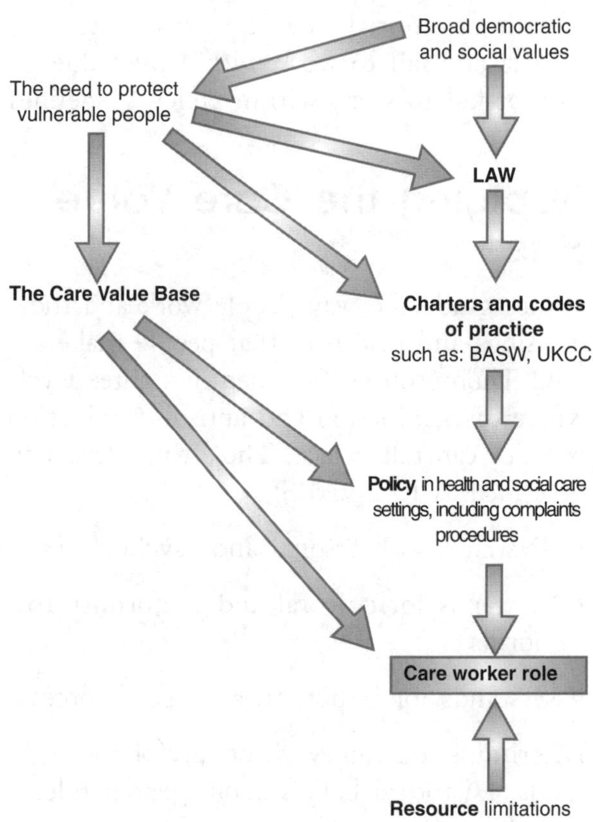


**Figure 1.26** Anti-discrimination influences on client care

## Codes of practice and charters of rights

Details of BASW and UKCC Codes of Practice have been discussed previously in this chapter. It is important to note that codes of practice and laws cannot protect clients directly. Figure 1.26 outlines the way in which the law, charters, value bases and codes of practice may influence client care.

The law, charters, policy and the care value base all influence the duties and role of care staff. The law influences the policies that organisations develop and policy influences practice – provided that there are systems to monitor the quality of practice. What really happens in practice is also influenced by the resources available to carers. If staff are short of time or stressed, then they may cut corners and fail to work within the value base or fail to work within policy guidelines.

## Applying the Care Value Base

Values guide the way people work and the decisions and priorities that people make. Neil Thompson (1997) identifies three levels where discrimination and anti-discrimination practice can take place. These three levels are described as P, C and S:

- P stands for personal and psychological
- C stands for cultural and conformity to norms
- S stands for structural and social forces.

Discrimination can work on any of the three levels. Historical beliefs about gender role, and about the superiority of ethnic groups, influences the social and political structures in which we live. Some organisations may

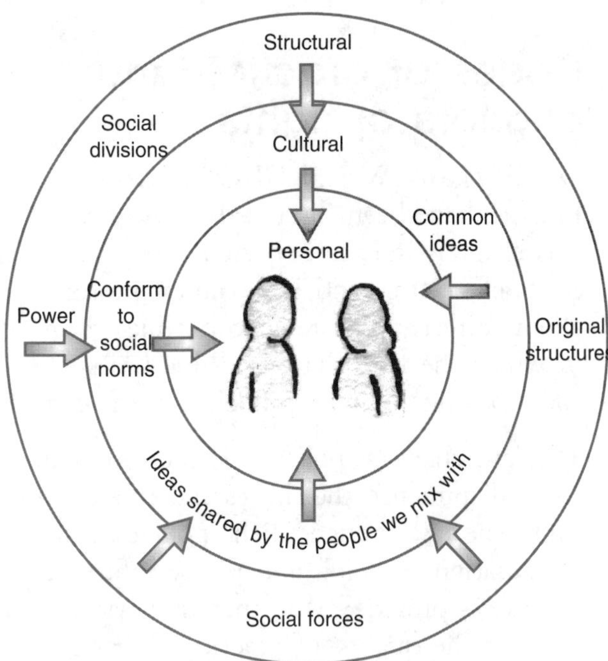


**Figure 1.27 Different levels of discrimination: P, C and S**

still value male employees more highly than women. Men may find it easier to get promotion because organisations have built-in or structural systems that make it easier for men to succeed. On the cultural level we mix with groups of people who share values and ways of behaving. A great deal of discrimination happens because people conform to the expectations of others. People might for instance join in jokes about a particular minority, not because they hold personal prejudices but because they want to fit in with others. On a personal level our own beliefs are often translated into our verbal and non-verbal behaviour. Our personal practice has a direct and immediate effect on others.

Thompson (1997) makes the point that individual workers can make a major difference to the quality of a client's life by checking their own assumptions and their own behaviour. On a personal level, working within the value base can ensure that care workers do not directly damage others. People have the power to choose how they interact with others.

On a wider cultural level individuals can 'make a difference', but it can be difficult to influence how others think and behave. Individuals can analyse what is happening and can challenge others to try to change group norms and values. Organisations can introduce management and quality systems which aim to ensure that workplace norms and expectations fit the value base for care. Where quality systems incorporate care values the cultural level of behaviour may soon become non-oppressive.

On the very widest structural level individuals often feel that they have little influence. Setting up general quality standards and systems is a task for government, and the standards and the resources which services have to operate within are strongly influenced by political views and values. Individuals may need to join pressure groups (see Chapter 5) or become involved in political debate to influence this level of structural discrimination.

In summary, individuals can make a great difference to other people if they work within the care value base. Organisations can make a great difference if the care value base becomes part of their quality procedures. On a structural level, resources and quality systems ought to exemplify the value base if the quality of life for clients is a genuine concern of those in power.

## Quality assurance

All care services need to work to standards and have a system for measuring that they are meeting standards. The health care system has audits which check that services meet quality standards, while social services have inspection units which register and inspect services. Standards are influenced by laws, subsequent regulations, codes of conduct and values.

All organisations such as homes, day centres or community services, need a system to monitor how effectively services are being delivered and whether customers are having their needs met. Organisations may have their own quality monitoring systems. At a local level, quality assurance groups may seek to clarify, prioritise or set standards. Ellis and Whittington (1998) explain quality assurance as a cycle or circular process which starts with setting standards (see Figure 1.28).

Promoting equality in care might be one area of quality assurance work where standards might be set. Current achievement might be measured, improvements planned and action taken to improve performance.

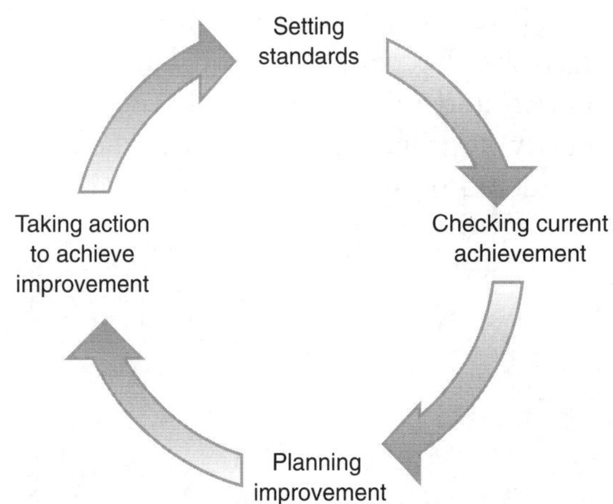


**Figure 1.28 The quality cycle (adapted from Ellis and Whittington, 1998)**

Areas to consider might include:

- the availability of policies on equal opportunity, confidentiality, harassment, health and safety
- staff training and understanding of policies
- the policies and procedures used to ensure equality of opportunity for staff, such as staff selection and interview procedures
- the availability of staff supervision and support so that there is a process for assisting individual staff to become effective at promoting equality
- management systems and structure for promoting quality. For example, are clients or their pressure groups or advocates involved in reviewing the effectiveness of the service they receive?
- is there a system for regular quality review of a service?
- staff attitudes, i.e. do staff work within the values of understanding rights and responsibilities, valuing diversity and confidentiality?
- staff rights respected; for example, staff have a right to be notified when an

employer wishes access to their health records. Procedures for maintaining health and safety include the need to notify appropriate authorities when accidents or serious illnesses occur.

### Think it over

Prepare a series of questions to ask when you visit a care service. Try to find out what policies on equal opportunities and confidentiality are available. What staff supervision and training is provided to support equal opportunities? Do management systems include a quality assurance system? Do staff support the rights of clients? Do members of staff support each other with attitudes that show value for diversity?

# Unit 1 Assessment

Unit 1 will be assessed through an external test. To prepare for this test you should undertake a study of one or more health, social care or early years settings. Your investigations should explore ways in which clients might be vulnerable and the ways care settings seek to meet clients' needs and promote their rights. Investigations should explore how codes of practice or charters are used in practice. Your studies of care settings should explore how key legislation influences clients' or workers' rights and how settings support the rights of both clients and workers.

## For an E grade

To pass the unit and achieve an E grade you will need to be prepared to:

1 Explain the possible damage that discrimination could cause to clients in a given setting.

2 Explain how policies, codes of practice and legislation are used to promote clients' rights (including confidentiality).

3 Identify ways in which staff can convey respect and promote client rights in a given setting.

4 Explain what non-discriminatory practice might involve in relation to practical care work.

To help prepare yourself for a test it may be useful to make a list of some of the risks to physical, social and emotional well-being that discrimination may cause. Use the section on the care value base and on the effects of discrimination on page 8 to help create your own explanation of discrimination. Use these sections to create a list of rights and of ideas for valuing diversity and maintaining confidentiality in order to work in a non-discriminatory way.

You might also like to list the key features of Acts of Parliament like the Sex Discrimination Act and the Children's Act. Use Figure 00 to explore how legislation might result in policies which promote clients' rights.

To help revise for the test you may also like to make a list of ways in which staff can take practical steps to promote clients' rights and convey respect. Use the section on the care value base to help you with this task and also look at Unit 2 – some of the skills involved in communication will be very important if care workers are to convey respect.

## For a C grade

You will need to know about legislation, codes of practice and charters to pass the test. In order to achieve a higher grade your work must show **three** additional things

1 **An analysis of how organisations may support workers in promoting clients' rights and evaluate the effectiveness of the support.**

You could do this by visiting care settings and asking senior staff a number of prepared questions on the following points:

- Equal opportunities policies
- Codes of practice
- Professional values
- Staff views on clients' rights
- Staff training policies
- Staff supervision policies.

After discussing these areas with staff on placements, it would be useful to discuss your findings with colleagues, teachers or tutors. You are more likely to develop 'evaluative skills' through discussion than through simply trying to memorise notes. Even if the settings you experience are not the same as case studies in the test, your experience of analysing what happens in practice may help you to analyse case studies in a test.

Another idea to help toward achieving a high grade is to make sure you have analysed case studies through written answers or through discussion, working out ways in which workers can support clients' rights.

2 **An analysis of why users of care services, children, adults with disabilities, older people, and people with physical and mental health needs, may be vulnerable to infringement of their rights.**

You will need to discuss how knowledge, social networks, social status and wealth influence the power that people hold. People with limited power and limited opportunities for communication may be vulnerable. Certain groups of people defined by ethnicity, gender, age, sexuality and class may also be more vulnerable than others. Your explanation of vulnerability might link with your knowledge of discrimination.

3 **An analysis of the benefits to clients of any day-to-day practice**

Laws and codes of practice do not necessarily have a direct influence on day-to-day practice. As well as listing examples of non-discriminatory practice, such as showing respect, offering choice and building an understanding of others' beliefs and needs, you should also be able to explain the benefits that these practices may bring to clients.

## For an A grade

Your work must show **two** additional aspects:

1 **You will need to be able to analyse the effectiveness of equal opportunities legislation in influencing care workers' attitudes and behaviour.**

Figure 1.26 provides a starting point for thinking about this issue. Legislation by itself does not create a quality service. There has to be the resources, finance and personnel to run the service. Managers and staff have to be committed to appropriate policies and to the use of appropriate values when making complicated moment-by-moment decisions. Inspection agencies have to use criteria which measure resources, policies, procedures and outcomes. Detailed discussion with staff who work in care settings might help you develop a view on the effectiveness of current legislation and systems for delivering a quality service. When you have formulated your own view you will need to be able to justify what you say with reference to your knowledge of the law and of procedures within care settings.

2 **You must be able to offer your own explanation of how care workers can improve their practice in promoting equal opportunities and clients' rights.**

You might like to quote Neil Thompson's (1997) analysis to help with this task. Thompson identifies different levels that practitioners can work at. Within a theoretical framework such as Thompson's, you might like to explore how staff training, supervision, quality inspection and interpersonal skills might be used in order to improve practice. Perhaps every worker can improve individual practice (assuming they are not severely stressed). Developing effective procedures may depend on good levels of resourcing and well-planned management. You might like to cross-reference theory from Unit 2

(Interpersonal Skills) and Unit 5 (Service Structures) to help you prepare for achievement at this level.

## Test

Read the following short passage and then answer the questions that follow.

> On a visit to a local nursery some students made the following observations:
>
> The centre was brightly decorated and there was evidence of artwork to celebrate spring. There were displays of items associated with different religions and artwork depicting people from different ethnic backgrounds and styles of clothing. When the students took notes on activities they noted that stories read to children were multi-national in origin. Staff explained that they had a policy of introducing children to stories from other cultures as well as the cultures represented by the children who attended.
>
> One area of artwork depicted a hospital scene, with a male doctor and female nurses. Female characters appeared to be caring for young boys and girls who might be ill.

### Questions

1 Identify at least two examples of good practice which promote non-discriminatory practice in the details above.

2 Identify at least one example of stereotyping in the details above.

3 In what ways might young children be vulnerable to discriminatory attitudes and beliefs?

4 What consequences could follow if children are constantly exposed to discriminatory or prejudiced attitudes?

5 List two positive ways in which staff might promote clients' rights in the setting discussed above.

6 What codes of practice and policies would you expect to find in the above setting in relation to promoting clients' rights and confidentiality?

7 The Children Act 1989 established the 'paramountcy principle'. Explain briefly what the paramountcy principle means when people discuss the needs of vulnerable children.

Read the following short passage and then answer the questions that follow.

> On a visit to a home which provided care for six adults with disability, a student observed the following:
>
> - Staff always asked the residents for their views and wishes before undertaking any kind of personal care or assistance.
> - Residents had different routines for getting up and going to bed.
> - All the male residents needed help with shaving, but some had chosen to shave with an electric razor whilst others needed 'safety razors'.
> - Staff would sometimes talk to the student about a client whilst the client was present in the room.
> - Residents were often asked their opinion about routine in the home.
> - Residents were encouraged to join in household activities but were not pressurised into helping staff with daily living activities.

UNIT I ASSESSMENT

**8** Identify two examples of good practice which promote the rights of clients in the details above.

**9** Identify one example where clients' rights might be infringed by the staff in the details above.

**10** In what ways might adults with learning disabilities be vulnerable to discriminatory attitudes and beliefs?

**11** Outline the ethical issue which might be involved if a resident chose to eat an unhealthy and excessive diet which caused them to put on weight and threaten their physical health. Under what circumstances might staff justify trying to persuade the resident to go on a diet?

**12** What consequences might follow from failing to maintain confidentiality when providing services to people with learning disabilities?

**13** Justify two ideas for improving the quality of care available to people with learning disabilities.

The following details were noted on a placement visit to a home for older people:

There were eighteen residents in the home; each resident had their own room apart from one couple who shared a double room. The rooms were arranged in units. One unit was known as a 'high dependency unit' and the residents in this unit had difficulties with orientation and memory perhaps due to Alzheimer's disease. Each resident was assigned a key worker, who was supposed to get to know him or her.

The staff often seemed pressured and worked across the different units in the building. Some staff reported that they had had very little training and didn't really know anything about Alzheimer's disease. Some staff also said that they knew very little about the people that they were caring for. Most staff seemed to think that there was too much work for them to be able to sit and talk to the residents. The manager of the home stated that there was time in the evening to talk, but residents were often unable to join in conversations. The home had to concentrate on physical care because that was what the residents' relatives expected.

**14** What aspects of the care value base are not being met in the story above?

**15** In what ways might the residents in the setting above be vulnerable?

**16** It is likely that the older people in the story above received less attention to their social and emotional needs than the adult residents in the previous story. Explain what sort of general discrimination might have resulted in this difference.

**17** Explain two ways in which residents' rights could be promoted by the staff in the setting above.

**18** Residents in the high-dependency unit might often express the wish to leave the building. Under what circumstances would the staff be ethically justified in trying to prevent them from leaving?

**19** Provide an analysis of the effectiveness of equal opportunities legislation in influencing the quality of care for older people.

**20** List three policies or other written documents you might expect a home for older people to make available in order to promote the rights of both staff and residents.

## Answers

1 Artwork was designed to celebrate spring and not a religious festival like Easter which might not apply to all the children. Where religion was celebrated it was multi-faith – including many religions. People of different ethnicity and styles of clothing were present. Stories were multi-cultural.

2 Doctors were assumed to be male and nurses were assumed to be female.

3 Children require a setting which shows a positive value for their own ethnicity, culture, gender and religion. Settings which emphasise one set of characteristics or beliefs may devalue or fail to value individuals. Where individuals are not valued this may influence the development of self-esteem or even the degree of emotional security that a child experiences.

4 Discrimination may damage a child's sense of self-confidence, self-worth or self-esteem. A child's emotional and social development may be damaged because of discrimination.

5
- Maintaining confidentiality – being careful not to disclose information which parents had given to the centre.
- Providing an appropriate range of choices of food and activities to meet varied cultural and individual needs.
- Being careful to value diversity in all activities and conversations with both children and parents, and show positive value to every child through interpersonal behaviour.

6 Policies on security of information, policies on safety, equal opportunities policies, perhaps a statement of values, ethics or professional code of conduct. A local charter defining the expectations which clients might have.

7 The paramountcy principle means that the needs of the child come first and take priority over the needs of others such as parents or relatives, or what is convenient for health or care workers.

8 Staff provide choice, i.e. with assisted shaving, routines, going to bed etc., personal care. Staff respect the wishes and dignity of residents. Residents are included in daily living tasks but not pressurised against their wishes. Residents have autonomy and are empowered to make choices.

9 Staff devalue residents by talking about them to others. This may infringe residents' rights to dignity, respect or confidentiality.

10 People may make assumptions that they are not capable of, or do not need to make choices or control their own lives. Emotional needs for safety or belonging may be ignored. Older people may impose their own views, wishes or assumptions on them. A lack of value may result in feelings of low self-worth, fear, withdrawal, helplessness and poor quality of life.

11 Increased body weight may threaten physical health, but removing choice and control may threaten emotional well-being. The final decision would be influenced by the principle of a right to autonomy or 'choice'. The exact technical nature of the risks the resident faced, the likely consequences of different staff actions and the fairness or consistency of staff behaviour.

If the resident was in serious risk of illness or death then the staff might decide to 'take over' and try to persuade the resident to diet. If there is only a low risk then the principle of choice might be seen as more important than assumptions about healthy body size.

**12** Failure to maintain confidentiality might result in a lack of trust, placing a client at physical or emotional risk, making a person feel devalued or not respected.

**13** Ideas should include reference to principles of improving choice, valuing diversity, improving control of daily living, showing respect and maintaining dignity, multi-cultural needs, meeting social and emotional needs and therefore increasing residents' sense of self-worth.

Ideas might include action on an interpersonal or communication level, or on a social or political level which will result in the principles above. Ideas might refer to meeting a range of human needs and use a theory such as Maslow's hierarchy to justify the importance of meeting specific needs.

**14** Residents' rights may not be respected. Residents may be being stereotyped as incapable of talking or of expressing their wishes or choices. Residents' rights to have their social and emotional needs considered may be ignored if the staff cannot find the time to talk to them. Diversity is unlikely to be valued as the staff are unable to get to know the background to and needs of the residents.

**15** Residents may not be treated as individuals as staff do not have time to get to know them. Personal needs and beliefs may be ignored. Some residents may feel emotionally threatened because their self-esteem or self-worth may be lost in such a situation. If residents cannot talk to staff that may make it difficult to maintain self-esteem.

**16** Ageism – the belief that older people have fewer needs or that little can be done for them. Ageism is sometimes expressed in the view that older people are not worth caring for.

**17** Staff might try to offer individual choices to residents with respect to every care task or daily living activity. Staff might show respect for residents' beliefs and identity in their conversational work. Staff might be careful to maintain confidentiality when dealing with records or in individual conversations. Staff might build relationships with residents in order to work out ways in which they can meet social and emotional needs.

**18** The ethical issues involved include:

- The need to assess the degree of risk that a resident might be in. This assessment will depend on knowledge of the actual circumstances.
- An assessment of the consequences – the resident may come to physical harm if they leave the building, but the resident may suffer emotional harm if they are prevented from leaving.
- Consistency – the residents' human rights must be respected.
- The principle of promoting autonomy – residents have a right to choice.

One solution to all of these issues might be that a member of staff should go out with the resident. The resident would then be safe but his or her rights and needs would be met. A lack of staffing may prevent this, but this practical problem may result in the residents' rights being infringed.

**19** Equal opportunities legislation established rights against discrimination on the grounds of race, gender or diability. It is unlikely that residents in the story above could profit directly from the legislation. The legislation does set up general principles, which might inform local charters or policies within the home. Quality care is likely to be understood as care which values the differing needs of individuals. The legislation may have little direct benefit for older people but it may help to establish principles that will benefit older people.

**20** An equal opportunities policy, a local charter of rights, a code of practice, values and ethics, NVQ standards, a confidentiality policy, a guide to the home, a policy on risk assessment, employment or induction guides.

## References and recommended further reading


Ellis, R. & Whittington, D. (1998) *Quality assurance in social care* Arnold

*Home life* (1984) Centre for Policy on Ageing, The Dorset Press

Seedhouse, D. (1988) *Ethics the heart of health care* John Wiley

*Social Trends (2000)* The Stationery Office

Thompson, N. (1997) *Anti-discriminatory practice* 2nd edn. Macmillan


### Recommended further reading


Thompson, N. (1997) *Anti-discrimatory practice* 2nd edn. Macmillan


## Relevant websites

Legislation – www.hmso.gov.uk/acts

DSS – www.dss.gov.uk

'Opportunity for All' – www.dss.gov.uk/ha/pubs/poverty/sum/suma.htm

Age Concern – www.ace.org.uk

Salvation Army – www.salvationarmy.org.uk

BASW – www.basw.co.uk

UKCC – www.ukcc.org.uk

Equal Opportunities Commission – www.eoc.org.uk

Commission for Racial Equality – www.cre.gov.uk

National Disability Council – www.disability-council.gov.uk

## Fast Facts

**Attitude** Socially-learned reactions to and likes and dislikes of people, objects or situations.

**Autonomy** Having independence and control over local or personal issues. In the context of care work, autonomy implies control of decisions over daily living activities.

**Belief** Ideas which we draw upon to make sense of our own particular view of the world.

**Black** A term used to describe physical characteristics, e.g. skin colour and racial features. The term has also been used in a political context to include all people who are oppressed by racism and discrimination because of skin colour or ethnic and cultural background.

**Children Act 1989** An Act of Parliament providing children with the right to be protected from 'significant harm'.

**Clients' rights** Rights to be different, free from discrimination, have confidentiality, choice, dignity, safety and security, and the development of personal potential.

**Confidentiality** The right of clients to have private information about themselves restricted to people who have an accepted need to know.

**Consequentialism** See Utilitarianism.

**Covert discrimination** Can include unthinking exclusion and unconscious discriminatory behaviour. People who commit acts of covert discrimination may not always fully understand their actions.

**Culture** A collection of ideas and habits shared by a given group, i.e. the norms and value base for the group. These help to reinforce the identity of the group, making it different from other groups. Individuals learn the roles acceptable to others within their culture.

**Data Protection Acts 1984, 1998** Acts of Parliament which give people a right to see information held on them, and rights to confidentiality and accuracy of information.

**Disability** The consequences of an impairment or other individual difference in a given social setting. Disability is socially determined; an impairment may have serious social consequences or not – it depends how people respond. For example, 'left-handedness' was a disability in past centuries because left-handed people were banned from certain jobs. Nowadays there is little prejudice against left-handed people and so the disability has disappeared although the difference remains.

**Discrimination** To be able to distinguish between things. In health and social care, it refers to a decision to deny one group the same rights as another.

**Discrimination, direct** Very open and obvious methods of disadvantaging a person or group of people, e.g. name calling, refusing to employ someone because of their age or religion etc.

**Discrimination, indirect** Subtle ways of disadvantaging an individual or group, e.g. not providing access for people in wheelchairs, or selecting people only from certain housing areas, in order to discriminate.

**Disempower** To deny clients the opportunity to take control of their life. To deny choice, to withhold information so the client is unable to make an informed choice. The opposite of empowerment.

**Empathy** A conscious effort to try to see the world as another person sees it. Empathy is an attempt to gain a closer understanding of another's feelings.

**Empiricism** Knowledge gained through experience.

**Empowerment** Encouraging an individual to take control of own life. This is achieved by sharing information with the client, so that they may make informed choices, and by working within the care value base.

**Equal opportunity** Aims to ensure that all people are afforded equal access to services and have equal rights in law and society. Ensuring that all have an equal right to develop to their full potential.

**Equal Pay Act 1970** An Act of Parliament which made it unlawful for employers to discriminate between men and women in relation to their pay and conditions of work.

**Ethics** The moral codes which form the basis for decision making and, therefore, the behaviour of workers in a given profession.

**Ethnic group** A group who share the same cultural tradition, perhaps a common ancestry or geographical place of origin. The group may share a common language, literature, music etc.

**Ethnic minority** A commonly used term in Britain to describe groups from the black community. The term also covers such groups as Chinese, Greek, Turkish people, etc. This broad term covers a range of factors e.g. race, religion, culture and language.

**Eurocentric** Viewing the world solely from a white European value base. This does not address issues raised within other cultures and may assume the superiority of European culture.

**Gender** Gender consists of the differences between males and females based on cultural or social expectations. Gender roles may appear to be biologically determined and 'natural', but are susceptible to change and may differ between societies and over time. An example of this would be the changing role of women in the workforce.

**Health and Safety at Work Act (HASAWA) 1974** An Act of Parliament placing responsibilities on employers and employees to create a safe workplace. The original Act has been updated and supplemented by many later sets of regulations and guidelines.

**Hypothesis** A projection or idea which is proposed and then tested out to see if the idea is valid or not.

**Identity** Put simply, a person's identity is how they see themselves and make sense of their life in relation to other people and society.

**Impairment** Physical damage or restrictions to the functioning of the mind or body. An impairment can result in a disability in social circumstances which do not enable an individual to compensate for their physical differences.

**Kantianism** The philosophy of Immanuel Kant whereby duty means that the same rules apply to all people. It is an essential duty always to tell the truth.

**Marginalise** In health and social care terms it is to push a group to the outer edge of society and social concern, and so disadvantage them. Such groups may be oppressed due to age, ability, gender, race, religion or social class.

**Maslow's hierarchy** The psychologist Abraham Maslow's description of human needs as belonging to the categories of physical, safety, love and belonging, self-esteem and self-actualisation. Quality care does not address only physical and safety needs. Higher level needs are also important if people are to have quality of life.

**Mental Health Act 1983** An Act of Parliament providing for compulsory restriction of people to hospital if they are mentally ill. The Act restricts the freedom of individuals who are considered ill.

**NHS and Community Care Act 1990** An Act of Parliament intended to uphold the principle that people are best cared for in their own homes, or in other familiar surroundings, rather than being admitted into residential care as a matter of policy.

**Norms** The accepted attitudes and values which underpin the behaviour of a particular social group, i.e. the 'rules' by which the group functions.

**Overt discrimination** Deliberate behaviour, such as deliberate exclusion, bullying, harassment, violence, or verbal abuse.

**Peer group** A group who share a common purpose or who are in a similar situation. For example, a youth club or a study group may have members of different ages but all have come together for a specific purpose.

**Policies** Formal written statements explaining what to do within an organisation or work-setting.

**Positive action** A positive step which aims to benefit individuals or groups who face discrimination, e.g. employing an interpreter to assist a student with hearing impairment in the classroom. In this way the student is not disadvantaged by the hearing loss.

**Prejudice** An attitude which is based on pre-judgements made about others, leading to discrimination. Prejudice is often based on ignorance and stereotyped views of an individual or group.

**Primary socialisation** The socialisation that takes place during early childhood when the rules and norms of the society into which an individual is born are acquired. Through the family a child learns the patterns of acceptable behaviour expected by their social group. The attitudes and values of the culture of that society are also formed.

**Race** The idea of a group based on perceived biological differences between people. In practice, a person is assigned to a particular race on the basis of the subjective impressions of others (ethnicity), not on the basis of measurable biological differences.

**Race Relations Act 1976** An Act of Parliament which makes discrimination on the basis of race illegal.

**Racial discrimination** Unequal treatment on the grounds of being a member of a particular racial group.

**Racial prejudice** An unfavourable attitude towards another because they belong to a particular race. This attitude may be based on negative stereotypes of that particular race.

**Racism** Attitudes and procedures (economic, political, social and cultural) which advocate and seek to maintain the superiority of one racial group or groups over others.

**Religion** The term used to refer to traditions or to personal spiritual beliefs, or both. People grow up with different religious traditions.

**Responsibilities** Society's values create rights for people – but rights are rarely without boundaries. People have responsibilities as well as rights. Rights are balanced with responsibilities.

**Secondary socialisation** Wider experience of the world outside the home exposes the child to different attitudes and values in society. The main agents of secondary socialisation are the media, education and peer groups.

**Security** Feeling physically and emotionally safe. Security policies and procedures are necessary to ensure the safety of staff, clients and their possessions.

**Self-actualisation** The highest level of development in Maslow's hierarchy. It means fulfilling your potential and achieving everything you need to achieve.

**Self-esteem** How well or how badly a person feels about himself or herself. High self-esteem may help a person to feel happy and confident. Low self-esteem may lead to depression and unhappiness.

**Sex** Sexual characteristics are the biological determined differences between males and females, such as the ability to father children, give birth and suckle children, etc. These differences are determined at birth and not generally susceptible to change.

**Sex Discrimination Act 1975** An Act of Parliament designed to prevent discrimination on the basis of gender.

**Sexism** Attitudes and procedures (including economic, political, social and cultural factors) which seek to maintain the superiority of one gender over the other.

**Social context** A particular social setting in which individuals have a preconceived notion about acceptable behaviour. There is clear definition of the roles and the behaviour associated with those roles in this setting. For example, in a hospital ward, the nurse is expected to behave in a caring and professional manner.

**Social role** The 'part' that an individual plays in a given situation. The accepted behaviour expected by others of that role, e.g. a college student being ready to learn, asking questions etc.

**Social status** The value a group places on a particular social role, giving credibility and respect. For example: the leader of a teenage group, because they can organise others or perhaps control the group through fear; a judge, because of the knowledge they hold and the power to uphold the laws of society. Status may be due to money or possessions and will vary depending on the culture of groups within society.

**Stereotype** A way of grouping people, objects or events together, attributing individuals with the same qualities and characteristics. Stereotyping can help the individual to make sense of the world by making predictions easier. Stereotyping may have positive or negative consequences.

**Utilitarianism** A philosophy originally developed by Jeremy Bentham and John Stuart Mill. It holds that a morally right act is one which benefits the greatest number of people.

**Values** Learned principles or thought systems which enable individuals to choose between alternatives and make decisions. Values guide behaviour in relation to what is judged to be 'valuable'. Values are learned in a cultural context and will develop in relation to the beliefs and norms which exist within a cultural group.

**Vulnerability** Being at risk of some kind of harm – not being protected from risk and harm.

Unit 2

# Communicating in health and social care

**Good communication skills are an essential tool for health and social care professionals, as they are needed to help develop relationships with people and to show individuals that they are valued. Effective communication skills also have implications for people's well-being.**

**This unit is organised in five sections. You will learn about:**

- **the types of interaction that require skilled communication, and why communication skills are important for valuing people**
- **effective communication**
- **communication skills in groups**
- **ways to evaluate your own communication skills**
- **maintaining client confidentiality.**

**The unit concludes with advice on providing assessment evidence for Unit 2.**

## 2.1 Types of interaction

Health and care work brings care workers into contact with people who may be lonely, anxious, devalued, discriminated against, emotionally vulnerable, or unable to express their thoughts and feelings. Communication skills provide an essential tool that care workers can use to meet the needs of vulnerable people. Good communication skills are also vitally important to ensure effective work with other professionals, relatives and within teams in care. Communication in a care setting is about much more than simply giving or receiving information.

### Think it over

Below are five situations where health or care staff will need to communicate with vulnerable people. All of these people have a range of needs which health or care staff need to respond to during their conversation.

### Five Case Studies

1. Mrs Whitaker is 84 years old, and has led an independent and successful life. She is about to be interviewed by a social worker in order to assess her care needs. She knows that she can no longer cope easily at home because of her arthritis and poor memory. Mrs Whitaker says that she feels 'useless' and that her life is ending now. Mrs Whitaker feels distressed that she is having to 'be

assessed'. She had hoped that her daughter and son-in-law would support her so that she did not 'have to want for anything'.

2. Karam is in hospital waiting to undergo a serious operation. He has discussed the technical nature of the operation with the surgeon who will be responsible. Karam has been supported by his family, but now he is alone. Karam tries to look calm but really he is anxious and worried. He calls to a nurse hoping that the conversation will help him to relax and feel safer.

3. Samuel is five years old and is starting at a new school. Samuel's parents have just moved into the area and so Samuel is joining a group of children who know each other. Samuel's mother has just left him and everyone in the room looks strange. Samuel feels frightened and alone; he begins to cry as a classroom assistant comes over to talk to him.

4. Leona is 28 and spends some of her time living with her parents and some of her time in a home for people with learning disability. Today she has been invited to a meeting to discuss 'her future'. Her parents and care workers are at the meeting. Leona explains that she wants to get a high paying job and buy a big house. Leona finds it difficult to understand why others at the meeting do not seem to support her in her ambition.

5. Arata is a member of a local youth group. Together with her friends she has come up with an idea for organising a 'girls only' exercise group during the week. But not all the members of the group support Arata's idea. When they get together there are arguments about organising and running such group. Arata hopes that one of the staff will be able to lead the group to help sort out what they can do.

## Human needs

One way of understanding the different types of human needs is through the work of Abraham Maslow (1908–70). Maslow's theory was that the goal of human life was personal growth, i.e. to develop personal ability and potential. However, before a person can fully develop his or her potential there are levels of need, called deficiency needs, which first have to be met. Maslow's levels of needs are often set out as a hierarchy in a pyramid as below (Figure 2.1). The important role of communication is described against each level of need.

### Think it over

Each of the five case studies above can be analysed in relation to the person's needs and the type of interaction required to meet that need. Can you identify one need in each case and suggest an appropriate type of interaction.

**Mrs Whitaker** The social worker assessing Mrs Whitaker will want to find out about her physical needs and will ask questions about her health. However, Mrs Whitaker feels threatened just because of the assessment. The social worker will need to

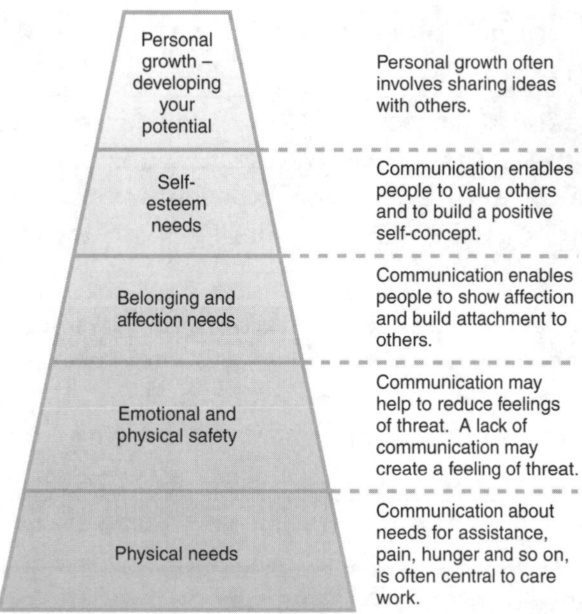


**Figure 2.1 Communication within Maslow's levels of need**

use communication skills to try to meet Mrs Whitaker's need for emotional safety. Mrs Whitaker may be feeling rejected by her family. At some stage, care staff may need to build a relationship to help explore this need. Communications skills will be essential to enable this. The social worker assessing Mrs Whitaker will be very concerned to talk and act in a way that improves her sense of self-worth and esteem. The social worker must communicate a sense of value towards Mrs Whitaker in order to be effective.

---

**Karam** The nurse working with Karam will be concerned to check his physical needs with respect to pain, anxiety and need for physical assistance. In addition to physical needs Karam feels threatened, and communication may help him. His family have supported him but they are not available now. The nurse may be able to help him to think about their support. Facing major surgery may threaten Karam's security and self-concept. The nurse may be able to communicate value and respect toward him.

---

**Samuel** The classroom assistant working with Samuel will have to work with his emotional needs. Samuel feels threatened, alone and not sure how to cope with the new experience of starting school with a group of strange children. Using conversation skills the classroom assistant will help Samuel to feel safe, and that he 'belongs' with the new group.

---

**Leona** Staff at the case conference will need to consider how to work with her to meet her social and self-esteem needs, as well as her physical and safety needs. It is important that staff do not threaten her self-esteem and that communication carries a sense of value to Leona.

---

**Arata** Arata has self-esteem, belonging and emotional safety needs, all linked with her proposal for a girls-only group. The youth worker will need to be sensitive to her cultural and gender perspective. Group discussion will need to be skilfully led, in order to meet Arata's needs alongside the needs of others in the group.

## Why effective communication is important

Health and care work is not just about meeting physical needs. Care work is about the quality of a person's life. Care workers do not just need skills to collect or pass on information. Effective communication in care work is needed in order to improve the quality of people's lives by addressing a range of needs. Effective communication is also about communication with relatives, colleagues and other professionals to create a safe, welcoming and valuing work environment.

## Communication and the value base in care

The NVQ standards in Care, 1992 to 1998, included the need to 'Support Through Effective Communication', as an element of the value base for care work. The current value base (see Chapter 1) has simplified the number of elements to be assessed. Effective communication may still be seen as a right which clients may expect and a responsibility which carers should meet. Effective communication is vital if staff are to foster people's equality, diversity and rights.

## Informal interaction

Health and care work involves constant communication with others. Even when staff are not talking, their body language will be influencing others around them. Some examples of informal interactions are shown in Figure 2.2.

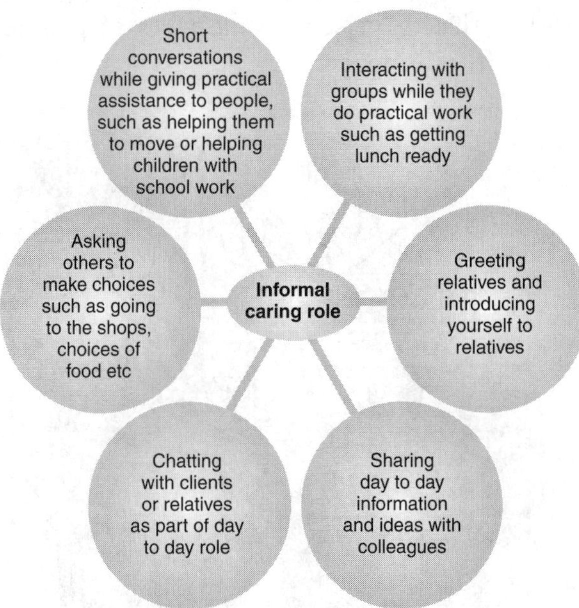


**Figure 2.2 Informal interactions in care**

The way care staff undertake informal communication is very important. Informal communication should make others feel respected and valued if care workers are working within the value base for care.

### Professional roles

Actors have to learn the 'parts' they play in films and plays; these parts are called 'roles'. Professional care workers also have a role to play. Many sociologists argue that our social behaviour can be understood in terms of 'roles' that people play in real life. Other people have expectations of care workers and these expectations influence the way carers act.

**Think it over**

What expectations of a care worker might exist in a residential setting? Who creates the 'role set' or set of people with expectations that influence interaction in care? Examine the diagram below and decide if there are any more roles that could influence care worker behaviour in a setting you have seen.

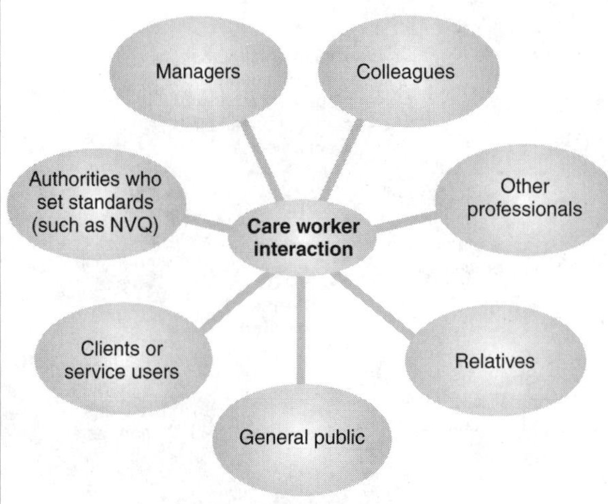


**Figure 2.3 A set of people of who create role expectations for care workers**

Although informal interaction is often unplanned, care workers must respond in ways which are appropriate both to their role and to the quality standards set out in agency policy and the care value base. If a care worker is feeling tired or angry about something in their private life, it would not be 'professional' to let their feelings influence interaction with vulnerable clients. Carers need a range of practical and 'emotional' skills to help them maintain their role. These skills are explained in section two of this chapter.

## Formal interaction

Nurses, social workers and other care workers need to use a range of communication skills in order to carry out formal procedures. Detailed analysis of communication skills can be found in the next section. Some examples of formal interaction are set out below (Figure 2.4). All these interactions require appropriate verbal and non-verbal skills. They require workers to work within an appropriate framework of values. Some situations also require 'emotional' skills or special skills in working with people with communication differences.

Formal interaction

- Explaining procedures such as surgical operations, how to apply for a service, how to appeal or complain about a decision
- Leading a planned group activity, such as a visit or reminiscence group. Teaching a skill
- Reporting accidents to managers
- Handing over details of work to new colleagues
- Negotiating with others during a case conference to discuss care plans
- Assessing need as part of the care planning process

**Figure 2.4 Examples of formal interaction**

# 2.2 Effective communication

This section explains the factors and skills which promote effective communication in care. Examples of damaging or inhibiting factors are also explained.

## Physical factors which influence communication

Effective communication depends on people being able to see, hear and receive messages. Although this may seem just common sense, physical barriers to communication often exist in care settings. Care settings in hospitals and homes may sometimes be noisy or badly lit. People with hearing disabilities may be disadvantaged because of background noise and difficulty in seeing the faces of people who are talking.

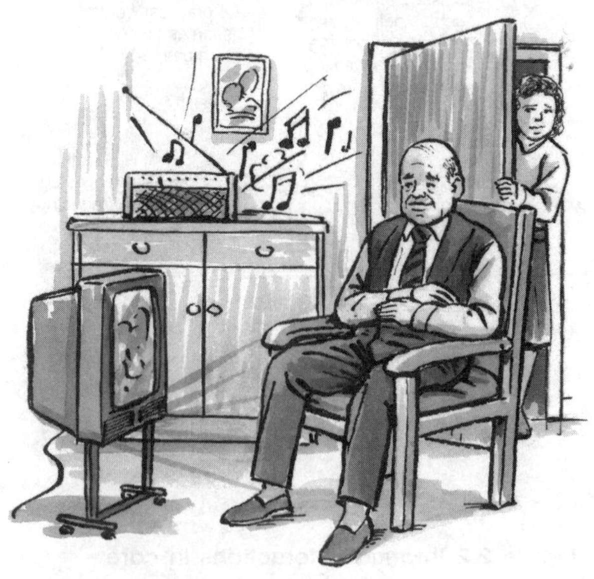

**Noise and restricted vision can make communication difficult**

### Minimising physical barriers to communication

Below are some ideas for checking that physical barriers do not inhibit communication:

- make sure that others can see your face and particularly your eyes and lips
- check that the setting is not too noisy
- make sure that the setting is appropriate to the conversation you hope to have. A private confidential setting is needed for many formal care interactions
- plan ahead to minimise distractions and interruptions. Formal interactions might require a pre-booked room where you can be free of distractions and interruptions.

Room in use
please do not enter

## Non-verbal communication

When we meet and talk with people, we will usually be using two language systems. We will use a verbal or spoken language and non-verbal or body language.

Effective communication in care work requires care workers to be able to analyse their own and other people's non-verbal behaviour.

Our body language sends messages to other people – often without us deliberately meaning to send these messages. Some of the most important body areas that send messages are shown in Figure 2.5.

### The eyes

We can often guess the feelings and

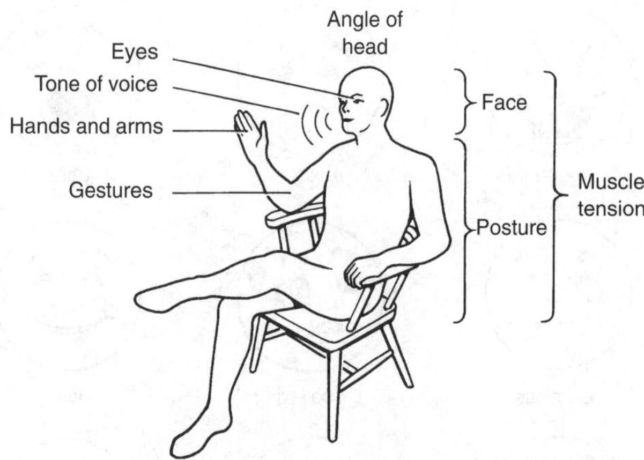


**Figure 2.5 Our body language sends messages to other people**

thoughts that another person has by looking at their eyes. One poet called the eye 'the window of the soul'. We can sometimes understand the thoughts and feelings of another person by eye to eye contact. Our eyes get wider when we are excited, attracted to, or interested in someone else. A fixed stare may send the messages that someone is angry. Looking away is often interpreted as being bored or not interested in European culture.

### The face

Our faces can convey very complex messages and we can read them easily – even in diagram form.

People's faces often indicate their emotional state. A person who is depressed may signal this emotion with eyes that look down – there may be tension in the face and the mouth will be closed. The muscles in the person's shoulders are likely to be relaxed but the face and neck may show tension.

A happy person will have 'wide eyes' that make contact with you – and the whole face will smile. When people are excited

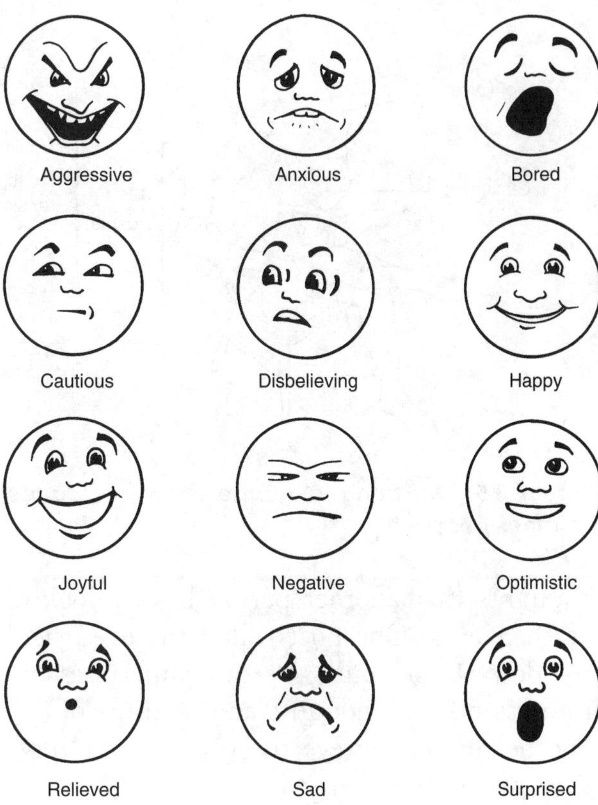


**Figure 2.6 The face expresses emotion**

they will move their arms and hands to signal their excitement.

### Voice tone

It's not just what we say, but the way that we say it. If we talk quickly in a loud voice with a fixed voice tone, people may see us as angry. A calm, slow voice with varying tone may send a message of being friendly.

### Body movement

The way we walk, move our head, sit, cross our legs and arms and so on, may send messages about whether we are tired, happy, sad or bored.

### Posture

The way we sit or stand can send messages. Sitting with crossed arms can mean 'I'm not taking any notice'. Leaning can send the message that you are relaxed or bored. Leaning forward can show interest. The body postures shown below all convey messages.

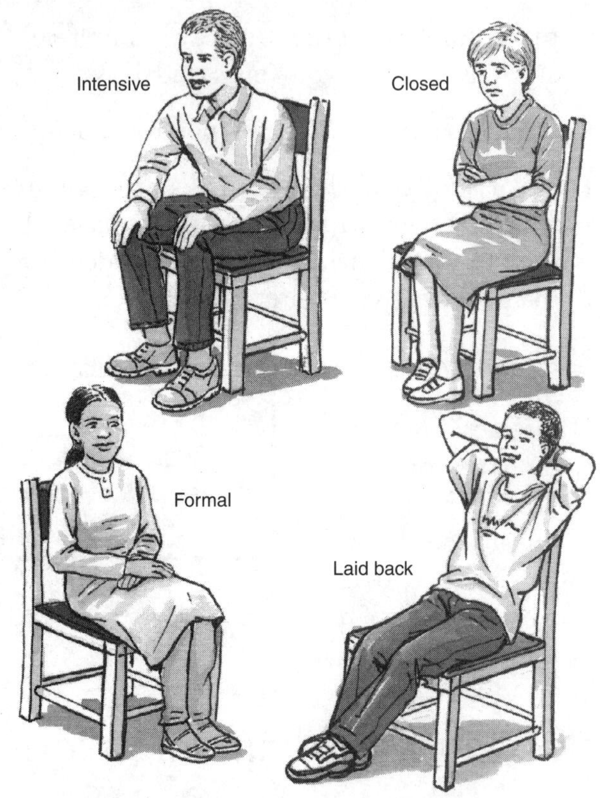


**Figure 2.7 Body postures that send messages**

### Muscle tension

The tension in our feet, hands and fingers can tell others how relaxed or how tense we are. If people are very tense their shoulders might stiffen, their face muscles might tighten and they might sit or stand rigidly. A tense face might have a firmly closed mouth with lips and jaws clenched tight. A tense person might breathe quickly and become hot.

### Gestures

Gestures are hand and arm movements that can help us to understand what a person is saying. Some gestures carry a meaning of their own. Some common gestures are shown below.

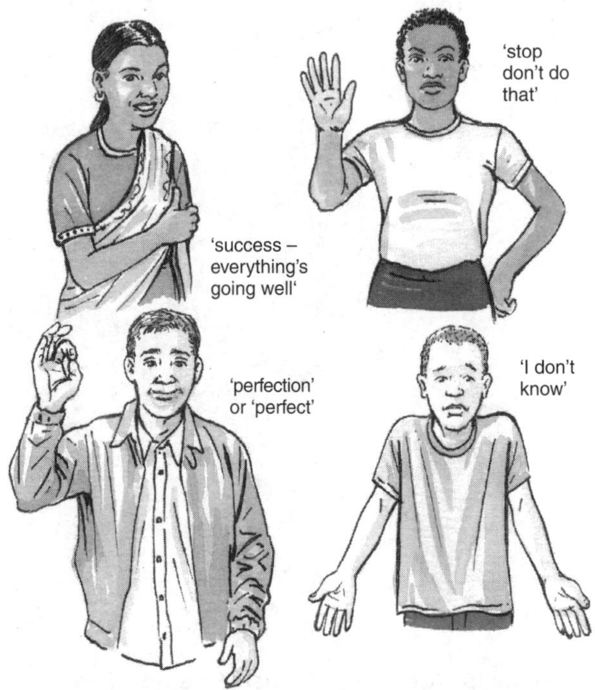


Figure 2.8 Some gestures common in Britain

## Touch

Touching another person can send messages of care, affection, power over them, or sexual interest. The social setting and other body language usually helps people to understand what touch might mean. Carers should not make assumptions about touch. Even holding someone's hand might be seen as trying to dominate them!

## Proximity

The space between people can sometimes show how friendly or 'intimate' the conversation is. Different cultures have different behaviours with respect to space between people who are talking.

In Britain there are expectations or 'norms' as to how close you should be when you talk to others. When talking to strangers we may keep an arm's-length apart. The ritual of shaking hands indicates that you have been introduced – you may come closer. When you are friendly with someone you may accept them being closer to you. Relatives and partners may not be restricted in how close they can come (but some fathers and adult sons may have unwritten but firm rules on proximity).

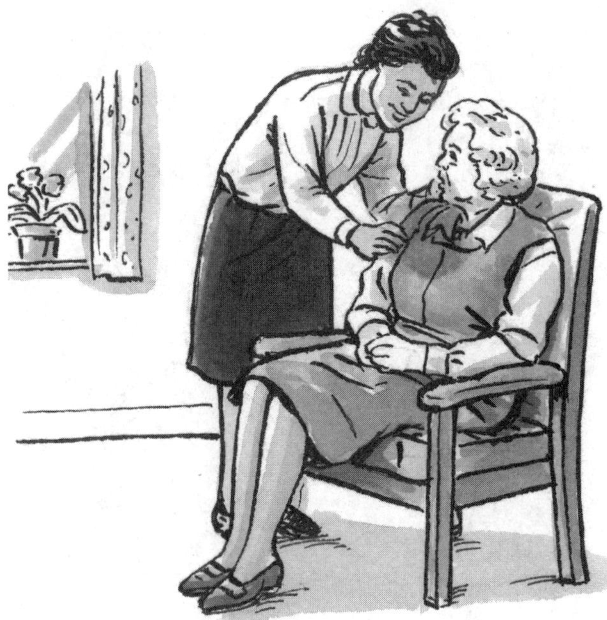

Carers can risk being perceived as rude or aggressive if they violate the personal space of others

Proximity is a very important issue in care work. Many clients have a sense of personal space. If a care worker assumes it is all right to enter a client's personal space without asking or explaining, he or she may be seen as being dominating or aggressive.

## Face-to-face positions (orientation)

Standing or sitting eye-to-eye can send a message of being formal or being angry. A slight angle can create a more relaxed and friendly feeling.

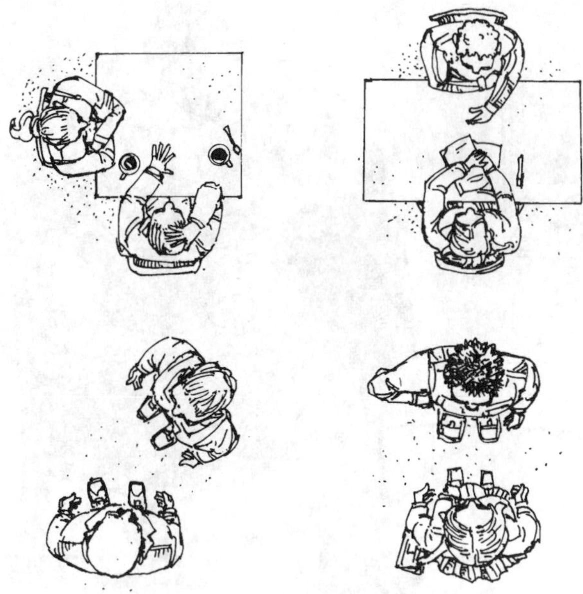

Figure 2.9 Face-to-face interaction

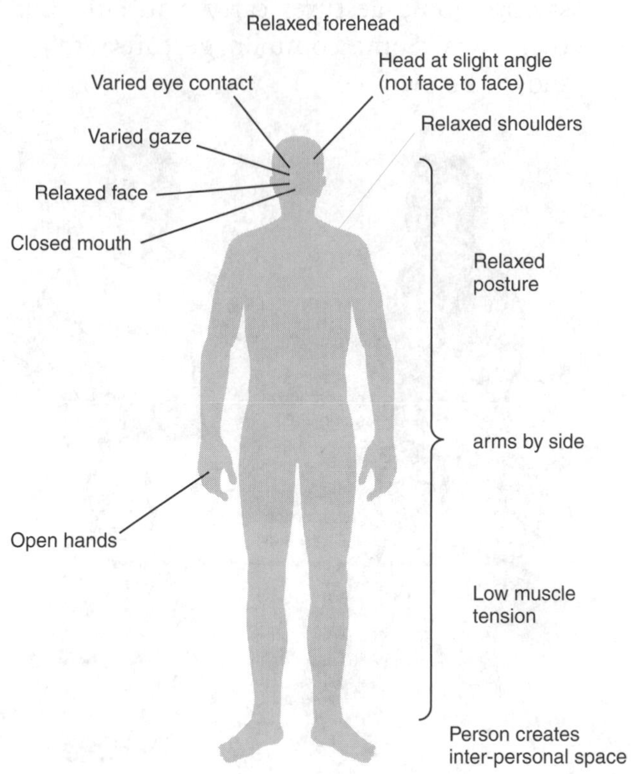


Figure 2.10 Non-verbal signs of being calm

## Emotional work

Most people who receive health or social care services are emotionally vulnerable. People may feel threatened or depressed. Communication is often aimed at meeting emotional needs. Carers will need to communicate a sense of calmness, being relaxed but responsive to the person that they are working with. If carers are tense or distressed themselves, then they are likely to increase the feelings of threat that a client has.

Non-verbal behaviour that conveys calmness is shown in Figure 2.10.

As well as being relaxed but responsive, care workers will need to use verbal skills to create an emotionally safe and constructive context for communication. The specialised skills for creating emotional safety were first identified by Carl Rogers (1902-1987).

Originally these skills were seen as a basis for counselling relationships, but they have since become adopted as a basis for any befriending or supportive relationship. There are three conditions for a caring supportive conversation and these are that the carer must show (or convey) a sense of warmth, understanding and sincerity to the other person. These conditions sometimes have other names:

- warmth is sometimes called acceptance
- understanding was originally called empathy
- sincerity was originally called genuineness.

## Conveying warmth

Conveying warmth means being seen as a warm, accepting person. In order to influence another person to view you this way you will need to demonstrate that you do not stereotype and label others. You will need to demonstrate that you do not judge other people as good or bad, right or wrong. This is sometimes referred to as a non-judgmental attitude. Warmth means not comparing people to see who is best!

Conveying warmth means being willing to listen to others. It means being able to prove that you are listening to a client because you can remember what they have said to you. Warmth involves using **reflective listening**. That is, you give your attention to the client when they talk, and remember what they say. You can then **reflect** the words back again.

| | |
|---|---|
| *Client* | 'I hate it here, you don't know what it's like, there's no one to talk to, they're all too busy, no one cares about me.' |
| *Carer* | 'I suppose everyone is busy and you feel that no one cares.' |
| *Client* | 'That's right, they don't – you aren't so bad, but you won't be here tomorrow.' |
| *Carer* | 'Well that's right, I can't come in tomorrow but we could talk for a while now if you would like that.' |

The carer is able to show the client that they are listening by repeating some of the things that the client has said. The repetition is not 'parrot fashion' because the carer has used their own way of speaking. The carer has also avoided being judgmental. When the client said that no one cared, the carer did not argue. The carer might have felt like saying, 'How can you say that – don't you know how hard we work for you? You want to think yourself lucky, there's plenty of people who would be pleased to be here, other people don't complain'. But such advice to think yourself lucky and make comparison with other people is judgmental; it does not value the client, it is not warm. If the carer had said these things it would have blocked the conversation. *Warmth* makes it safe for the client to express their feelings. Warmth means that the carer could disagree with what a client has said, but the client should feel safe that they will not be discriminated against or put down.

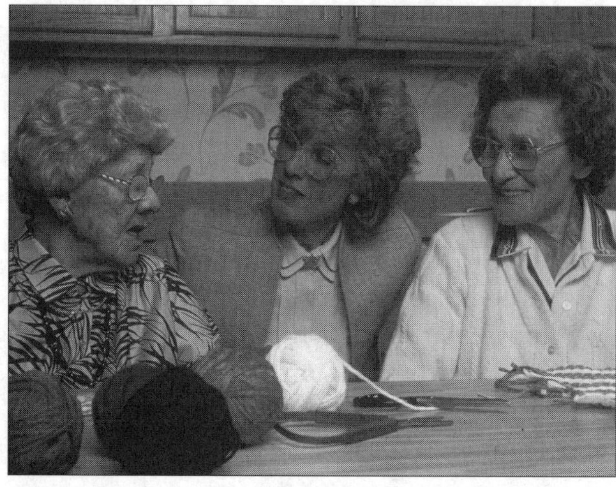

Figure 2.11 Warmth involves using reflective listening

In developing the skill of showing warmth, it is important not to judge. Carers must accept that clients have the right to be the way they are, and to make their own choices. While you may disapprove of a client's behaviour, you must show that you do not dislike them as an individual person. This is particularly important when working with clients with challenging behaviour. It is essential that clients know it is the behaviour which is disliked, not them as a person.

## Conveying understanding

Understanding involves learning about a person's individual identity and beliefs. Carl Rogers saw the idea of understanding or empathy as 'the ability to experience another person's world as if it was your own world'; the key part being the 'as if'. We always keep an idea of our own world and we know that the clients have different experiences from our own. It is important to try to really understand clients' thoughts and feelings.

Reflective listening provides a useful tool to help carers to gradually learn about their clients. By keeping a conversation going, the client may feel that they are understood; the carer is warm and non-judgmental, so it becomes safe to tell the carer something about their life. If the carer checks that they understand the client, the client may feel valued and so is encouraged to talk more. The more the client talks, the more the carer has a chance to learn about their views.

*Client* 'So anyway, I said to the doctor look these pills are only making me worse, I don't want them.'

*Carer* 'So you told him to stop them.'

*Client* 'That's right, I don't believe in pills – you end up rattling round with all that lot inside you – if you're meant to get better you will, that's what I say.'

*Carer* 'Have you always believed that pills don't help?'

*Client* 'Yes, well since I was young, I put my faith in God.'

By listening and conveying warmth the carer is being given the privilege of learning about the client's religious views and perhaps even needs. Understanding can grow from a conversation which conveys value for the client.

If you can get to understand your clients a sense of trust may develop. If the client is understood and not judged they may consider it safe to share thoughts and worries with their carer.

## Conveying sincerity

Being sincere means being open about what you say and the way that you speak. It means not acting, not using set phrases or professional styles which are not really your own. In some ways being sincere means simply being yourself, being honest and real! However, being 'real' has to involve being non-judgemental, trying to understand people rather than trying to give people advice. If being honest means giving other people your advice – don't do it! However, when you listen and learn about other people, do use your own normal language. Think about ways you might describe yourself and occasionally you can share details of your life with clients. Sometimes it is necessary to share your thoughts to keep a conversation going. Sharing information from your own life might help to convey your sincerity or genuineness in some situations.

Look at the conversation below:

*Client* 'But what's the point in talking to you, I mean you don't really care, it's just your job.'

*Carer* 'It is my job, but I do care about you, and I would be pleased to talk with you. I chose this work because I care and because I can make the time to listen if you want to talk about it.'

### Supportive skills

Understanding, warmth and sincerity have to be combined in order to provide a safe, supportive setting.

Learning to create a supportive relationship with clients will involve practice and a great deal of self-monitoring and reflection. It will be necessary to get feedback from colleagues, supervisors and most importantly clients, when you practise conveying warmth, understanding and sincerity. You may be able to tell if your communication is effective because the client may reflect your behaviour. That is, if you are warm and understanding and the client comes to trust you; then you may find that the client is warm and friendly back toward you. If you are honest and sincere, your clients may be honest and sincere with you. The quality of a supportive relationship is that it can become a two-way process. You may find working with clients more enjoyable because you become skilled at warmth, understanding and sincerity.

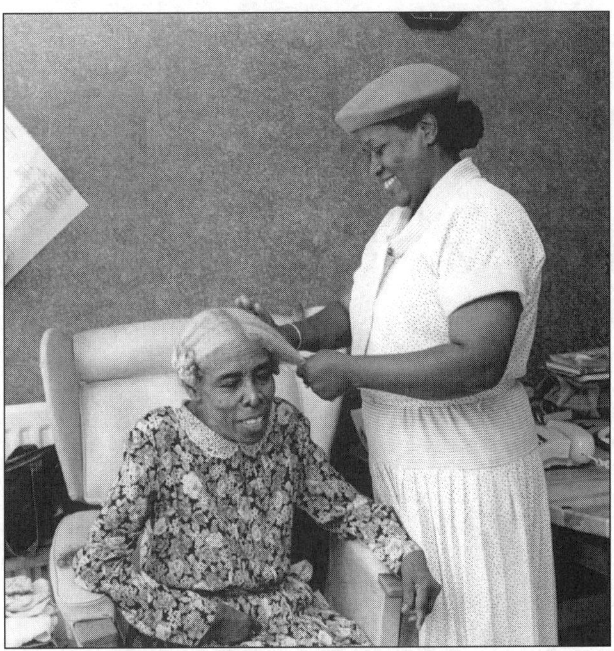

Client and carer in supportive relationship

The following ideas may help to develop supportive skills.

1 Work with a friend. Take turns in imagining that you are upset or sad while the other person uses reflective listening skills. Tape record the conversation. Play the tape back and evaluate your performance in terms of warmth, understanding and sincerity.

2 Watch videos of conversational skills or counselling situations where warmth, understanding and sincerity are demonstrated. Discuss how this is effective and how you might develop your own conversational skills.

3 Think about your own conversations with clients and keep a log book to reflect on your own skills development.

4 Practise being warm, understanding and sincere with your supervisor or tutor – ask them for feedback!

5 Work on supportive behaviour as part of a group project. Practise being supportive while undertaking some problem-solving work.

## Social factors and values

Building an understanding of another person requires skill, but it also requires carers to understand the social factors and values necessary for effective work. Learning about other people can be emotionally demanding. Some people may find that learning about different cultures and lifestyles is stressful. Workers' own attitudes, beliefs and assumptions can be challenged when we realise the range of possibilities that exist. The emotions of carers may block their ability to use communication skills to build an understanding of others. It is for this reason that care workers need to focus on the Care Value Base and 'foster the quality and diversity of people'. Effective communication involves positive commitment to valuing the differences in others. Valuing diversity in others will make it possible to use warmth, understanding and sincerity to show self-awareness and respect for others.

Skilled carers have to get to know the people they work with in order to avoid making false assumptions. In getting to know an individual, carers will also need to understand the ways that class, race, age, gender and other social categories influence the person. A person's culture may include all the social groups they belong to.

There are many different ethnic groups in the world, many different religions, many different cultural values, variations in gender role, and so on. Individuals may belong to the same ethnic group yet belong to different religions or class groups. Knowing someone's religion will not necessarily tell you all of that person's beliefs, or general culture.

You can pick up background knowledge on different ethnic and religious customs, but it is impossible to study all the differences that might exist for individual clients. The best way to learn about diversity is to listen and communicate with people who lead different lives from ourselves. As well as working within the Value Base for Care, carers should value the practice of evaluating and developing their own communication skills. The assessment of this unit focuses on this skill.

## Communication and culture

Non-verbal communication is a language. There are many languages in the world and they do not all have the same concepts and

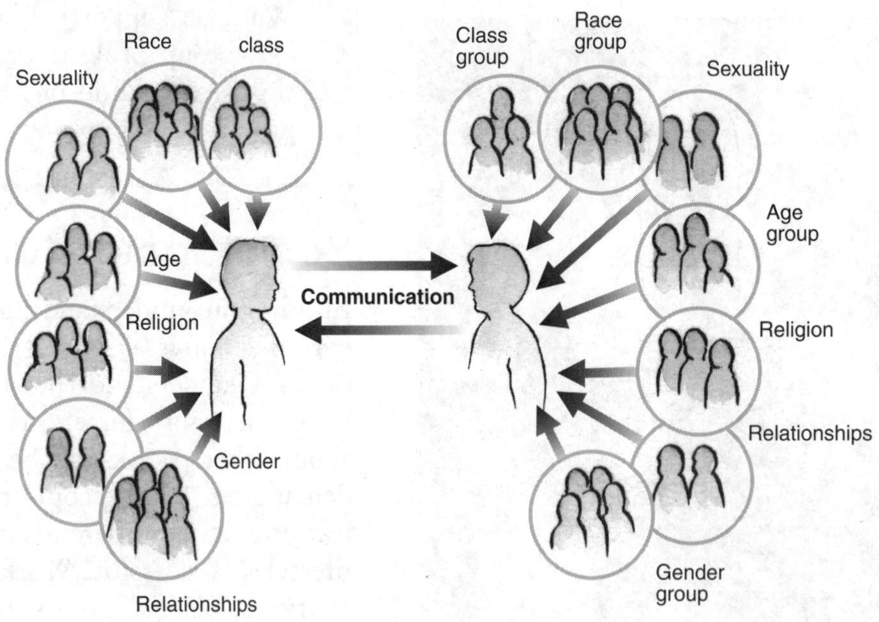


**Figure 2.12 The groups a person belongs to will influence his or her beliefs and behaviour**

sounds. Non-verbal communication is not the same everywhere.

For example, in Britain the hand gesture with palm up and facing forward, means, 'Stop, don't do that.' In Greece it can mean, 'You are dirt' and is a very rude gesture.

Why do the same physical movements have different meanings? The answer lies in culture. One explanation for the hand signs is that the British version of the palm-and-fingers gesture means, 'I arrest you, you must not do it'; whereas the Greek interpretation goes back to medieval times when criminals had dirt rubbed in their faces to show how much people despised them.

Without in-depth studies of history and culture, it is confusing to consider why gestures mean what they do. No one knows all the history and all the cultural possibilities of body language and non-verbal communication. But it is vitally important that carers should always remember that people have different cultural backgrounds. The carer's system of non-verbal communication may not carry the same meanings to everyone. We can easily misinterpret another person's non-verbal messages.

Sometimes cultural differences are very marked. White British people are often seen as 'unusual' or odd when they go outside Europe, because they keep a large personal space around them. Other people are not allowed to come too near when they speak, or to touch them. In many other cultures, standing close is normal and good manners – touching an arm or shoulder is just usual behaviour. However, some British people feel threatened by such non-verbal behaviour because it is not what they have grown up with. For some people, strangers who come too close or who touch are trying to dominate or have power over them. They become afraid or defensive. However, things work out when this need for space and distance is understood and allowed for by people from other cultures.

From a caring viewpoint, respect for other people's culture is the right attitude. People learn different ways of behaving, and good carers will try to understand the different ways in which people use non-verbal messages. For instance, past research in the USA suggests that white and black Americans may have used different non-verbal signals when they listened. It suggests that some black Americans may tend not to look much at the speaker. This can be interpreted as a mark of respect – by looking away it demonstrates that you are really thinking hard about the message. Unfortunately, not all white people understood this cultural difference in non-verbal communication. Some individuals misunderstood and assumed that this non-verbal behaviour meant exactly what it would mean if they had done it. That is, it would mean they were not listening – the opposite of what was happening!

## Learning the cultural differences

There is an almost infinite variety of meanings that can be given to any type of eye contact, facial expression, posture or gesture. Every culture develops its own special systems of meanings. Carers have to understand and show respect and value for all these different systems of sending messages. But how can you ever learn them all?

In fact, no one can learn every possible system of non-verbal message, but it is possible to learn about the ones people you are with are using! It is possible to do this by first noticing and remembering what others do – what non-verbal messages they are sending. The next step is to make an intelligent guess as to what messages the person is trying to give you. Finally, check your understanding (your guesses) with the person: ask polite questions as well as watching the kind of reactions you get. So, at the heart of skilled interpersonal interaction is the ability to watch other people, remember what they do, guess what actions might mean and then check out your guesses with the person. Remember:

- never rely on your own guesses, because often these turn into assumptions
- if you don't check out assumptions with people, you may end up misunderstanding them
- misunderstandings can lead to discrimination.

**Think it over**

Imagine you are working with an older person. Whenever you start to speak to her she always looks at the floor and never makes eye-contact. Why is this?

Your first thought is that she might be sad or that you make her sad. Having made such an assumption, you might not want to work with this person – she is too depressing and you do not seem to get on. You might decide that you do not like her. But you could ask: 'How do you feel today; would you like me to get you anything?' By checking what she feels, you could test your own understanding. She might say she feels well and is quite happy, and then suggest something you could do for her. This means that she cannot be depressed.

Why else would someone look at the floor rather than at you?

1 It could be a cultural value. She may feel it is not proper to look at you.

2 She may not be able to see you clearly, so she prefers not to try to look at you.

3 She may just choose not to conform to your expectations. Looking at the floor may be important to some other emotional feeling that she has.

So it would be unfair to assume that she was difficult or depressed just because she did not look at you when you talked to her.

Good caring is the art of getting to understand people – not acting on unchecked assumptions. So non-verbal messages should never be relied on; they should always be checked. Non-verbal messages can mean different things depending on the circumstances of the people who send them. But all messages are like this. Words can be looked up in a dictionary, and yet words do not always carry exactly the same meaning.

As well as looking at the 'whole picture' of people's words, their non-verbal messages and where they are, it is also necessary to understand their culture, their individuality and how they see their social situation. This is why caring is such a skilled area of work. People can improve their skills constantly through experience, and through linking new ideas to their experience. The main thing is always to check assumptions. It is important to remember that it is easy to misunderstand others. By checking ideas it is possible to reduce the risks of being uncaring or discriminatory.

## Culture, age and gender

A person's understanding of him or herself will be strongly influenced by past personal history and current social context.

Socialisation into the rules of a culture has a major part to play in the way individuals form their self-concept.

Perceptions of age-appropriate behaviour and gender-appropriate behaviour are strongly influenced by culture. Culture is the term used to describe the norms and values which belong to an identifiable social group. People are socialised into the norms and values of a culture; they learn the socially accepted rules of their group. Group norms and values – the 'rules' for behaviour – vary between different religious, ethnic, class, gender and age groups.

Norms and values which influence interpersonal interaction vary a great deal between different class groups and different regions of Britain. Not only do norms of interaction vary, but they also constantly evolve and change. It might be possible to invent a dictionary of rules for understanding the meanings of verbal and non-verbal behaviours; but such a dictionary would need constant revision for it to be accurate.

## Case study: Miss Tucknell

Florence Tucknell was born in 1912. When she was young there was a cultural norm that only close friends and family would call her by her first name. She was Miss Tucknell to everyone else. For a stranger to call her 'Florence' would be a sign of disrespect, a sign that they thought they were socially superior or more powerful than her. When Florence went into a respite care home for a week she was upset that everyone used first names. She knows that this is what goes on nowadays, but this was not how she was brought up to behave.

Miss Tucknell was very pleased to be greeted by her key worker who introduced herself by saying, 'I'm Anthea Shakespeare, may I ask your name?'. 'Miss Tucknell, please.' 'Shall I call you Miss Tucknell then?' 'Yes please.' 'Miss Tucknell was annoyed with one of the other staff who said, 'Hello Flo, I've come to take you into lunch'. Miss Tucknell avoids this care worker whenever she can.

## Case study: Martin Howarth

Martin Howarth was born in the north of England in 1949. He recently moved to the south-east of England and took a job as a care worker. Martin was shocked to find that many of his younger female colleagues were complaining about his behaviour. Martin has been socialised into the norm of calling women 'Flower' or even 'Petal.' When Martin used these terms he was expecting to communicate approval, comradeship and warmth. Martin believed that these were universal terms of endearment, i.e. 'You are likeable, we're all working together, we get on – don't we?'. His new colleagues in the south had never been referred to as 'Flower' before and saw it as sexist and degrading: 'You are saying that I am weak, short-lived and that all that matters about my existence is my degree of sexual attractiveness!' Martin soon learned that age, gender and region affect how words are understood. Words change their value with time.

People of different age groups have usually been socialised into different norms with respect to interpersonal behaviour.

Age norms and gender norms may also interact.

## Verbal skills

Effective communication always involves a process of listening. This process is sometimes referred to as a communication cycle. This cycle involves:

- hearing what another person says
- watching the other person's non-verbal messages
- having emotional feelings
- beginning to understand the other person
- sending a message back to the other person.

## Listening skills

We can often understand other people's emotions just by watching their non-verbal communication; but we can't always understand someone's thoughts without good listening skills.

Listening is not the same as simply hearing the sounds that people make when they talk. Listening skills involve hearing another person's words, thinking about what they mean and then thinking what to say back to the other person. Sometimes this process is called 'active listening' and sometimes 'reflective listening', because the person's conversation is reflected back (like the reflection in a mirror) in order to check understanding. As well as thinking carefully and remembering what a client says, good listeners will make sure that their non-verbal behaviour shows interest.

Skilled listening involves several stages:

1 Looking interested and ready to listen

2 Hearing what is said

3 Remembering what is said

4 Checking understanding with the other person.

### Checking our understanding

It is usually easier to understand people who are similar to ourselves. We can learn more about people who are different from us by checking our understanding of what we have heard. Checking understanding involves hearing what the other person says and asking questions. Another way of doing this is to put what a person has just said into your own words and say it back to

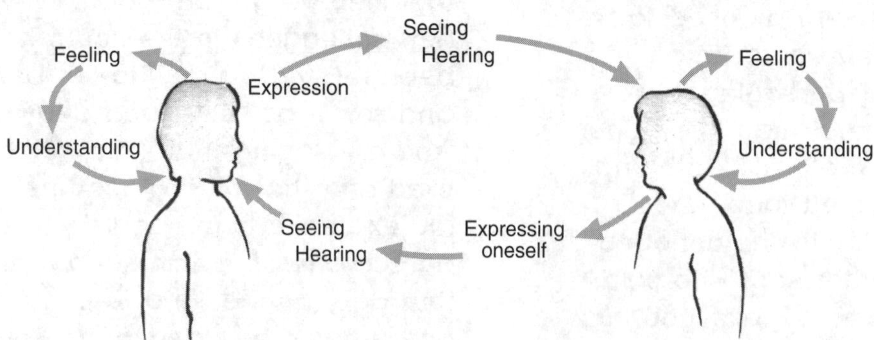


**Figure 2.13 The communication cycle involves more than just talking**

them; we can then find out if we did understand what they said.

When we listen to the complicated details of other people's lives, we often begin to form mental pictures based on what they tell us. It is important to check these mental pictures to make sure that we are understanding correctly. It can be very hard to remember correctly what people tell us if we don't check how our ideas are developing.

Good listening involves thinking about what we hear while we are listening and checking our understanding as the conversation goes along. Sometimes this idea of checking our understanding is called 'reflection', because we are reflecting the other person's ideas.

Good listening can feel like really hard work. Instead of just being around when people speak, we have to build up an understanding of the clients around us. However, although listening is hard work, people who are attracted to work in care usually enjoy learning about other people and their lives.

## Keeping a conversation going

A popular game in the past was to try to keep a plate spinning on the end of a stick – you have to keep turning the stick to keep the plate spinning, otherwise it will fall off! It can be the same with conversations. It can be hard to get to know people unless you can keep a conversation going.

Starting a conversation is often easy. We ask someone how they are today, we introduce ourselves or we ask a question. If we remember, we can mention things that have been talked about before, such as, 'How did you get on at the dentist yesterday?'.

Once a conversation has started, the trick is to keep it going long enough. Skills which help with this are turn taking, using non-verbal communication to show interest, being good at asking questions, using prompts and using silence at the right times.

Turn-taking conversations involve taking turns to listen and talk. If you are trying to get to know a client you will probably do

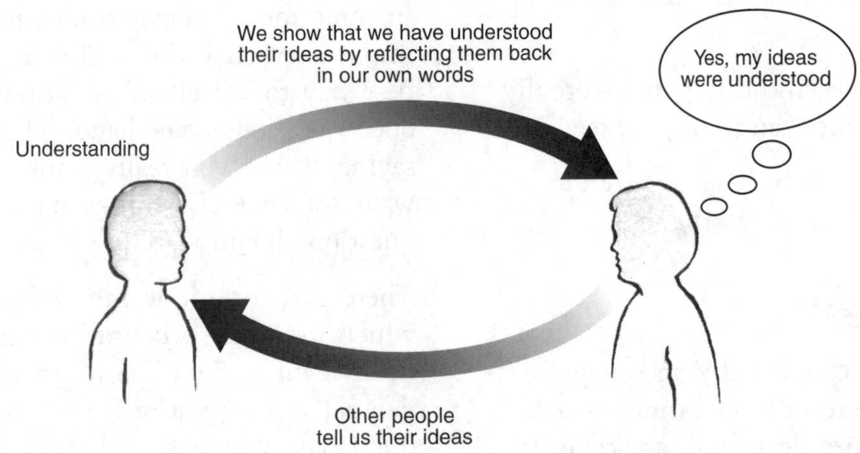


Figure 2.14 Good listening is crucial to understanding – especially in a care setting

less talking and more listening. People need to take turns for a conversation to work. People normally show when they want you to talk by slowing down the rate at which they speak their last few words, changing the tone of the voice slightly and looking away from you. The person will then stop speaking and look directly at you. If you are sensitive to these messages you will be ready to ask a question or say something which keeps the conversation going.

Another important skill is looking interested in what a client is saying. Looking interested is one way we can show respect – carers should be interested in what clients say because learning about others is part of the professional skill of a carer. So carers should show interest even if the client is talking about things which they would find boring in private life.

Showing interest involves giving the other person your full attention. Non-verbal messages which usually do this include:

- eye contact – looking at the other person's eyes
- smiling – looking friendly rather than 'cold' or frozen in expression
- hand movements and gestures that show interest
- slight head nods, indicating non-verbally 'I see,' or 'I understand,' or 'I agree.'

Showing interest can be a good way of keeping another person talking.

## Asking questions

Some questions do not really encourage people to talk. Some do. Questions which don't encourage people to talk are called **closed questions**. Closed questions are not very useful when trying to get to know people. Questions like, 'How old are you?' are 'closed'. They are closed because there is only one, right, simple answer the person can give: 'I'm 84', and so on. Closed questions don't lead on to discussion. 'Do you like butter?' is a closed question – the person can only say yes or no. 'Are you feeling well today?' is a closed question – the person may only say yes or no.

**Open questions** on the other hand are open ended. Instead of giving a yes/no answer, the person is encouraged to think and discuss their thoughts. A question like, 'How do you feel about the food here?' means that the other person has to think about the food and then discuss it.

Open questions keep the conversation going. Sometimes closed questions can block a conversation and cause it to stop.

The more we know about someone the more we can be sensitive about the type of questions that we ask. Some people don't mind questions about their feelings or opinions, but do dislike questions which ask for personal information. Getting to know people often takes time and usually involves a number of short conversations rather than one long conversation.

In some formal conversations it can be important to ask direct closed questions. The best way to ask closed questions is to ask open questions beforehand. There is an old saying that if you really want to find out what someone else thinks then, 'Every closed question should start life as an open one'.

There is a technique called **funnelling**, which uses this principle in formal interviewing. First the interviewer asks general open questions, then narrower questions, then a closed question. The answer to the closed question can be followed up using probes and prompts.

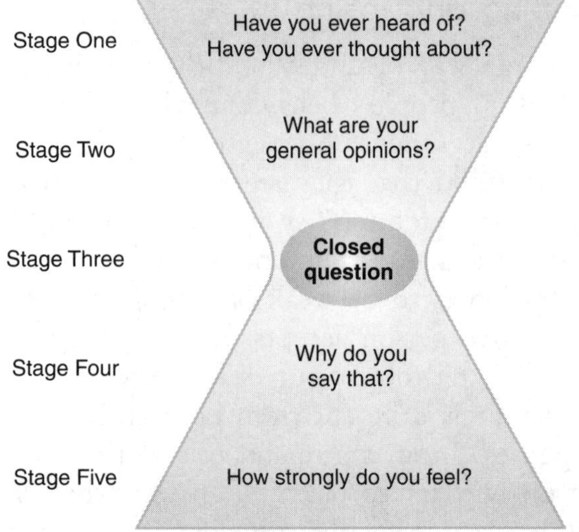


Funneling: Open questions should lead into the closed question. After the closed question probes and prompts may help to clarify a response. Funneling makes it possible for every closed question to start off as a series of open questions.

**Figure 2.15 The funnelling technique**

For example, a care worker might be trying to find out about the life history of an older client. Perhaps the care worker wants to ask, 'Were you interested in music?' It can be 'cold' and even aggressive to just fire questions like this at people. Instead, the question could be funnelled.

*Carer* What was it like in the evenings before television came along? [*open question*]

*Client* Well, we used to get together and make our own entertainment.

*Carer* So what sort of activities did you do? [*open question*]

*Client* Oh, gossip, talking to neighbours, sing-songs.

*Carer* Were you interested in music? [*closed question*]

*Client* Well a bit – I used to have piano lessons – but we couldn't afford a piano at home.

Funnelling is a skill which enables carers to lead into questions 'gently'; it is a great alternative to asking too many closed questions.

### Silence

One definition of friends is 'people who can sit together and feel comfortable in silence'. Sometimes a pause in conversation can make people feel embarrassed – it looks as if you weren't listening or interested. Sometimes a silent pause can mean 'let's think' or 'I need time to think'. Silent pauses can be all right as long as non-verbal messages which show respect and interest are given. Silence doesn't always stop the conversation. Some carers use pauses in a conversation to show that they are listening and thinking about what the client has said.

## Recap

If you need to keep a conversation going you can:

- use non-verbal behaviour like smiling and nodding your head to express interest
- use short periods of silence to prompt the other person to talk
- paraphrase or reflect back what the other person has said so that they will confirm that you have understood them
- ask direct questions
- use probes and prompts to follow-up your questions.

### Probes and prompts

A probe is a very short question, such as, 'Can you tell me more?'. This kind of short question usually follows on from an answer that the other person has given. Probes are used to 'dig deeper' into the person's answer; they probe or investigate what the other person has said.

Prompts are short questions or words which you offer to the other person in order to prompt them to answer. Questions such as, 'So was it enjoyable or not?', 'Would you do it again?' might prompt a person to keep talking. Sometimes a prompt might just be a suggested answer – 'More than 50?' might be a prompt if you had just asked how many clients a carer worked with in a year and they seemed uncertain.

Probes and prompts are both useful techniques to improve questioning skills, when you are trying to keep a conversation going.

## Assertive skills

Some people may seem shy and worried, they say little and avoid contact with people they don't know. Other people may want people to be afraid of them, they may try to dominate and control others. Fear and aggression are two of the basic emotions that we experience. It is easy to give into our basic emotions and either become submissive or aggressive when we feel stressed. Assertion is an advanced skill which involves controlling the basic emotions involved in running away or fighting. Assertion involves a mental attitude of trying to negotiate, trying to solve problems rather than giving in to emotional impulses.

### Winning and losing

A simple way of understanding assertion is to look at people's behaviour when they have an argument. An aggressive person will demand that they are right and other people are wrong. They will want to win while others lose. The opposite of aggression is to be weak or submissive. A submissive person accepts that they will lose, get told off or put down. Assertive behaviour is different from both these responses. In an argument an assertive person will try to reach an answer where no one has to lose or be 'put down'. Assertion is a skill where 'win-win' situations can happen – no one has to be the loser. For example, suppose a client or service user is angry because their carer is late:

| | |
|---|---|
| *Client:* | 'You're late again – I'm not putting up with it – I'm going to make sure you lose your job'. |
| *Aggressive response:* | 'Don't you talk to me like that – you're lucky I see you at all – if you don't like what I do then find yourself another service'. |
| *Submissive response:* | 'I'm terribly sorry, I promise I won't be late again'. |
| *Assertive response:* | 'I'm sorry that you're angry, but I really couldn't help it, please let me explain why I had to be late today'. |

The assertive response aims to meet the emotional needs of both people without anyone being the loser. The aggressive response tries to meet the needs of the worker and not the client – it aims to give the worker power and keep the client vulnerable. The submissive response may allow the client to control and dominate the worker. Assertive skills can help enable carers to cope with difficult and challenging situations.

To be assertive a person usually has to be able to:

- understand the situation that they are in – including facts, details and other people's perceptions
- control personal emotions and stay calm
- act assertively using the right non-verbal behaviour
- act assertively using the right words and statements.

Learning to stay calm and use the right verbal and non-verbal behaviour is a skill which can be developed by watching other experienced professionals and copying their performance. Role play and reflection practice can also help to develop assertive skills. Some verbal and non-verbal behaviours involved in assertion are summarised in the table below.

Assertive skills are important in any situation where people have to solve problems, i.e. in work, domestic and social situations! Carers working with the five people described at the beginning of this chapter would want to achieve a 'win-win' situation where the best possible outcome was achieved. Carers want to help clients to speak out clearly about their views. It is important that vulnerable people are 'empowered' to control their lives. At the same time, rights and responsibilities have to be thought through. A working care plan or group outcome may not always include everything a client wants. Effective communication in care involves the skills listed under assertive behaviour in Table 2.1 below.

| Aggressive behaviour | Assertive behaviour | Submissive behaviour |
|---|---|---|
| *Main emotion*: anger | *Main emotion*: staying in control of own actions | *Main emotion*: fear |
| Wanting your own way | Negotiating with others | Letting others win |
| Making demands | Trying to solve problems | Agreeing with others |
| Not listening to others | Aiming that no one has to lose | Not putting your views across |
| 'Putting other people down' | Listening to others | Looking afraid |
| Trying to win | Showing respect for others | Speaking quietly or not speaking at all |
| Shouting or talking very loudly | Keeping a clear, calm voice | **Submissive non-verbal behaviour** including: looking down, not looking at others, looking frightened, tense muscles. |
| **Threatening non-verbal behaviour** including: fixed eye contact, tense muscles, waving or folding hands and arms, looking angry. | **Normal non-verbal behaviour** including : varied eye contact, relaxed face muscles, looking 'in control', keeping hands and arms at your side | |

**Table 2.1** Some differences between aggressive, assertive and submissive behaviour

## Empowerment

Assertive skills may help to create an atmosphere where vulnerable people do not lose out. Effective communication involves making sure that clients and service users are empowered.

Smale *et al.* (1993) contrast a historical way of working with the idea of empowerment. In the past, carers, social workers or nurses would often regard themselves as experts on people. Professionals would assess a client's needs and then present the client with a possible range of services to meet the carer's view of the client's needs. The power in this situation all lies with the carer. The carer learns about the client, the carer decides what his or her needs are then the carer might set about 'helping' the client. The client becomes a passive 'patient', someone who shows patience while undergoing treatment.

Smale *et al.* (1993) propose that carers should always work from the principle that 'people are, and always will be, the expert on themselves' (page 13). While people may not be expert on their own biochemistry and may need treatment for biological illness, people themselves will be the experts of their own social, emotional and cognitive needs. The idea is that power should be given to the clients, that clients should be empowered to make their own decisions about their own lives. In principle this sounds fine, but many clients receive social care because they are not able to make or not confident in making their own decisions.

If the carer can build an understanding with a client, however, if the carer can empathise with a client, then the carer and client can work together to solve problems. This approach links with the idea of self-advocacy, where the worker enables a client to speak for himself or herself.

Very often, meeting clients' needs may depend not only on interacting with clients but also interacting with relatives or friends in the clients' social 'network'. Where clients are not able to express their own beliefs, or communicate about their personal and cultural identity, it may be important for the care worker to discuss problems with relatives to get information about the client. Rather, the care worker is trying to understand the viewpoint of the relatives and the client. A relative may understand the client's personal or cultural identity in a way that the care worker does not. A relative may be in a position to speak for the client or act as an advocate for the client. For example, a wife may be able to explain the needs of her husband who has dementia. The wife may also be able to provide information about her husband's beliefs and previous lifestyle. If the care worker can talk to the wife, then he or she may be able to learn ideas for communicating effectively with her husband. Learning about the husband's life might enable the care worker to ensure that routine, diet, social activities and so on fit with the husband's past identity and lifestyle.

The principle of empowerment implies that the client's problems are solved through building an understanding between the client and the care worker. The client's problems are not solved by professionals or care staff on their own. The principle of not keeping power solely with the staff, but empowering clients to control their lives, will follow from the principles involved in the Care value base.

### Think it over

Below is an example of a disempowering interaction. It takes place at lunch-time in the lounge of a rest home with other residents listening.

| | |
|---|---|
| *Carer* | Come on Bill, it's time for lunch. What's the matter, don't you want any? |
| *Resident* | What's the time? |
| *Carer* | 12 o'clock, come on now, look lively. |
| *Resident* | But I'm not hungry. |
| *Carer* | You're not? Well, you don't have to eat, you know. But why don't you just come along with me, your appetite will come back, I'm sure it will! |
| *Resident* | What's for dinner? |
| *Carer* | Can't you remember? You had a menu yesterday. |
| *Resident* | I never did – I don't remember it. |
| *Carer* | Well, don't worry yourself, we'll give you something, you're not fussy are you? |
| *Resident* | I'll not eat pork and I'll not eat all that sweetcorn rubbish – chicken food, that's what that is. I want decent food. |
| *Carer* | Well, just leave anything you don't like. Look – here we are – just sit here. |
| *Resident* | But this isn't where I usually sit. |
| *Carer* | Well, it's all change today. Have a change, Bill, do you good. Now don't start on me! |

## An empowering interaction

A verbal interaction in this care setting which fulfilled the value base requirements might have gone something like:

| | |
|---|---|
| *Carer* | It's lunch time, Mr Sidwell, do you want me to help you to the dining room? |
| *Resident* | What's the time, then? |
| *Carer* | It's 12 o'clock. Do you want lunch yet? |
| *Resident* | I'm not really hungry. What's the dinner anyway? |
| *Carer* | Well. I'll just check with the menu. Ah yes, you could have an egg salad, ham salad or the cooked choice. |
| *Resident* | Egg salad would be all right – there's none of that rubbish in it – that sweetcorn, is there? |
| *Carer* | I'll make sure there's no sweetcorn – but why do you dislike it so much? |
| *Resident* | It's rubbish, we used to feed it to pigs and chickens in the war – I'm not being treated like that now. I don't see why I should put up with it. |
| *Carer* | Oh, I didn't know it used to be fed to animals. We don't do that nowadays. |
| *Resident* | Well, there's some strange things nowadays; help me over there will you, that's where I want to sit. |
| *Carer* | Yes, of course – then I'll get your lunch for you. |

In this interaction there is evidence that the carer wants to empower the client. The client has the power to choose whether he wants to go in for lunch or not and whether he wants help or not. The client's questions are answered with respect and there is no suggestion of the carer having a right to control or take power over the client. As well as providing a choice for the client, the carer is careful to listen to the client. The carer reflects the statement about sweetcorn: 'I'll make sure there's no sweetcorn – but why do you dislike it so much?' The carer is actively interested in the client and is trying to build an understanding of his needs. The carer is rewarded by finding out the answer – sweetcorn is only fit for animals, according to the client. The client's dignity would be offended if it was offered to him.

By carefully asking the right questions the carer is working in an anti-discriminatory way – and avoids making inappropriate assumptions. The carer is also able to demonstrate respect for the client's beliefs and to support and value the client with effective communication. The client's right to confidentiality and privacy is not infringed.

The key issue which makes this an empowering interaction is the fact that the carer seems to give power to the client rather than disempowering or taking power from the client.

The principle of empowerment follows from working within the Care value base. Empowerment is an important goal of all caring interaction.

## Communication difficulties

Communication can become blocked if individual difficulties and differences are not understood. There are three main ways that communication becomes blocked:

1 A person cannot see, hear or receive the message.

2 A person cannot make sense of the message.

3 A person misunderstands the message.

Examples of the first kind of block, where people do not receive the communication, include visual disabilities, hearing disabilities, and environmental problems such as poor lighting, noisy environments, and speaking from too far away.

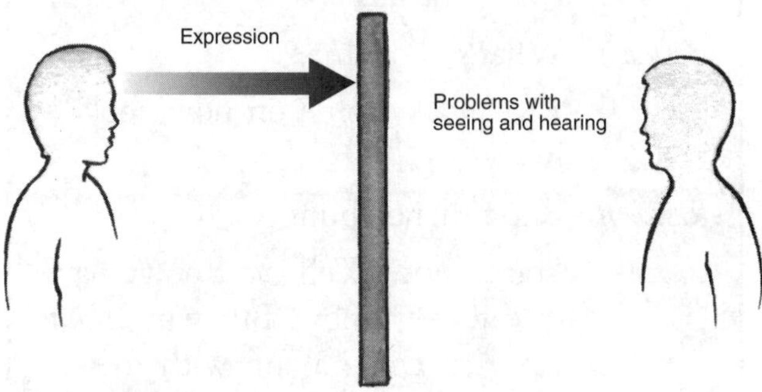


**Figure 2.16 Environmental problems like noise and poor light can create communication barriers**

Examples where people may not be able to make sense of the message include:

- the use of different languages, including signed languages
- the use of different terms in language, such as jargon (technical language), slang (different people using different terms), or dialect (different people making different sounds)
- physical and intellectual disabilities, such as being ill, or suffering memory loss, or leaning disability.

Reasons for misunderstanding a message include:

- cultural influences – different cultures interpret non-verbal and verbal messages, and humour, in different ways

- assumptions about people – about race, gender, disability and other groupings
- labelling or stereotyping of others
- social context – statements and behaviour that are understood by friends and family may not be understood by strangers
- emotional barriers – a worker's own emotional needs may stop them from wanting to know about others
- emotional differences – very angry or very happy people may misinterpret communication from others.

Effective communication requires care workers to evaluate the possible barriers to communication and find ways of overcoming these barriers. The section on evaluating communication at the end of this chapter reviews this idea.

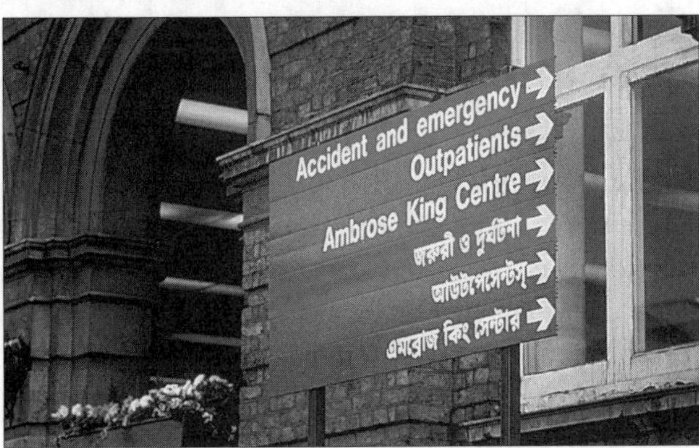


**Language barriers can be overcome by using signs in more than one language**

## Ways of overcoming difficulties in communication

It is always important in care work to learn as much as possible about other people. It is useful to know that some people may have their own 'preferred forms of interaction'. This may include a reliance on non-verbal messages, sign language, lip-reading, use of description, slang phrases, choice of room or location for a conversation and so on.

Everyone has communication needs of some kind. Needs to do with disability are sometimes referred to as 'special needs'. Some people with a disability object to the term 'special needs', as it appears to emphasise difference rather than value diversity. Below are some ideas for overcoming barriers to communication.

### Visual disability

It can be helpful to:

- use language to describe things
- assist people to touch things (e.g. touch your face to recognise you)
- explain details that sighted people might take for granted
- check what people can see (many registered blind people can see shapes, or tell light from dark)
- check glasses, other aids and equipment.

### Hearing disability

It helps communication if you:

- don't shout; keep to normal clear speech and make sure your face is visible for people who can lip-read
- show pictures, or write messages
- learn to sign (for people who use signed languages)
- ask for help from or employ a communicator or interpreter for signed languages
- check hearing aids and equipment.

### Environmental constraints

You could:

- check and improve lighting
- reduce noise
- move to a quieter or better lit room
- move to smaller groups to see and hear more easily
- check seating.

### Language differences

It can help if you:

- communicate using pictures, diagrams and non-verbal signs
- use translators or interpreters
- are careful not to make assumptions or stereotype
- increase your knowledge of jargon, slang and dialects
- re-word your messages – find different ways of saying things
- speak in short, clear sentences.

### Physical and intellectual disabilities

A number of different factors can assist in communication. It can be a good idea to:

- increase your knowledge of disabilities
- use picture and signs as well as clear, simple speech
- be calm and patient
- set up group meetings where people can share interests, experiences or reminiscences
- check that people do not become isolated.

### Misunderstandings

These can be common in all kinds of interactions – personal and domestic as well as work-related! You can:

- try to increase your knowledge of different cultures
- watch out for different cultural interpretations
- avoid making assumptions about or discriminating against people who are different
- use reflective listening techniques to check that your understanding is correct
- stay calm and try to calm people who are angry or excited
- be sensitive to different social settings and the form of communication that would be most appropriate in different contexts.

## Emotional barriers which can inhibit communication

Sometimes it is very difficult to listen to and communicate with others. Clients often have very major emotional needs, they are afraid or depressed because of the stresses they are experiencing. Listening involves learning about frightening and depressing situations. Carers sometimes avoid listening to avoid unpleasant emotional feelings.

Communication can be inhibited because:

- carers are tired – listening takes mental energy
- carers are emotionally stressed by the needs of clients
- carers do not understand the culture or context of others
- carers make assumptions about others or label or stereotype others.

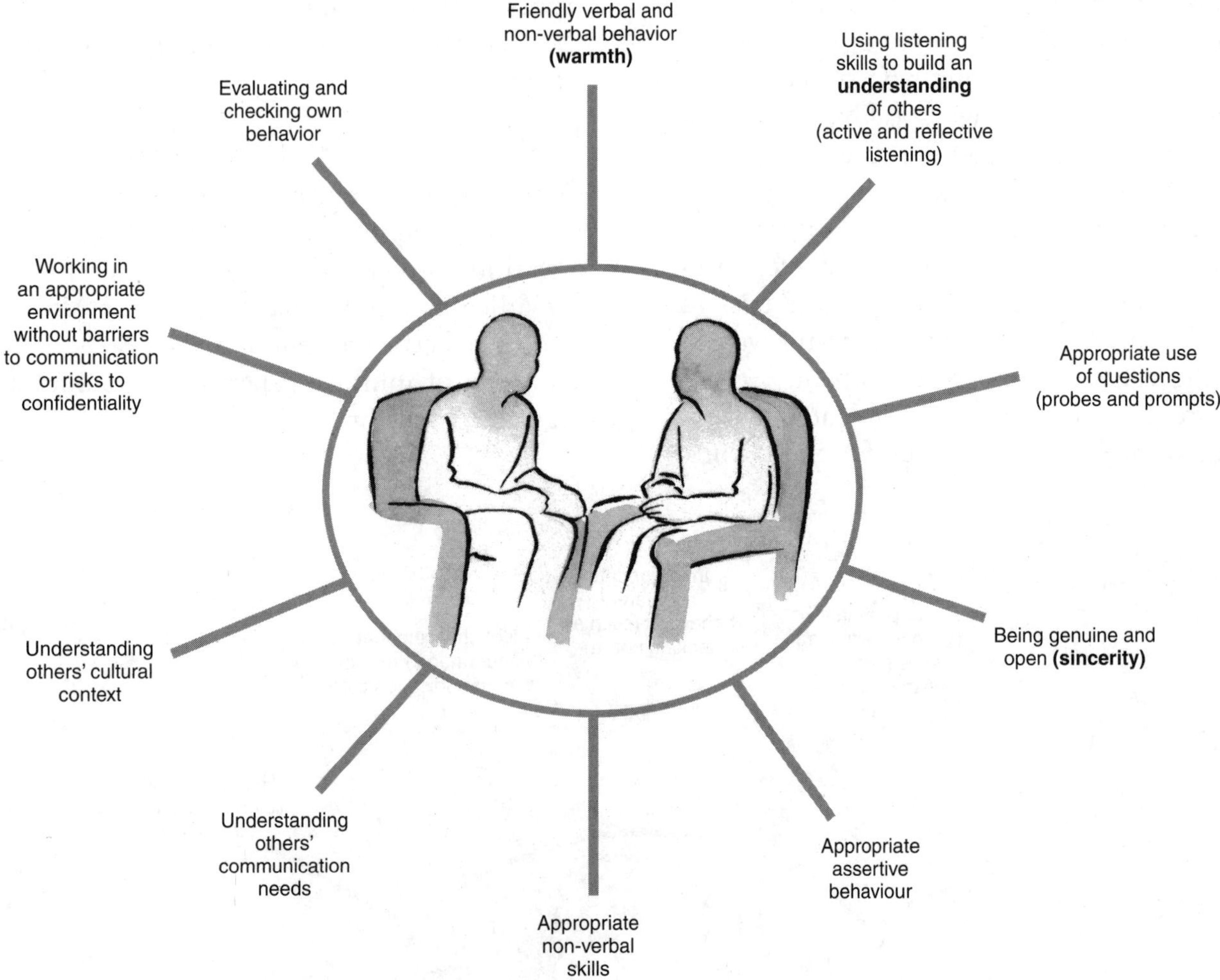


**Figure 2.17 Factors which enhance communication**

## Labelling and stereotyping

People who have difficulty hearing or seeing are sometimes assumed to be awkward or mentally limited. Older people are sometimes seen as demented or confused if they do not answer questions appropriately.

People can also be labelled or stereotyped when they use different language systems. Some people will shout at those who don't speak the same language, as if increasing the volume would help. People who sign to communicate are sometimes thought to be odd or to have learning difficulties, because they don't respond to written or spoken English.

Cultural differences can also lead to labelling and stereotyping. Someone may use gestures and eye contact to show respect, but another person may misinterpret the messages as aggression or disrespect.

## Advocacy

Sometimes, when people have a very serious learning disability or an illness (such as dementia), it is not possible to communicate with them. In such situations care services will often employ an advocate. An advocate is someone who speaks for someone else. A lawyer speaking for a client in a courtroom is working as an advocate for that person and will argue the client's case. In care work, a volunteer might try to get to know someone who has dementia or a learning disability. The volunteer tries to communicate the client's needs and wants – as the volunteer understands them. Advocates should be independent of the staff team and so can argue for the client's rights without being constrained by what the staff think is easiest or cheapest to do.

## Ineffective communication

Communication can be inhibited by carers not appropriately using the knowledge and techniques described in this section. Prejudice and emotional barriers can also inhibit effective communication. A summary of inhibiting factors is set out in Figure 2.18 below.

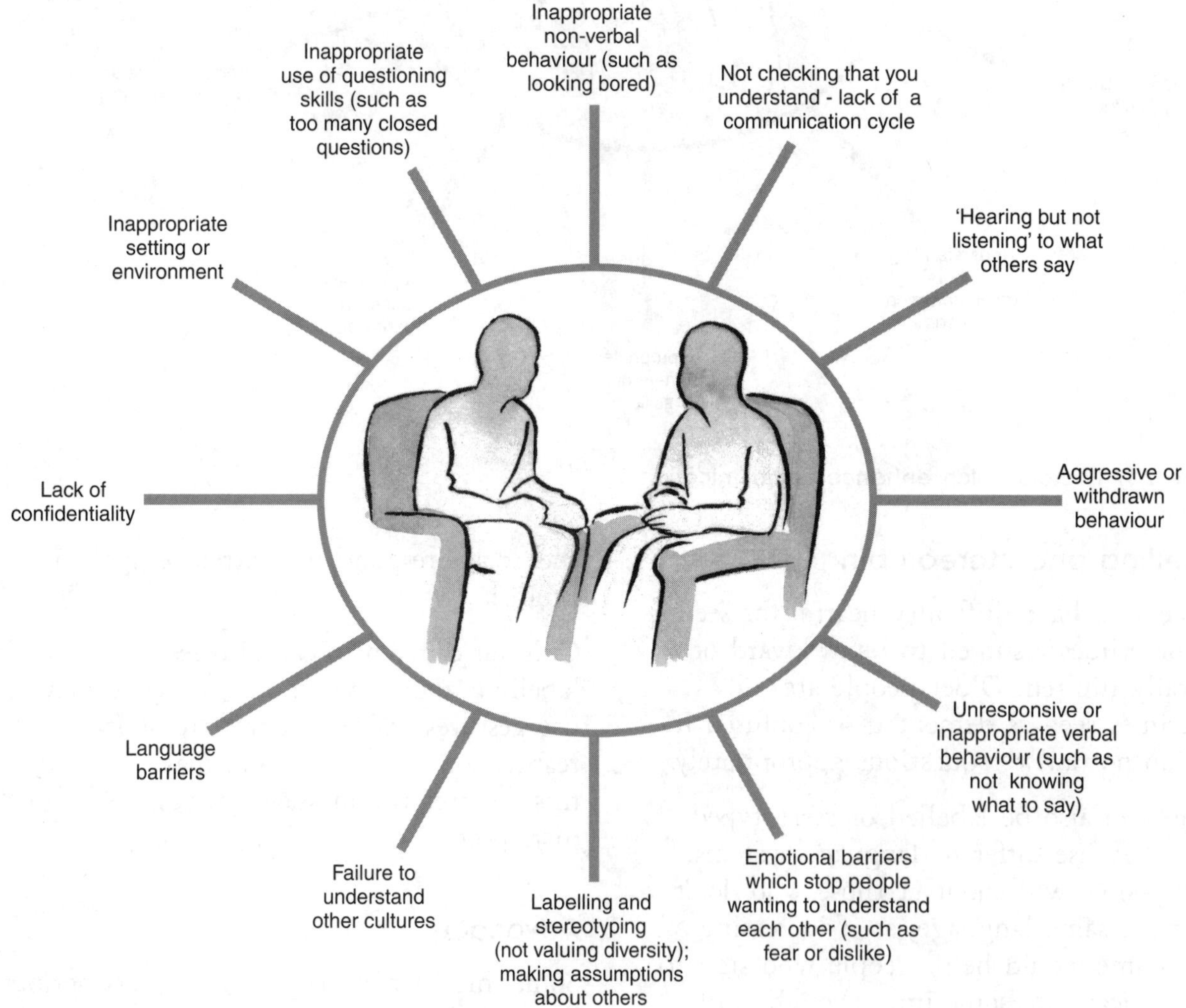


**Figure 2.18 Factors which inhibit communication**

### The consequences of ineffective communication

> **Think it over**
>
> Nowadays, social services are well aware of the need to meet people's social, cultural and emotional needs. But situations such as the case study reported below did happen in the past. Do you think that there could still be a risk of these things happening today?

## Case study

Mr Mansel is 84 and moved into a rest home after having a stroke. Mr Mansel grew up in Jamaica but moved to Britain 50 years ago. Unfortunately he has been placed in a home some distance from his friends and receives few visits. None of the staff understand Mr Mansel's history or cultural background. The home has a number of staff vacancies and is currently short staffed. Staff have little time to talk to Mr Mansel. The stroke has affected Mr Mansel's speech and staff find communication difficult and time consuming. Other residents in the home have communication differences including hearing disabilities and disorientation and memory loss. Some residents avoid Mr Mansel and appear to label him as different from themselves. Mr Mansel feels isolated and distressed.

Ineffective communication, such as Mr Mansel is experiencing, can immediately result in:

- a loss of self-esteem – you feel you can't be worth much if people don't communicate with you
- a loss of purpose in life – you may feel excluded or alienated from others if you cannot communicate
- a loss of support – you may find life difficult to cope with if your social and emotional needs are not met
- a feeling of being threatened – if people do not communicate you may not be able to predict what is likely to happen.

These problems may result in a belief that we can no longer control our life circumstances.

One of the major risks facing Mr Mansel is that of **learned helplessness.** Martin Seligman (1975) published a theory of learned helplessness which explains how a loss of control over our life circumstances can result in a process of learning to become withdrawn, depressed and helpless.

Helplessness starts when a person learns that no matter what they do they cannot control what is going to happen. People can develop a general helpless attitude to daily living when major needs like communication are 'out of control'.

According to Seligman, the first stages in the process of becoming helpless are to react with frustration and anger. In the case study above, Mr Mansel may become aggressive, perhaps shouting at others or damaging property. In the past, such problems were often regarded as being due to 'confusion', 'age', or dementia. Seligman explains that aggression can be a last attempt to control – when nothing else works you can lose your temper. In a 'stressed' care environment Mr Mansel's anger is unlikely to get him the attention he needs. Instead he may be labelled as disturbed or difficult and isolated further.

The next step in the process is learning to 'give-up'. Giving up saves energy. Withdrawal from trying to communicate may be the best coping strategy. Being 'withdrawn' can protect a person. Mr Mansel cannot get his social and self-esteem needs met but there may be a sense of safety in not attempting to communicate. Ineffective communication may not matter so much if you come to expect no communication at all.

## Think it over

Have you ever visited a care setting where people appear depressed and withdrawn? Sometimes physical illness and the problems of coping with change may cause depression. Could the process of 'learning to withdraw' and become helpless also account for some of these problems?

The process of learning to become helpless does not stop with withdrawal. If a person cannot predict what is likely to happen to them then they are likely to become anxious. The stress of anxiety can cause a deeper level of withdrawal, a withdrawal into depression. Seligman argued that helplessness and anxiety could result in clinical depression due to changes in brain chemistry. A lack of communication could be enough to cause anxiety. Mr Mansel may not know what is happening around him or what to expect from staff. If he feels unable to respond to discrimination and exclusion he may experience anxiety and withdrawal. Serious mental ill-health may result.

Finally, Seligman believed that severe depression resulting from learned helplessness could be fatal. This may be particularly true when an individual is in poor health.

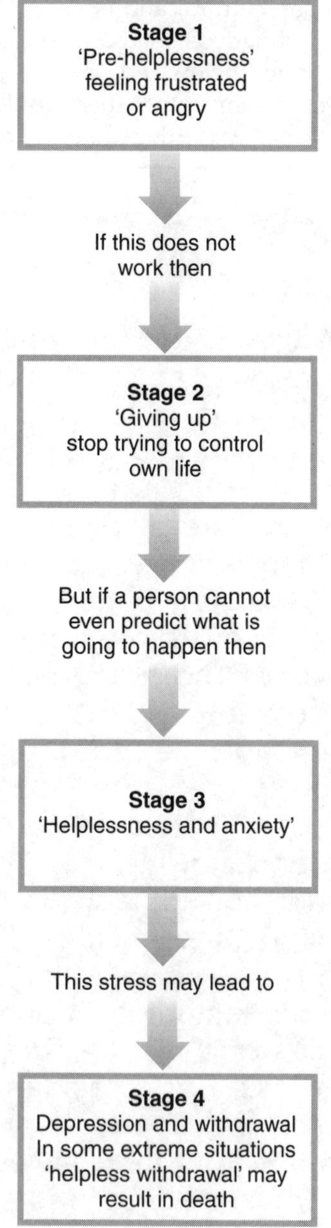


**Figure 2.19 The process of learned helplessness**

Effective communication is therefore not just a right which clients may expect – not just a quality of care issue. Effective communication is necessary to protect the mental well-being of vulnerable people. Poor communication can be understood as a form of abuse. If Seligman's theory is correct then it is possible to argue that this abuse may be enough to cause death.

## 2.3 Communication skills in groups

### Types of groups

In everyday language 'group' can mean a collection or set of things, so any collection of people could be counted as a group. For example, a group of people might be waiting to cross the road. These people have not spoken to each other, they may not even have communicated non-verbally – they are simply together in the same place at the same time. They are a group in the everyday sense of the word, but not in the special sense of 'group' that is often used in health and social care work.

In caring, working with a group implies that the people belong together and would identify themselves as belonging to a group. Groups have a sense of belonging which gives the members a 'group feeling'. This could be described as group identity.

Social scientists sometimes use the term 'primary group' to mean people who know each other and feel they belong together. The term 'secondary group' is used when people simply have something in common with each other.

Primary groups in care usually share the following features:

- people know each other
- there is a 'feeling of belonging' shared by people in the group
- people have a common purpose or reason for coming together
- people share a set of beliefs or norms.

Some groups seem to 'just come together', but other groups require a lot of skilled leadership and effort before people are able to work together.

### Group stages

Many theorists have studied the way people start to work together. Before a sense of belonging can develop in a group, people need to learn about each other. Most groups seem to go through some sort of struggle before people finally unite and work effectively together.

One of the best known theorists to explain the stages that groups often run through is Tuckman (1965). Tuckman suggests that most groups go through a process involving four stages before they can become effective.

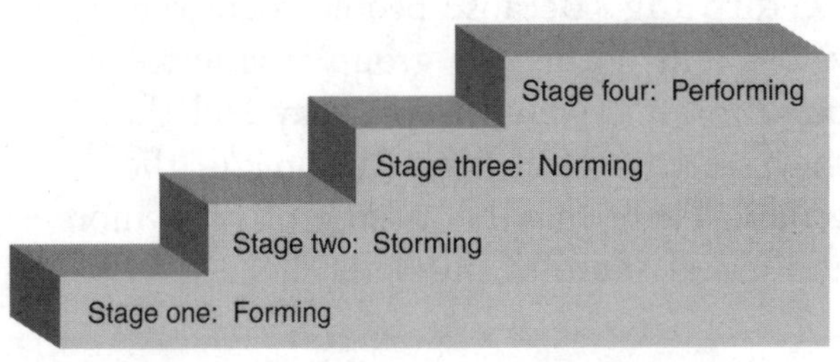


**Figure 2.20 Tuckman's four stages of group formation**

### An outline explanation of group formation

**Forming** When people first get together there is likely to be an introductory stage. People may be unsure why they are attending a meeting. The purpose of the group may not be clear. People may have little commitment to the group and there may be no clear value system. Stereotyping and prejudice may be expressed.

**Storming** There may be 'power struggles' within the group. Different individuals may contest each other for the leadership of the group. There may be arguments about how the group should work, who should do the tasks and so on. Groups can fail at this stage and individuals can decide to drop out because they do not feel comfortable with other people in the group. Staff teams sometimes split into sub groups who refuse to communicate with each other, if they become stuck in the storming stage.

**Norming** At this stage group members develop a set of common beliefs and values. People are likely to begin to trust each other and develop clear roles. 'Norms' ae shared expectations which group members have of each other. Norms enable people to work together as a group.

**Performing** Because people share the same values and norms the group is able to perform effectively. People may feel that they are comfortable and belong in the group. There may be a sense of high morale and a real sense of purpose.

## Communication in groups

Just looking at the way people sit or stand can sometimes give an indication of whether a group is at the 'performing stage' or whether it is not working effectively or working as a group. Seating patterns can have a major influence on how a group works.

When working with a discussion group it is very important that everyone can see and hear one another. Non-verbal communication will be important, and if people cannot see everybody's faces this will not be possible. Usually, chairs are placed in a circle when planning a discussion group. In a circle everyone can get non-verbal messages from everyone else.

Organising a group to sit in a circle may suggest that everyone is equal, that everyone is expected to communicate with everyone else. This freedom to communicate is also linked with creating a feeling of belonging: 'We can all share together – this is our group!' (Figure 2.21a).

Other patterns of seating will send different messages. Teachers might sit in the middle of a half-circle. This sends the message, 'We are all equal and we can all communicate with each other, but the teacher is going to do most of the communicating!' (Figure 2.21b).

At a formal lecture, people sit in rows. This sends the message 'The lecturer will talk to you. You can ask questions but you should not talk to one another!' (Figure 2.21c).

Some less formal seating arrangements can be chosen to create blocks. Sometimes a desk or table acts as a block. For example, in Figure 2.21d, the two people on their own might be sending the message 'We are not sure we want to be with this group'. The table can make them feel separate, 'We'll join in only if we feel like it'.

Sometimes space can be used to create a gulf. In Figure 2.21e, person A cannot see person C properly – so the two of them are unable to exchange non-verbal messages. Person A sits 'square on' to person F.

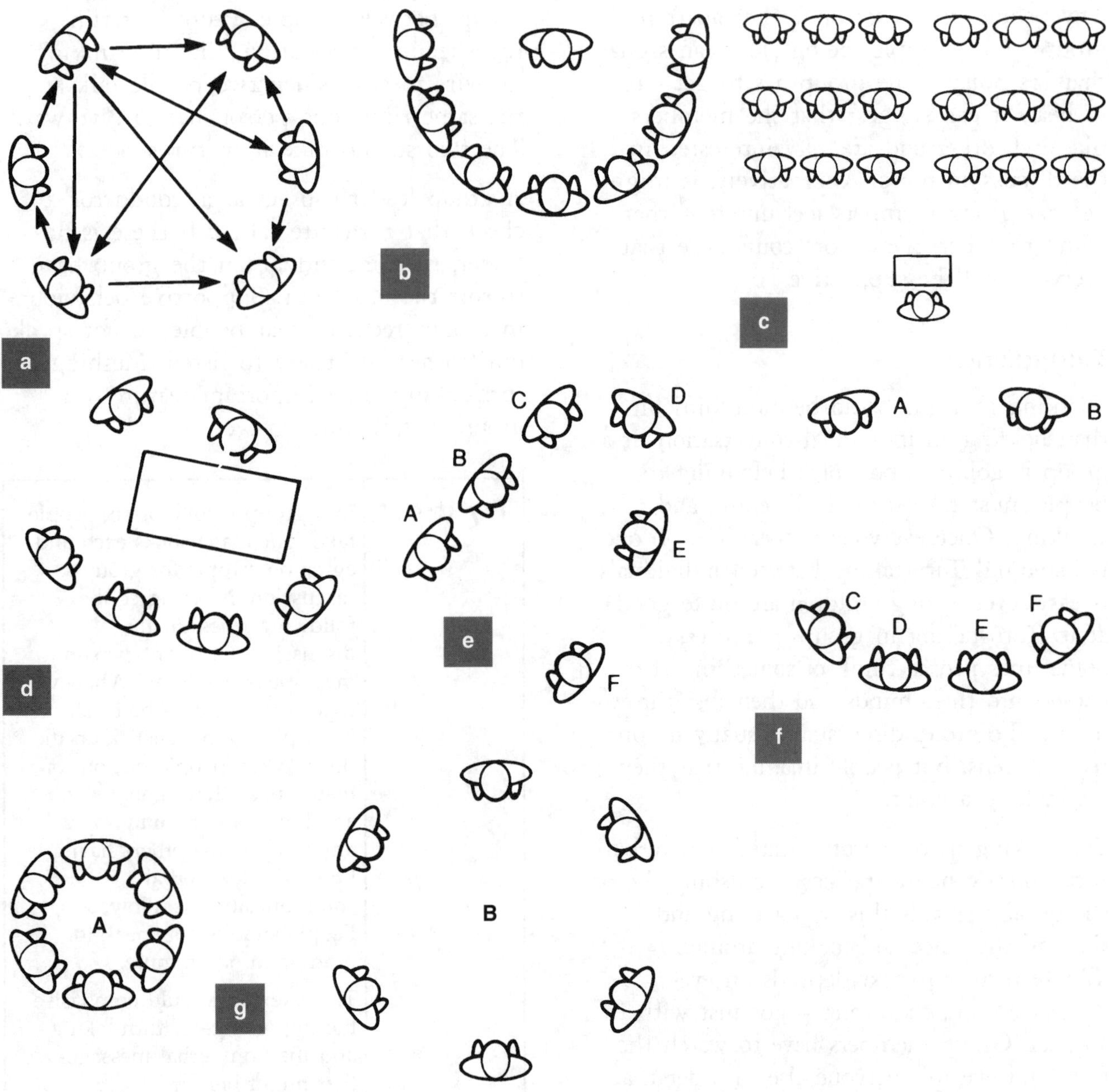


**Figure 2.21 Seven patterns of interaction**

Perhaps A does not want to talk to C. Perhaps F and A do not trust each other. The layout of seats makes it look as though there could be tension or reluctance in this group.

Space can also signal social distance – see Figure 2.21f. A and B are keeping their distance from the rest of the group. There could be many reasons,[1] but perhaps they are sending the message 'We do not really belong with you four!'

Another consideration is whether a group of people is sitting close together or spaced out. In Figure 2.21g, group A are huddled together, whereas group B are more spaced apart. There might be a number of reasons why people get closer or further apart in groups. For example, being close can signal that it's noisy – the group has to get close to hear. It can suggest that the members like each other and are very interested in the discussion topic. Alternatively, it might be that group members feel unsafe – that being together gives more confidence that everyone will be supportive.

### Turn-taking

Working in a group can be more difficult than holding an individual conversation. If a group is going to be worth belonging to, people must take turns in listening and speaking. Once everyone is speaking, no one is listening! Turn-taking between individuals is easy; even young children are quite good at it. Turn-taking in groups is not easy. Sometimes people think of something that comes into their minds and then just throw it into the group discussion. Usually no one really listens, but people imagine that they are making a point.

Turn-taking involves complicated non-verbal behaviour. When a speaker is finishing, he or she usually signals this by lowering and slowing the voice and looking around. Whose turn it is next depends on eye-contact around the group – not just with the speaker. Group members have to watch the faces and eyes of everyone else in order that just one person takes over and speaks in turn. If people get excited or tense, then they usually add gestures to their other non-verbal messages to signal forcefully that they want to speak next. Sometimes people will put their hand out or nod their head to say (non-verbally): 'Look, it's my turn next!'

Eventually turn-taking goes wrong, and two or more people start talking at once. This is called a failure to 'mesh'. Meshing means that conversation flows easily around the group, between people. People interlink together in conversation, like interlinking in 'wire mesh'. When two people talk at the same time, one person has to give way. The two should take it in turns.

A group leader can act as a 'conductor' to check that turns are taken. If there is no leader, then individuals in the group have to sort the order out. Supportive behaviour in groups requires that people do not speak until others are ready to listen. Meshing or turn-taking is an important feature of a group that is working well.

| **Try it out** | In a group of five or six people, take four matchsticks each and agree on a topic for group discussion. Next, agree the following rules for the discussion. Only one person may speak at a time. Whenever that person speaks he or she must place a matchstick on the floor. When people run out of matchsticks they cannot say anything. No one may say anything unless others have finished. Non-verbal communication is allowed. People should not speak for more than one minute.<br><br>This exercise should emphasise the importance of turn-taking and the non-verbal messages that might help it. |
|---|---|

In the matchstick game above you will find that conversation becomes difficult. Sometimes people discover that they have forgotten what they wanted to say by the time they have put down their matchstick. This is because we often join in with the conversation in a group whenever we feel like it. We respond to what other people have said, but we have not thought out our own ideas to the point of being able to say them clearly. If the group goes quiet and people look at us, we forget what we were going to say!

## Getting care groups to work

Most care groups have a purpose or task to work on. Children get together to play games, adults may get together in recreational groups. Groups often need a focus – a game to play, an activity to join in or a topic to discuss. Consider the following observations on group behaviour.

1 If individuals are going to join in a supportive group meeting, then someone will need to introduce the activity and start the conversation. From time to time, when the conversation wanders, someone will need to steer it back to the right topic.

2 Occasionally group members will need to clarify, or make sense of, what is being said.

3 Throughout the group meeting people will need to exchange ideas on the activity or topic being discussed.

4 Towards the end of a meeting, group members will need to agree on what has happened or what the group has decided. The group will come to some kind of conclusions.

### Enhancing the group experience

As well as performing their tasks, groups have to be 'maintained'. Group maintenance consists of encouraging a sense of belonging and keeping the whole meeting enjoyable. The following are some behaviours to maintain and enhance group discussion in a caring setting.

- laughter can help to relieve tension and create a warm, friendly feeling that everyone can join in
- show interest in the people in the group – learn about the 'identity' of group members
- be 'warm' and show respect and value when listening to people who are different from yourself or who have had different life experiences. This behaviour makes it safe to be in the group
- express feelings honestly and with sincerity. This will help others to understand your identity. Help others to understand you as well as trying to understand others
- take responsibility for everyone having a chance to speak and contribute. Some people may need to be encouraged or invited to speak, some people may need organising, so that turn-taking works!
- if necessary, get people to explain what they have said, and to talk through disagreements. Group members need to feel that their shared values will make it possible to arrive at solutions when people disagree.

A group leader must keep reflecting on what is happening in the group. Does the group need to come back to the task? Is this the right time for a funny story? Should I make it clear that I am listening and that I value what is being said by this person? Every other group member who really wants the group to work will also monitor how the group is getting on with its task.

Remember:

1 Groups often need to keep working on a task.

2 Keep a sense of belonging going.

3 Make sure each individual is supported and valued.

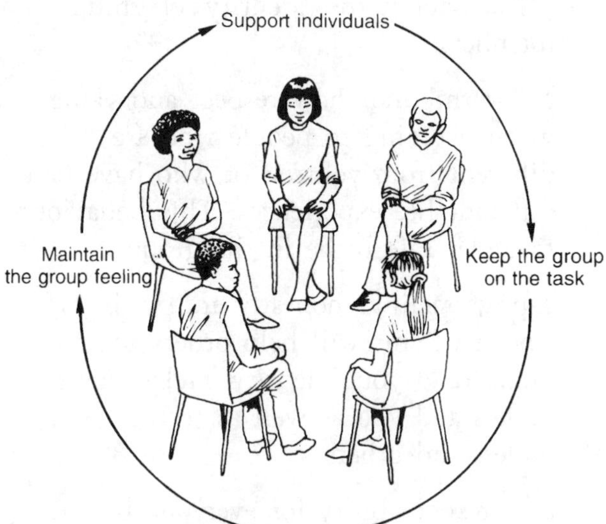


**Figure 2.22 The dynamics of a care group**

## Participation patterns

Whether a group is working effectively or whether there are problems may become clearer if the participation pattern of people in the group is observed. The participation pattern for a group records how communication works between people; for instance, the group may have a leader who delivers one-way communication to others

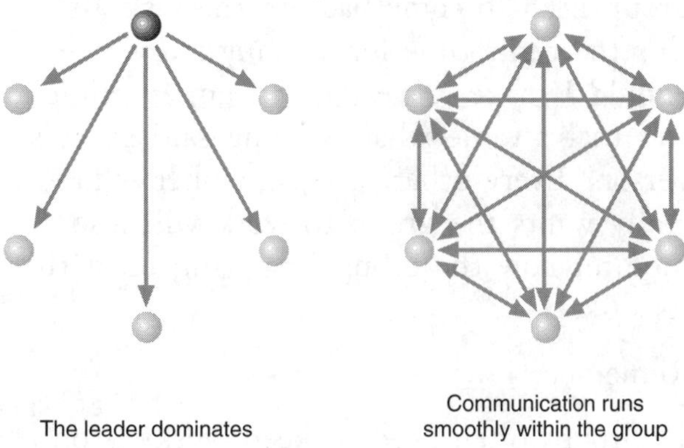


**Figure 2.23 Two patterns of participation**

for much of the meeting. This pattern may suggest that the group is not ready or able to work independently. A working group is more likely to have a general participation pattern where everyone interacts with and includes everyone else.

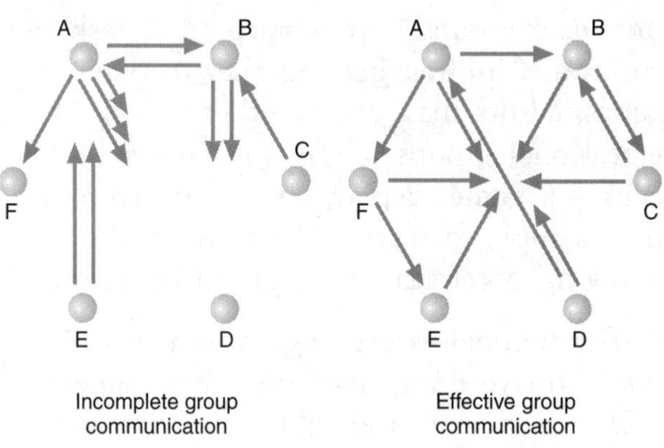


**Figure 2.24 Group participation**

One way of working out a participation pattern is to keep a record of who is talking and who is responding to them. The two diagrams above record the major statements made by people and who they were aimed at over a ten-minute period.

In Figure 2.24, the arrows which stop in the middle symbolise communication to the group as a whole, with no eye contact or speech focused on a single individual. Arrows which go to an individual symbolise communication with that person directly. The effective group contains a mixture of general communication to the group and some communication between individuals. What makes this pattern look effective is that everyone is involved with communicating within the group.

The incomplete group communication diagram shows that D was excluded from communication, C only communicated with B, and only A and B communicated to the whole group. The reason for this pattern was that A and B were contesting with each other for control of the group which was at the 'storming stage' of development.

> **Think it over**
>
> What would happen if you drew a participation pattern for a group that you were involved in? How would your own 'lines of communication' with others look?

## Group values

Effective group participation patterns are most likely to be found in groups which share the same norms and values. In care work the 'value base' of valuing equality and diversity, promoting the rights, responsibility and right to confidentiality of others, should provide a basis for groups to develop their 'ground rules' or norms around.

In practice, sharing the care value base is likely to mean that group members will encourage one another to speak; after all, everyone has an equal right to speak out and be included in the group. Group members will try to understand and value differences between people. This means that people will show respect and value for one another. Group members may also be concerned to develop their skills and make contributions to discussions which help the group to work effectively.

### Inhibiting group interaction

If people do not share caring values then it is quite likely that some people may try to dominate the group. Sometimes people 'pair' with others who think the same way, to fight for control of a group. People can block the progress of a discussion with irrelevant or other deliberate distractions aimed at disrupting a discussion. Sometimes people may become withdrawn and ignore the group if they don't feel they belong. Groups have to develop shared beliefs and a feeling of 'belonging' if they are to work effectively.

Some group situations are easier to communicate in than others. If you mix with people who share the same beliefs and values it may be easy to work with them. Valuing diversity involves learning about differences in other people. It can sometimes be easier to use one-to-one communication to learn about others than to try to do this in a group discussion. The communication cycle works more easily between two people than within a group.

Group discussion such as at a case conference can sometimes be difficult for individuals. Some reasons for finding discussion difficult are listed below:

- not knowing the beliefs and values of the others
- not understanding the purpose of a meeting
- feeling different from others in the group
- not feeling confident of communication skills
- feeling threatened by other members (perhaps they may stereotype or label you)
- feeling powerless and believing that others control the group.

> **Think it over**
>
> This chapter starts with the stories of Leona and Arata, who both have to experience difficult group discussions. What help will they each need in order to cope with a case conference or a group where their ideas may not be accepted?

Care workers often need to take a leadership role with groups in order to protect people who feel threatened or vulnerable within a group. Being a leader means taking the initiative to start the work of the group and also focusing the group on the values and beliefs which will enable it to work effectively. Professional carers will make special efforts to welcome people into group discussion and will try to make sure that others do not experience discrimination or exclusion when they are in a group. The care value base should guide the behaviour of health and care staff whenever groups meet.

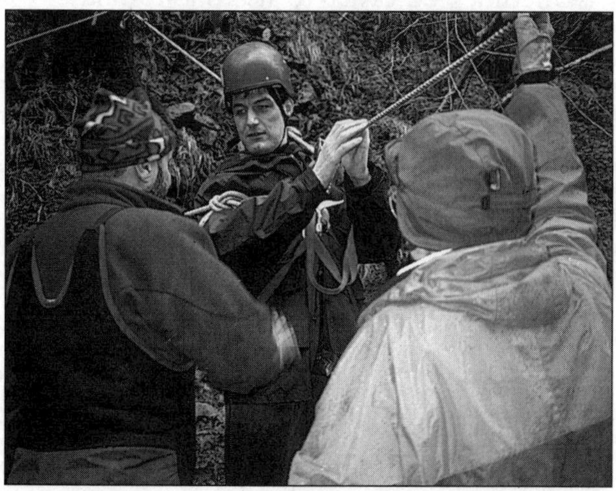

Being a leader means taking the initiative

## Observing and evaluating group behaviour

A theorist called Bales put forward the idea of classifying the behaviour of people in groups. Bales (1970) suggested that observers could understand and analyse what was happening in a group by using an interaction analysis of individual members' behaviour. An interaction analysis involves classifying the way people behave using defined categories. Bales' categories are outlined below.

Using categories can be a useful way of getting insight into how an individual is influencing the work and the emotional maintenance (or feeling) involved in group communication. Studying individual communication may take a lot of time however. It is also possible to design a grid which can be used minute by minute to try to categorise the task and maintenance behaviours occurring in groups. An example relevant to the standards in this unit is offered in Figure 2.25.

Table 2.2 Bale's categories of behaviour classification

| | |
|---|---|
| **Group Task** | **Gives suggestion (including taking the lead)**<br>Gives opinion (including feelings and wishes)<br>Gives information (including clarifying and confirming)<br>Asks for information<br>Asks for opinion<br>Asks for suggestion |
| **Group Maintenance**<br>(called 'Social-emotional Area' by Bales) | Seems friendly<br>Dramatises<br>Agrees<br>Disagrees<br>Shows tension<br>Seems unfriendly |

| | Behaviour seen in each individual | | | | | | | | | |
|---|---|---|---|---|---|---|---|---|---|---|
| | 1 | 2 | 3 | 4 | 5 | 6 | 7 | 8 | 9 | 10 |
| **Group task:** | | | | | | | | | | |
| Starting discussion | | | | | | | | | | |
| Giving information | | | | | | | | | | |
| Asking for information | | | | | | | | | | |
| Clarifying discussion | | | | | | | | | | |
| Summarising discussion | | | | | | | | | | |
| **Group maintainance:** | | | | | | | | | | |
| Humour | | | | | | | | | | |
| Expressing group feelings | | | | | | | | | | |
| Including other people in discussion | | | | | | | | | | |
| Being supportive (using supportive skills) | | | | | | | | | | |
| **Behaviour which blocks group communication:** | | | | | | | | | | |
| Excluding others | | | | | | | | | | |
| Withdrawing | | | | | | | | | | |
| Aggression | | | | | | | | | | |
| Distracting or blocking discussion | | | | | | | | | | |
| Attention seeking and dominating discussion | | | | | | | | | | |

**Figure 2.25 A profile to monitor group behaviour**

## Planning, managing and concluding a group activity

Successful group activities require careful planning and management. Consider Alesha's experience here.

Alesha wants to involve a small group of adults who have learning disabilities in a cookery class. The idea is not to train the group to make cakes, but to provide an enjoyable social experience which the group could join in with and maintain their social skills. Before she could start, Alesha would need to plan. She would need to plan what ingredients to buy, and her own preparation of the ingredients, before the session began. She would also need to organise the use of an oven for baking cakes, etc.

As well as this, Alesha would need to plan how to support the group. Who does or doesn't get on with others? Who might be

**Try it out** Another idea for studying group behaviour is to use the fish-bowl method of observation.

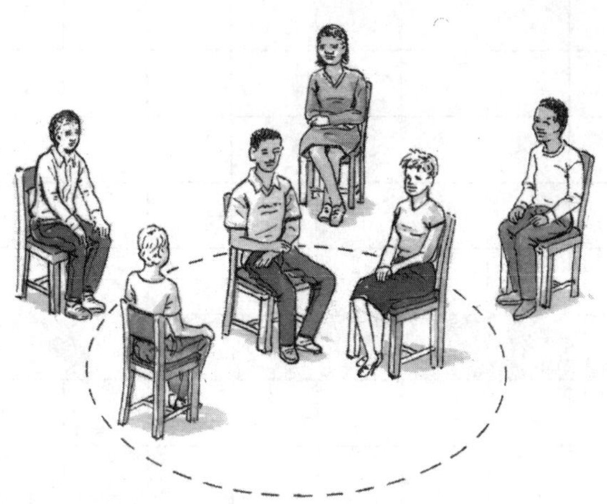

Figure 2.26 The fish-bowl method

The people in the middle are being watched – they probably feel like goldfish in a bowl! They will need to trust you if the observation is going to work. They discuss something important while you sit on the outside to listen and watch. What will you monitor? A wide range of things can be monitored, but to start with you might like to watch:

1 Non-verbal messages – how do people organise the turn-taking? How does eye-contact work?

2 Questions – how good are people at asking other people for their ideas?

3 Giving opinions – do people ask one another for their views and share ideas?

4 The pace of conversation – how do people speak? Are there any silences?

After five minutes or so of listening and watching, the group should stop and people should share what happened. Did the people in the group remember what the people outside saw and heard? After discussing the monitoring, the group on the inside of the fish-bowl should change places with the observers.

able to help with tasks? How could she interest and motivate everyone? How would she keep the atmosphere enjoyable? All this planning would depend on Alesha's ability to use her imagination, perhaps to picture the group and work out how to organise the session.

Alesha would need to ensure that the tasks were enjoyable and appropriate to each individual. Before moving on to do the activity, she could also get feedback on the plans from a senior member of staff – just to check that the activities were appropriate.

Doing the session would not necessarily be straightforward. Alesha would need to monitor how the session was going: did the verbal and non-verbal messages from her group suggest that they were enjoying themselves? Alesha would need feedback, so she could ask the group members what they thought. Another member of staff might help her by joining in and providing feedback. While leading the cookery session Alesha would also be observing or taking in what is happening.

After the session is over Alesha would need to evaluate what had happened. Evaluation would depend on imagination. The evaluation would enable Alesha to make recommendations to improve her work in the future by thinking her work over before, during and after the cookery session. Alesha is thus able to develop her own self-awareness and sense of skill.

A process of planning, doing and reviewing may enable individuals to understand how their own skills influence others. The ability to imagine and understand how an individual's behaviour will influence outcomes lies at the heart of getting a group activity to work.

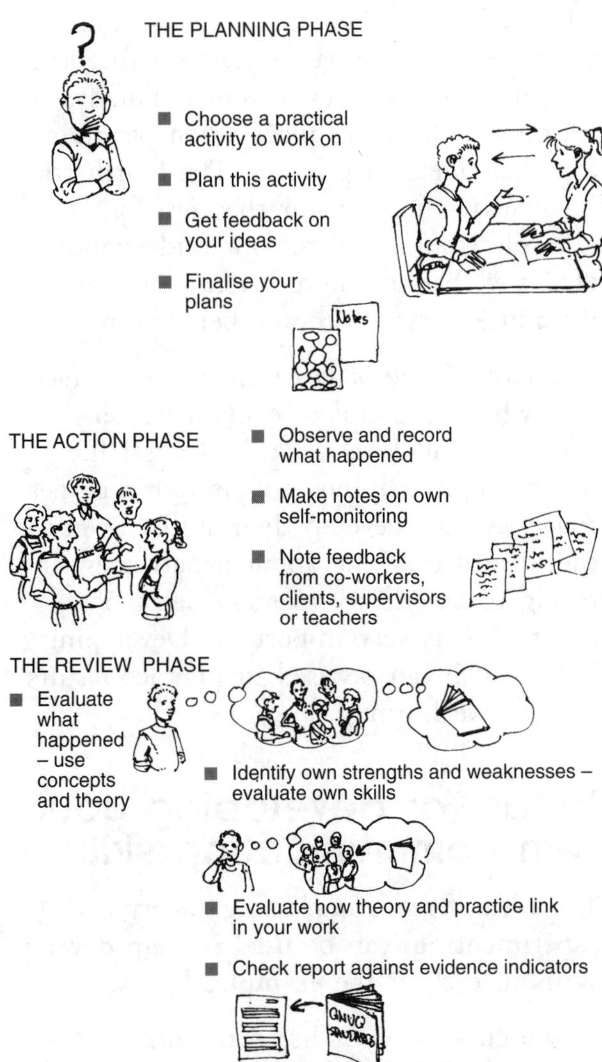


**Figure 2.27 Three phases in getting an activity to work**

## 2.4 Evaluating communication skills

Few people develop effective communication skills just by reading about them. There are three main ways that people learn to develop skills.

1 Trial and error. Experience of communication provides opportunities to improve skills by remembering techniques that seem to work and not repeating behaviours that don't seem to work. The problems with the trial and error method include:

- it is not appropriate to try ideas out on vulnerable people.
- trial and error often doesn't work when complex skills are involved.

2 Watching others and copying their behaviour. Watching examples of skilled communication provides us with ideas that we can use.

3 Learning to evaluate our own behaviour. Evaluation involves self-assessment and thinking through ways to develop skills.

Professional carers, such as nurses and social workers, are trained to develop evaluation skills because self-assessment may help them to continuously develop and improve their skills. Some theorists, such as Kurt Lewin and David Kolb, have tried to explain the steps that might be involved in evaluating personal practice. Over 50 years ago Kurt Lewin suggested that practical learning might involve a four-stage process of **planning, acting, observing** and

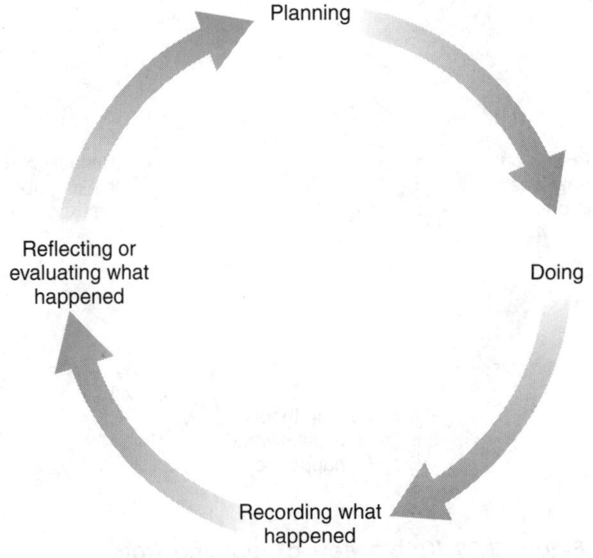


**Figure 2.28 The practical learning process**

**reflecting.** Planning involves imagination and working out what needs to be done. Acting means *doing* – trying something out. Observing means taking note of what happened – perhaps getting feedback from others. Reflecting means using imagination to think something through.

David Kolb (1984) developed Lewin's ideas and put forward a slightly different four-stage explanation of learning from experience. In 'Kolb's Cycle' learning can be seen as developing from experience. We have an experience of communicating – perhaps we are introducing ourselves to a client. If practical experience is to result in learning, then an individual will need to reflect on, or evaluate that experience. Reflection involves thinking through what happened; did the conversation go well, did the other person trust me? The third stage is to make up theories which explain why things worked or didn't work. This is where textbook theory can be useful. Theory can help to explain events and to predict what will work. Perhaps a conversation went well because we understood the other person's non-verbal expressions? Finally, learning really takes place when people try out their ideas in practice. The fourth stage involves testing out our theories; for example thinking about our understanding of non-verbal communication as we introduce ourselves to another person.

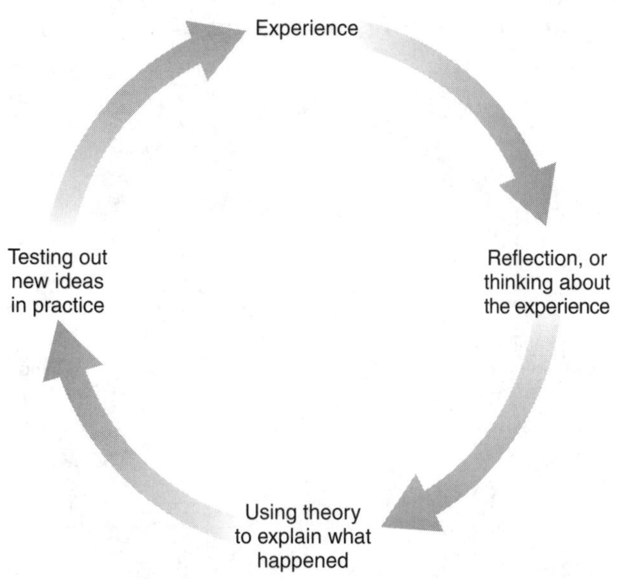


**Figure 2.29 Kolb's view of learning from experience involves the four stages described above**

The Kolb Cycle of Learning is an abstract idea which is useful to explain how a person might develop skills. In real life many people may not go through four neat stages as they develop their skills. Even so, the idea of thinking about experiences, and trying to use theory to make sense of experience, is very important. Developing ideas which can be used in practice results in effective learning.

## Ideas for developing your own communication skills

The idea of reflecting, using theory and experimenting, can be used to help develop skills in each of the examples below.

- Watch a video or listen to audio recordings of professional communication and think about what you have seen. Discuss the skills you have seen with others – try to explain what is happening. Try to practise important skills in a follow-up role-play.
- Ask friends or colleagues to observe your skills with others, i.e. use **peer assessment.** Listen to their ideas on what was effective and how your skills could be improved. Think about their ideas and use concepts discussed in this chapter to plan how you could improve your skills. Use your new ideas in a future conversation.

- Watch a video or listen to an audio recording of yourself. Use **self-assessment** to analyse your behaviour using the concepts explained in this chapter. Plan ways of improving your effectiveness and try these new ideas out in an appropriate conversation.
- Try to think about the effect your verbal and non-verbal behaviour has on others while you are talking and listening. When you have a 'free moment' think back on what happened. Try to explain your thoughts using the concepts in this chapter. Work out other ways you could have behaved. Try to use new ideas in future conversations.

Developing skills involves more than just having some experience and more than just knowing some theory. Experience and theory have to be linked together for learning to work. The following process based on Lewin's and Kolb's ideas may explain the idea of linking theory and practice.

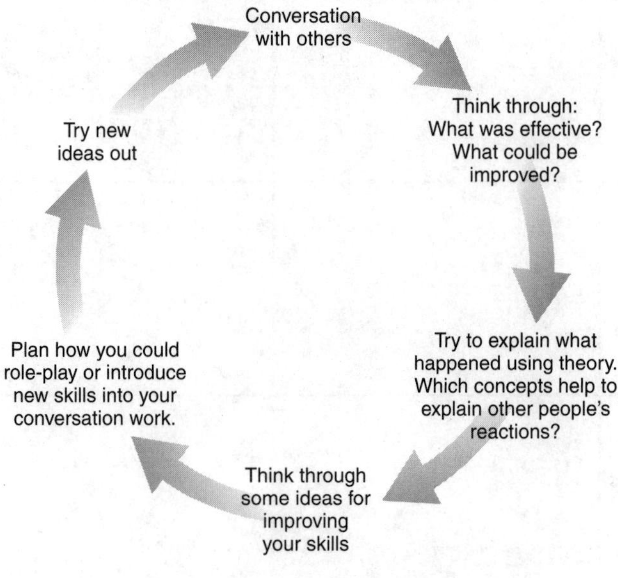


**Figure 2.30 Linking theory and practice to develop learning**

In order to evaluate your own communication skills it can be useful to think through the detail of your own performance. Key concepts to check are listed in Table 2.3 which follows. When you watch real or videotaped communication you could look for evidence of effective behaviour under each of these headings. When judging effectiveness you should think about the purpose of the communication and the responses of other people involved. Effective communication in care contexts will result in other people understanding the communication and also feeling valued and respected. Some conversations involve the need to create emotional safety. People who feel emotionally safe will probably respond by behaving in an understanding, warm and sincere manner.

You might like to use a rating scale to help evaluate the use of the skills areas below. A possible scale might be:

1 = Very effective and appropriate use of the skill

2 = Some appropriate use of the skill

3 = Area not applicable or relevant

4 = Some ineffective or inappropriate behaviour

5 = General inappropriate or ineffective behaviour

| | Rating scale<br>Mark 1, 2, 3, 4 or 5 | Evidence seen |
|---|---|---|
| **Non-verbal communication**<br>Eye contact<br>Facial expression<br>Angle of head<br>Tone of voice<br>Position of hands and arms<br>Gestures<br>Posture<br>Muscle tension<br>Touch<br>Proximity<br>Dress and appearance | | |
| **Verbal communication: listening skills**<br>Encouragement<br>Reflection<br>Use of prompts<br>Conversational skills<br>Questioning<br>Use of silence<br>Clarity<br>Pace of conversation<br>Turn taking | | |
| **Creating emotional safety**<br>Understanding<br>Warmth<br>Sincerity<br>Appropriate responsiveness and calmness | | |
| **Attention to values**<br>Rapport<br>Respect for diversity in others<br>Appropriate choice of language<br>Understanding the influence of culture and gender on communication | | |
| **The quality of the environment for communication**<br>Physical barriers to communication<br>Privacy<br>Maintaining confidentiality | | |

Table 2.3 Analysing communication

## 2.5 Maintaining client confidentiality

Confidentiality is an important right for all clients. It is important because:

- clients may not trust a carer if the carer does not keep information confidential
- clients may not feel valued or able to keep their self-esteem if their private details are shared with others
- clients' safety may be put at risk if details of their property or their habits are widely known
- a professional service that maintains respect for individuals must keep private information confidential
- there are legal requirements to keep personal records confidential.

**Trust** is important. If you know that your carer won't pass things on, you may feel able to tell him or her what you really think and feel.

**Self-esteem** is involved, because if your carer promises to keep things confidential, it shows that he or she respects and values you; it shows that you matter.

**Safety** is an issue, because you may have to leave your home empty at times. If people know where you keep your money and when you are out, someone may be tempted to break in. Carers need to keep personal details confidential to protect clients' property and personal safety.

Medical practitioners and lawyers have always strictly observed confidentiality as part of their professional role. If clients are to receive a professional service, care workers must copy this example.

### The legal context of confidentiality

Confidentiality is a basic human right, and it is so important that it has become a specific issue in the value base for care. The Data Protection Acts 1984 and 1998, the Access to Personal Files Act 1987 and the Access to Health Records Act 1990, make it a legal requirement that Health and Social Care agencies keep client details confidential.

A new Data Protection Act was passed in 1998, this Act updates the law on confidentiality of information. All records about clients which are filed will be seen as data, whether they are held electronically or on paper.

The 1998 Act provides individuals with a range of rights including:

- the right to know what information is held and to see and correct the information if necessary
- the right to refuse to provide information
- the right that data should be accurate and up-to-date
- the right that information should not be kept for longer than necessary
- the right to confidentiality – that the information should not be accessible to unauthorised people.

### Clients' wishes

It is important to know what a client wants to be kept confidential. Clients may not wish their relatives and friends to know about their finances or their medical details, or to know about their day-to-day domestic details. Wherever possible, care workers should discuss what they can and cannot pass on to other people. Sometimes a resident in care or a patient in hospital might want to talk to their relatives directly rather than have a care worker or nurse talk to them.

It is important to know a client's wishes and not simply to answer any question that is put to you.

Information should only be given to people who have a 'need to know'. Colleagues, supervisors and managers may need to know what has happened with individual clients. Otherwise, carers should maintain a client's confidentiality when talking to other people such as neighbours, unless the client has given them permission to speak. Carers have to be careful what they say and to whom they say it.

## Security of information

Carers have to answer phone calls and meet strangers who ask for information. Unless you are sure about a person's identity, never pass on confidential details such as a client's address. If pressed, explain that it is your policy (or the organisation's policy) not to give confidential information.

For example, you might receive a phone call from a social worker requesting information. If you do not know the social worker, you should always say that you will phone him or her back at the office with the information. That way you can check the caller is genuine. You cannot be sure of identification over the phone. Your caller could be lying.

Equally, if a visitor came into the building and made enquiries about a client, it would be vital that you had proof of his or her identity and that you were sure the person had a right and need to know before you disclosed anything about your client. If in doubt, you could ask the visitor to meet the client or to speak to the manager.

Written and computer-based records should also be kept in a secure place where they cannot be read by unauthorised people. This usually means in a locked office or locked cupboard, or an electronic system protected by a password.

## The boundaries of confidentiality

It is not always easy to work out the boundaries of confidentiality.

### Think it over

You are working with older people in a rest home. You have built a relationship with one of the residents who likes and trusts you. One evening he says, 'I can trust you can't I? If I tell you a secret, you will keep it confidential, won't you? Only I've been saving all my tablets – I've got these pains and I don't want to go on. When the time is right, I'm going to take all of the tablets and kill myself. I wanted you to know why I'm going to do it'.

Would you follow the value of confidentiality unquestioningly and keep the resident's secret? Would you let him commit suicide, or would you decide it was right to break confidentiality?

In the case of a potential suicide, the answer is that confidentiality should be broken. The manager of the home needs to know about the tablets. The reason is that confidentiality has a limit or a boundary to it. If you are told that someone may do harm to themselves or to others, then this information lies outside of the boundary of confidentiality. The carer's role means that they must report the danger.

Carers have a duty to protect the health and well-being of clients. This responsibility can conflict with the need to keep things confidential, but the duty to protect the client's life is more important than the general principle of maintaining confidentiality.

Another reason for breaking confidentiality is that carers have rights too. How would you feel if a resident put you in the situation where you knew he or she intended to commit suicide, but then tried to make you powerless to do anything? Is this fair on you? You might also be at risk professionally – you might lose your job, or fail to get a good reference if you do not protect the health and safety of clients. You have a right to protect yourself, and this right has to be considered when making decisions with respect to the boundaries of confidentiality.

### The right not to know!

Sometimes a client might start to tell you about a particular worry, for example, that he or she gets picked on or about a serious family problem. You realise that you may have to pass on the information. Rather than listening to the details and then worrying about confidentiality, you could decide to raise the issue with the client: 'Well, look, this sounds as if your social worker should know about it. I think you should tell him, but if you tell me all about it, I may not be able to keep it confidential. Are you sure you want to tell me the details?' In a situation like this, the client can decide to tell you everything knowing that it may not be kept confidential. Or he or she may prefer that the situation should be kept confidential, and therefore stop the conversation.

## Dilemmas

Sometimes the issue of confidentiality is not straightforward. Consider the problems raised below.

### Think it over

1 Suppose you work with an older person who tells you, 'My son-in-law takes my pension every week, but don't tell anyone. He might stop my daughter from visiting me and I couldn't bear that.'

You need to ask yourself whether there is a risk of harm to the older person or to others. You might decide that the older person is at risk – she is being financially abused. The older person is vulnerable to her son-in-law's behaviour and the situation would need careful handling. You would have to be very careful who you spoke to about this problem. Your manager might be the only person you could share the information with.

2 Suppose a young child tells you that his adult brother may have stolen some money. Is there a risk of harm to the child or others?

There does not seem to be a risk for the child or any obvious risk of future harm to others. The information you have been given may not even be correct. Unless you have more information, it may be best not to repeat stories that you hear from clients.

3 Suppose an adult tells you that she is seriously worried about her marriage and thinks she may have to get a divorce.

Is there a risk of harm to the adult or others? Again, there is no risk – the adult may become very upset later, but the information should be kept confidential.

4 Suppose a patient in hospital tells you that he is in severe pain, but that he wants you not to let anyone know.

Is there a risk of harm to the patient or to others? There might be. The pain could be a sign that some serious problem is developing, or it might just be in the client's mind. This is a difficult situation.

We can usually work out what to do when issues are straightforward. Very often, however, real-life problems are not simple or straightforward. Even the examples above become less clear cut if more detail is added to them. For example:

1 The older person lives with her son-in-law and her allegation cannot be proved.

2 The police have just interviewed you about thefts which are associated with assaults in the area.

3 The adult tells you that she feels suicidal.

When situations are not straightforward, it is important to explore them with colleagues and managers. In order to avoid breaking confidentiality, you might be able to describe a situation without actually identifying a client.

Decisions about confidentiality can be very complex – the important thing to understand is that the care role has boundaries and that not all information can be kept confidential.

## Ensuring confidentiality

Every care setting will have its own policies and procedures which are aimed at preventing mistakes when it comes to confidentiality. For example, some conversations should only take place in rooms where no one can overhear them. There should be a range of security measures to make sure information stays confidential and does not become lost or inappropriately altered. See Unit 6 page 486 for information on the Data Protection Act.

**Manual records** should be:

- kept in a locked room or a locked cupboard to which only authorised staff have access
- kept in a particular secure room or area, to avoid the risk of their being lost or left where others might see them
- filed using a system such as an alphabetical one so that they can be found easily
- included in a policy as to who should update or change details.

(It may also be good practice to record the initials of the person who made the records and the date of any changes.)

Where **electronic records** are involved there should be:

- a back-up copy in case the original is lost or damaged
- a password security check to ensure that only appropriate staff have access
- a policy on the printing of details so that hard copies do not get lost, or seen by others
- a policy on who is authorised to update or change records. The recording system must prevent information being altered or lost by accident
- a system for printing out faxed documents in an appropriate confidential area and a system to prevent inappropriate people having access to confidential material
- a procedure for checking fax numbers before they are transmitted.

# Unit 2 Assessment

You will need to produce a report which explores your own communication skills in a health, social care or early years setting. This report might be based on work you have done in a placement, or perhaps on discussions you have had during visits to care settings. You will also need to produce records of effective communication in:

- one-to-one interactions with a client.
- one group interaction with clients who are different from the clients you communicated with in the one-to-one interactions.

The report must review the communication skills you demonstrated in your interactions. You might like to use the rating scale on page 116 to help you with the individual one-to-one task. You might like to use this rating scale and the group observation profile (Figure 2.25) to help you review your group communication skills.

## Influences and barriers

The report must also explain the context of the interactions and other factors which influenced communication. You need to explain how you avoided barriers which might block communication. Figures 2.17 and 2.18 might provide a useful starting point to help plan your writing on these issues. It might also be useful to re-read the sections on barriers to communication, group formation and patterns of communication (Figures 2.21, 2.23 and 2.24).

## Valuing people

Your report must explain how effective communication can contribute towards valuing people as individuals. Before writing this section it may be important to re-read the section on culture, empowerment and emotional work. Figure 2.17 may also provide a useful starting point to help with this section.

## Confidentiality

Your report must explain how client confidentiality can be maintained. While on visits or on placements you may have noticed how conversations take place and how records are kept. Thinking about the settings that staff–client conversations took place in, were they confidential? Use the points raised on pages 00 and 00 in order to assess the security of confidential information.

## For a C grade

You need to complete the tasks above but in addition you must also:

1 Develop your report on your communication skills so that it provides evidence of the ability to analyse issues. You need to produce a review of the effectiveness of your interaction skills. This review must explain how you may have improved your interaction skills. To achieve this you might like to rate how your skills were before you studied for this unit and how your skills have developed through study and practical work since then. Use the section on evaluating communication skills and perhaps the rating scale on page 116 to help you review your own effectiveness.

2 Your report on 'valuing people as individuals' must include an analysis of the implications of inappropriate communication for the health and well-being of clients in a chosen care setting. Figure 2.18 provides an overview of inappropriate communication. This diagram may provide a starting point to

help explain how poor communication could result in a loss of self-esteem, a loss of purpose, a loss of support, threat or even learned helplessness. You may choose to explain how poor communication could lead to unmet needs as set out in Figure 2.1. You may want to make links with the issue of clients' rights and care values as explained in Unit 1. Poor communication and insensitivity to others may result in discrimination and abuse. At C grade you need to make links between care workers' behaviour and important areas of theory.

## For an A grade

At this grade you will need to complete the tasks and the analyses that are required for the lower grades and you will also need to evaluate your experience as follows:

3 Your report on communication skills must provide a detailed and in-depth evaluation of your practical work. Your report will demonstrate that you have been able to both understand and use a wide range of theory on verbal and non-verbal communication together with other ideas contained in this chapter. At this level it is not enough to just describe ideas, you must show that you can really use theory in practical work with other people. You could do this by describing the way individuals or groups behaved and then explaining and evaluating behaviour using your knowledge.

4 Your report on communication skills should also provide a realistic action plan for improving your group and one-to-one communication skills. Some people like to use official-looking action plan forms to help with planning. If you do choose to develop a 'form' you could base it on the rating scale set out on page 116. You also need to explain how this form is really going to help you to develop. At A grade level it will be important to use the theory of learning cycles (see Figures 2.29 and 2.30) to help you explain how you can plan your own development. You should also use the ideas of watching, discussing and peer and self-assessment to help you design a plan which is worth an A grade.

5 Your section on valuing people should include your evaluation of the extent to which appropriate communication skills are demonstrated in a chosen care setting. You must make realistic recommendations for improving your interactions. At A grade level you must be careful to provide evidence and give reasons as to why communication was effective or ineffective on given occasions that you observed. It is not good enough just to have an opinion. You must justify your opinions by explaining how certain interactions met people's needs or failed to meet people's needs. You must explain how communication met emotional and social needs or else failed to meet them. You should report your observation of clients' reactions as this may give you the evidence you need to justify the statements that you make.

Recommendations may include the need for more training or supervision. If you make these recommendations be careful to explain in detail what is needed. You may believe that people need training in supportive skills, or in recognising barriers to communication, or in being sensitive to cultural needs. If more time is needed to work with people you need to explain what skills could be used if staff had more time. At A grade it is important to provide a detailed evaluation of issues in order to prove that you understand theory and that you have spent time thinking about how it could work in practice.

# Unit 2 Test

Check your knowledge of theory using the following test.

Read the short conversation set out below between a nurse and patient in a hospital setting and then answer the questions which follow.

| | |
|---|---|
| Nurse: | Hello, how are you this morning? |
| Patient: | I'm not feeling well, I've got pain in my back. |
| Nurse: | Did your relatives visit yesterday? |
| Patient: | Er, no I haven't seen them. |
| Nurse: | I've just got to check your chart now. |
| Patient: | Can you do something for my pain please? |
| Nurse: | I'll ask the doctor later. |
| Patient: | But I asked for something yesterday and never saw the doctor. |
| Nurse: | Well they are all very busy you know. |
| Patient: | But that is no use to me is it, can't you do something now? |
| Nurse: | Don't get worked up now. I'll see what I can do but we are all very busy you know! |

## Questions

1 Identify some of the inhibiting factors which may prevent this conversation from meeting the client's needs.

2 List three types or levels of need that the patient may have had in a hospital setting.

3 Why are closed questions often inappropriate in caring conversations?

4 Identify one barrier to effective communication in the conversation above.

5 Name two consequences that may follow for the patient if they are constantly treated the same way as in this conversation and they are in hospital for a length of time.

6 Explain the difference between listening and just hearing.

7 List three important qualities that a supportive conversation should include.

8 If a group of people is to work effectively for a reasonable period of time name two key aspects of group interpersonal communication that you would be able to observe between members.

9 List at least four barriers which could inhibit communication in a group context.

10 List three reasons why it is important to maintain confidentiality in health or social settings.

## Answers

1 Inhibiting factors include:

- Short closed questions, a lack of supportive behaviour, including no attempt to build an understanding, and a lack of warmth ('I'll see the doctor later').
- No effective use of a communication cycle, including checking understanding.
- Little evidence of listening skills – the patient's statements about pain are not responded to.

- Possible aggressive responses such as 'don't get worked up now'.
- Being unresponsive to client needs.

2 **a** Physical needs including pain.
**b** Safety needs such as 'Why am I in pain, how serious is this, what will happen'.
**c** Emotional needs, including the need to feel a sense that other people do care about what happens, and a sense of belonging.
**d** Self-esteem needs – being important enough to be taken seriously and not ignored.

3 Closed questions do not help to keep a conversation going. Closed questions often fail to convey warmth or be supportive, and may block conversation.

4 Emotional barriers – the nurse may have wanted to stay detached from the needs of the patient.

5 Unmet physical need – the person stays in pain.

- Unmet safety and emotional needs involving loss of self-esteem, insecurity, feeling threatened.
- Learned helplessness – learning to withdraw and giving up trying to influence others' behaviour.
- Depression – due to loss of control or lowered self-esteem.

6 Listening involves a communication cycle where the listener checks their understanding with the speaker and reflects back what they have heard. Listening is an active process or skill, which contributes to understanding. Hearing involves just receiving sound or information. It is possible to hear what a person says without indicating that you were listening or that you want to understand what another person is saying.

7 A supportive conversation should convey understanding, warmth and sincerity.

8 Group communication would involve keeping people working on the **task** and meeting social and emotional needs through group **maintenance** behaviours.

9 Barriers include:

- Group interaction patterns may exclude individuals.
- Emotional barriers such as not wanting to understand.
- Labelling, stereotyping and prejudice.
- Language barriers including jargon.
- Not following non-verbal systems, such as not knowing when to speak.
- Physical disabilities which are not responded to – such as hearing or visual disabilities.
- Poor listening skills.

10 Confidentiality is important because:

- It maintains a sense of trust.
- It may help to preserve a client's self-esteem.
- It helps to meet physical and emotional safety needs.
- Professional services have to be confidential to be professional.
- Confidentiality is a legal requirement.

# References and recommended further reading

Bales, R. (1970) *Personality and interpersonal behaviour* Holt, Rinehart & Winston

Johnson D. and Johnson F. (1997) *Joining together: Group theory and group skills (6th edition)* Allyn & Bacon

Kolb, D. (1984) *Experiential learning: Experience as the source of learning and development* Prentice Hall

Maslow, A.H. (1970) *Motivation and personality* (2nd edition) Harper & Row

Rogers, C.R. (1951) *Client centred therapy* Houston

Tuckman, B. (1965) 'Development sequence in small groups' in *Psychological Bulletin*, Vol 63, No 6

Seligman, M. (1975) *Helplessness* W.H. Freeman and Co.

Smale, G. *et al*, (1993) *Empowerment, assessment, care management and the skilled worker* NISW: HMSO

Thompson N (1996) *People skills* Macmillan Press

# Fast Facts

**Advocacy** Arguing a case for another. In law an advocate argues a legal case for a client. In care work an advocate tries to understand and argue from a client's perspective. Advocates should be independent of care providers.

**Assertiveness** The skill of negotiating for your own needs whilst respecting the needs of others. Avoiding the tendency to 'fight or to run'. Clearly explaining your own case.

**Auditory** The form of communication taken in through the ears (hearing).

**Body language** This is the language of non-verbal communication, messages we send with the body. It consists of signs that other people can read in the way our body looks, or the way it moves. Non-verbal communication has a slightly wider meaning than body language. 'Non-verbal' covers everything which is not actual words (for example, tone of voice). Body language focuses on the way the body, face, eyes, hands etc. look and move.

**Body movements** The speed and type of people's movements can send a vast range of messages. We can interpret tension, anger, attraction, happiness and many other emotions by watching how people move their hands, eyes, head and body.

**Boundaries** A boundary may represent a line that you may go up to, but must not cross. Boundaries divide areas into different sections. In practical care work, boundaries define the limits of a carer's role.

**Buffering** Partners, friends and family may help to protect a person from the full stress of life changes and conflicts. Michael Argyle called this protection 'buffering'.

**Communication difficulties** Blocks or barriers which prevent communication. Examples might include blocks which prevent people from receiving a message, or making sense of a message or understanding a message.

**Communication Cycle** The process of building an understanding of what another person is communicating.

**Confidentiality** A care value and part of the NVQ value base. Confidentiality means keeping information that you have about others to yourself; only sharing it with individuals who have a 'need to know'.

**Culture** The customs and ways of thinking that people learn define their culture. It is the social learning that influences how people understand themselves, and so has a very important influence on how people explain their own individuality. Differences in culture lead to non-verbal messages being interpreted in different ways.

**Data Protection Acts 1984, 1998** Provide people with legal rights with respect to the confidentiality of information.

**Dependence** Having to rely on others in order to maintain physical, social or emotional well-being. People can also become dependent on drugs and aids to daily living.

**Devaluing** Stereotyping the views and beliefs of others as worthless or ridiculous. Devaluing a person's culture and beliefs can undermine his or her personal development.

**Discrimination** Treating a person or group in a different way from how others are treated. Discrimination can be either negative or positive; but when used on its own, the word usually refers to negative discrimination, which is to treat certain people less well than others.

**Distance** Distance is one of the things to look for when trying to interpret other people's non-verbal messages. Distance has no fixed meaning, but in some cultures, standing or sitting close can mean: affection or love, anger or aggression, fear, or difficulty in hearing one another. Standing or sitting back might mean feeling comfortable or feeling separate. The cultural setting and other communications help us to work out the best interpretation.

**Emotional support** A general term, used to include listening and conversational work, to support other people's individuality and self-esteem.

**Empowerment** Giving power to others. Using your situation to enable other people to make their own decisions and to control their own lives.

**Eye contact** This happens when people's eyes 'contact' each other and send non-verbal messages. Eye contact is important in both individual and group communication. Turn-taking in conversation often relies on eye contact. Messages of interest, attraction, affection, hostility and many other emotions can be sent by eye contact alone.

**Facial expression** The face is an important area of the body for sending non-verbal messages. Even line diagrams can convey instant meaning to people. Facial expression is often easier to control than our eyes. Much non-verbal communication using the face is conscious if not always deliberate. People think about their faces and control them.

**Feedback** Getting information from others which is 'fed' to you to help you learn, adjust and develop your skills.

**Funnelling** A system for organising questions so that closed or focussed questions always 'lead up to', using general open questions to prepare the respondent.

**Gaze** Allowing the eyes to meet with other people's eyes and exchange looks. Gaze is part of the non-verbal system of eye contact which is a central component of non-verbal communication.

**Gestures** These are non-verbal messages sent (mainly) with the arms, hands and fingers. Gestures are especially sensitive to cultural interpretation. A hand-signal can mean 'everything is fine' in one culture, and can be a serious insult in another.

**Groups** In social care a 'group of people' means people who feel that they belong together. They will share some common purpose, common culture, or common values.

**Group formation** Groups take time to build a sense of belonging. A collection of people will probably be very cautious at first. There is often tension until people feel that they belong – that they share common values.

Once people feel that they all belong together, the group may work well.

**Group maintenance** The social needs of group members when they are working. Maintenance activities create an appropriate social atmosphere to enable members to work effectively.

**Group task** The work or activities that a group of people have come together to do.

**Group values** These are shared beliefs which everyone agrees with or supports. Respect and value for other people's individuality, using supportive communication, preventing discrimination and encouraging choice and control in others are caring values.

**Independence** Freedom from dependence on others. The right to choose and control one's own lifestyle.

**Individuality** This is a general term covering the sense of self that people develop from culture, religion, gender, age, race, social circumstances and their own physical and intellectual nature. Individuality is everything that makes the individual special. Recognising individuality is a necessary starting point for creating equality or a feeling of being equal. Recognising individuality involves not making assumptions about people.

**Interest** Communicating interest is a step on the way to building an understanding of other people during conversation.

**Interpersonal interaction** Interpersonal interaction includes every type of communication between people.

**Labelling** Identifying individuals as members of a particular group, whether or not they see themselves as members. Labelling is linked to stereotyping, and people are expected to conform to the behaviour associated with the stereotype with which they have been labelled.

**Learned helplessness** The process of learning to give up and withdraw when a person comes to learn that they cannot control important life events.

**Learning** Any change in what you are capable of doing which is not due to impairment, growth or some other purely physical process.

**Listening skills** The ability to build an understanding of another person's views when expressed verbally. Listening skills may include reflective listening, questioning skills, ability to understand non-verbal behaviour, ability to show respect for others, use of silence and self-monitoring skills.

**Meshing** When the contributions to a conversation link in a smooth and effective way, they are said to mesh. They fit together like links in a 'wire mesh' fence.

**Mirroring** Not to be confused with reflecting. Mirroring is when a person copies another person's non-verbal messages. A person who is attracted to someone may copy his or her way of sitting or standing when talking. For example, a person may cross his or her legs if the other person has crossed legs. Successful mirroring sends the message: 'I like you'.

**Monitoring own behaviour** This is a really important skill for developing caring abilities. Monitoring involves reflecting on your own behaviour and on the reactions of other people. It involves thinking about what is happening within group or individual communication.

**Muscle tension** This is one type of non-verbal message. Tension can communicate messages about the other person's emotions, especially when linked with body posture. It is something else to look for when trying to understand other people.

**Non-verbal signals** Using our eyes, faces and bodies to send signals. Messages which do not involve words. Tone of voice is often regarded as non-verbal, because verbal relates only to the words used in a message.

**Observational skills** Observation of others will involve trying to understand their appearance, verbal and non-verbal communication. Observational skills may imply the ability to monitor own and others' behaviour.

**Orientation** Organising your own or others' positions in the space available. The way people face or look when communicating. (Orientation relates to direction.)

**Pace of communication** The speed of a person's conversation. Speech that is too fast or too slow can be hard to understand. Some people may require you to speak more slowly than normal so that they can understand your everyday speech.

**Participation patterns** Ways of recording interaction within a group.

**Peer assessment** Being assessed by people in the same situation as yourself – other students assessing you, or other work colleagues.

**Personal space** This is an area of space which an individual tries to keep other people out of. It can be seen as the distance between people when they communicate with one another. Like many non-verbal messages, distance is used in different ways by different cultures. How closely people stand will depend on their culture, their feelings for one another and the physical and social situation.

**Pitch** The degree of high or low tone in someone's voice. A high-pitched voice is used in baby talk.

**Posture** This is the way a person positions his or her body. Posture usually sends messages about the individual's degree of tension or relaxation. It can also send all sorts of social messages, such as 'I'm really interested', 'I don't want to be here', and so on.

**Proximity** (see **Personal Space**)

**Questioning** This is an important skill for keeping a conversation going. Questions can be open or closed.
A closed question is where the kind of answer required is simple and fixed. 'How old are you?' is a closed question because the answer has to be a number – once you've said it there is little else to say. 'How do you feel about your age?' is open because the other person could say almost anything – how long they speak for is 'open'. Giving a short quick number is a 'closed' reply. Closed questions are of limited use in working with people. Open questions are often much more valuable for building an understanding.

**Reflective listening** This is a care skill which involves either using your own words to repeat what another person said, or repeating the words exactly, or using non-verbal messages with silence. The idea of reflection is to use conversation like a mirror, so that the other person can see his or her own thoughts reflected. They can then be altered more easily.

**Responding skills** Use of verbal and non-verbal communication to respond to others. Responses may use reflective listening, questioning and skills focused on understanding the other person.

**Role boundaries** Boundaries to the commitment or duties involved in a 'caring relationship'.

**Self-confidence** An individual's confidence in his or her own ability to achieve something or to cope with a situation. Self-confidence may influence and be influenced by self-esteem.

**Self-disclosure** This happens when we tell other people about our own experiences, thoughts and feelings. Some self-disclosure can be useful when trying to understand others. It can create a sense of trust.

**Self-esteem** How well or badly a person feels about himself or herself. High self-esteem may help a person to feel happy and confident. Low self-esteem may lead to depression and unhappiness.

**Self-image** The kind of person we think we are. If there is a big gap between our ideal self and our self-image we are likely to have a low self-esteem.

**Sensory contact** Touch, smell, vision, hearing or other sensations which give us information about other people.

**Silence** Silence is a useful part of some conversations. Sometimes silence is better than just talking to fill a gap. It can provide an opportunity for feelings to be expressed non-verbally.

**Sincerity** This involves being real and honest in what we say to others. Without sincerity, warmth and understanding, relationships usually break down or 'go wrong'. Honesty with clients is an important part of relationship and supportive work.

**Social context** A setting where social influences affect an individual's learning and development.

**Social role** The behaviour adopted by individuals when they are in social situations. Group norms and individual status help to define a role such as mother, sister, engineer etc.

**Status** A measure of the power or prestige of a person. Status helps to define how people are treated by others and how they see themselves.

**Stereotyping** Judging an individual to be a certain type of person by his or her appearance or behaviour. A stereotype is not a description of a real person. It is a collection of characteristics which members of a particular group are expected to possess. People who have been stereotyped are expected to behave as 'typical' members of the group to which they have been assigned.

**Stress** A physical condition. Symptoms may include tiredness, irritability, lack of clear thinking, difficulties in sleeping and physical illness.

**Submissiveness** Feeling that others' needs are more important than your own, giving in to them so as to avoid trouble.

**Supportive skills** Warmth, understanding and sincerity can be used together to create a safe, caring conversation.

**Tactile** Something which can be touched.

**Tone of voice** Voice tone is the sound of the voice, rather than the words that are spoken. The tone of someone's voice can send messages about attraction, anger, sympathy and other emotions. Because voice tone is separate from spoken words, it is classed as 'non-verbal'. The sound of our voice is separate from the word messages we send.

**Touch** This is another way of sending non-verbal messages. Touch can be a very important way of saying 'I care', or 'I am with you'. Touch can be interpreted in various ways. It can send messages of power and dominance, and can be sexual as well as caring. The important thing is how a person understands touch, not what you intend.

**Understanding** An important goal of caring is to learn about other people's individuality. It is necessary to build some understanding so that you correctly communicate respect and value.

**Value base** A system of values to guide the care profession. Values summarised on the NVQ 'O' Unit are valuing diversity, promoting rights and responsibilities and maintaining confidentiality.

**Values** Values are learned through systems which enable individuals to make choices and decisions. Values may guide communication skills.

**Valuing others** Promoting a sense of self-esteem in other people.

**Verbal communication** Spoken messages – messages which use words – are 'verbal'. The opposite is non-verbal communication, which means messages sent without words. Non-verbal language is often harder to understand than verbal language.

**Warmth** A supportive skill which displays the ability to be non-judgemental and to listen to clients. Warmth can help to create a safe conversational atmosphere which may lead to a sense of trust.

# Physical aspects of health

Unit 3

**This unit is concerned with the major organ systems of the body and their basic anatomy and physiology. This includes the recording of body measurements and the accurate analysis of the results.**

**You will learn about:**

- **human body systems: physiology and anatomy**
- **homeostasis, whereby the body maintains a stable environment**
- **how physiological measurements of individuals in care settings are taken**
- **the importance of safe practice and how to reduce potential health and safety risks**
- **the analysis and accuracy of results when taking physiological measurements – applying science in a care context.**

## Introduction

This unit introduces you to the anatomy and physiology of the most important organ systems of the body. No one body system can function in isolation: all are dependent on at least one other system and often more than one. Inter-relationships between body systems are important in care because diagnosis, treatment and care must relate to the whole client and should not focus on one system only. For example, a client with a broken leg who is waiting for an operation to pin her leg is bedridden; this could cause the blood in a leg vein to clot and part of this may break off to obstruct the lungs or brain causing serious complications or even death.

As well as covering inter-relationships, this chapter also investigates the control mechanisms that operate to keep the internal environment within a limited range of extremes. For example, the temperature of the inside of the body must be kept from fluctuating with the external climate because the enzymes controlling all the chemical reactions inside the body slow down or stop working at low or high temperatures. People are not aware of these control systems – they happen automatically – but they can go wrong, as in hypothermia and heat stroke. Control of the internal environment of the body is called **homeostasis**.

In order to monitor the internal environment and to try to understand what is happening inside the body, carers can take physiological measurements such as pulse rates, breathing rates, blood pressure and body temperature. Some measurements can be taken without using specialist equipment and are part of the daily routine for many carers. Other measurements need equipment, such as sphygmomanometers to measure blood pressure and thermometers for measuring body temperatures. Some measurements can be taken both manually and by special equipment that is more likely these days to have electronic displays.

This chapter explains the use of equipment to take physiological measurements from clients. However, figures from measurements will be of no use without knowing the expected normal range of the data or the implications of figures outside the normal range. This is why this chapter covers the expected range of measurements and deviations from normal.

To complete Unit 3 you must collect data with safe practice, you should be able to judge the accuracy of your figures and be able to demonstrate patterns through graphical displays and subsequent analysis.

# 3.1 Physiology and anatomy

## The respiratory system

There are two definitions crucial to your understanding of the respiratory system. These definitions are as follows:

- respiration: this is the release of energy from the breakdown of food molecules
- energy: which is best described as a stored ability to do work.

### Aerobic and anaerobic respiration

There are two types of respiration – aerobic and anaerobic. **Aerobic** respiration is the type usually carried out by our body cells and involves the use of oxygen from the air around us. It is very efficient and produces a lot of energy for work by the body, such as pumping blood around the body, digesting food and walking.

**Anaerobic** respiration takes place when the muscle cells are working so hard that the amount of oxygen required to release the energy cannot be taken in sufficient quantities by the lungs and air passages to carry out aerobic respiration. It can be thought of as a temporary emergency short-cut for the body. It is much less efficient than aerobic respiration and produces less energy; it also causes toxic waste products, such as lactic acid, that can only be allowed to accumulate for a short period. Running at maximum speed for a few minutes uses energy mainly produced anaerobically, while running longer races – such as the 1500 metres or even the marathon – means that energy must be produced by aerobic respiration. This is why athletes tend to specialise in races of particular distances.

It is aerobic respiration which takes place most of the time. The link between the respiratory system and respiration is described below.

The respiratory system comprises the anatomical structures and the physiological processes that take the vital oxygen into the body and transport it to the body cells where aerobic respiration can be carried out and, at the same time, eliminate its waste products. Respiration and energy release can *only* take place inside body cells.

The word equation for aerobic respiration is:

Food (glucose sugar) + oxygen
= energy + carbon dioxide + water

The chemical equation for respiration is:

$$C_6H_{12}O_6 + 6O_2 + = 6CO_2 + 6H_2O$$

$C_6H_{12}O_6$ Represents one molecule of glucose sugar, $6O_2$ and $6CO_2$ is six molecules of oxygen and carbon dioxide and, finally, $6H_2O$ is six molecules of water.

Carbon dioxide and water are waste products and need to be eliminated from the body.

The study of the process of respiration is facilitated by subdivision into four distinct parts:

- breathing
- gaseous exchange
- transport in the blood
- cell respiration.

## Breathing

The chest or thorax is an airtight box containing the lungs and their tubes, the bronchi. There are two lungs (right and left), each with its own bronchus, which unite to form the windpipe or trachea. The trachea joins the back of the throat or pharynx, which connects with both mouth and nose, which are of course open to external air. All these tubes are lined with mucus-secreting cells and have either C-shaped rings or small plates of cartilage in their walls to prevent collapse. Mucus is the sticky white jelly-like material used to lubricate and trap dust particles that can enter by external passages.

The lungs themselves have a thin, outer covering of membrane called the pleura and are located behind the chest wall which is also internally lined with pleura. Between the two layers of pleura is a thin film of moisture, which exerts surface tension, so allowing the two layers to slide up and down but not allowing them to pull apart easily. This means that when the chest wall moves, the lungs are usually pulled with them.

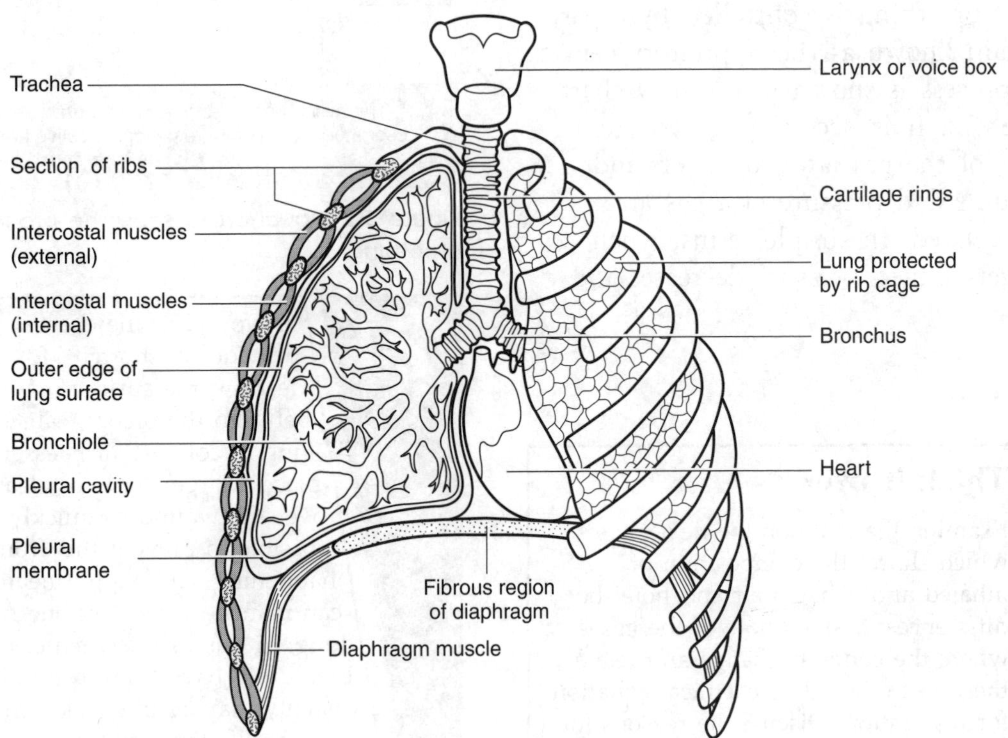


**Figure 3.1 Section through the thorax to show the respiratory organs**

## Think it over

Read the preceding paragraph again and study the diagram of the chest. You will have heard of the condition known as pleurisy and might know that there are two types – 'wet' and 'dry' pleurisy. It can be painful to breathe if you have pleurisy. What do you think has happened to the chest of a client who has pleurisy?

Forming the wall of the chest, outside the pleura, is the bony rib cage with two sets of oblique muscles joining them together – these are known as the intercostal muscles (*inter* means between; *costal* means ribs). A sheet of muscle called the diaphragm forms the floor of the chest. The diaphragm is dome-shaped, with the highest part in the centre and the edges firmly attached to the lowest ribs. The chest is an airtight cavity with the trachea being the only way for air to enter.

Rhythmic breathing is controlled by a part of the brain known as the respiratory centre and the process is shown in the flow chart in Figure 3.2. It is necessary for you to know one of the gas laws to understand this. Volume and pressure of a gas are inversely related. In simple terms, when volume gets larger, pressure decreases and vice versa.

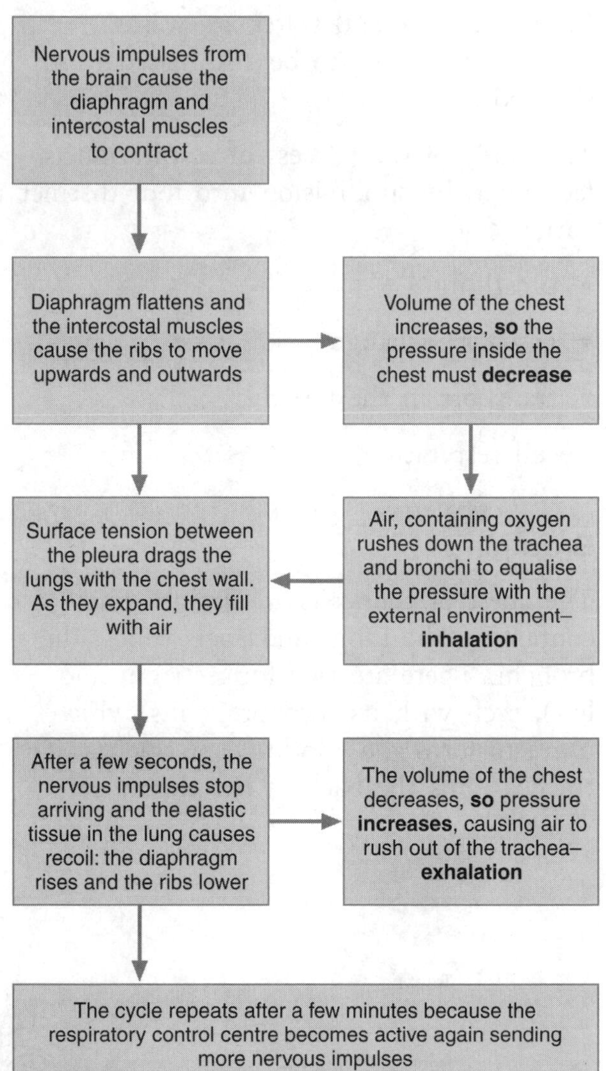


**Figure 3.2 Flowchart to show the process of breathing**

## Think it over

Examine the table on the next page which shows the composition of inhaled and exhaled air and note the differences. Make a note of the gases where the contents change and relate these to the word or chemical equation for respiration. Discuss the reasons for the changes with a partner or tutor.

?

A wound in the chest wall provides a 'shortcut' for air and destroys the surface tension between the pleura, causing the lung to collapse. It is essential to place a large sterile or clean pad over the wound as quickly as possible to prevent this from happening. Although a healthy person can manage with only one functioning lung, in this case oxygen-carrying blood will have been lost and the casualty may be in shock – making the situation life-threatening.

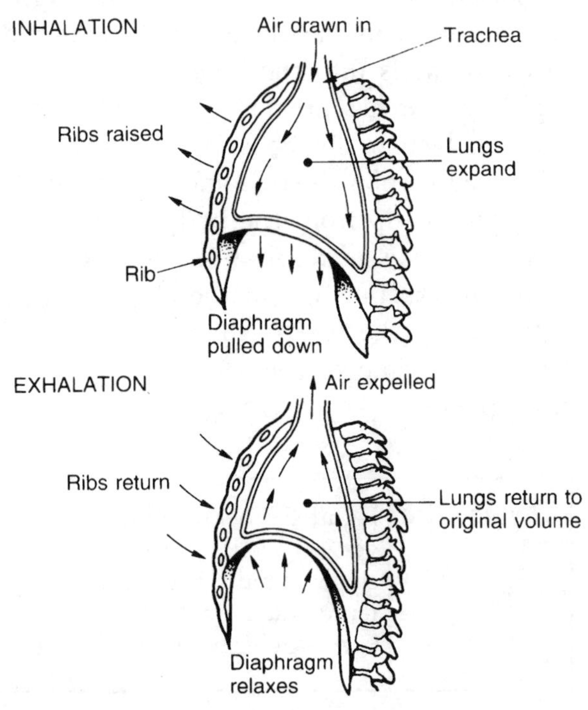


Figure 3.3 Changes during inhalation and exhalation

## Gaseous exchange

Inside the lungs, smaller and smaller branches of the bronchi, called bronchioles, open into thousands of air sacs, each consisting of a cluster of alveoli. Each air sac with its alveoli and bronchiole looks rather like a bunch of grapes on a stem.

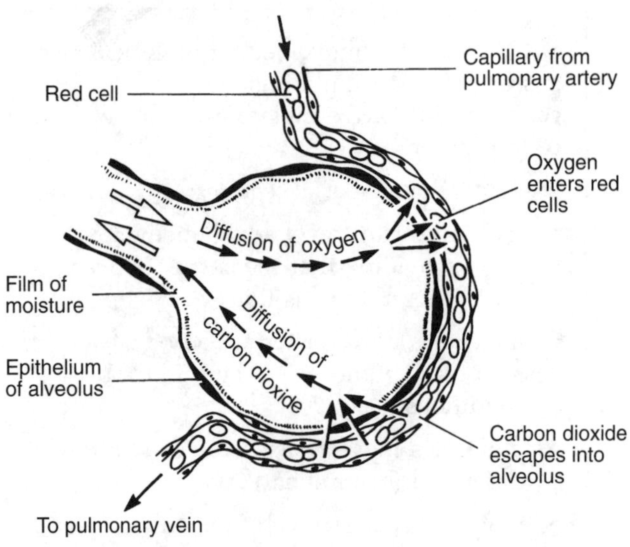


Figure 3.4 Gaseous exchange in the alveoli

The wall of each alveolus is only one cell thick and surrounded on its outside by tiny blood vessels called capillaries – these, too, have walls only one cell thick. The air in each alveolus is separated from the blood in the capillary by very thin walls, only two flat cells thick. A film of moisture in which the respiratory gases dissolve lines each alveolus. The walls of the alveoli contain elastic fibres capable of expansion and recoil.

The process by which gases exchange across these walls is called **diffusion** (see box).

| Gases present in the air | Composition of inhaled air | Composition of exhaled air |
|---|---|---|
| Nitrogen | approximately 80% | approximately 80% |
| Oxygen | 20% | 16% |
| Carbon dioxide | trace – 0.04% | 4% |
| Water vapour | varies with climate | saturated |

Table 3.1 The differences in the compositions of inhaled and exhaled air

**Diffusion** is the movement of molecules of a gas or a liquid from a region of high concentration of the molecules to one of low concentration.

There are some special features:

- molecules can travel across membranes or cells, providing that the barrier between the concentrations is thin
- molecules move faster at body temperature and slow down in cooler conditions
- molecules move faster if the concentration difference (or gradient) is high
- more molecules travel if the surface area is greater; this is why diffusion sites around the body carry projections or waves
- diffusion slows down over a period of time (because the concentration difference decreases) unless the diffused molecules are removed at the low concentration and fresh supplies of new molecules maintain the high concentration.

## Think it over

Imagine how it would be if 90 per cent of your class or group stood at one end of the room and 10 per cent at the other, with everyone moving randomly around the room to music. Someone stops the music after ten minutes. Would you still have the same proportion of people in different parts of the room? Of course you would not, people would be much more evenly distributed. That is what diffusion is about: an 'equalling up' of moving molecules which were unevenly distributed in the first place. Place a line of chairs in the middle of the room and it would not make any difference to the result, it would just take longer to cross the barrier. Build a wall across the room (don't try this at home!) and it would make a difference – the barrier is now too thick to cross.

Dissolved oxygen will pass from the high concentration in the alveolar air across the two thin walls into the blood in the capillary that has previously unloaded most of its oxygen to the cells of the body. Dissolved carbon dioxide and water have been picked up from the body cells as waste products of respiration and are high in the blood, but low in the alveolar air, so they pass in the reverse direction. Exhalation removes them into the atmosphere.

| **Try it out** | Figure 3.5 below shows a vertical section through the chest. Identify the features represented by the letters A to G and describe their purpose. |
|---|---|

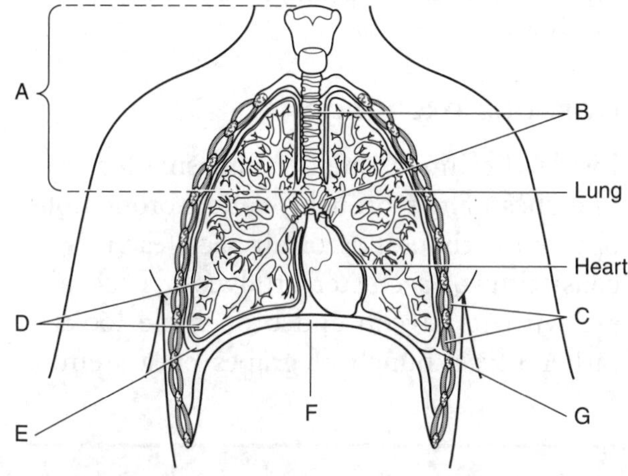


**Figure 3.5 Vertical section through the chest**

You can show practically that there is very little carbon dioxide in the atmosphere and considerably more so in exhaled air by the 'lime water' experiment. You can also show that oxygen is used up during respiration by the gas jar and candle experiment.

**Try it out**

You will need a gas jar, a stop clock, piece of clean rubber tubing, glass plate and a spoon attached to a gas jar lid that is able to hold a small candle, (a diagram of the apparatus is shown in Figure 3.6).

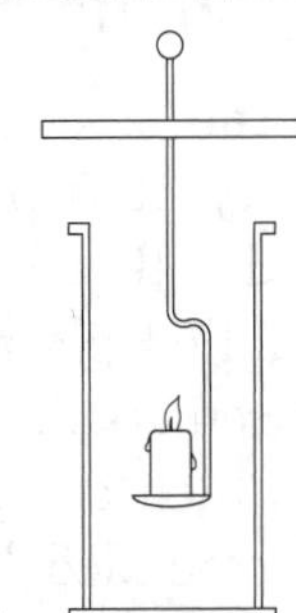

Figure 3.6 Apparatus to show that oxygen is used up during respiration

An empty gas jar contains atmospheric air, which is the same as inhaled air. Light the candle and lower into the gas jar, starting the stop clock as soon as the lid closes off the gas jar. Stop the clock as soon as the candle goes out and record the number of seconds that the candle burned. Repeat five times, ensuring that the gas jar is filled with fresh air every time. Calculate the mean time during which the candle burned.

Holding the gas jar upside down, place one end of the rubber tubing inside it and exhale firmly into it several times. Slide the tubing out and cover the inverted gas jar with the glass plate before turning upright. The gas jar is now filled with exhaled air. Repeat the procedure with the lighted candle and the stop clock, being careful to slide the glass plate off just as the candle is entering. Calculate the mean of five timed recordings as before.

You should find that the timing for exhaled air is much shorter than for inhaled air. Burning or combustion can only occur when oxygen is present, so the times represent the quantities of oxygen present. If the time for inhaled air represents 20 per cent of oxygen, find out what percent of oxygen is represented by the timing for exhaled air.

**Try it out**

Set up the laboratory glassware as shown, taking particular note of the way in which the tubes are arranged in the flasks. You can use either hydrogen carbonate indicator or the more traditional lime water in the flasks. Attach clips that open and close at points 1 and 2 or use your fingers to nip the rubber tubing together. Closing the tubing at point 2, breathe in through the mouthpiece and note the air from the atmosphere bubbling through flask A. Breathe out through the mouthpiece while closing at point 1. This time the exhaled air will bubble through flask B. Repeat this about five times. You should notice that flask A remains the same colour but flask B changes colour. Both lime water and hydrogen carbonate indicator demonstrate the presence of carbon dioxide with a colour change. You have successfully shown that atmosphere air contains very little carbon dioxide whereas exhaled air contains much more. Respiration produces carbon dioxide.

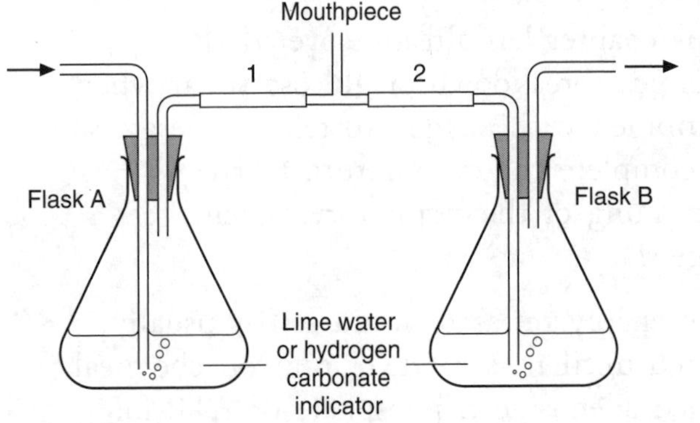


Figure 3.7 Apparatus used to show that carbon dioxide is produced by respiration

## Transport of gases in the blood

When oxygen enters the blood in the lung (or pulmonary) capillary, it is immediately taken up by red blood cells which lie in the liquid part of blood called plasma. Red blood cells contain a remarkable pigment called haemoglobin, which combines avidly with oxygen when surrounded by the high concentration of oxygen found in the lung, but also releases the oxygen in the environment with a low concentration of oxygen surrounding body cells. The cells are continuously using up oxygen in the process of respiration and producing waste carbon dioxide and water in the process. Diffusion takes place again! This time, carbon dioxide and water diffuse from the cells into the plasma of the blood capillary and are carried away by blood vessels to the lungs for elimination. Oxygen is delivered to the 'hungry' cells for use in respiration.

## Cell respiration (also known as tissue respiration)

This chapter has already covered the chemical breakdown of glucose sugar when combined with oxygen to release energy, so to complete the cycle return to the beginning of the respiratory system, see page 2.

The energy released into a cell is usually stored until it is needed, in a cell chemical called adenosine triphosphate or ATP for short. When the energy is required for work ATP breaks down to make adenosine diphosphate (ADP) and energy is released. This ADP is then recycled and used to store more energy from respiration. This is rather like charging a rechargeable battery from the mains electricity supply. The advantage of this system is that there is always a ready supply of energy within the cell.

We have already seen that anaerobic respiration is a less efficient way of producing energy; it occurs within muscle cells only during strenuous exercise when breathing cannot occur fast enough to supply enough oxygen. The waste product formed during anaerobic respiration is called lactic acid and an individual can only tolerate a certain amount of this material before the exercise has to stop due to fatigue. Athletic training can improve critical levels of lactic acid tolerance, but limitations still exist.

### Think it over

Next time you watch trained athletes run a 100 metre-race notice that there are very few, if any, breaths until after the race – they are running anaerobically! Longer distance runners cannot do this.

## Lung volumes

The last part of any inhaled air fills up the bronchi, trachea, throat and nose – none of which have suitable characteristics for gaseous exchange, so the actual amount of air which undergoes gaseous exchange is much smaller than that breathed in. For the average person, this so-called dead space air is approximately 150cm$^3$.

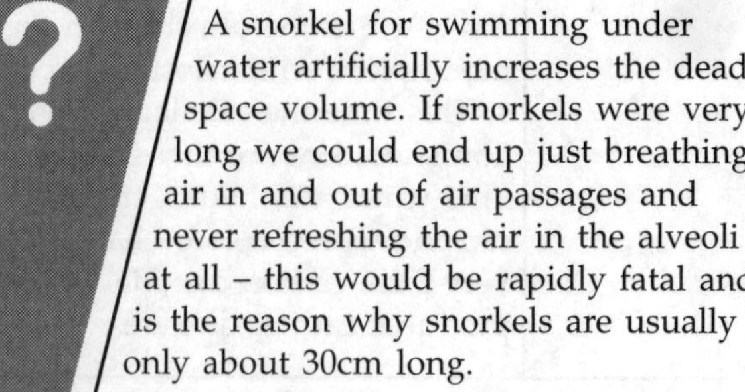

A snorkel for swimming under water artificially increases the dead space volume. If snorkels were very long we could end up just breathing air in and out of air passages and never refreshing the air in the alveoli at all – this would be rapidly fatal and is the reason why snorkels are usually only about 30cm long.

*Tidal volume* is the volume of air which is taken in during one breath. At rest this is approximately 500cm$^3$, so the amount of air actually reaching the alveoli is (500–150) cm$^3$ per breath. During activity, this volume can rise considerably. The number of breaths taken in one minute is the respiratory or breathing rate.

*Pulmonary ventilation* is the volume of air taken in each minute and is calculated by multiplying the tidal volume by the respiratory rate. For example, 16 breaths per minute $\times$ 500 cm$^3$ tidal volume = a pulmonary ventilation of 8dm$^3$/min. Units of cubic decimetres (dm$^3$) are the new units used instead of litres, but they are exactly the same volume, namely 1000 cm$^3$.

*Vital capacity* is the maximum volume of air that can be exhaled after a maximum inhalation, and clearly will vary according to chest size and health. This is why males generally have higher lung volumes than females and adult lung volumes are larger than those of children. Generally, adults have vital capacities ranging from 4.5 to 6 dm$^3$.

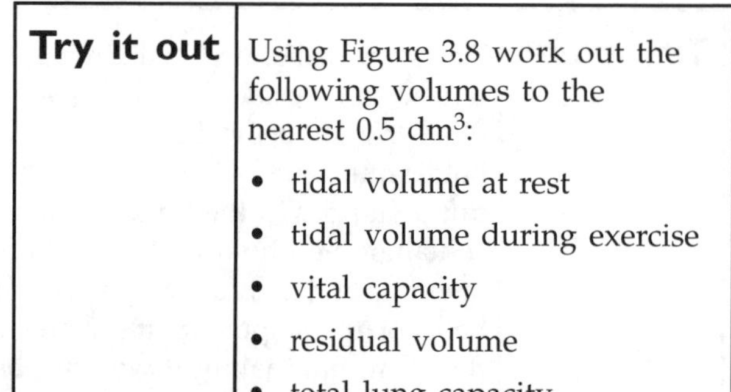

| **Try it out** | Using Figure 3.8 work out the following volumes to the nearest 0.5 dm$^3$:<br>• tidal volume at rest<br>• tidal volume during exercise<br>• vital capacity<br>• residual volume<br>• total lung capacity. |
|---|---|

After the most forceful exhalation, the lungs still contain air – called the residual volume – so the total lung capacity is the sum of the residual volume and the vital capacity. If we are asked to take a deep breath, this is the inspiratory reserve volume and similarly a forced exhalation is the expiratory reserve volume. A spirometer chart to show these lung volumes is shown in Figure 3.8.

If a spirometer is not available, you can use a large water trough or bucket, rubber

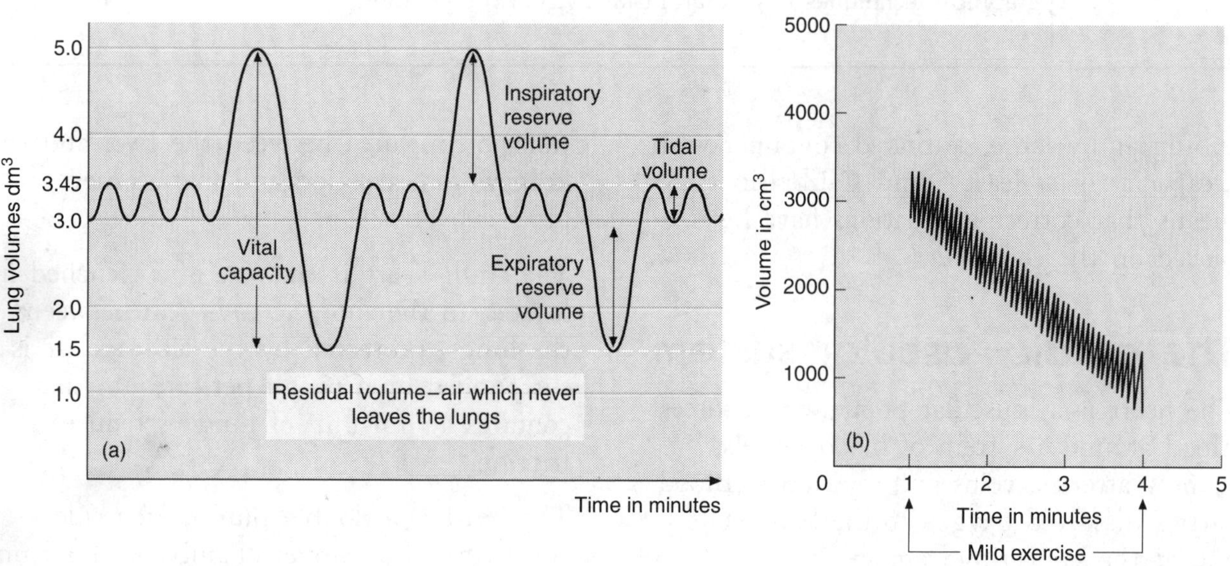


Figure 3.8 Spirometer chart to display lung volumes.

**Try it out**

Turn your calibrated container filled with water upside down in a water-filled trough, being careful either to hold your hand over the opening or put a stopper in the neck of the container. Still holding the container opening under water, remove your hand or the stopper. Some water will flow out, but mainly it will still be filled with water. Read and record the level of the water.

Push a length of rubber tubing through the container opening until it pushes through into the space above the water. Take as deep a breath as you can and exhale into the rubber tubing. Take care, water may flow over the trough! Now, read and record the water level in the container again. The difference between these two levels will indicate your *vital capacity*.

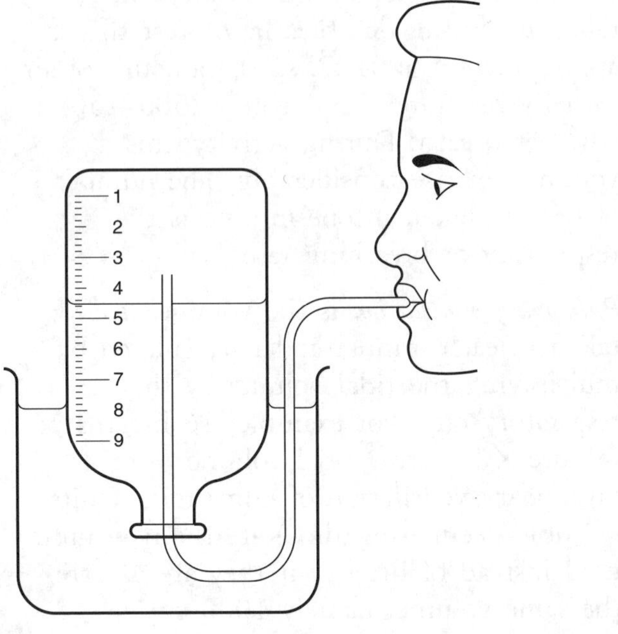


Using a simple laboratory-style spirometer

Repeat the experiment, but this time breathe in and out quietly. Get your partner to record the readings of inspiration and expiration. This is the *tidal volume*.

**Note on analysis**

If you are part of a group performing any of these techniques, you will be able to collect a number of readings and display them in the form of a statistical chart and use graphical techniques to give an instant visual presentation.

tubing and a large calibrated container with a capacity of at least $5dm^3$. Calibration means that correct graduations have been placed on the container.

## The cardio-vascular system

The heart is a muscular pump which forces blood around a system of blood vessels, namely arteries, veins and capillaries. Blood carries dissolved oxygen to the body cells and at the same time removes carbon dioxide and water. However, blood also distributes heat, hormones, nutrients and enzymes around the body as well as transporting urea between the liver and the kidneys for excretion and many other products.

The adult heart is the size of a clenched fist located in the thoracic cavity in between the lungs, protected by the rib cage. It is surrounded by a tough pericardium that contains a thin film of fluid to reduce friction.

The heart is a double pump, each side consisting of an upper chamber (the atrium) and a lower chamber (the ventricle). The right-sided pump contains deoxygenated blood and is totally separate from the left

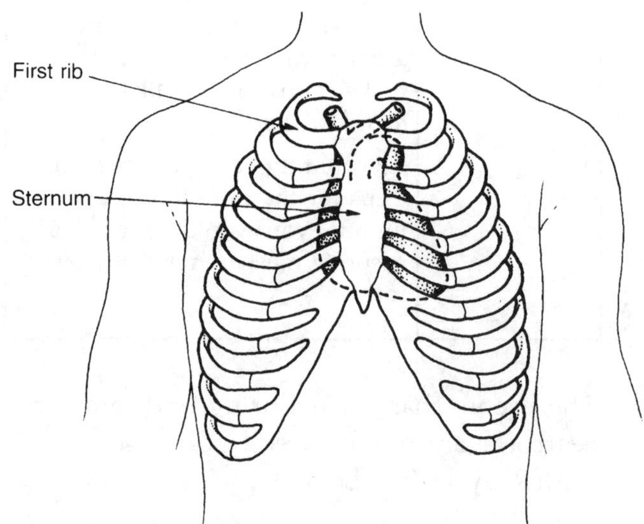


**Figure 3.9 The position of the heart**

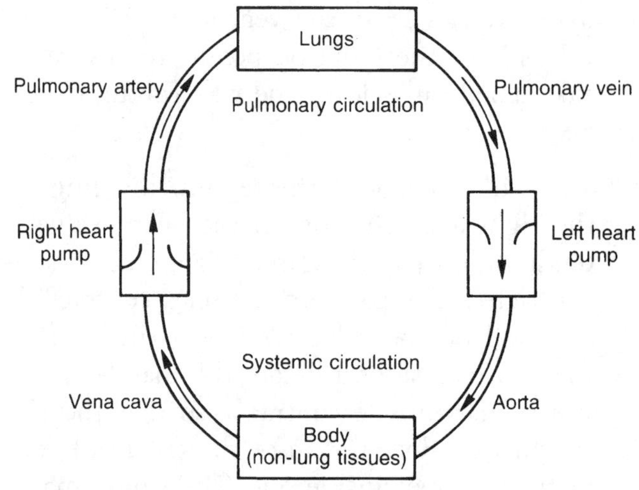


**Figure 3.10 Double circulation: blood flows through the heart twice in one circuit**

side that contains oxygenated blood. Each chamber has a major blood vessel either entering or leaving the heart. The atria (plural of atrium) carry veins pouring blood into them and the ventricles bear arteries that carry blood away from the heart.

> ? It is helpful to remember that atria have veins, ventricles have arteries: A and V in each case, never two As or two Vs.

The right pump receives blood from the body tissues, having off-loaded its oxygen, and pumps the blood to the lungs for re-oxygenation. The left pump receives blood from the lungs, fully loaded with oxygen, and distributes it to the body tissue. You will notice that the blood travels twice through the heart in one circuit around the body. This is known as a double circulation. Figure 3.10 illustrates this, but notice how the right and left halves have been separated.

One circulation is to and from the lungs and is known as the pulmonary circulation. Whenever you see or hear the word pulmonary you will know that it is referring to the lungs; so the artery taking blood from the right ventricle is the pulmonary artery and the vein returning blood from the lungs to the left side of the heart is the pulmonary vein(s), in fact there are four of these. The other circulation is called the systemic circulation because it carries blood to and from the body systems, except the lungs of course!

The main artery of the body is the aorta which leaves the left ventricle, and the main vein returning blood to the right atrium is the vena cava. There are two divisions of this vein, the superior and inferior vena cavae returning blood from the head/neck and remainder of the trunk respectively.

The semi-lunar valves are located where the main arteries leave the ventricles. All these valves have the same purpose – to ensure that blood only flows one way through the heart.

You will also notice the septum dividing the right and left sides of the heart, valve tendons and papillary muscles in the ventricles. The papillary muscles contract and pull on the valve tendons a tiny fraction of a second before the main ventricular muscle contracts, so that the contraction does not force the tricuspid and bicuspid valves inside out. The valves make noises when they close, but not when they are open (rather like clapping your hands) and these noises are the heart sounds that doctors listen for with a stethoscope.

| **Try it out** | Ask to borrow a stethoscope and listen to either your own or a partner's heart sounds. They make sounds rather like *lubb, dup, lubb, dup.*<br>By counting each pair of lubb, dups for the duration of one minute, you would have a very accurate measurement of heart rate. |
|---|---|

The events that occur during one complete heartbeat are more correctly called the cardiac cycle (see below).

## Think it over

Study the labelled diagram of the heart (Figure 3.11) and find all the major blood vessels you have studied.

You will need to examine the diagram of the heart again to see four valves labelled. Two of these, the tricuspid and bicuspid, are located at the junctions of the atrium and ventricle on each side.

You can remember these because the TRIcuspid valve is on the RIghT side, (a rearrangement of the letters) so that other side, the left, must be the bicuspid valve.

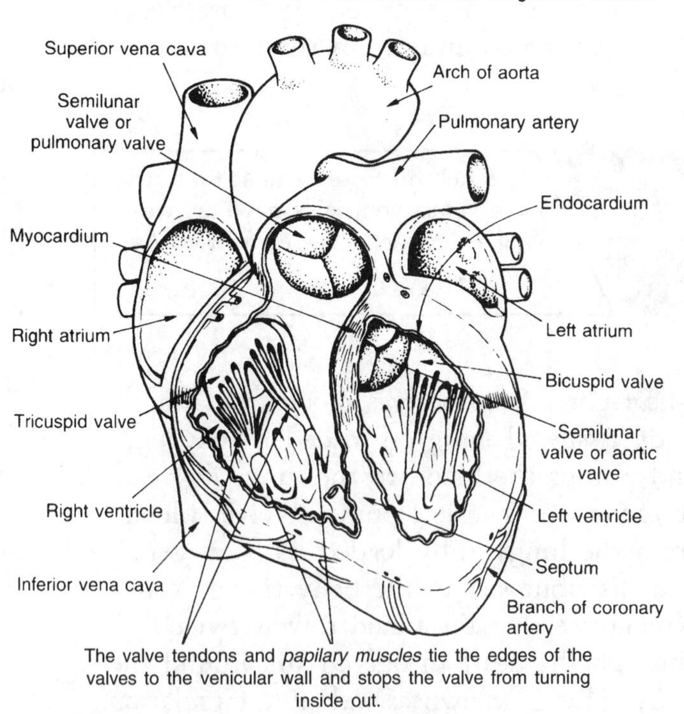


**Figure 3.11 A section through the heart**

?

Heart murmurs are extra sounds heard between the normal heart sounds, some are significant and indicate heart problems, while others carry no significance. They are usually the result of disturbed blood flow.

## The cardiac cycle

If the heart-rate, at rest, is counted at around 70 beats each minute, then the time for each beat is 1 ÷ 70 minutes or 60 ÷ 70 seconds. This works out as approximately 0.8 seconds for each beat of the heart.

If this is represented by 8 small squares, each to the value of 0.1 second, then we can produce a diagram as shown in Figure 3.12. If we wish to show events happening in the atria and ventricles during this period, we can have two 'timelines'. The shaded squares represent when the cardiac muscle is contracting and the plain squares, relaxation. Contraction phases are called *systole* or *systolic periods* and relaxation periods *diastole* or *diastolic periods*. (See Figure 3.12.) These names are also used for the two figures in a blood pressure measurement.

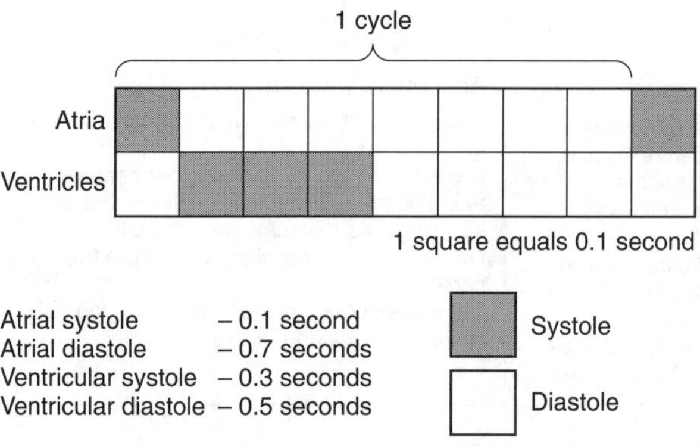


**Figure 3.12 Timed events in the cardiac cycle: allocations of systole and diastole**

The events in the cardiac cycle can be described as follows:

1 Atria contract, blood is pushed into ventricles under pressure.

2 Ventricles bulge with blood, pressure forces the tricuspid and bicuspid valves shut. This causes the first heart sound to be heard with a stethoscope; it sounds like 'lub'. Atria relax and begin to fill with blood.

3 Ventricles begin contraction, pressure in blood rises and forces open the aortic and pulmonary valves.

4 Systole in the ventricles pushes blood in to the aorta and pulmonary artery. These are elastic walled and begin to expand.

5 Ventricles begin to relax and blood falls back with the effect of gravity for a few moments and catches in the pockets of the semi-lunar valves of the aorta and

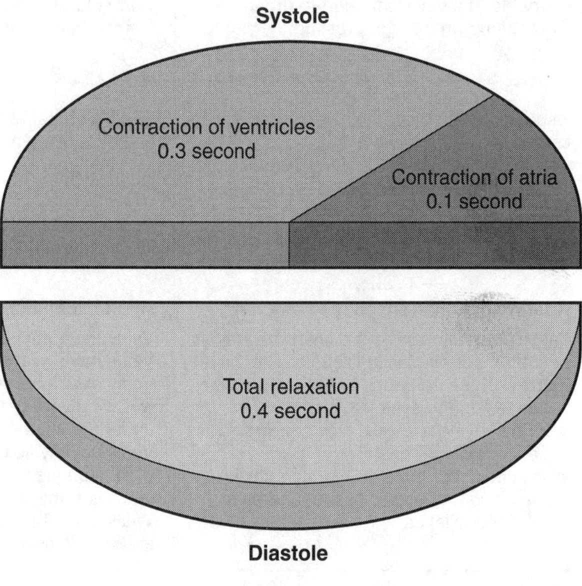


**Figure 3.13 Cardiac cycle: at rest**

pulmonary artery, pressing them together and closing off the opening. This causes the second heart sound which, through a stethoscope, sounds like 'dupp'.

6 Tricuspid and bicuspid valves are forced open and blood rushes from the filled atria into the ventricles during their diastolic phase. On being filled to about 70 per cent capacity, atrial systole occurs and the heart has completed the cycle at the point where it started.

*Note*: in a healthy heart, both the two atria and the two ventricles contract simultaneously.

## Blood vessels

These tubes, together with the heart, make up the circulatory system. The main types of blood vessel are:

- arteries
- veins
- capillaries.

Each type has functional and anatomical differences which are summarised in Table 3.2.

Each organ has an arterial and a venous supply bringing blood to the organ and taking blood away respectively. The link vessels supplying the cells of the tissues of the organ are the *capillaries*. A protein-free plasma filtrate driven out of the leaky (selectively permeable) capillaries becomes the tissue or interstitial fluid which supplies the cells. It is through the blood and tissue fluid that raw materials for respiration, hormones, enzymes, etc. get to the cell organelles. This is also the route for communication, as the circulatory system must go to all organs.

| Arteries | Veins | Capillaries |
|---|---|---|
| **Functional differences**<br>Carry blood away from heart to organs<br>Carry blood under high pressure | **Functional differences**<br>Carry blood to heart from the organs<br>Carry blood under low pressure | **Functional differences**<br>Connect arteries to veins<br>Arterioles and capillaries cause greatest drop in pressure due to overcoming the friction of blood passing through small vessels. |
| Usually contain blood high in oxygen, low in carbon dioxide and water<br>*What are the exceptions?*<br>Large arteries close to the heart help the intermittent flow from the ventricles become a continuous flow through the circulation. | Usually contain blood low in oxygen, high in carbon dioxide and water | Delivers protein-free plasma filtrate high in oxygen to cells and collects up respiratory waste products of carbon dioxide and water. |
| **Anatomical differences (see diagram)**<br>Large arteries close to the heart are almost entirely made of elastic tissue to expand and recoil with the outpouring of blood from the ventricles during systole.<br>Arteries have thick walls with corrugated lining and round lumens.<br>Walls consist of three layers, endothelial lining, muscle and elastic tissue, and outer tough fibrous layer. | **Anatomical differences**<br>Veins have thinner walls than arteries<br>Veins have oval spaces in centre (lumina)<br>Veins over a certain diameter contain valves which prevent blood flowing backwards under the influence of gravity.<br>Veins usually lie between skeletal muscles which squeeze blood flow onwards during muscular activity.<br>Walls have three coats but far less muscle and elastic tissue and more fibrous tissue. | **Anatomical differences**<br>Capillaries have walls which are only one cell thick.<br>Capillaries have leaky walls (permeable) enabling small molecular nutrients and dissolved gases to exchange with cells.<br>No cell can lie more than a few cells from a capillary.<br>Capillaries often smaller than red blood cells which must distort to pass through. |

**Table 3.2 Functional and anatomical differences between arteries, veins and capillaries**

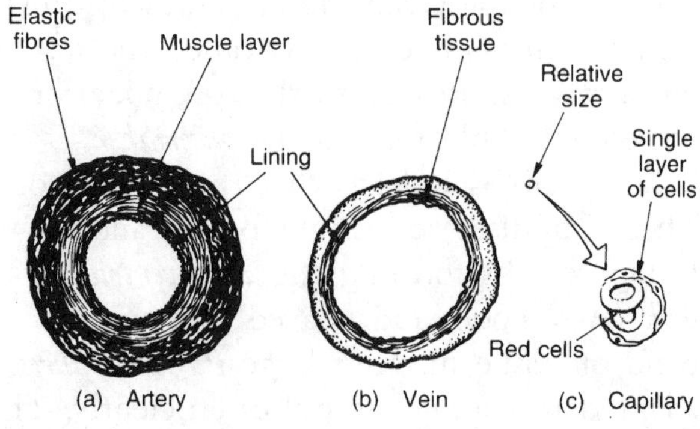


**Figure 3.14 Blood vessels, transverse sections**

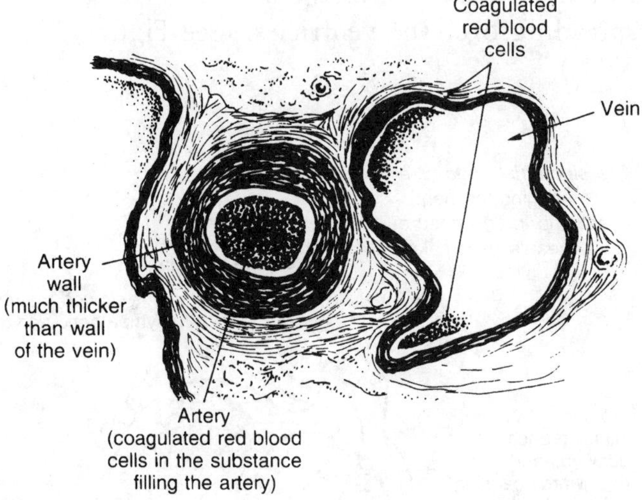


**Figure 3.15 Transverse section through a vein and an artery**

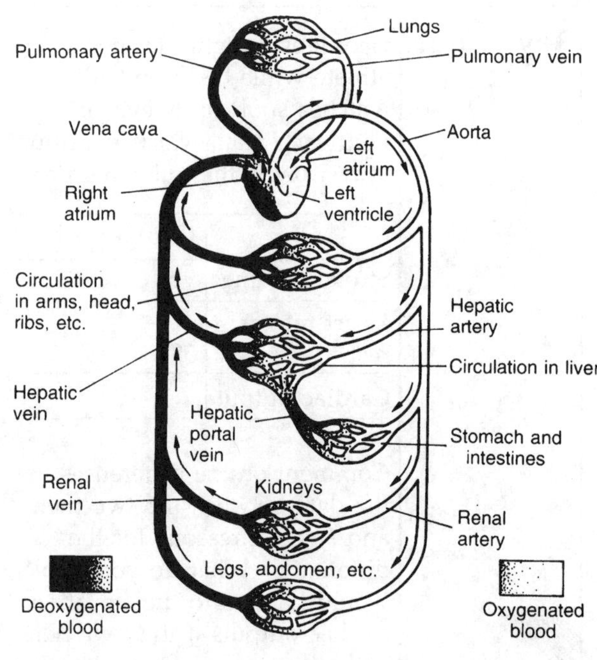


**Figure 3.16 The human circulatory system**

## Cardiac output

Each ventricle has a capacity of approximately 70 $cm^3$ of blood. This is called the stroke volume as it is the quantity expelled at each beat of the heart. With moderate exercise and stressful circumstances the stroke volume can increase to 110 $cm^3$ or as high as 140 $cm^3$ in strenuous activity! Heart rate at rest varies a great deal, but in untrained people it is usually between 60 and 80 beats per minute. Cardiac output is the volume of blood expelled in one minute so is the result of heart rate multiplied by stroke volume.

**Try it out**

George is a highly trained athlete while his friend Ali watches sport on television. Find each man's cardiac output at rest using the following data:

| | George | Ali |
|---|---|---|
| Stroke volume | 90 | 70 |
| Heart rate at rest | 58 | 70 |
| Cardiac output | | |

Comment on the differences in the data between the two men and suggest reasons for the differences. What do you think would happen to their relative cardiac outputs if the two men had to run vigorously to catch a bus?

## Cardiac muscle

The muscle which makes up the heart walls is not found anywhere else in the body. The muscle fibres form a branching network along which nervous impulses pass with great speed. One remarkable feature of cardiac muscle is its ability to contract rhythmically without being supplied by nervous impulses, this is called *myogenicity*. When isolated from a nerve supply, the atrial muscle contracts at a faster rate than the ventricular muscle; however, in a healthy heart both rates of contraction are governed by the autonomic nervous system (see page 159).

## Nervous conduction through the heart

A cluster of special cells lie in the upper part of the right atrium and every few moments they become excited, sending nerve impulses across the branching network of the atrial muscle fibres to cause contraction. This cluster is called the *sino-atrial node* (shortened to the S-A node) or more commonly termed the *pacemaker*, because this is indeed what these cells do. These impulses are caught by yet another group of cells forming the *atrio-ventricular node* (A-V node) and relayed to a special band of tissue made of large *Purkinje fibres*, adapted to conduct impulses efficiently. The A-V node delays the transmission to allow the atria to complete their beat. The Purkinje fibres form the *Bundle of His* (or A-V bundle) which crosses the fibrous ring separating atria and ventricles, and then divides into *left* and *right bundle branches* running either side of the septum before spreading over the ventricles. (See Figure 3.17.)

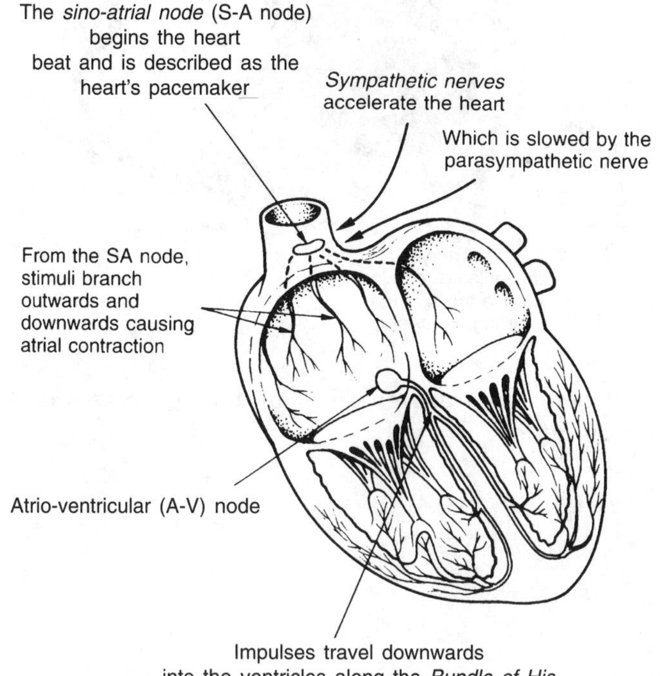


**Figure 3.17 The heart's conduction system**

Impulse conduction is very fast so that the two ventricles beat together to force the blood around the body organs.

If the conduction system fails, artificial pacemakers can now be fitted which supply electrical stimuli from their batteries to stimulate the cardiac muscle direct.

## Nervous control

Despite this elaborate conduction system, the heart also has a nervous control to allow for an almost instant response to the dangers and stresses of everyday life. There are two sets of nerves constantly making a play for control over the heart's rate by influencing the S-A node, which is only rarely allowed to beat at its own pace. Both nervous commands form part of the *autonomic nervous system* (see page 159) which co-ordinates and controls the internal organs (or viscera) of the body. One set continuously tries to calm the heart down, slowing its pace and reducing the strength of the beat. This is the *parasympathetic* branch of the autonomic nervous system, which unceasingly aims for peace and contentment. The other branch is the *sympathetic*, aiming for increased strength of heartbeats and a stirring of pace. It is called into action during muscular work and stress (see Figure 3.17). The sympathetic branch is closely associated with the release of the hormone *adrenaline*.

## Pulse

A pulse can be felt whenever an artery crosses over a bone, thus there are many places in the body where pulses can be felt. The most common places for feeling a pulse are at the wrist and in the neck. The wrist pulse is felt below the thumb on the inner side of both arms and the neck pulses on either side of the trachea inside the strap muscle of the neck. See page 176 for monitoring pulse rates.

| **Try it out** | Practise finding your own and your partner's wrist and neck pulses and record the number of beats in 15 seconds. Multiply by 4 to obtain the rate per minute. |
|---|---|

## Blood pressure

Blood pressure (BP) is the pressure exerted by the blood on the walls of the blood vessels and is generated by the contraction of the ventricles during the heartbeat. The new units for measuring BP are kilopascals (kPa), but you will find that most establishments still record in the older traditional units of millimetres of mercury. Information on measuring blood pressure can be found on page 182.

A blood pressure reading looks like a fraction, but it is not. It is two figures separated by a line; the upper figure represents systolic BP at the height of ventricular systole while the lower diastolic figure is the pressure when the ventricles are relaxed.

The highest BP is found in the aorta, large and medium arteries and after that there is a gradual drop in pressure throughout the circulation, falling to zero as the blood returns to the right atrium.

The arterioles account for the greatest drop in BP as the blood flows through them. They have muscular walls that can contract (producing vasoconstriction) or relax (vasodilation) and this is under the control of the vasomotor centre in the brain. Vascoconstriction causes BP to rise, but the arterioles are not the only factor involved in controlling BP (see below).

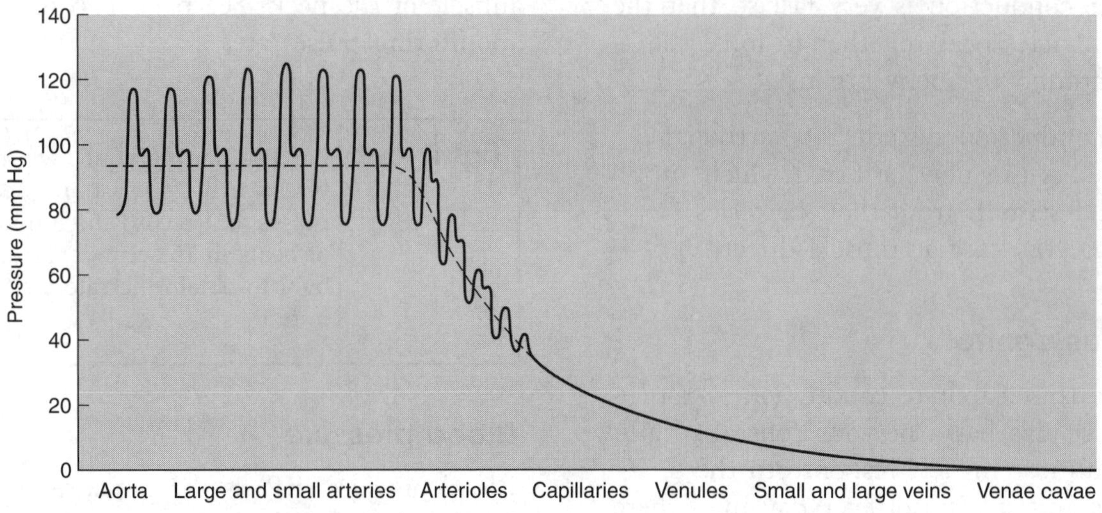


**Figure 3.18 Graph to show blood pressure in the main vessels of the circulation**

### Think it over

Imagine that you are lying in bed, your head, heart and legs are in the horizontal plane and your heart is delivering blood to every part of your body. Then the alarm clock rings and you leap out of bed to get ready for work. Your head is now much higher than your heart and your legs are far lower. If your BP did not change to drive blood up to your head, you would faint, becoming horizontal again. Changing BP depends on a combination of adjustments of blood volume, resistance from the arterioles (vascular resistance), stroke volume and heart rate.

## Blood volume

It might appear surprising that blood volume can change and so influence blood pressure. The spleen acts as a reservoir of blood and can add more blood to the system when necessary. The veins, also, being thin walled can allow blood to pool in the lower legs. See below on venous return.

## Blood flow

This is the volume of blood which flows through a tissue in a period of time – usually millilitres per second. The speed or velocity of blood flow is inversely proportional to the cross-sectional area of the blood vessels it is flowing through. The aorta has a wide lumen but it is only one single vessel, whereas there are millions of capillaries with a huge cross-sectional area between them although they are microscopic. This means that blood flow through the aorta (40cm per second), large arteries and veins is rapid whereas blood flow through the capillaries is very slow, in fact less than one centimetre per second.

### Think it over

Why is it important that blood flows only slowly through capillaries?

## Venous return

This is the return of blood from the capillaries back to the right atrium of the heart. As we have seen in Figure 3.18 the pressure in capillaries, venules and veins is quite low. Although this pressure difference is small it is usually enough to keep blood moving and so maintain cardiac output, but two additional boosts are provided by:

- the skeletal muscle pump: veins in the lower limbs also contain valves opening only to allow blood to flow towards the heart. As the veins are thin-walled and located between skeletal muscle groups, blood is prevented from falling back to these valves when the contracting leg muscles squeeze the veins
- the respiratory pump: we have already seen that to effect inhalation a negative pressure is produced in the thorax by the descending diaphragm muscle. At the same time this causes a positive pressure in the abdomen below. Consequently blood moves from the abdominal veins to the thoracic veins down the pressure gradient.

In these ways, blood is returned to the heart to complete the systemic circulation.

## Blood

Blood consists of straw-coloured plasma in which several types of cells are carried. Plasma is mainly water in which various substances are dissolved, such as gases like oxygen and carbon dioxide, nutrients like glucose and amino acids, salts, enzymes and hormones. There is also a combination of important proteins collectively known as plasma proteins; these have roles in blood clotting, transport, defence and osmosis.

The most numerous cells in the plasma are red blood cells (erythrocytes) which are bi-

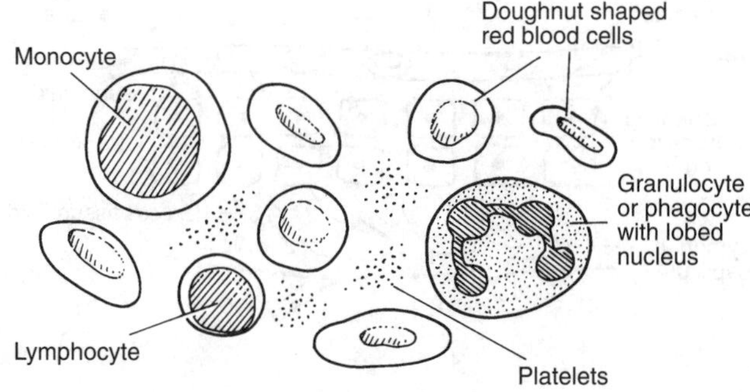


**Figure 3.19 Diagram of blood to show different blood cells**

concave in shape, very small and packed with iron-containing haemoglobin that is responsible for combining with oxygen from the lungs. In the mature state, these cells have lost their nuclei (and consequently their power to divide) in order to have a larger surface area and more haemoglobin. They have a limited life of approximately 120 days.

White cells or leucocytes are larger cells, which are less numerous and have various roles in defending the body against invasion. There are several types, but the most numerous are the granulocytes or polymorphs that are capable of engulfing foreign material such as bacteria and carbon particles. Granulocytes carry lobed nuclei and granules scattered throughout the cell material. Large monocytes are also efficient at engulfing foreign material and both granulocytes and monocytes are able to leave the circulation and travel through tissue.

Lymphocytes are smaller cells containing round nuclei and clear cytoplasm. They assist in the production of antibodies which form part of the plasma proteins.
Thrombocytes or platelets are not full cells but products of the fragmentation of much larger cells. They play a vital role in blood clotting.

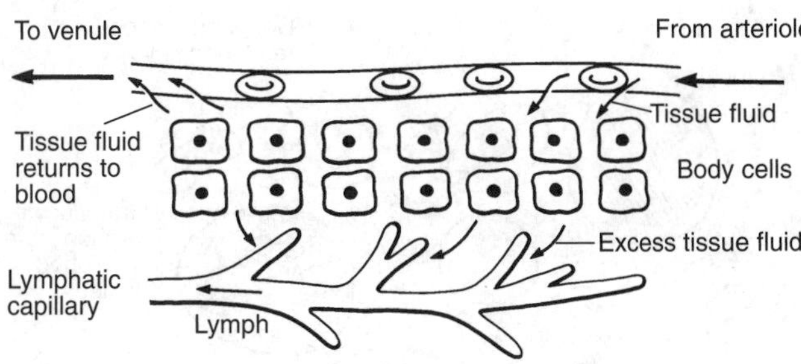


**Figure 3.20 The relationship between blood capillaries, cells and lymphatic capillaries (lymph vessels)**

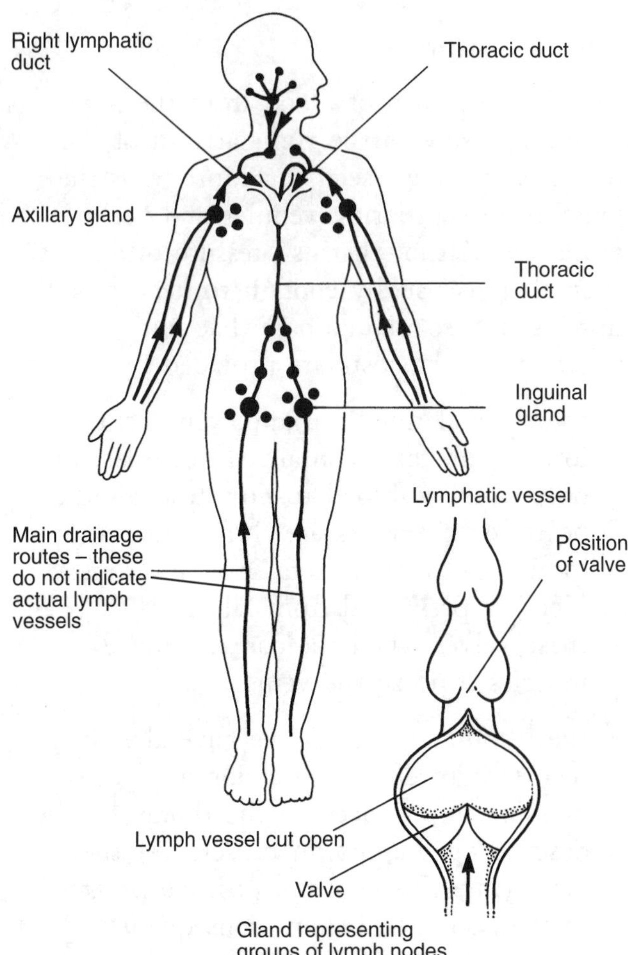


**Figure 3.21 The position of the main lymph nodes and vessels**

## Lymphatic system

The lymphatic system also forms part of the cardio-vascular system. The lymphatic system begins as closed-ended *lymphatic capillaries* which lie in the spaces between cells (see Figure 3.20). They unite to form larger and larger vessels passing upwards eventually to join the great veins in the neck. At several points in this lymphatic circulation, the lymph fluid passes through small nodules known as *lymph nodes*, which are scattered about the body in groups (see Figure 3.21). Lymph nodes contain lymphocytes and macrophages which destroy any microbes which have entered the lymphatic vessels from the tissue spaces. They do this by initiating the antigen-antibody response (sometimes called the *immune response*) and by *phagocytosis* (digestion of microbes), which destroys the microbes.

# The digestive system

The purpose of digestion is to change the large complex molecules that make up our food into small soluble molecules which are capable of being absorbed through the wall of the gut into the bloodstream, in order to be used for energy in respiration and other raw materials. You will probably already be familiar with the main chemical components of food as shown in Table 3.3 on the next page.

**Note**: protein, carbohydrate and fat form the bulk of our diets and are called **macronutrients**; vitamins and minerals are only required in tiny amounts and are called **micronutrients**.

In order to break the macronutrients down into small molecules, various parts of the digestive system produce biological catalysts called **enzymes**. Enzymes are specific to the material they break down and most names of enzymes end in *–ase*, so they are easily recognisable.

| Chemical component in food | Types of food containing this component | Purpose of this type of food | End product of digestion as small soluble molecule |
|---|---|---|---|
| Protein | meat, fish, milk, cheese, eggs, soya bean | to provide raw materials for making new cells and repairing damaged cells | amino acids |
| Carbohydrate | bread, rice, pasta, sugar, cereals, cakes, sweets | to provide energy for respiration | simple sugars such as glucose |
| Fats (lipids) | butter, margarine, oils such as sunflower and olive oil, milk, cream, eggs | to protect vital organs and insulate the body, to carry some vitamins<br>to provide raw materials for hormones (steroids) and cell membranes | fatty acids and glycerol |
| Vitamins | green vegetables, fruits, milk, fish liver oils, cereals, nuts | do not provide kilojoules for energy, but are essential to many chemical processes in the body | not required |
| Mineral salts | similar to vitamins | take part in chemical reactions, form important body fluids and pigments like haemoglobin | not required |
| Fibre | cereals, bread, fruits and vegetables | prevent constipation, assist in preventing bowel disorders, give feeling of fullness so curbs appetite | not digested |
| Water | various foods and drink | allow body fluids to flow, provide solvent for other chemicals, helps regulate body temperature and eliminate waste products of metabolism | absorbed into the bloodstream without change |

**Table 3.3 The chemical components of food**

Relatively few molecules of enzyme are required to break down many food molecules as enzymes themselves are not used up in the reactions. Enzymes are sensitive to temperature, working best around body temperature, and they are also sensitive to the pH of their surroundings. Some, like gastric protease, prefer acid conditions, some like lipase prefer alkaline conditions while salivary amylase prefers a neutral pH7.

The digestive system is a tube that extends from the mouth to the anus; it is dilated, folded and puckered in the various parts of its length. You will need to learn the names of the regions, their main purpose and the outcome of their activities. The whole structure is also known as the alimentary canal.

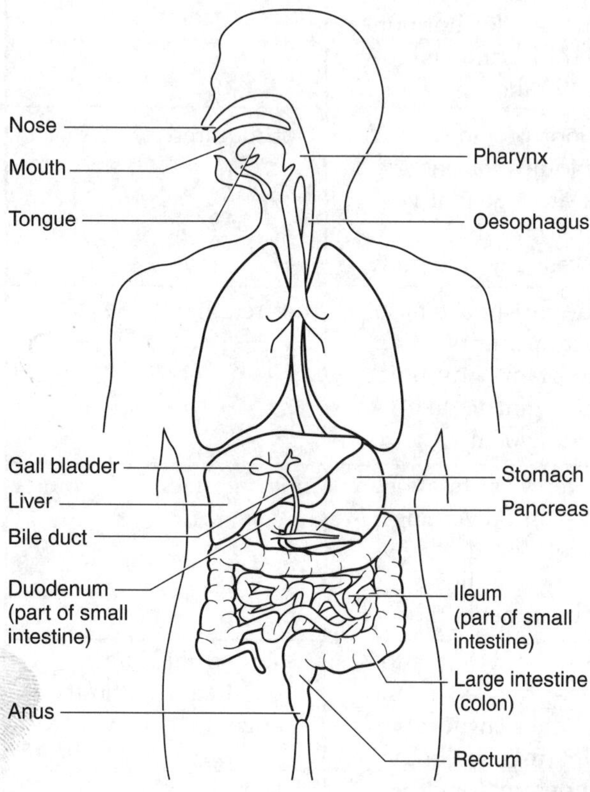


**Figure 3.22 The alimentary canal**

*Ingestion* is the act of food being taken into the mouth, here it is mixed with saliva, chewed and rolled into a small ball suitable for swallowing (a *bolus*). Saliva contains an enzyme called salivary amylase and this starts the process of breaking down carbohydrate starch. Many people do not chew their food for long these days as food is well cooked and refined so the amylase has only a short time to work before the bolus passes quickly down the oesophagus into the stomach.

### In the stomach

Food stays in the stomach for up to three hours and the strong muscles in the wall of the stomach churn the food into a loose paste called *chyme*. During this time, gastric glands in the stomach produce (gastric) protease often called pepsin which is poured onto food and this begins to break down proteins. Unlike the amylase, that prefers neutral conditions, pepsin favours acid conditions and hydrochloric acid also from the gastric juice is secreted on to the food simultaneously. The acid activates the pepsin to work and also helps to kill bacteria in raw foods. In babies, another enzyme, called rennin, is produced to solidify and digest milk proteins. The pH of the stomach contents falls to 1-2.

### The small intestine

Protein and carbohydrate have started to break down by the time food leaves the stomach to enter the small intestine. Two very important organs pour juices on to the chyme in the first part of the small intestine to help further breakdown.

- The liver pours bile on to the chyme. Although bile does not contain enzymes, it contains important bile salts which reduce dietary fat into tiny globules (emulsification). Bile also contains pigments that are the waste products from degraded haemoglobin released from worn-out red blood cells.

- The pancreas pours an enzyme-rich juice onto food that continues the breakdown of all three major food components:
  - protease or trypsin that acts on proteins
  - amylase that continues the breakdown of starch
  - lipase that digests fats, which have been emulsified by liver bile.
- An abundance of alkaline salts raise the pH of the gut contents in this region to 7-8 as the pancreatic enzymes work best in an alkaline medium.

| **Try it out** | Mix about 2 $cm^3$ of oil with about 4 $cm^3$ of water and let it stand for a few minutes. You will see the oil float to the top and form a layer. Repeat, but this time add a small amount of bile salts (if you do not have bile salt, add a little detergent such as washing up liquid, that has a similar effect), shake and leave again. This time, you will notice that the fat remains in small globules and the solution looks milky. The effect of bile salts is to increase the surface area of the fat so that the enzyme lipase can work efficiently. |
|---|---|

The intestinal wall itself contains glands which produce enzyme-rich juices, such as:

- maltase (maltose sugar from malt to glucose)
- lactase (lactose sugar from milk to glucose and galactose)
- sucrase (sucrose cane sugar to glucose and fructose)
- dipeptidase (dipeptides to individual amino acids)

These work either on the surface or inside the epithelial cells.

The rest of the small intestine is concerned with the absorption of the end-product of digestion into the bloodstream. As well as being very long and folded, the inside wall contains thousands of tiny projections to increase the internal surface area for absorption. These are called *villi*, and each is thinwalled (one cell thick) and well supplied with both a capillary network and a branch of the lymphatic system called a lacteal. In addition, each lining epithelial cell contains hundreds of tiny microvilli which can only be seen through an electron microscope. An enormous increase in surface area is created by the villi and microvilli, ensuring fast and efficient absorption of nutrients (Figure 3.23).

The end-products of protein and carbohydrate digestion, namely glucose and other monosaccharide sugars and amino acids, diffuse through the walls of the villi into the blood capillaries, while the fatty acids and glycerol pass into the lacteals. (This means 'like milk', remember the exercise with the oil and the result, milky looking!) Lacteals and lymphatics unite into larger vessels and discharge eventually into the large veins close to the heart. It is a circuitous way for fat products to enter the blood, but avoids the discharge of a lot of potentially harmful fat direct into the bloodstream (see page 150, the lymphatic system).

Amino acids and simple sugars, such as glucose, pass directly into the capillaries of the villi and these join up to form the hepatic portal vein that carries these

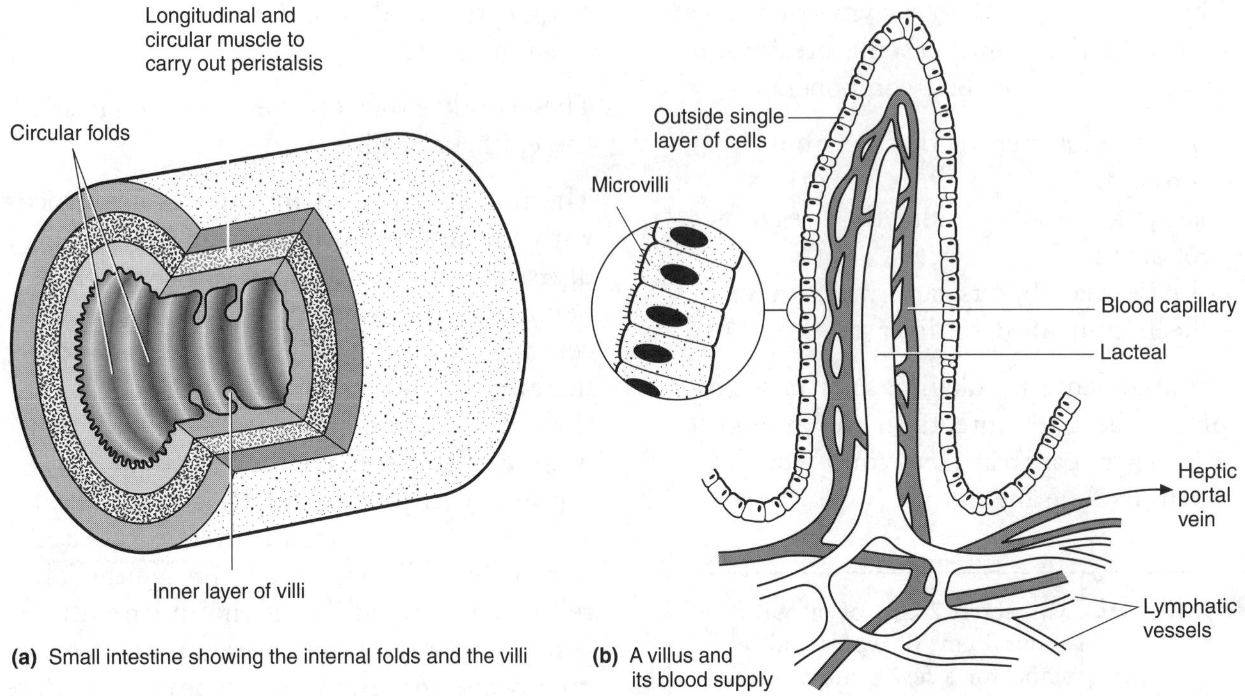


**Figure 3.23 The small intestine contains thousands of villi and microvilli**

products to the liver and breaks up into liver capillaries (see Figure 3.16 The human circulatory system, page 145). A portal vein is one that starts and ends in capillaries, unlike most other blood vessels which have capillaries at only one end.

The end-products of digestion have been absorbed in to the blood and are transported either to cells, if the raw materials are required immediately, or to storage depots around the body or broken down.

## The liver

One of the largest storage organs in the body is the liver. Glucose is turned into glycogen to be stored here and in the muscles. A hormone called insulin is responsible for this (see page 169). When the glycogen stores are full, excess glucose is converted to fat and insulin is again responsible for this conversion. Amino acids, surplus to the needs of the body, cannot be stored and the liver breaks them down in a process called **deamination**.

Amino acids (and their parent proteins) are nitrogen-containing compounds, and the nitrogen part is detached and converted into a substance called **urea** that is excreted from the blood by the kidneys (see page 156). The rest of the molecule can be used for energy. The liver also stores fat-soluble vitamins until they are required.

### Think it over

In the western world, most people consume excess protein in their diet and it is degraded through deamination into urea, making extra work for livers and kidneys; in underdeveloped countries, however, protein foods are in short supply and many people suffer serious health problems because of protein deprivation.

Mineral salts dissolve into ions in the digestive juices and are absorbed into the blood along with amino acids and glucose. Water-soluble vitamins follow the same route, but fat-soluble vitamins are transported with the fatty acids and glycerol via the lymphatic system to the liver.

Fatty acids are converted to triglycerides and used to:

- make external and internal cell membranes along with protein molecules
- manufacture steroid hormones
- protect delicate body organs against knocks (fat becomes liquid at body temperature)
- form a long term store of energy underneath the skin and around organs
- insulate the body against heat loss.

Fibre/cellulose is not absorbed at all and passes out as part of the body motions or faeces.

### Think it over

When the alimentary canal is irritated by toxins (poisons) from bacteria such as Salmonella, the food is rushed along the gut too fast for much watery juice to be reabsorbed and so the faeces are far more fluid, a condition we call diarrhoea. The irritation may also cause vomiting upwards. This loss of water can cause serious dehydration problems, particularly serious in babies and the elderly who have inefficient water balance systems.

Monitoring the nature, colour and consistency of faeces and vomit can be important with some clients. Loss of blood from either end of the gut indicates a medical problem such as gastric ulcer, haemorrhoids, colitis, polyps or cancer of the bowel. If the blood loss is high up in the intestine, the blood itself becomes partially digested and the faeces appear black, this is called melaena. Loss of blood from the gut should always be investigated.

## The large intestine

As food passes along the alimentary canal, the digestive glands have poured large volumes of enzyme-rich juices onto the food. The body cannot afford to lose this quantity of essential water, so the purpose of the large intestine is to return this water into the blood by re-absorption. By the time the food residue has reached the last part of the large intestine, known as the rectum, a semi-solid motion has been formed. Faeces contain cellulose, dead bacteria and scraped-off gut lining cells. It is coloured brown by the bile pigments.

?

There are more than 25 000 cases of cancer of the large intestine each year in the UK, accounting for 20 per cent of all deaths from cancer. The disease is much more common in western countries and current thinking is that diets which are high in red meat and fat and low in fibre content are probably to blame. There is also a genetic factor, with siblings and children of affected victims being more likely than the average person to contract the condition. Contrary to public opinion, this type of cancer can produce no pain until late in the disease. Changes in the production of faeces, bowel habits and blood mixed in with the faeces are more likely to alert attention to the condition than pain.

| Try it out | Make yourself a table to show the different regions of the alimentary tract, the digestive secretions, enzymes produced and their effects. |
|---|---|

## The renal system

We have already looked at the process of deamination of amino acids by the liver to produce urea that enters the blood stream. One of the chief functions of the renal system is to remove this, together with surplus water and salts, from the body in a process called **excretion.**

Excretion is the elimination of the waste products of metabolism. As well as the kidneys and liver, the other main organs of excretion are the skin and lungs, removing water and carbon dioxide.

| Try it out | Make a table to show the main organs of excretion, excretory products and their sources of origin. |
|---|---|

The renal system consists of two kidneys and the tubes leading from them to the bladder called the ureters, the bladder and the urethra. The only difference between males and females is that the urethra in the male is longer and also serves as part of the reproductive system as it is used to convey semen (spermatozoa and gland secretions) during copulation. Short renal arteries leave the aorta to enter each kidney and renal veins carry the blood from the kidneys to the inferior vena cava. The kidneys are dark red in colour because they receive one quarter of the cardiac output.

### The kidneys

Each kidney holds approximately one million microscopic units called nephrons that are responsible for producing urine. Urine travels to the bladder down the ureters and is voided at regular intervals from the bladder via the urethra.

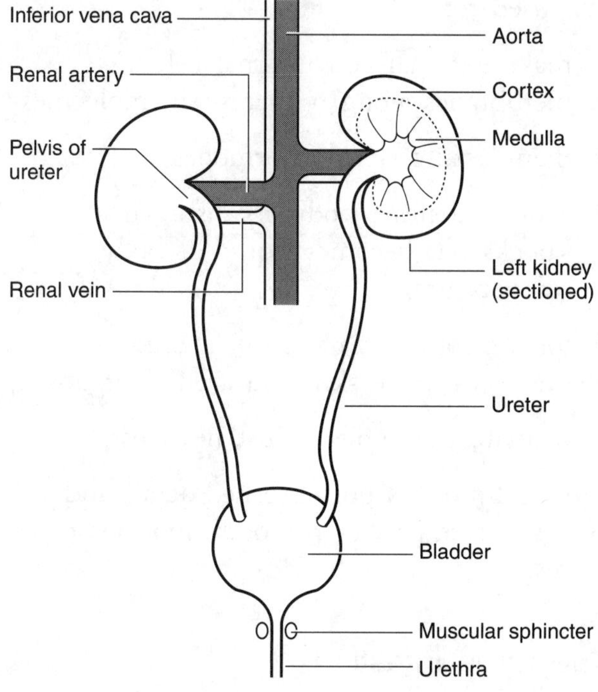


**Figure 3.24 Diagram of the renal system**

The renal artery enters the kidney and breaks up into many tiny capillaries that form knots called *glomeruli*, held tightly inside the first cup-shaped part of the nephrons – the Bowman's capsule. The capillary, which exits from each glomerulus, is narrower than that which entered, resulting in a 'traffic jam' of blood and raised pressure. The pressure is responsible for forcing out about 10 per cent of the plasma through the one-cell thick wall of the Bowman's capsule and glomerulus to enter the cavity of the Bowman's capsule.

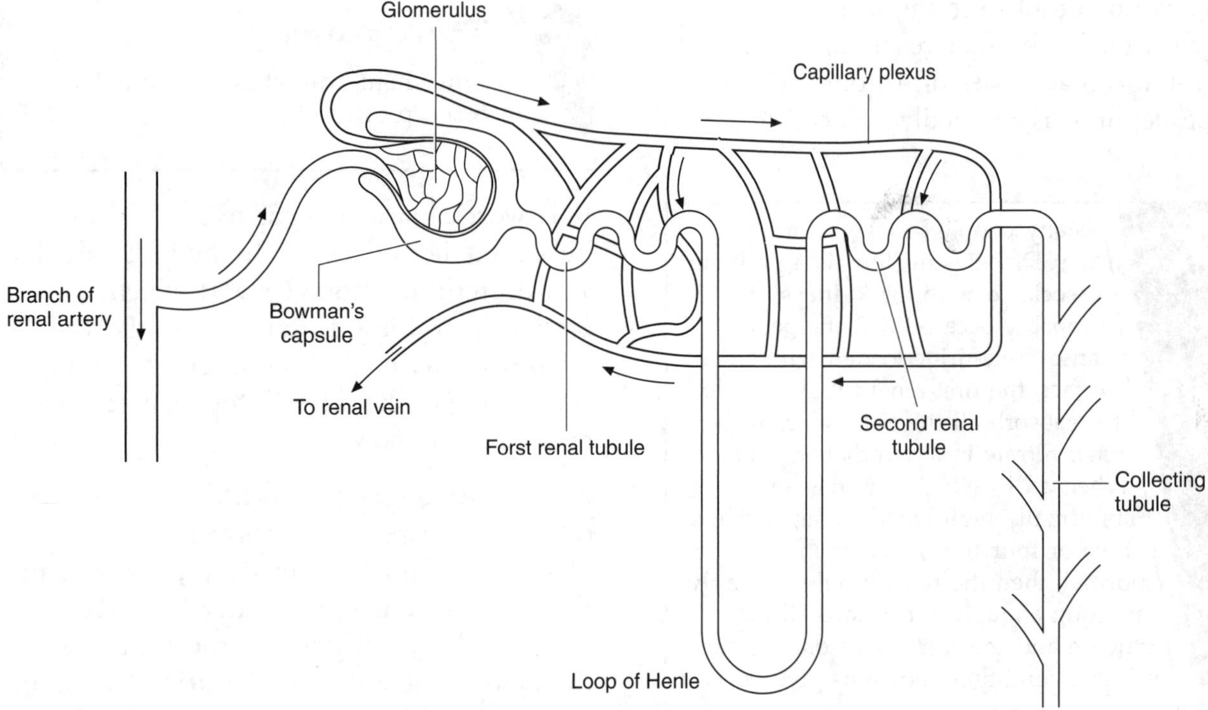


**Figure 3.25 Diagram to show the structure of a nephron**

Note that blood cells and plasma proteins are too large to be filtered and remain in the blood. This process is called ultrafiltration and it is dependent on the fairly small glomerular pressure.

> **Think it over**
>
> If an individual suffers from a haemorrhage or severe shock, their BP falls due to a lack of circulating blood; this leads to a fall in glomerular pressure and a decrease in the amount of renal filtrate produced. Why is this an advantage in the short term?

The fluid is called glomerular or renal filtrate and it is not yet urine. It consists of water, urea, salts, glucose, amino acids and other dissolved materials. Many of these are useful to the body and cannot be wasted, so the rest of the nephron is concerned with re-absorption of useful materials and tailoring the composition of urine to suit the needs of the body at any given time.

> **Think it over**
>
> John has a cardiac output of 5.75dm3/min. How much renal filtrate will he produce in his kidney nephrons in one hour?

We have already looked at the need for food and the fact that glucose and amino acids are used for energy, growth and repair, so they must be saved and returned to the blood. The first coiled part of the nephron tubule is closely surrounded by a capillary network, and is concerned with re-absorption of all glucose, all amino acids, 88 per cent of water and salts, particularly sodium and chloride ions, as these are important chemicals of body fluids.

There is no contol over the selective reabsorption in the first renal tubule and the volume that passes on through the rest of the nephron is markedly reduced.

?

Many people believe incorrectly that Diabetes mellitus is a problem associated with the kidneys, probably because diabetic people can excrete urine loaded with sugar. In fact, the first renal tubule is able to reabsorb all the glucose from the renal filtrate in a non-diabetic person. When a diabetic person has an abnormally high blood sugar, perhaps three or four times greater than normal, then the renal tubule is simply not long enough to reabsorb all the glucose and the rest passes on into the urine, a condition known as glycosuria.

The renal filtrate passes on to the loop of Henlé and is now much reduced in volume, containing water, salts and urea. The concentration of urea has now increased significantly because of the reduced volume. This part of the nephron carries out a special task of producing a high sodium concentration in the surrounding medulla and is responsible for concentrating urine. The second part of the renal tubule after the loop of Henlé tailors the water and salt concentrations to suit the body's circumstances, and it requires the assistance of the endocrine system in managing this.

**Diuresis** means a copious flow of urine and there are many natural substances which act as *diuretics*, such as tea and alcohol. You may have heard of a client or a relative who takes 'water' tablets; these are diuretic medicines and are often prescribed for people with a high BP.

**Think it over**

Why should diuretics help to reduce blood pressure?

It is worth knowing that one of the most important hormones in the body is called anti-diuretic hormone (ADH) which is produced by the pituitary gland and the hypothalamus in the brain. The name of this hormone should tell you that it helps to reduce the flow urine.

As the filtrate passes down the second renal tubule the water is reabsorbed into the blood if antidiuretic hormone is present in the bloodstream. If the water has been reabsorbed then it has left the filtrate, so the amount of water in the urine has been reduced and the volume is smaller. ADH is produced when body water is getting short and therefore the blood is more concentrated than it should be. You will find more about water regulation on page 168 under homeostasis.

A hormone from the adrenal cortex called *aldosterone* similarly controls the amount of sodium in the body.

The filtrate runs through the area known as the medulla and you will recall that this is an area where sodium has built up to a high concentration. Surplus water leaves the filtrate by **osmosis** in this area.

The definition of osmosis is: the movement of water molecules from a region of high concentration (of water molecules) to a low concentration (of water molecules) through a partially permeable membrane.

This might at first seem confusing but remember that if you have many water molecules then there is a smaller number of other molecules, in ordinary terms the solution is a weak one. A more concentrated solution has fewer water molecules and more of other types.

?

Osmosis is a special case of diffusion, only concerned with water molecules, and it takes place through a partially permeable membrane such as the cell membranes of the tubular cells.

### Urination

Once the relevant hormones have controlled the filtrate content, the fluid is known as urine and it flows from the tip of each kidney pyramid through the pelvis of the ureter, down the ureter itself to collect in the bladder. As the bladder approaches 70 per cent capacity, nervous impulses are sent to the brain and an individual feels the need to urinate. At a convenient time, the bladder muscle contracts, sphincters relax and urine is forced out through the urethra to the exterior. If the warning signals are continually ignored then the bladder will empty itself automatically. This is what happens in babies before their nervous systems and muscular co-ordination are sophisticated enough to provide control. It can also happen in older people who may have suffered strokes or nervous and muscular degeneration so that they have lost control. Losing control over urination is termed incontinence.

The kidneys of some people fail to work effectively (renal failure) and they must either have regular dialysis to remove the waste products by a kidney machine or have a kidney transplant.

## The nervous system

This system is the fastest means of communication in the human body, used to control, co-ordinate and inform organs of change. The nervous system consists of:

- the central nervous system (brain and spinal cord)
- peripheral nerves (cranial and spinal nerves)
- the autonomic nervous system.

All consist of nerve cells (or neurones), their fibres and supporting cells (neuroglia).

### The central nervous system

Neurones bringing nerve impulses from sensory receptors to the central nervous system (CNS) are *sensory neurones* and those bringing impulses from the CNS to effect change are *motor neurones*. Where neurones link these, they are known as *relay*, *connector* or *internuncial neurones*. Information from external sources such as the skin receptors responding to environmental temperature change, pain, pressure, touch, light, sound, taste, smell, etc. are said to be under the influence of the *somatic nervous system* (CNS and peripheral nerves). Changes within the body, such as alteration of heart and breathing rate, rhythmic contractile activity of smooth muscle, are under the control of the autonomic nervous system.

There are large numbers of sensory receptors of different types in the human body, each type responding to a particular type of stimulation. Some reach our conscious levels, like pain, change of external temperature, etc., while many others are continually monitoring at a subconscious level, such as changes in blood pressure, flow of digestive juices, etc.

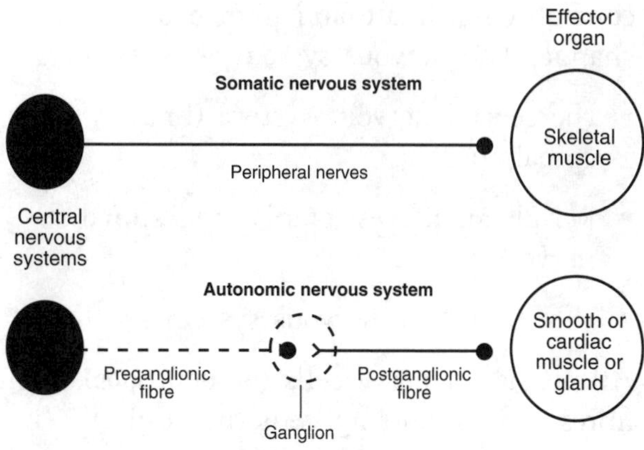


**Figure 3.26 The somatic and autonomic nervous system**

A stimulus may be defined as a change in environment which activates sensory neurones. The role of sensory neurones is to respond to such a stimulus and convert it to nerve impulses. This process is known as *transduction* and sensory receptors function as *transducers*. It must be emphasised at this point that all impulses are similar. In other words, impulses derived from pain receptors are no different from impulses, say, from a change in temperature. How then, are we able to tell the difference? The subsequent pathway and destination of those impulses cause us to interpret them differently. For example, light impulses activate photoreceptors in the light sensitive retina of the eye and impulses travel to the hindmost part of the brain, the *occipital cortex*, to be interpreted as pictures – we describe this as seeing or visualising. Impulses from sound receptors in the organ of Corti (the audioreception part of the ear) travel to a completely different part of the brain, the *temporal lobe*, to be interpreted as sound. The actual impulses are identical. It is possible in theory to 'transplant' the nerve carrying the impulses from the organ of Corti to the occipital lobe and have sounds interpreted as vision, and vice versa. So, if you rang a bell in such circumstances, the ringing could be interpreted visually, though it probably would appear as a series of flashing lights rather than an organised scene. This produces another problem – how do we know whether a stimulus is slight or marked if the outcome is the same? Each impulse, once produced, has exactly the same magnitude as the next impulse, i.e. there are no small or large impulses. Differentiation of information comes through in the spacing and frequency of impulses. This can be seen in Figure 3.27.

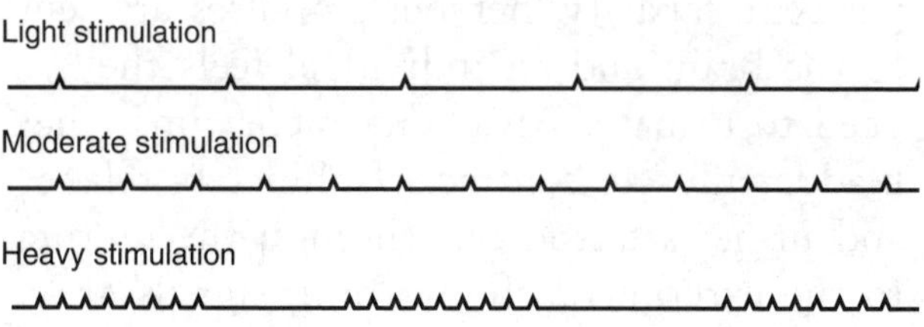


**Figure 3.27 Differences in spacing and frequency of impulses**

The nerve impulse, also known as an *action potential*, is a wave of electrical excitation produced by stimulations of a neurone. The stimulus results in changes in ionic concentrations. This wave of excitation travels down the neurone until it reaches the branched endings known as *synaptic knobs*. Once there, a minute break in protoplasmic continuity between neurones or neurone/gland or muscle interface must be overcome. The tiny gap between excitable cells like this is called a *synaptic cleft* and is filled with extracellular fluid. At synapses, impulses cause the release of neurotransmitter molecules to flood the cleft, diffuse across and attach to specific receptors on the next (or post-synaptic) neurone's cell membrane. Once the receptors are 'filled' sufficiently, a further wave of excitement is triggered down the post-synaptic neurone.

It can be seen from this description that a wave of electrical excitation becomes transformed into chemical signals across synapses and converted back to electrical phenomena in the next cell.

It is interesting and vital to note that impulses are able to travel in only one direction across a synapse as the facilities for producing neurotransmitters are present only at the expanded endings of the first (or pre-synaptic) neurone.

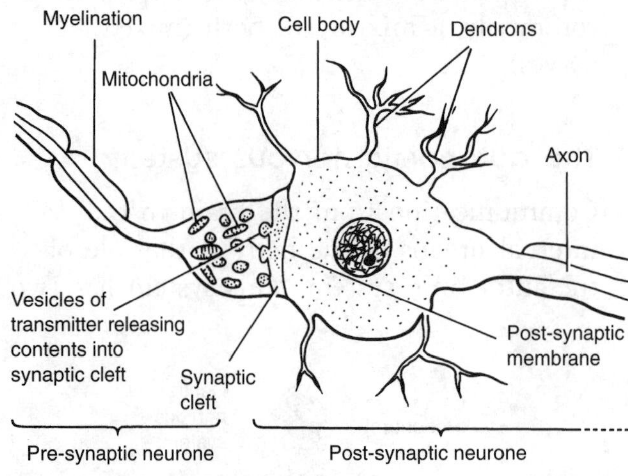


**Figure 3.28 A synapse**

Neurotransmitter chemicals form the main vehicle for drug action on the nervous system. Any inhibitor of the transmitter must slow down the action of impulses crossing the synapse and vice versa. Once released the transmitter is broken down fairly rapidly (or impulses begin to merge) and the products of the breakdown are recycled into neurotransmitter molecules again using energy from ATP in the neurones' mitochondria. This process takes time and, if there has been continued stimulation over a steady period, neuronal fatigue might occur due to depletion of neurotransmitter molecules. There may be hundreds of synapses impinging on one neurone.

Usually several synaptic endings need to release transmitters at the same time for a nerve impulse to be set up in the post-synaptic cell (*spatial summation*). When one synaptic ending receives impulses several times in rapid succession, these also may be added together to create a post-synaptic impulse and this is known as *temporal summation* (see Figure 3.29). Impulses generated by weak stimuli may not be adequate to summate either in space or time, so the impulse gets no further than the first synapse.

In this way, sensory overload is avoided – we are not constantly aware of the feel of our clothes on our skin, for instance and the feel of chairs, patterns of noise, etc. do not pass into the memory part of the brain. If selection from the constant bombardment of our senses did not occur, human brains would be enormous. Synapses therefore act

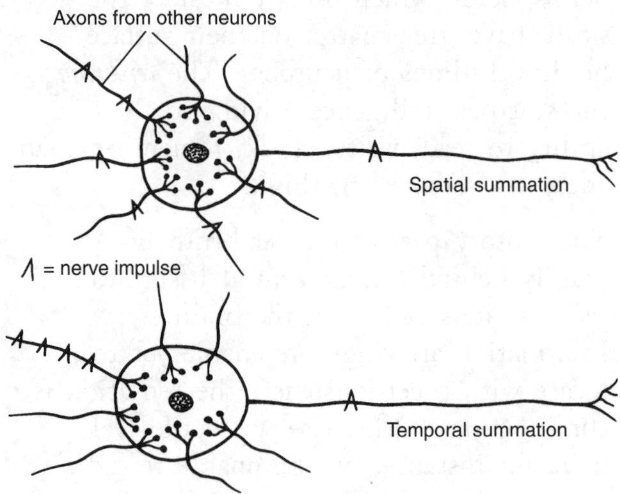


**Figure 3.29 Spatial and temporal summation**

as 'goalkeepers' of information, passing on only the essential in communication and co-ordination.

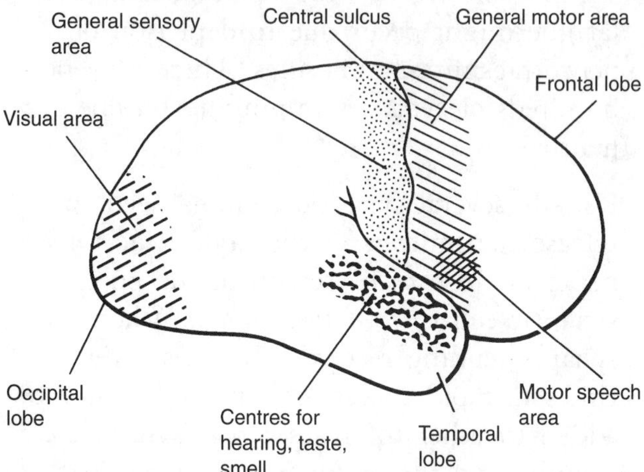


**Figure 3.30 The functional areas of the brain**

## The brain

The greatest bulk of neurones used in communication function in the brain. There are two types of matter in the brain, *grey* and *white matter*. Grey matter contains the vital cell bodies of the neurones, while white matter consists of the tracts of fibres, in practice axons and dendrons, on their way to and from other parts of the brain or other organs. The large cerebral hemispheres, which occupy most of the skull, have grey matter on their surface holding billions of neurones. The *cerebrum* is the seat of intelligence, giving us the ability to read, write, speak, remember, plan ahead and, above all, think.

The sensory part of the cerebrum lies mainly behind a large central fissure (or *sulcus* as it is called) in the brain. Information arriving here enables us to locate with precision where the sensation is coming from. Otherwise we would feel pain, for instance, but be unable to locate exactly where the pain was coming from. The intact sensory area of the cortex is essential for this. Centres for speech, hearing, taste and smell lie below the general sensory area in a protruding side lobe – the *temporal lobe*. The visual area lies at the back of the brain. (See Figure 3.30.)

The motor area of the brain lies in front of the central sulcus in the cerebrum. Stimulation in this area leads to muscle contraction in a specific location on the opposite side of the body. Conversion of speech into thoughts and thoughts into speech take place in an area close to the temporal lobe, but within the motor area. Transference of impulses between the CNS and other parts of the body uses the routes provided by the peripheral nerves (Figure 3.31). These are collections of axons (motor nerves), dendrons (sensory nerves) or, more commonly, a mixture of both (mixed nerves).

## The autonomic nervous system

Communication from the brain to the internal organs of the body is the role of the autonomic system. This system has two

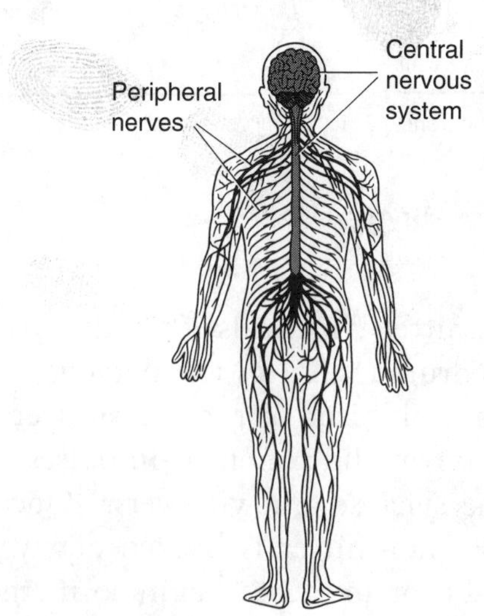


**Figure 3.31 The central nervous system and peripheral nerves**

distinct parts known as the *sympathetic* and *parasympathetic branches*. These serve to act rather like a brake, slowing down, or as an accelerator, speeding activities up. Unfortunately, it is not possible to say that the sympathetic is the accelerator and so on, because both systems carry out a combination of activities. There is some value, however, in considering the role of each system and this can lead to a satisfactory understanding.

The role of the sympathetic nervous system is to prepare the body for emergencies, commonly known as *fright*, *flight* and *fight* reactions. This is a response built to enable survival from predators and is not wholly suitable for modern-day living, but unfortunately we have to live with it. The main activities of the sympathetic system are:

- releasing more energy-rich glucose from storage
- providing more oxygen to unlock the glucose energy
- distributing the energy, providing raw materials to muscles and a few other places
- bypassing most organs not useful in an emergency, such as skin and the alimentary canal
- activating any other activity useful in an emergency, such as sweat secretion, making skin slippery to predators and aiding cooling
- enhancing the activity of the nervous system by harnessing hormonal communication as well.

As you will see from Figure 3.33 these functions involve the cardio-respiratory system to a great extent. The parasympathetic system, by contrast, is activated more during peace and contentment, calming the heart and breathing rates, yet speeding up digestive processes.

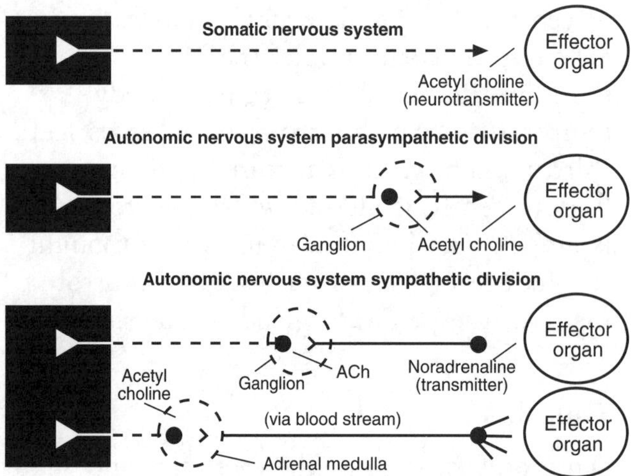


**Figure 3.32 The sympathetic and parasympathetic systems of the autonomic nervous system**

| | Sympathetic nervous system | Parasympathetic nervous system |
|---|---|---|
| 1 | Leaves thoracic and lumbar sections of spinal cord | Leaves cranial and sacral regions of the central nervous system |
| 2 | Short pre-ganglionic neurones and long post-ganglionic neurones | Long pre-ganglionic neurones and short post-ganglionic neurones |
| 3 | Ganglionic chain at the side of the spinal cord | Ganglions in the walls of organs |
| 4 | Associated with fight, fright and flight response | Associated with peace and contentment |
| 5 | Closely linked with medulla of adrenal gland | Not linked in this way |

**Figure 3.33 The differences between the sympathetic and parasympathetic nervous systems**

## The hypothalamus

The hypothalamus lies between the thalamus and the pituitary gland. It contains several groups of neurones collected in centres that regulate important features for survival. For example, the thermoregulation centre regulates body temperature, the thirst centre makes us feel thirsty when water is required and the feeding centre is alerted when the stomach is empty. The hypothalamus is also thought to produce hormones itself and to control many of the pituitary gland hormones.

## The skin

Sense organs, such as the eyes, ears and tongue are collections of sensory receptors specially adapted to detecting particular stimuli. One of the most important sense organs in the body is the skin.

Our intact skin forms a most effective barrier between the complex internal environment within the body and the external environment that teems with micro-organisms, poisons, harmful rays and physical dangers such as sharp points and rough surfaces. We even harness harmless micro-organisms to live on the surface of the skin, to act as guardians, preventing more harmful disease-causing micro-organisms called pathogens from 'squatting' there and causing disease. If these are removed by antiseptics or other chemical means, there is the danger of removing this protective barrier. Washing regularly with hot, soapy water removes many harmless bacteria and keeps their population in check as bacteria double their numbers every 20 minutes!

> **Think it over**
>
> One of the most important ways of preventing infection is regular hand washing particularly after going to the toilet, handling raw food, stroking pets, dealing with wounds etc.

The external surface of the skin is protected by layers of dead cells that form both waterproof and bacteria-proof barriers. If the skin is damaged, pathogens may enter and cause infection.

> **Think it over**
>
> How many times has your skin surface become infected when the surface is intact? The 'dead cell' barrier is very effective.

Once the skin surface is breached, the white cells in the blood become very active and engage in phagocytosis (engulfing and digesting the bacteria) and the production of antibodies that neutralise the invading micro-organisms. Skin contains numerous types of nerve endings capable of detecting changes in external temperature, touch, pressure and pain. The finger tips (and a baby's tongue) are one of the most sensitive areas of the body and contain large numbers of sensory nerve endings. The back of the trunk and back of the hand contains far fewer and is less sensitive.

| **Try it out** | Choose a partner and test the sensitivity of the fingertips and back of the hand by pressing *lightly* with either one or two compass or sharp pencil points when he or she is blindfolded. Ask your partner to say how many points he or she can feel and record the accuracy of their answers. The points should be only 3 to 5 mm apart. |
|---|---|

As well as defending the body and acting as a sense organ, the skin has an extremely important part to play in regulating our body temperature – see page 168 on homeostasis.

## Endocrine system

This system interlocks and works with the nervous system to provide communication and co-ordination throughout the human body. Whereas the nervous system is based on waves of excitation passing down specialised neurones, the endocrine system consists of several glands secreting chemicals known as *hormones* to effect change. Hormones, literally meaning 'to urge on', are secreted directly in to the bloodstream and use the circulatory system as a route for distribution. A common analogy often made is that the nervous system is like a telephone system, fast and efficient but only able to go if the correct wiring is available, whereas the endocrine system is like the postal system, much slower but able to get to every cell. Figure 3.34 summarises the differences between the two systems.

| Nervous system | Endocrine system |
|---|---|
| Electro-chemical phenomena form 'message' – action potentials or nerve impulses | Chemical molecules for 'message' – known as hormones |
| Travels down nerve fibres | Travels in blood stream |
| Has rapid transmission | Much slower transmission |
| Travels to cells supplied only by nerve fibres | Travels to all cells in body |

**Figure 3.34 The differences between the nervous system and the endocrine system**

## Hormones

Hormones can be steroids (derived from cholesterol), proteins or products of proteins (peptides, amines). They affect certain cells which are fitted with cell membrane receptors for that particular hormone, either directly through an enzyme-based system or via the nucleic acids in the nucleus. Most hormones are secreted in short bursts with little or no secretion in between. Under stimulation the bursts become more frequent, so raising the blood concentration of that particular hormone. In the absence of stimulation, the bursts become less frequent and the blood hormone levels decrease. This is part of a feedback process, see page 163.

Hormones are generally used where the effect is long-term or where time is not an important factor, such as growth and control of reproduction. Figure 3.35 shows the location of the major endocrine glands.

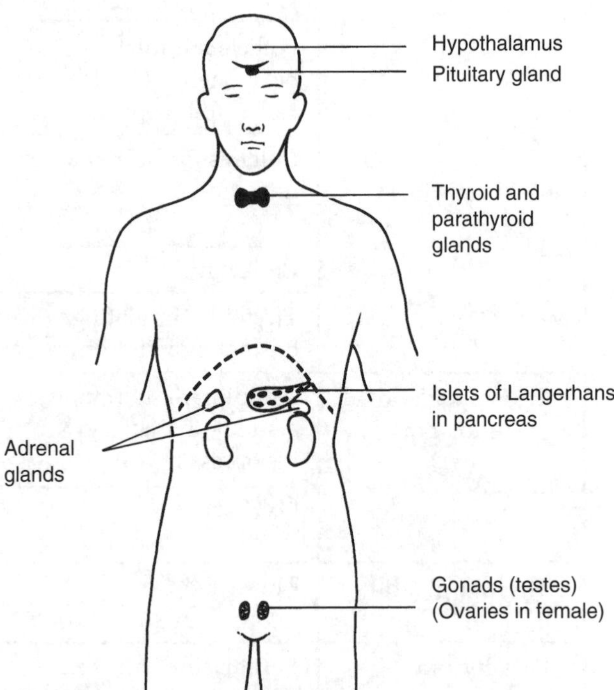


**Figure 3.35 The main endocrine glands in the body.**

The basic functions of hormones are:

- control of most stages of reproduction
- significant role in growth and development
- assistance with smooth and cardiac muscle contraction
- regulation of metabolism, including energy release
- control of extracellular fluid volume and composition
- maintenance of homeostasis, even in emergency situations.

## The endocrine system

Table 3.4 shows the major hormones and their actions.

| Endocrine gland | Major hormones | Summary of the actions of the hormones |
|---|---|---|
| Hypothalamus also part of the brain | Releasing and inhibitory factors that control other endocrine glands | Stimulation and inhibition of many glands, particularly the pituitary gland |
| Pituitary gland – anterior part | Growth hormone | Skeletal, muscular and soft tissue growth |
| | Adrenocorticotrophic hormone (ACTH) also known as corticotropin | Stimulation of the hormone cortisol from the adrenal cortex |
| | Follicle stimulating hormone (FSH) also called follitropin | Stimulates the production of gametes from the gonads |
| | Luteinising hormone or lutropin | Causes ovulation and the formation of the corpus luteum in females. Causes testosterone to be secreted from the testis in males |
| | Prolactin | Stimulates breastmilk formation after childbirth |
| | Thyroid stimulating hormone or thyrotropin | Stimulates the thyroid gland to produce thyroxine |
| Pituitary gland – posterior part | Antidiuretic hormone also known as vasopressin | Causes water reabsorption in the second renal tubules and collecting ducts. |
| | Oxytocin | Causes rhythmical contractions of uterine muscle in childbirth |
| Thyroid gland | Thyroxine | Regulates growth and development and controls the basic metabolic rate |
| Parathyroid glands | Parathyrin | Controls calcium in blood and body tissues |
| Adrenal glands – the medulla | Adrenaline and noradrenaline | Stimulates the fright, flight and fight response to stress. Involved in the regulation of blood sugar |
| Adrenal glands – the cortex | Cortisol | Involved in regulating blood sugar and repair of body organs damaged in degenerative diseases |
| Pancreas (islets of Langerhans) | Insulin<br>Glucagon | Regulation of blood sugars |
| Ovaries | Oestrogen and progesterone | Growth and development of primary and secondary sexual organs and female secondary sexual characteristics |
| Testes | Testosterone | Growth and development of primary and secondary sexual organs and male secondary sexual characteristics |

Table 3.4 The major hormones and their actions

## Interaction of body systems

Human body systems do not work in isolation; they must interact with one another to ensure effective metabolism.

The cardiovascular system and respiratory systems work together to circulate oxygenated blood throughout the body and to remove the waste carbon dioxide and water produced during cell respiration. The nervous system, through the autonomic nerves, governs the rate at which the heart beats and the chest moves in breathing. Without a supply of oxygenated blood all body systems cease to function. The cardiovascular system is the transport route for hormones, urea and nutrients so links with the endocrine, renal and digestive systems.

The internal body organs have nerve supplies from the autonomic nervous system to speed up their actions or slow them down and almost every cell in the body is controlled by the actions of hormones, particularly insulin and thyroxine.

The digestive system is clearly linked with the endocrine system through insulin, cortisol and adrenaline which work in concert to regulate blood sugar in accordance with everyday activities. For example, when a person is digesting lunch, a rising blood sugar stimulates the production of insulin from the pancreas which, in turn lowers the blood sugar by converting it to glycogen in the liver and muscles. Two hours later, while the person is playing a game of squash, blood sugar drops. Adrenaline and glucagon are secreted to stimulate the conversion of glycogen back to glucose to elevate blood sugar to normal levels. During the game, the activity of the cardiovascular and respiratory systems will increase to drive more oxygenated blood to the muscles, raise BP, heart rate and breathing rate. The nervous system will be highly active in forming strategies to beat the opponent, contracting muscles to move and strike the ball and closing down the blood supply to unnecessary organs during the stress of the game. As the game proceeds, heat which is generated by skeletal muscles will stimulate the thermoregulation centre in the brain which will cause the sweat glands to become active and the skin capillaries to dilate – producing a hot, flushed wet skin that will lose heat to the environment. Loss of water in sweat will cause more ADH to be secreted and the kidneys will produce more concentrated urine. Every body system we have covered is therefore involved in this after-lunch game of squash!

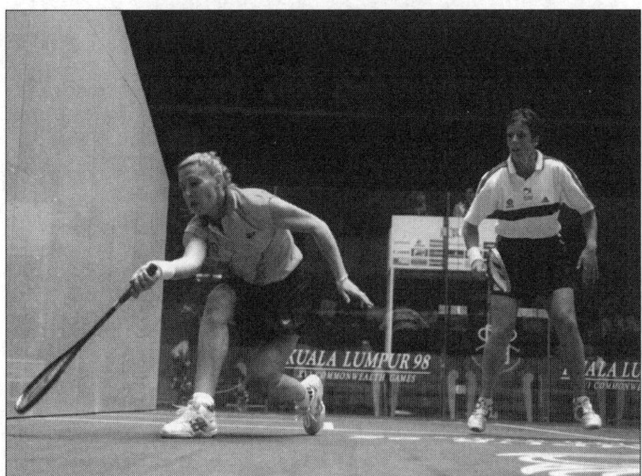


**Many human body systems are interacting together to allow these squash players to keep on playing**

| **Try it out** | Make a list or flow chart of the interaction between the systems if the squash players drink a pint of orange squash after the game is over. |
|---|---|

| **Try it out** | You could skim read the body systems again, selecting information that relates to another body system and make patterned diagrams to show interactions that you can use in your assessment evidence. |
|---|---|

## 3.2 Homeostasis

This is the process by which the human body maintains a constant internal environment despite external changes. Body organs can only maintain their functions efficiently within a narrow range of conditions such as temperature, acidity, blood pressure and so on. When a condition varies from its set point for working optimally, automatic regulatory mechanisms are activated to counteract the disturbance and re-establish the set point. This is homeostasis: it is the process that maintains the constancy or stability of the body's internal environment.

In order to accomplish this, regardless of which body system is involved, there is the need for *receptors* to detect changes in the external environment, a *control centre* (usually in the brain) to receive and act on the information from the receptors and *effectors* to act to bring the system back to normal. This is known as the *negative feedback* effect as the change is always dampened down or lessened to return the system to normal.

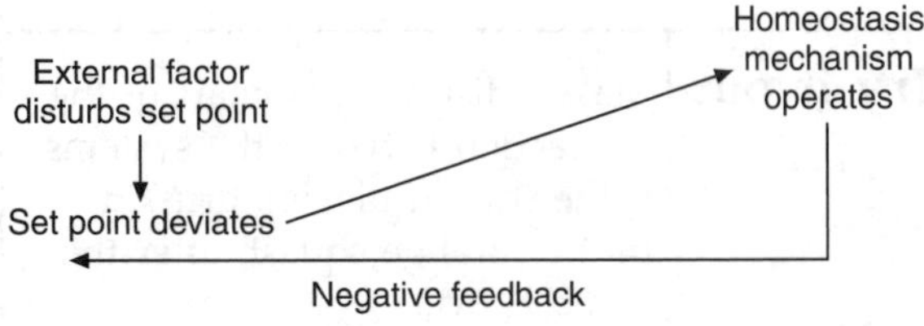


**Figure 3.36 Negative feedback in homeostasis**

Negative feedback effects are the most common types of homeostatic control.

*Positive feedback* effects are very rare in human physiology, because they stimulate greater deviations from normal and eventually result in a 'bust' situation. Childbirth, involving the continued stimulation of uterine muscle, is an example of positive feedback, resulting in 'bust' – the birth or expulsion of the foetus. We will be concerned wholly with negative feedback situations in this unit.

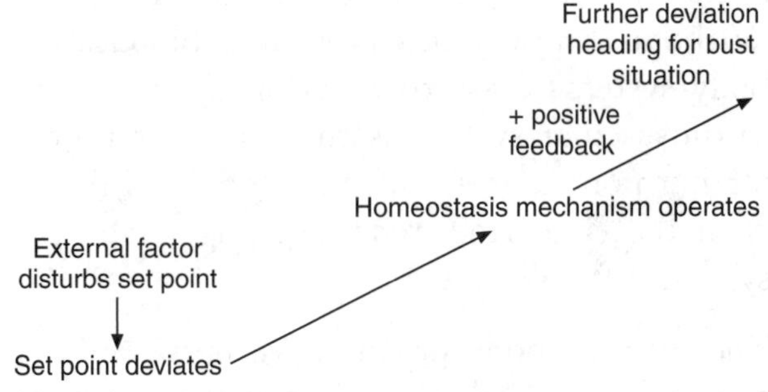


**Figure 3.37 Positive feedback in homeostasis**

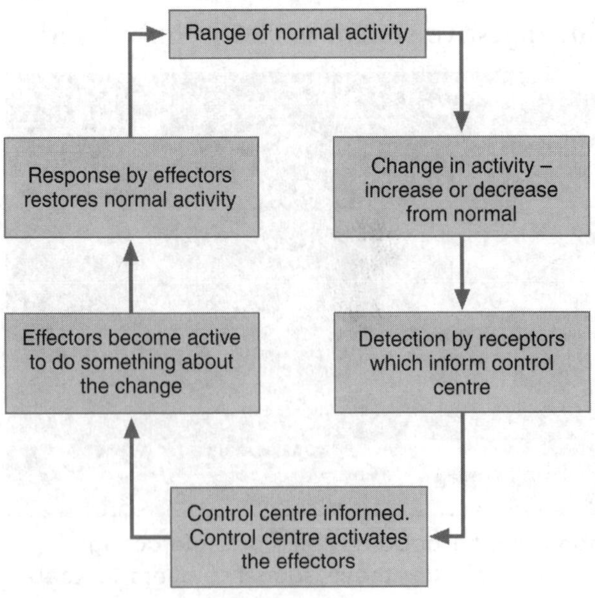


**Figure 3.38 The stages of homeostasis and negative feedback**

The flow chart in Figure 3.38 illustrates how receptors, the control centre and effectors operate to restore normal activity.

Important homeostatic mechanisms within the body are:

- maintaining blood glucose level
- body temperature regulation
- maintaining heart rate
- maintaining respiratory rate
- regulating water balance.

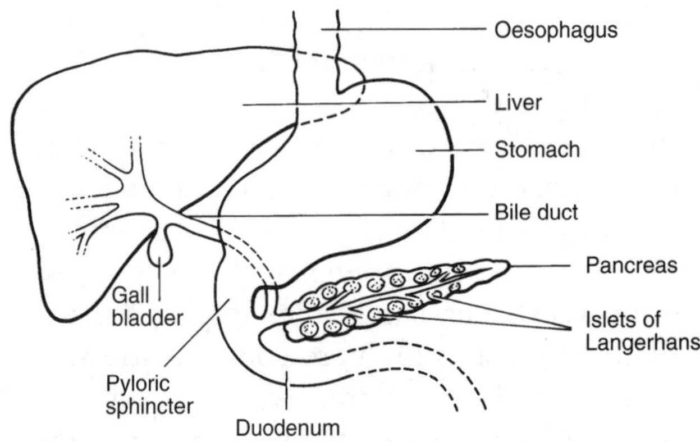


**Figure 3.39 The pancreas and islets of Langerhans**

## Maintaining blood glucose level

In the first part of this chapter we looked at the need for body cells to have a constant supply of energy to enable them to perform their functions. Energy is provided chiefly by glucose dissolved in the plasma of blood that is forced out of capillaries to make tissue fluid. Body cells cannot survive if they are not continually bathed in tissue fluid that supplies oxygen, glucose and many other essential substances. However, given that the source of glucose is food but meals are taken at periodic intervals throughout the day, and for most people not at night, there must be a homeostatic control mechanism which regulates the constant supply of blood glucose.

Glucose does not pass very readily through cell membranes to enter cells. It needs a 'helping push' from a hormone, *insulin,* released from clusters of cells (*the islets of Langerhans*) scattered throughout the pancreas which lies slightly below and behind the stomach (see Figure 3.39).

There are several types of cells in the islets of Langerhans, but the two major types are *alpha* and *beta cells* responsible for insulin secretion. During and after a meal, the digestive system breaks down complex carbohydrates to produce glucose which is absorbed through the gut lining into the bloodstream. As the level of glucose in the blood rises, the islets are stimulated to produce insulin which acts to reduce blood glucose level. As the level falls towards normal, the stimulation is inhibited – a clear example of negative feedback.

Insulin causes blood glucose level to fall by making it easier for the entry of glucose cells through the cell membranes. In addition, it converts glucose into a storage compound, *glycogen*. It is particularly good at doing this with skeletal muscle fibres and liver cells. Minor roles also involve increasing protein and lipid synthesis. Once inside cells, the glucose is either oxidised in respiration and converted to glycogen for storage, or (if glycogen stores are full) converted to fat.

When blood glucose needs to be replenished from the 'store', another islet hormone, *glucagon* (this time from the alpha cells), reverses the actions of insulin and tops up the blood glucose by converting glycogen into glucose. Glucagon is also regulated by negative feedback, controlled by the falling level of blood glucose.

Glucagon is not alone in mobilising stored glucose. A very important hormone called *adrenaline* (released from the *adrenal medulla*, the central part of the adrenal glands, when the sympathetic branch of the autonomic system is stimulated) carries out the same function. Previous reference to the sympathetic nervous system emphasised its fight, fright and flight response to stress. One of the facets of this response is the release of large amounts of glucose into the bloodstream for energy. This occurs because adrenaline converts glycogen to glucose as well. A summary of these main actions is shown in Figure 3.40.

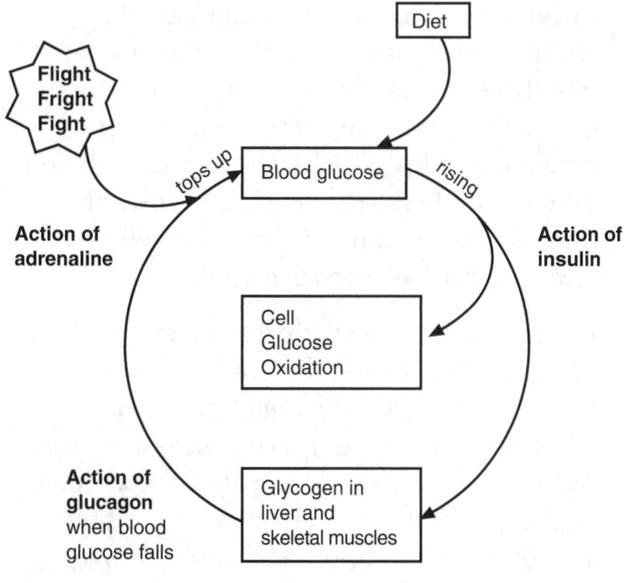


**Figure 3.40 A summary of the influences of blood glucose**

Control of blood glucose is a complex interplay of hormone actions, energy demands, state of health and outside influences. Only the major actions have been discussed here.

## Homeostatic regulation of body temperature

Humans are the only animals that can survive in both tropical and arctic conditions and this is largely due to negative feedback homeostasis mechanisms for thermo-regulation which means that under these conditions body temperature varies very little. The mechanism is shown in Figures 3.41 and 3.42.

At all times, the main aim of the thermo-regulatory systems is to maintain the vital organs of the human body (often referred to as the *core*) at a constant temperature, at the expense of the peripheral areas, chiefly the skin.

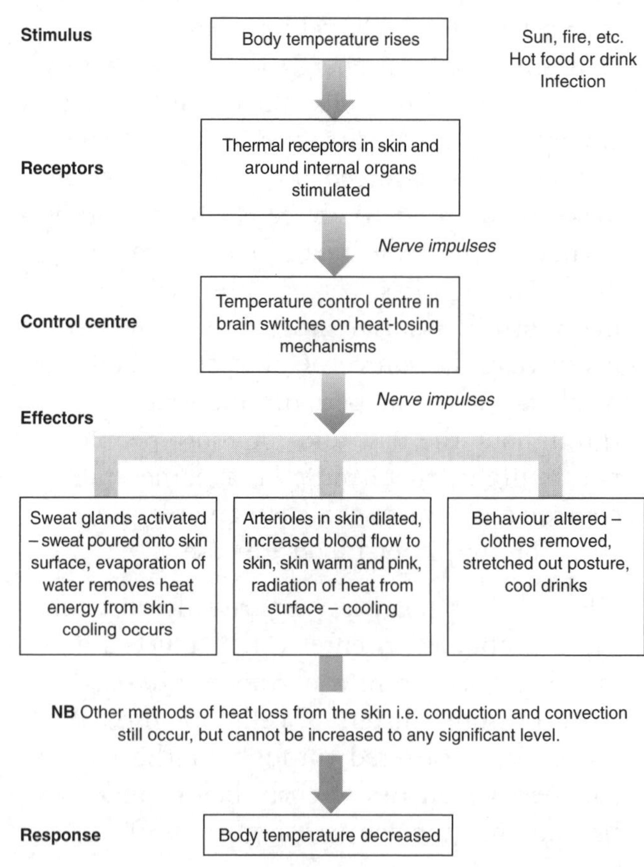


**Figure 3.41 The homoeostatic mechanism for regulating rising body temperature**

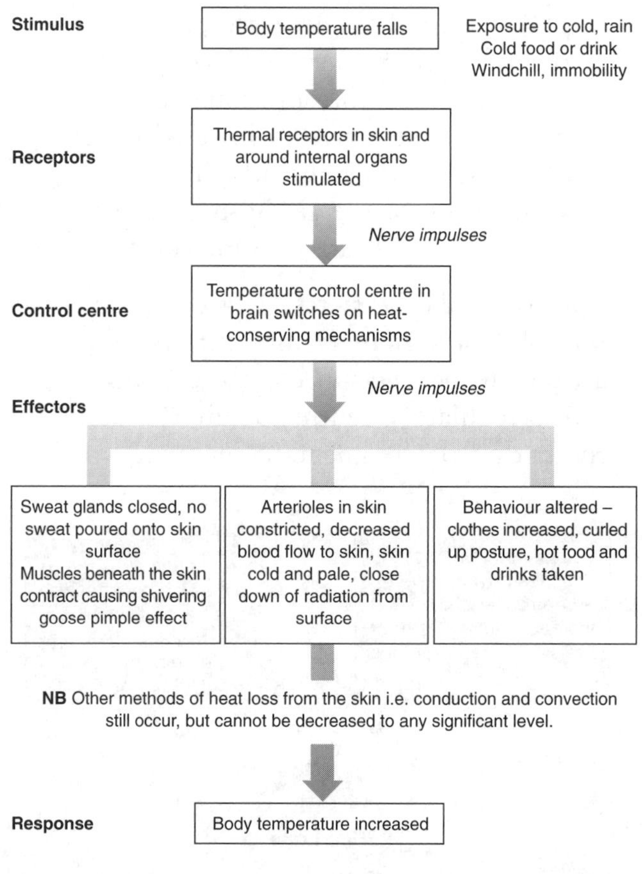


**Figure 3.42 The homoeostatic mechanism for regulating falling body temperature**

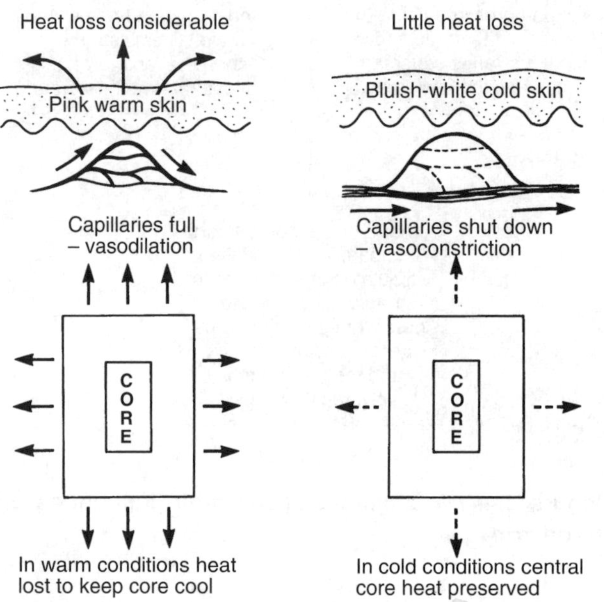


**Figure 3.43 Temperature regulation**

## Homeostatic regulation of heart rate

When any form of excitement, fear, stress or exercise is undertaken, the brain – acting as the control centre again – stimulates the release of adrenaline from the adrenal glands located on the top of each kidney. At the same time, it sends nervous impulses down the sympathetic branch of the nervous system to the heart and other organs. These actions cause the heart to beat both faster and stronger.

### Think it over

When you have been afraid or excited, have you suddenly become conscious of your heart 'pounding' away in your chest? Normally, we do not notice our heart beating, but under these circumstances, the increased rate and strength of each beat become really noticeable.

As a result, these faster stronger beats will send more blood bounding around the body – however, the blood is re-distributed between the organs and the muscles get the greatest share. The skin and digestive system receive very little blood, hence you will look pale and often feel nauseous. This is a primitive response designed to enable you to run away quickly or stand and fight, the so-called 'fight or flight' response. Blood pressure and breathing rates also rise, whereas secretions decrease making your mouth very dry and it can be quite difficult to swallow. Adrenaline is soon destroyed once the emergency is over; sympathetic nerve impulses die down and the parasympathetic impulses slow the heart rate back to normal.

## Autonomic nervous system

The sympathetic and parasympathetic branches collectively form part of the autonomic nervous system and they act rather like a brake and accelerator to the internal organs. The sympathetic is not always the accelerator and the parasympathetic the brake – sometimes they work the opposite way round on organs.

When there is no emergency the same two nerves tailor the heart rate to suit the circumstances. They are influenced by:

- increase in blood pressure. Receptors sensitive to stretch in the walls of major blood vessels such as the aorta and carotid artery are triggered when BP increases and they send impulses to the medulla of the brain. In the medulla there is a cardio-regulatory centre. Nervous impulses travel to the heart down the parasympathetic nerve called the vagus nerve and slow the heart rate. In the absence of stimulation, the reverse occurs and the sympathetic nerve impulses speed up heart rate.
- increased venous return. Stretch receptors in the major veins close to the heart are stimulated when there is more blood flowing into the right atrium and therefore an increase in BP. This type of receptor is known as a baroreceptor because it monitors pressure. In this case, heart rate needs to increase to move that blood quickly, so the sympathetic nerve to the heart sends more impulses to increase heart rate and strength
- increased carbon dioxide and low oxygen concentrations. Chemical receptors called chemoreceptors can be triggered by higher and lower concentrations of chemicals, such as oxygen, carbon dioxide, hydrogen ions (and consequently pH). Clusters of chemoreceptors exist in the walls of the aorta and the carotid arteries (called the aortic and carotid bodies) are sensitive to lowered oxygen and raised carbon dioxide. They cause stimulation of the cardio-regulatory centre and so heart rate increases.

Control of the heart rate is a complex interplay of various factors but the heart action can be fine-tuned by the brain cardio-regulatory centre to suit the needs of the body from moment to moment.

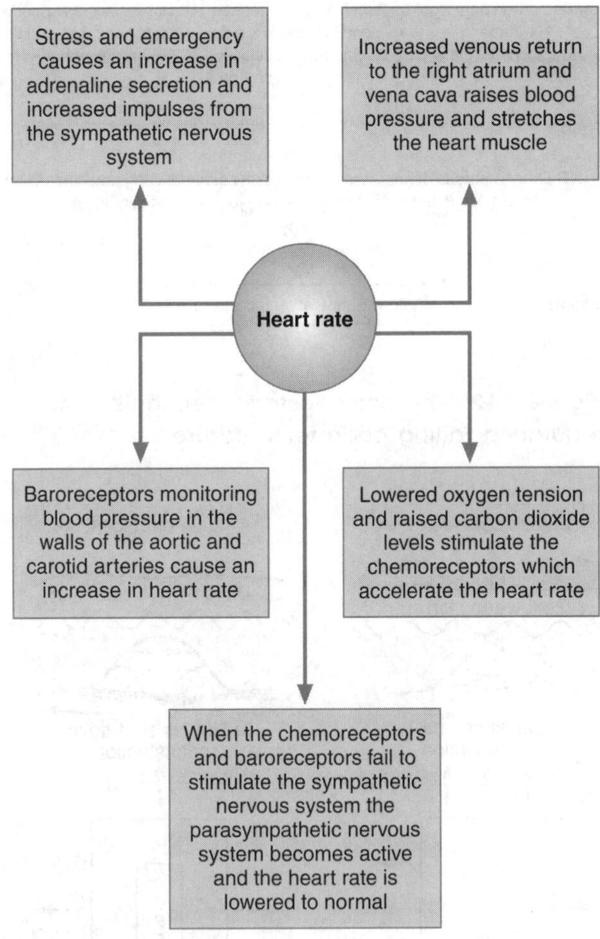


**Figure 3.44** A summary of the main influences on heart rate

## Homeostatic control of breathing rate

The medulla of the brain contains clusters of neurones which represent the respiratory centre; one cluster is responsible for inspiration and the other for expiration. In normal quiet breathing, the inspiratory centre is active for approximately two seconds followed by the expiratory centre activity for three seconds.

| **Try it out** | Calculate the normal breathing rate for an individual in normal quiet breathing with the above timings. |
|---|---|

We are all aware that we can suddenly hold our breath, take deeper breaths than normal or speed up the rate of breathing. Above the medulla in a part of the brain called the *pons* there are two further centres associated with respiration, these are:

- the pneumotaxic centre – this inhibits the inspiratory centre as the lungs fill with air, so allowing expiration to occur
- the apneustic centre that sends impulses to the inspiratory centre to prolong inspiration.

Earlier in the chapter expiration was described as an elastic recoil of the lungs and a relaxation of the intercostal muscles and the diaphragm. This is so in quiet breathing, but in forced expirations, such as blowing into a peak flow meter, expiratory centre neurones actually send impulses to the muscles causing expiration.

### Other influences on the control of breathing

Just as there is control of the rhythm of the heart so there are other influences on the control of breathing:

- Higher control from the cerebral cortex can give us voluntary control over breathing by influencing the apneustic centre.
- Stretch receptors located in the walls of the bronchi and bronchioles will inhibit the inspiratory centre when the lungs are over-filled (Hering-Breuer reflex).
- Chemoreceptors in the aortic and carotid bodies sensitive to increased hydrogen ions and carbon dioxide levels, as well as lowered oxygen tension, will stimulate the respiratory centre to cause deeper and faster breathing to wash out the increased chemicals and restore oxygen levels. The latter has to be a significant drop to exert an effect. When carbon dioxide increases, it ionises to produce hydrogen and hydrogen carbonate ions, so a rise in carbon dioxide is always partnered by a rise in hydrogen ion concentration and this lowers the pH of the blood.

| **Try it out** | Time your own quiet inspirations and expirations in seconds, after allowing time for them to settle down.<br>Then breathe forcibly and quickly about 8 or 9 times, as if you are breathing into a peak flow meter, and time how many seconds it takes to restore your inspiration. The time lapse is because you have washed carbon dioxide from your lungs and it must build up again to stimulate inspiration. |
|---|---|

The respiratory centre also exerts an influence over the cardiac centre.

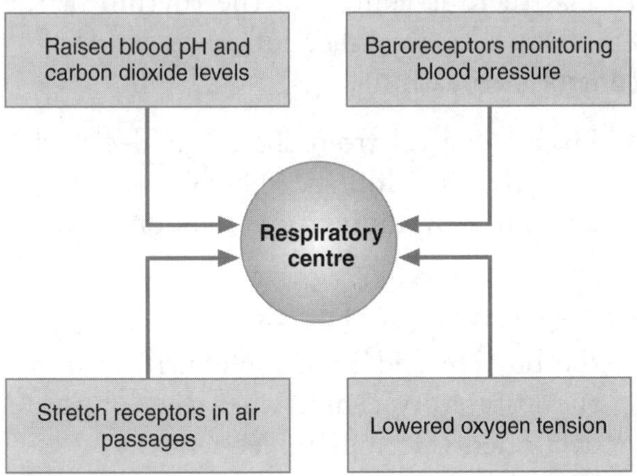


**Figure 3.45 The influences on the respiratory centre**

Muscular activity requires a great deal of energy; cells must respire more rapidly for the extra energy to be produced. More oxygen is consumed and as a result more carbon dioxide and water waste is manufactured.

The process shown in Figure 3.46 describes the sequence of events that occurs during exercise. The whole process relates back to the general concept of homeostasis, the receptors, control centre and effectors. The shaded box represents the normal and is a good place to start – *exercise* begins the deviation from normal.

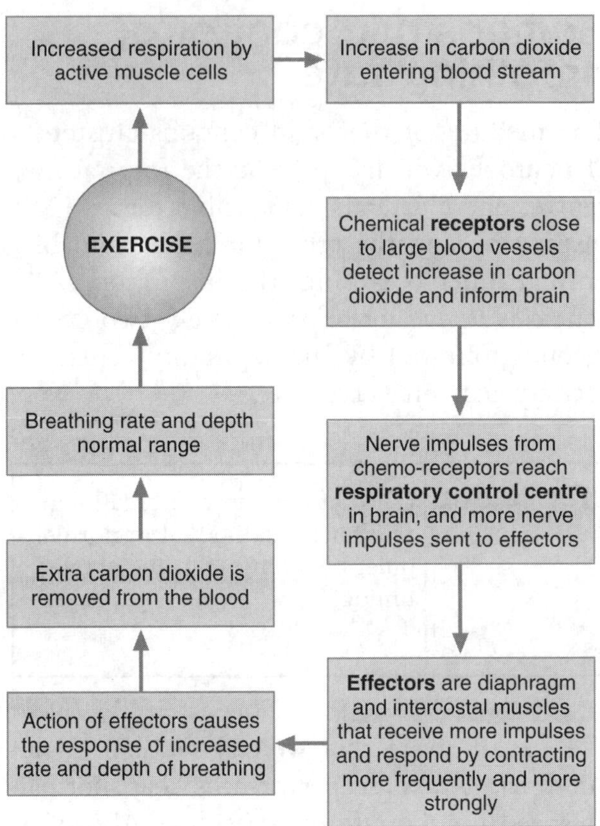


**Figure 3.46 Homeostatic control of breathing rate during exercise**

## Homeostatic control of water

### Homeostatic mechanisms regulating water levels

Most people are aware that the human body cannot survive for long without a supply of water. It is the most frequently occurring substance in the body, but like most other chemicals, its levels must be kept as constant as possible. Too little water leads to cell *dehydration* and too much to 'waterlogging' or *oedema*. Both conditions result in cell dysfunction and therefore there is a homeostatic mechanism for water regulation.

Water levels themselves are not detected by receptors, but the effect of water concentrations on *osmotic pressure* is. Special sensory receptors, called *osmoreceptors*, lie close to blood vessels in part of the brain called the *hypothalamus*. The hypothalamus is connected to a most important endocrine gland, the pituitary gland, by a short stalk. The gland itself is composed of two major areas – the anterior and posterior lobes of the pituitary gland. The osmoreceptors have long axons which run down the posterior pituitary stalk to end as synaptic knobs among the posterior pituitary cells.

When the osmoreceptors are stimulated by high osmotic pressure of blood (i.e. less water in blood so it is more concentrated) they rather surprisingly synthesise *antidiuretic hormone*, usually referred to as ADH, which is released from the cells of the posterior pituitary gland. Diuretics are substances which increase the flow of urine (many people refer to prescribed diuretics as 'water tablets') so antidiuretic describes a substance which decreases the flow of urine. (See page 156 on the renal system.)

The flow of urine from the minute nephrons in the kidneys can be increased by cutting down the volume of water reabsorbed back into the bloodstream in the last part of each nephron. If water is re-entering the blood, it cannot be exiting from the body in urine and vice versa! If the water concentration in blood is greater than normal, i.e. the blood is more dilute, then osmoreceptors are not stimulated, ADH secretion is markedly reduced, little reabsorption of water in the last part of the nephron occurs (they behave more like steel tubes) and the excess water is eliminated in the urine, thus returning osmotic pressure to normal.

Most water input is from food and drink, but about half a litre of water is made daily from the respiratory process. Although water can be lost in several ways from the body only two are significant in health – urine volume and sweating in hot weather.

The amount of water lost through sweating clearly depends on the external environment; but it can amount to several litres in hot countries. Sweat is a dilute salt solution, however only the water is evaporated in cooling the body and this is

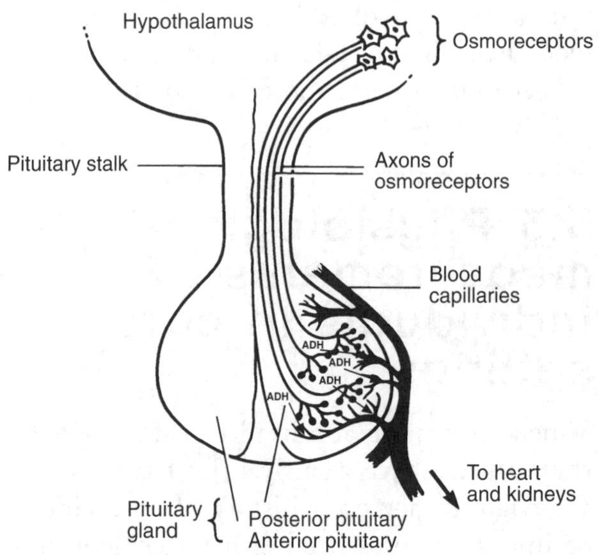


**Figure 3.47 ADH secretion**

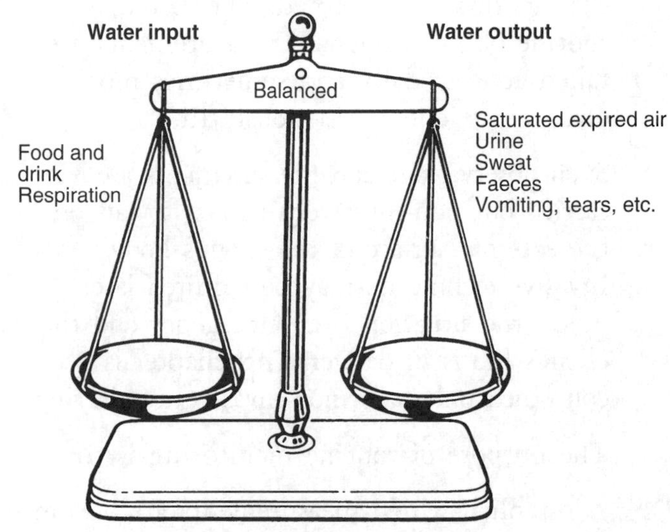


**Figure 3.48 The water balance**

the reason why skin tastes salty after sweating. Under such circumstances, the thirst centre is stimulated and people feel the urge to consume more fluid. After several days in a hot climate the body becomes depleted of salt and this is why people in hot climates are urged to take with them a supply of pleasantly flavoured salt tablets and to add more salt to their food. Even in the UK in a hot spell it may be necessary to add more salt to food in the summer time.

## 3.3 Physiological measurements of individuals in care settings

When clients are admitted to care settings they usually have a fairly brief letter from their family doctor, a history of an accident or injury or notes from either Accident and Emergency or an Outpatient clinic. To find out more information about a client a careful medical history and a routine examination is performed. Thereafter, routine observations and measurements are taken at least daily and sometimes more often if the client is seriously ill.

Such observations and measurements are carried out non-invasively, that is to say, on the external surface of the client's body. Invasive techniques may be required later unless the situation is an emergency and the client's life is in danger. This chapter is concerned only with non-invasive monitoring.

The purpose of routine monitoring is to:

- establish which measurements are within normal ranges
- find out which measurements are outside the normal ranges
- collect data from the client to establish their standard measurements
- make recommendations for the most suitable form of care for the client
- investigate which homeostatic control mechanisms are not working efficiently.

The routine measurements taken in care settings include:

- pulse rate
- body temperature
- blood pressure
- respiratory rate
- peak flow
- lung volumes.

The last two are features of pulmonary conditions and may not be carried out in individuals with non-pulmonary conditions.

In this section of the chapter, we will cover the types of equipment you might use, safe practice in using the equipment, accuracy and ways to reduce errors, possible health and safety risks and how to reduce them and the expected range of results. In addition, we will also cover the meaning of any deviations from the expected range of results.

Before taking any measurements from clients, you should explain carefully what you are going to do and check that this is satisfactory to them. Clients are people like you with feelings and anxieties. You will find that clients with high blood pressure will anxiously question the carer about the reading after having their BP measured.

### Taking a pulse as a measure of the heart rate

#### Pulse rate

The pulse rate is usually checked during a medical examination as it can give hints about a person's state of health. Other characteristics of the pulse can also be important, such as its strength, rhythm and the feel of the artery concerned.

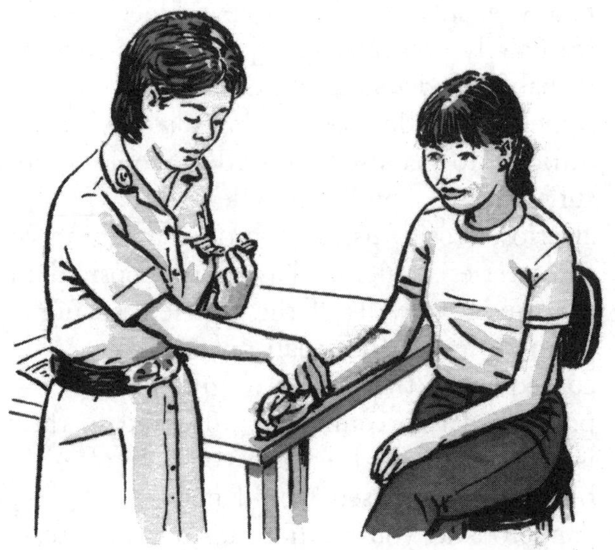

Taking a pulse

A pulse can be felt wherever an artery crosses a bone. The most usual place to feel for a pulse is at the wrist, just below the base of the thumb where the radial artery crosses the bones of the wrist. However, in an emergency, if the circulation is shutting down, the *carotid artery* is the main one to feel as this comes straight off the aorta which leads blood away from the heart. This pulse can be felt in the neck on either side of the windpipe. Pulses can also be felt in the groin (*femoral artery*), temple and upper surface of the foot.

A baby's pulse is often difficult to find and the brachial artery on the inner side of the upper arm is often easier to locate.

The pulse rate corresponds to the contraction of the ventricles of the heart, which forces blood through the arteries causing a shock wave which travels along the arterial system. The shock wave is the pulse that you are feeling. The blood actually travels more slowly.

## Taking a pulse as a measure of the heart rate

To take a pulse, press lightly against the artery wall with two or three fingers. Do not use the thumb, as this has a pulse of its own and you may find that you have counted your own pulse instead! You will also need a time-piece which is capable of reading seconds. Count the number of beats in a set period and multiply by the correct multiple to make up to 60 seconds, i.e. one minute. The minimum you must count for is 20 seconds, and in this case you would multiply by three to get the rate per minute.

The pulse rate is usually between 60 and 80 beats per minute.

| Causes of a faster than normal resting adult pulse rate | Causes of a slower than normal resting adult pulse rate |
|---|---|
| Being a baby or young child | Being a very fit adult |
| Exercise or exertion | Fainting |
| Fright | Compression of the brain |
| Haemorrhage | Some disorders of the heart |
| Fever (pyrexia) | |
| Some illnesses | |

Figure 3.49 The causes of variations in pulse rate

| **Try it out** | Take your own pulse or that of a friend:<br>• at rest (after at least ten minutes)<br>• after a short spell of minor activity such as waving your arms in the air<br>• after some strenuous activity like running on the spot for several minutes.<br>Check that a strenuous activity is all right for that person. Record your readings and convert to pulse rates per minute. |
|---|---|

Pulse readings can also be taken by digital monitors from a finger or wrist device and also from many modern digital blood pressure recorders. Some pulse rates are irregular and this may indicate a heart disorder so this must be brought to a supervisor's attention. Pulse rates can change significantly over a few seconds due to anxiety, excitement, embarrassment, movement or lighting a cigarette.

## Accuracy and potential sources of error

### An example

I measured John's pulse for 15 seconds and multiplied by 4 to find the rate per minute.

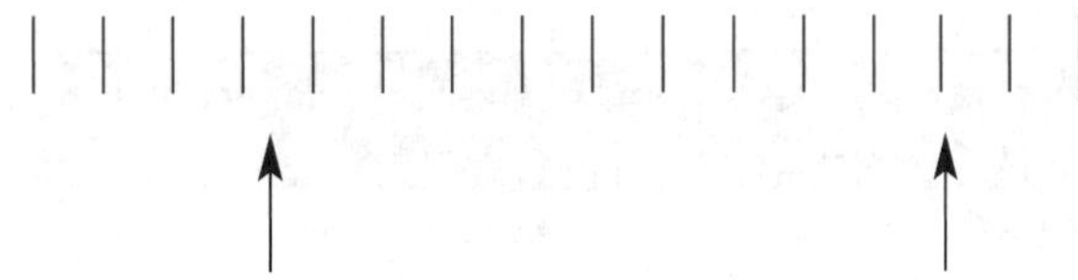

If the strokes above represent the beats of John's pulse and the two arrows the period of 15 seconds during which the count was made, there are 16 beats counted which multiplied up make his pulse rate to be 64 beats per minute. However, a little time was lost before the first beat occurred and the count was stopped immediately after the last beat, not half way in between as was started. John's heart rate is actually 65 beats per minute (measured for the whole minute) so we have lost one beat when multiplied up. One in 64 is an error of 1.6 per cent ($^1/_{64} \times 100$), i.e. not significant at all.

When a pulse is irregular, it can be very difficult to count and very easy to miss a beat; the error might rise to 5 per cent and still not be very significant. If you are inexperienced as well, you might have to take the pulse readings a few times to be reasonably accurate. Fast pulse rates such as in babies and young children (and sometimes, older people) can also be quite difficult to get used to. Older people often suffer from a condition called arteriosclerosis, also known as 'hardening of the arteries'. Calcium has been deposited in the muscular walls of the arteries causing them to feel harder than normal, consequently the fingers might need to press harder to count the pulse and so there is a potential for blocking the flow of blood. This in itself would not be dangerous as you are not closing the artery for many seconds, but it could lead to significant errors.

The level of accuracy of equipment stated in the manufacturer's handbook or instructions is usually said to be plus or minus 2.5 per cent. This means that if the pulse rate is recorded as 80 beats per minute, it will be in the range of 78 to 82 beats per minute.

## Safe practice when taking pulse readings

When you use electronic digital recorders you must check the manufacturer's instructions for safe practice and potential risks and find the level of accuracy. Different types of equipment may work in different ways, but all pieces of electrical equipment carry potential hazards – mainly of electrical shock and burns to both client and carer.

You must be constantly on the alert for:

- malfunction of equipment
- frayed flexes and trapped wires
- loose and faulty plugs and sockets.

This type of fault must be reported *immediately* – verbally and in writing; most large establishments have special forms for reporting faulty or damaged equipment. The equipment must be clearly identified as faulty with a notice and taken out of use. Only suitably qualified personnel should undertake investigation, modification, repair or permanent removal. No one should be asked to use faulty equipment in his or her job role.

## Body temperature

In order that the body can function optimally, the body temperature must be kept within narrow limits. Body temperature varies widely between people and even in the same person there can be variations as temperature is affected by sleep, eating and drinking, exercise and also the time of day. In most people, body temperature is lowest around 3 a.m. and highest around 6 p.m. In women, body temperature is affected by the menstrual cycle, being highest around ovulation and lowest during menstruation. In addition to all of this, body temperature varies according to the part of the body in which it is being measured.

### Recording body temperature

There are three common places for measuring body temperature:

- under the tongue in the mouth, called oral temperature
- in the armpit or axilla
- in the rectum – this raises anxiety and stress levels and is confined to seriously ill clients, unconscious clients or where the use of other sites is not possible.

Rectal temperatures are nearest to core temperatures but slow to change; they are generally higher than oral temperatures by up to half a degree Celsius. Axillary temperatures are roughly 0.3°C lower than oral temperatures. Normal body temperature is considered to be 37°C but this is too precise given the large number of influences on body temperature so a range of 36.5 to 37.2°C is acceptable.

### Types of thermometer

1 **Traditional clinical thermometers** consist of a mercury-filled bulb, a fine bored tube sealed at the other end and a scale measuring in degrees. Modern thermometers in the UK measure in degrees Celsius (this used to be called centigrade), older thermometers measured on a quite different Fahrenheit scale – now no longer in use. The wall of one side of the tube is specially thickened to form a magnifying lens so that the scale can be read more easily. The thermometer should be inserted for 10 minutes to reach its maximum level of

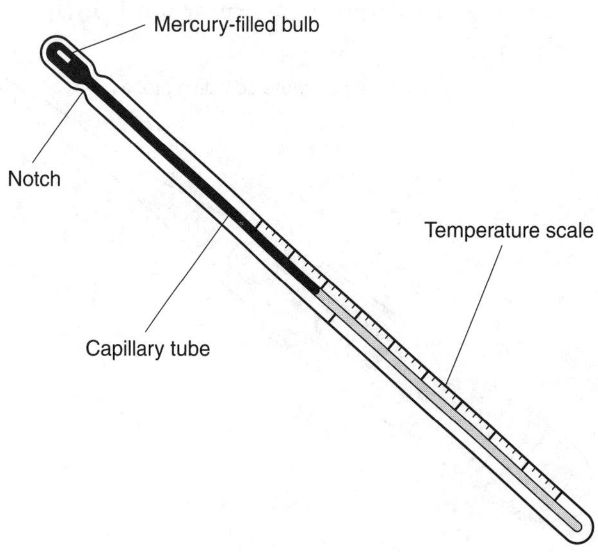


Figure 3.50 A clinical thermometer

mercury expansion and then removed. A kink in the tubing prevents the mercury from descending until the thermometer is shaken down into the bulb ready for the next recording. This type of thermometer can be used orally, in the axilla or in the rectum. However, there are now new guidelines on the use of this type of thermometer (see page 181 safe practice).

Different styles of this type of thermometer exist to measure oral, axillary and rectal temperatures and they are inexpensive to purchase; many people have this type in their own medicine cabinet at home.

2 **Ear thermometers**; these are also called infra-red light reflectance thermometers. This type of thermometer takes the reading from the eardrum by reflection of an infra-red beam of light from a probe in the ear canal. The probe has a disposable tip cover. They are the top choice in many doctors' surgeries and hospitals. Clearly, this type of thermometer is very quick to use and suitable for carers to carry around with them.

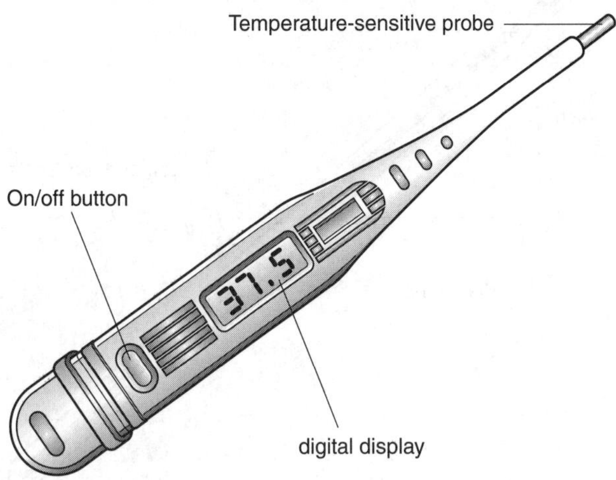


**Figure 3.51 An electronic digital thermometer**

3 **LCD strip** thermometers are available cheaply at any high street pharmacist (LCD stands for liquid crystal display), and parents of babies and young children are encouraged to keep one at home. They are disposable, very safe and easy to use, taking only a few minutes to detect a temperature.

4 **Electronic digital thermometers** use an electronic probe with a disposable cover attached to a digital readout display, taking only a few seconds to effect a reading. They are expensive to buy but particularly useful with young children who are not inclined to remain still for very long.

## Accuracy and potential sources of error

This varies according to the type of equipment that is being used. Taking an accurate body temperature is not as straightforward as it appears to be. There have been several studies concerned with the accuracy of temperature recordings (Blainey, 1974; Eoff and Joyce, 1981; Boylan and Brown, 1985; Durham *et al* 1986; Baker *et al* 1984). Durham *et al.* (1986) produced a table of the factors affecting oral and rectal temperatures. A summary is provided in Figure 3.52.

Once again, you will find the accuracy of the electronic digital thermometers in the manufacturer's instructions and they have not yet been identified as causing problems in this regard. The same cannot be said for ear thermometers and there are recorded comments about the accuracy of these currently on the world wide web see:

www.cnn.com/HEALTH/9809/28/ear.thermometer

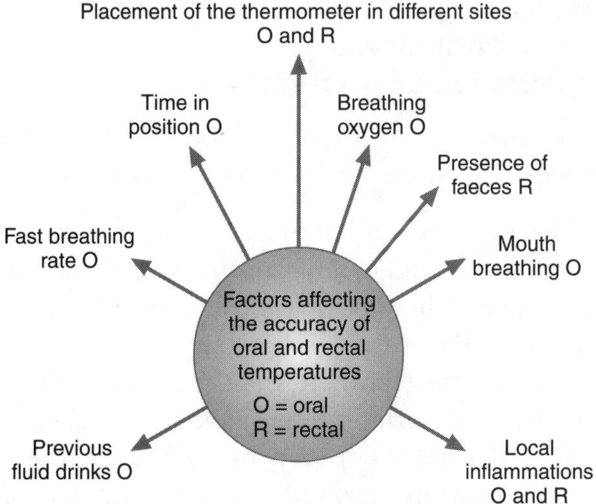


**Figure 3.52 A summary of factors affecting oral and rectal temperatures**

There appears to be the potential for gross inaccuracy in temperature recording in this type of equipment. One doctor commented on a difference of four degrees between the two ears on the same client, clients with very high temperatures recording normal temperatures and those without high temperatures recording fevers. He also found that moving less than half an inch (about one centimetre) gave two different temperature readings in the same ear of one client. Clearly, this relatively new type of equipment can produce very significant errors and more studies will be carried out.

LCD strips do not provide exact readings, but generally indicate when there is a raised body temperature.

## Potential health and safety risks and methods of reduction

Clinical thermometers must be sterilised before use in a reliable antiseptic solution that is changed regularly. However, mercury-containing equipment is potentially poisonous if the thermometer is broken or bitten and European legislation now requires the gradual elimination of all mercury-containing equipment. This is particularly important in equipment used to measure oral temperatures. Although still common in home medicine cabinets, you will find very few, if any, traditional clinical thermometers used in large care settings.

Ear thermometers, even with disposable covers on their probes, have been found to be contaminated with bacteria and half of those discovered could have had bacteria resistant to antibiotics. The danger here is of transmitting ear infections that could be difficult to treat. The only safe way of reducing this contamination would be to introduce cheap, disposable, easily fitted probes or use an alternative type of thermometer. There are no significant health and safety risks with LCD strips apart from their less than exact readings.

Electrical equipment hazards have been already covered, see page 178 pulse readings.

| **Try it out** | Find as many types of thermometer as you can and take simultaneous readings of your body temperature in the axilla with each piece of equipment. Compare their ease of use, body temperature reading and calculate their potential for error. Remember not to use mercury-containing equipment if you can avoid it and be aware of the emergency procedure if mercury is spilled. This is to cover the mercury with flowers of sulphur and evacuate the room. |
|---|---|

## Monitoring blood pressure

Blood pressure (BP) is the pressure exerted by the blood on the walls of the blood vessels.

There are three main ways to measure blood pressure:

1 By the traditional mercury sphygmomanometer, however you must remember that this equipment contains mercury and is being phased out under European legislation

2 By electronic digital recorders that frequently give pulse readings as well

3 By an invasive technique using a pressure transducer inserted directly into the bloodstream. You will not be using this method.

| **Try it out** | Write down the definition of blood pressure, the manner in which it is recorded, the meaning of both numbers and the purpose of monitoring blood pressure. |
|---|---|

Some modern sphygmomanometers have a built-in stethoscope for listening to the blood flow. Sphygmomanometers in the traditional form consist of a cloth cuff which encloses an air bladder connected to tubing and a rubber or plastic bulb used for pumping air into the bladder. The tubing connects to a measuring device or gauge – traditional ones still in use are filled with mercury.

### Measuring blood pressure using traditional mercury sphygmomanometers

You should only measure blood pressure if there is a trained person with you.

The cuff is wound round the upper arm with the bladder (which can be felt) located just above the elbow joint and facing forward. Place the stethoscope over the artery at the elbow, it should be quite flat to the skin surface. The bladder is inflated using the manual pump or bulb until the gauge measures around 200 units, measured in millimetres of mercury. This has the effect of blocking off the supply of blood to the arm, so clearly the inflation must not be left at this level for more than a few seconds.

The cuff is slowly deflated by turning a thumbscrew between the bulb and tubing, while listening carefully through the stethoscope. At the first sounds of blood rushing into the artery, read the gauge. This is known as the *systolic pressure* and it represents the contraction of the ventricles and the recoil of the elastic walls of the aorta as blood passes through. This is the highest level you will record and represents the *numerator* of the fraction depicting blood pressure.

Continuing to deflate the cuff slowly, the beats appear to get gradually louder and then suddenly begin to die away, this is usually described as a muffled sound. Once again, note the reading on the gauge. This is the *diastolic pressure* representing the pressure which exists between heart beats, and the load against which the heart has to work. The diastolic pressure is the more important value of the two, and forms the denominator of the fraction.

A healthy young adult has a blood pressure reading around 110/75 mm Hg, but an

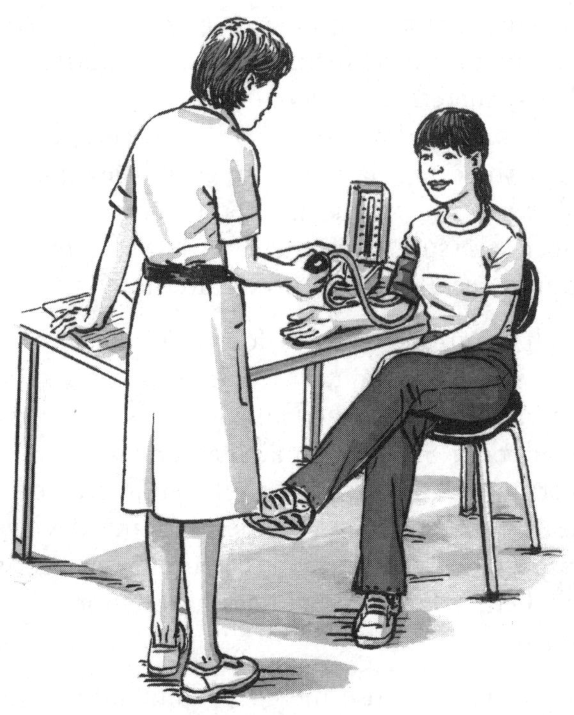

Taking a blood pressure recording

older person has higher blood pressure 130-140/90-100 mm Hg. Hg is the chemical symbol for mercury and is used to shorten the term 'millimetres of mercury'.

Blood pressure varies with activity and circumstance. It rises during pregnancy, exercise, smoking and being anxious about things. Blood pressure falls during sleep and relaxation. Abnormally high blood pressure is known as *hypertension* and low pressure is *hypotension*.

### Measuring blood pressure by electronic sphygmomanometers

The principles here are very similar, but they are easier to use. There is a microphone or transducer built into the cuff which connects to the electronic display. The cuff is inflated in the same way and slowly deflated. The readings appear on the digital display.

**Try it out**

Before you begin this activity:

- check that your partner has no medical history of heart or chest problems before undertaking more strenuous exercise
- use common sense in determining the exercise and limit the duration to five minutes – a suitable example would be stepping on and off a step about twenty times or running up a short flight of stairs.
- if you are in doubt about your partner's ability to carry out the exercise test, then either consult your tutor or choose another partner.

In the presence of a competent person, take and record blood pressure and pulse readings of a partner during:

- rest
- mild exercise
- severe exercise
- stress, such as before a test
- and after eating food.

Take the pulse readings every minute and continue until the resting rate has returned. Plot a graph of pulse against time and note the duration of the exercise on your graph.

Construct a bar chart to show the variation in blood pressure under different circumstances.

### Accuracy and potential sources of error

Anxiety causes a rise in BP, particularly the systolic figure and many clients become anxious when they have they BP measured. If the cuff is inflated too high it can become painful and this also raises BP. We have looked at the effect of the external temperature on vasoconstriction and vasodilatation of blood vessels. If a client feels hot then their blood vessels will be dilated and BP will be lower and vice versa in cold conditions.

Exercise and smoking increase BP, so it should not be measured immediately after these. The presence of arteriosclerosis will affect BP readings, as the vessel wall is not as flexible.

Using a mercury sphygmomanometer, it is possible that the carer may not inflate the cuff high enough at the outset, may not hear or interpret the sounds correctly and may deflate the cuff too quickly to be precise in the reading. It is often the case that a carer pre-judges what the BP should be and this pre-judgement interferes with the actual reading. The carer may get disturbed during taking the reading, or not position either the cuff or the stethoscope correctly. The deflation screw is often too hard to undo or too loose and the tubes may be compressed. The scope for error with this equipment can be small or very large; it depends on the experience, degree of care and concentration shown by the carer.

With electronic equipment, once again the cuff and microphone may not be positioned correctly or inflation may be imprecise. It is important in both cases that the client is sitting with the cuff at the same level of the heart. If the equipment is used correctly and it has no faults, the error is likely to be a small per cent and you will find this in the manufacturer's instructions as before.

### Potential health and safety risks and methods of reduction

You should be aware that COSHH (Control of Substances Hazardous to Health) regulations as part of the EU regulations include measures stipulating that all mercury-containing devices must be phased out. In care establishments, this includes thermometers and mercury sphygmomanometers. In order to comply with these regulations care establishments are replacing traditional temperature and blood pressure equipment with electronic digital recorders and other alternatives.

Such equipment has to follow accuracy guidelines and you will find relevant information in each manufacturer's handbook. Similarly, manufacturer's instructions must be carefully followed for health and safety guidelines and any device suspected of malfunction should be correctly labelled, taken out of use and sent for repair.

If you have to use mercury-containing equipment as there is no alternative, be extremely careful and know what to do if there is any leakage or spillage (see page 179 clinical thermometers). You should always have a suitably qualified person as a supervisor when you are using sphygmomanometers.

## Monitoring respiratory rates

To count the rate of breathing, watch your client carefully for each rise and fall of the chest that represents one whole breath. You may need to place your hand on the upper chest in the 'necklace' position, remembering that making contact with a client under these conditions tends to make breathing faster owing to nervousness or embarrassment. It is a good idea to watch the chest movements while pretending to be taking the pulse! You can also take breathing rates from a spirometer time trace. (See spirometer, page 139.)

A person can, voluntarily, alter his or her own breathing rate, that is the number of breaths per minute, but there is little reason for doing so. Mainly, alterations occur unconsciously due to the activity of the respiratory centre. Normal range for breathing is 8 to 17 breaths per minute at rest in a healthy person. This can rise to around 70 to 80 during strenuous exercise. In fact, anything that raises the general metabolism also raises the breathing rate. A baby breathes much faster than an adult does – approximately 30 to 40 breaths per minute – gradually slowing during childhood to reach the adult level around puberty.

Most medical conditions affecting the blood, such as anaemia, the lungs themselves, such as pneumonia, or the heart and cardio-vascular system, such as heart failure, increase breathing rate and may cause actual breathlessness. Damage to the brainstem due to a stroke or head injury may increase or reduce the rate of breathing and skeletal damage or anything that produces pain on breathing may also change the rate.

In care work, the rhythm of breathing is also important and the degree of shallowness or depth of each breath. You should notice whether the client produces noise on breathing such as a wheeze, bubbling sound, gasp or grunt. This may indicate narrowing of the air passages, infection in the respiratory passages or pain on breathing. Clients who suffer from chronic bronchitis and emphysema often, literally, haul their chests up to inhale, relying heavily on their sterno-mastoid muscles that run down the neck from below the ear to the sternum, and sometimes referred to as strap muscles. Any factors that have been described should be recorded.

?

Some people suffer from brief periods of acute anxiety known as panic attacks and the cause is usually unknown. During the attack, they experience a sense of breathing difficulty, dizziness, palpitations, sweating and faintness. Fast shallow breathing occurs, known as hyperventilation, and this makes the symptoms worse. Hyperventilation can be treated by placing a **paper** bag over the sufferer's mouth and nose for a **few** minutes. The carbon dioxide which builds up makes their breathing deeper.

| **Try it out** | With a partner carry out the same activity as you did for blood pressure and pulse readings, but this time monitor breathing rates. Plot a graph of breathing rate against time, indicating clearly on your graph where conditions changed, for example where exercise began and finished. Compare the rates of change with the pulse rate graph and BP bar chart. Write up your findings. |
|---|---|

### Accuracy and potential errors

For a trained observer, there is likely to be few errors, but an untrained carer might easily miss a breath or count both a rise and a fall as one breath; particularly if distracted or not concentrating. On a spirometer, the potential for error is much less. We have already mentioned how breathing is affected by nervousness or anxiety and this is more likely to affect the result than anything else. Clearly, you will need to check that the client has not just been moving quickly, smoking or has been influenced by any of the factors mentioned before in this section.

### Potential health and safety risks and methods of reduction

There is very low risk in observing a client's chest movements as long as the client is clearly informed and not anxious. There is no need to take precautions providing that the client has been informed and the atmosphere is non-threatening.

## Measuring peak flow

As well as monitoring breathing rate, peak flow measurement is becoming an important guide to pulmonary or lung function. Peak flow meters record the maximum speed of a person's exhalation and this is usually associated with the diameter of the respiratory tubes. Peak flow can be more accurately measured using the medical spirometer, and this should be used in the first measurement to get a base line. Also available are electronic peak flow meters, but their accuracy is in some doubt and they are very expensive.

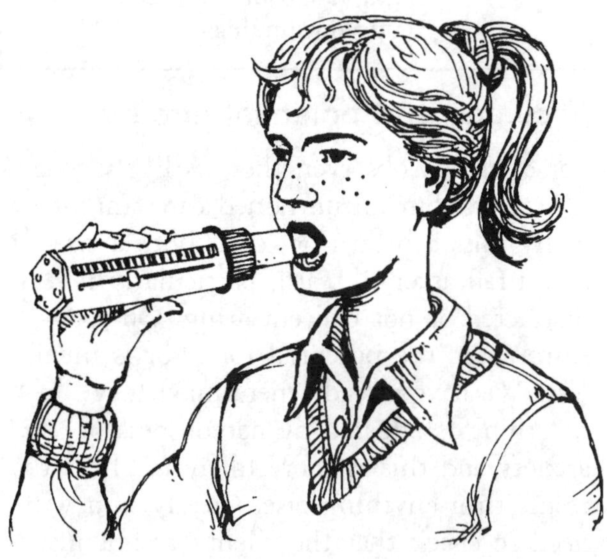

**Figure 3.53** A peak flow meter

A variety of small peak flow meters are available for home use. Smaller devices are available for use by small children.

Many children and adults with moderate to severe asthma use these devices to monitor their condition and therapy. Clients with chronic bronchitis and emphysema monitor their lung function in the same way. Clients requiring chest physiotherapy and athletes in training may also find the data useful.

The peak flow of the forced expiration (exhaling as rapidly as possible through the device) occurs in the first 100 milliseconds (one millisecond is one thousandth of a second) so a prolonged effort is not necessary. Normal range for men is 500 – 700 litres or $dm_3$ per minute, and for women 380 – 500 $dm_3$/min. Children will be proportionately less, depending on their height and chest size.

When a client has no symptoms of asthma, a standard or 'bench mark' can be obtained by spirometry and classed as the personal best. The portable device readings can then be calculated on a percentage of the personal best basis and used for monitoring. That is:

observed reading divided by personal best $\times$ 100

Clients with readings of 50 per cent or less are said to have severe asthma, and may be at risk of death in a severe attack. This class of reading is often said to be in the red danger zone. Clients with scores of 50 to 80 per cent are in the yellow or amber zone, classified as moderate asthmatics, and those between 80 and 100 per cent are mild asthmatics in the so-called green zone. Peak flow readings vary with age, sex, race, height, smoking history, respiratory muscle strength and effort. As they change with age, a new personal best should be established each year for monitoring standards.

Clients with good care supervision are asked to monitor their peak flow twice a day before any medication and record these readings in a diary alongside details of their medication. They take the diary to regular outpatient clinics for discussion with the appropriate medical supervisor.

### Asthma

Asthma is a common condition characterised by recurring attacks of breathlessness and wheezing due to a narrowing of the bronchioles. Attacks can be brought on by exercise, infection, dust, allergies, smoky atmospheres etc. The condition is becoming increasingly common in young people (most asthmatics have their first attack before the age of five years) and can start at any age; it also tends to run in families. The number of deaths during attacks is also rising, and this is why monitoring of potentially severe attacks is so important. Approximately 10 per cent of all school-age children in Britain have asthma and 5 per cent of the general population.

| **Try it out** | Carry out a survey to show how the incidence of asthma in your school or college compares with the national statistics. Refine your survey to show how many people with asthma in your organisation use peak flow meters for monitoring purposes – is their asthma classed as mild, moderate or severe? Do the individuals use their peak flow readings in association with their inhalers i.e. if the reading is lower than normal, do they take an extra puff of their inhalers? A well-designed questionnaire might produce some very interesting data, and provide contacts for your assessment! |
|---|---|

Recent studies in America have shown that client descriptions of symptoms such as wheezing, 'tight' chest and so on are notoriously unreliable in judging the severity of the narrowing of the bronchi (bronchospasm) and even doctors can underrate the severity of an attack.

### Accuracy and potential for error

All peak flow meters should meet specified guidelines for accuracy and precision, but variation between devices made by different manufacturers is unpredictable and clients are advised to use the same device for serial monitoring. Most devices can monitor up to 2 per cent change in peak flow; this is considered accurate enough for serial monitoring.

### Potential health and safety risks and methods of reduction

There is a potential for fungal contamination of portable peak flow devices and clients are encouraged to wash the device regularly with soap and water, according to the manufacturer's instructions. In addition, other precautions include the following:

- devices should be replaced every one to two years, and there is the possibility of failure before that time, giving misleading data
- forced exhalations into a peak flow meter can cause some clients to suffer an attack; these clients should not use peak flow meters
- inaccurate measurement may promote over-medication
- over-reliance on peak flow meters may lead to a delay in seeking medical treatment

- failure to obtain new annual personal best readings may lead to errors of judgement
- there is potential for unrecognised device malfunction
- when it is not possible to substitute spirometry for initial diagnosis.

You can gain more useful information from searching 'asthma' and 'peak flow meter' on the internet, particularly The Cleveland Clinic Foundation at:

http://www.ccf.prg/ed/online3.

| **Try it out** | For this activity, try to get at least three people who suffer from asthma, three smokers and three non-smoking non-asthmatic people who are reasonably fit. Check that it is safe for the people with asthma to use the peak flow meter. Take at least three readings and construct bar charts for comparison. You can either calculate the mean of the three readings and plot one bar chart or make three separate bar charts for each individual. Compare your findings. Taking the best mean of all samples, which should be the fit non-smokers and non-asthmatics, and regarding this value as 100 per cent, find the ratio of the other two means compared to this. |
|---|---|

More accurate measurements of breathing rate can be obtained using a spirometer (under supervision); this is called spirometry.

## Spirometry

The principle of a biological spirometer is quite simply breathing in and out of a volume of air trapped by a moveable box inverted over water. As inhalation occurs the box is depressed and re-elevated during exhalation; the up and down movement of the box is recorded by an ink pen on a moving drum covered in graph paper (called a kymograph) or displayed electronically. The moving gases between the person inhaling and exhaling and the air in the box are in a sealed system, and the subject does not move his or her mouth from the mouthpiece during the activity. During the activity a clip closes the subject's nose. There are several types of spirometer and you must use this equipment under supervision, having familiarised yourself with the manufacturer's instructions.

A chart from a subject using the spirometer to investigate lung volumes will appear similar to the one in Figure 3.8. See section on 'Lung volumes' page 138.

## Potential health and safety risks and methods of reduction

Only a few breaths can be taken with safety, as the box quickly becomes depleted of oxygen and filled with nitrogen and carbon dioxide. To reduce this hazard, the spirometer should have a continuous measured supply of oxygen piped in and a device for absorbing carbon dioxide gas. Strict supervision by a competent person is essential and the equipment must be fully functional with trained operators on hand. There must be no dangers of cross-infection, so mouthpieces should preferably be disposable or thoroughly cleaned with disinfectant between clients.

**Medical spirometers** are much more sophisticated and are electronic, portable, and client friendly with results readily available in printout format.

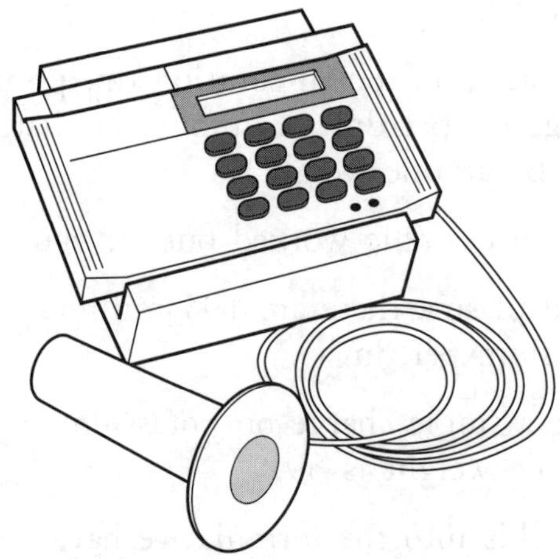

Figure 3.54 A medical spirometer

## Monitoring physiological data on blood sugar

Monitoring a person's blood sugar level can be very important – in the control of Diabetes mellitus, for example. **You will not be expected to do this** type of practical work, but understanding the procedures involved will help you to appreciate the homeostatic control of blood sugar.

Keeping blood sugar levels under control is crucial for people with Diabetes mellitus in order to help prevent eye, kidney and nerve damage. The traditional tests involve:

- sending blood samples to a laboratory for a special test
- using the finger stick test which uses a blood glucose meter to detect the levels – this is usually done at home.

Both these tests involve piercing the skin many times in a week, and this skin damage increases the chances of infection even when the skin surface is cleaned with antiseptic swabs first. Recently, non-invasive techniques have been devised:

- shining infrared light through a person's forearm or finger
- drawing glucose from the blood through the skin using a low-level electric current
- measuring glucose in saliva or tears.

These techniques are very new and you will be extremely fortunate if you have access to one of these.

You can find out more by surfing the web on measuring blood glucose levels; some useful web pages are:

www.niddk.nih.gov/health/diabetes/summary/noninmet/noninmet.htm

www.niddk.nih.gov/health/diabetes/ndep/control.material/handout/abcs.html

www.diabetic.org.uk/news/-arch-98/news13.htm

Sugar, abnormally excreted through urine, can be tested easily by using glucose strips, but all fluids should be handled with care using protective rubber gloves. Never carry out any of these procedures without permission or supervision until a suitably qualified person has trained you.

## Electrolyte concentrations

Other physiological data can involve determining the levels of different electrolyte concentrations in body fluids, particularly blood. Sodium and potassium ions are the main *cations* (see below) of the extracellular and intracellular fluids respectively.

An electrolyte is a substance that splits into ions (charged particles) when it is dissolved in water. These ions may carry positive or negative charges. The former are termed cations and the latter, anions. They are called that because if placed in between two electrode plates, known as cathodes and anodes, the electric current causes cations to move towards the cathode and anions to move towards the anode. This process is called electrolysis, hence the term electrolyte.

- Common cations in body fluids are: sodium, potassium, calcium, hydrogen,
- Common anions in body fluids are: chloride, hydrogen carbonate, phosphate

There are ranges for normal levels of most ions in body fluids. The units of ion concentration are milliequivalents per $dm_3$ ($meq/dm_3$). There is a formula for calculating the concentration of an ion. You will need to know the atomic weight of the ion, the number of milligrams in solution and the number of charges on the ion. For example, sodium, potassium and hydrogen have a single charge whereas calcium has two charges and they are written as follows:

Sodium – $Na^+$ potassium – $K^+$
hydrogen – $H^+$ calcium – $Ca^{2+}$

Atomic weights for these chemicals are:

| Name of ion | Atomic weight |
|---|---|
| Sodium | 23 |
| Potassium | 39 |
| Hydrogen | 1 |
| Calcium | 40 |

Other values can be found in the Periodic table in the top left-hand corner of each box, the Periodic table is a feature of most chemistry texts.

The formula for calculating the concentration of an ion in solution is the number of milligrams of the ion per $dm^3$ divided by the atomic weight of the ion multiplied by the number of charges on that ion. So:

Concentration of ion in solution ($meq/dm^3$) = milligrams per $dm^3$ × number of charges divided by atomic weight

Here is an example worked out for you:

In blood plasma there are 195 milligrams of potassium per $dm^3$.

There is a single charge on potassium and the atomic weight is 39.

Putting this into the formula we have:

Concentration of potassium ions in blood plasma = 195/39 × 1 = 5meq/$dm^3$

However, in intracellular fluid, there are 6033mg/$dm^3$, so –

Concentration of potassium ion in intracellular fluid = 6 033/39 × 1 = 157meq/$dm^3$.

This confirms that potassium is of major importance inside cells.

| Try it out | You can now work out for yourself the concentration of sodium in blood plasma and intracellular fluid and see the relative importance of sodium inside and outside cells.<br>Number of mg of sodium in blood plasma = 3496<br>Number of mg of sodium in intracellular fluid = 322<br>Atomic weight of sodium =23<br>Number of charges =1<br>Is sodium a major ion in intracellular fluid?<br>The answer is at the end of the chapter. |
|---|---|

## 3.4 Safe practice

When making observations or taking measurements from clients, it is vital to use equipment that is in good working order, safe techniques and safe procedures to ensure that no harm or injury can happen to either the client or you. Clients are generally sick or frail people who have enough pain and suffering to contend with, without adding more observations and tests. If a client refuses to have a measurement taken, do not employ coercion or force but inform your supervisor straight away and maintain pleasant communication with your client.

There may be many reasons that you do not understand for the client's refusal, which may only be a temporary setback anyway. The client may not understand the purpose of the measurement, someone may have carried out a similar procedure only ten minutes previously, the client may be confused, depressed, in pain or simply fed up with being disturbed.

Legislation exists to protect both employees and clients in health and social care settings. It is worth remembering how many newspaper headlines, TV documentaries and court cases you have heard about because a carer has made a mistake which has resulted in permanent injury or disability to a client. Hundreds of thousands of pounds have been paid to some clients by hospitals in compensation for negligent practice. However, every client would tell you that he or she would rather *not* have been injured and the money is of little consequence.

| Think it over | Have you ever spent some time in hospital or visited a friend or relative who has? The novelty quickly wears off, especially if you are feeling better. You may begin to worry about getting home and can feel quite tired. It is a long day in hospital, which starts quite early, and many people have a disturbed night's sleep because of the unfamiliar environment and strangers sleeping or not sleeping around them. You seem to be constantly interrupted and can get quite irritable, even if you are normally an easy-going person.<br>Try to empathise with your clients (put yourself in his or her shoes) and realise that you may know about their medical health but have no idea what personal problems they might have. |
|---|---|

### Health and Safety at Work Act

It is important that you know about the key features of the Health and Safety at Work Act 1974 (HASAW), which are as follows:

**employers must make all reasonable efforts to ensure the health, safety and welfare of all their employees by informing you:**

- how to carry out your job safely without risk to yourself and others
- of risks identified with the job, that may affect you
- what measures have been taken to protect you from the identified risks and how to use these measures
- how to get first aid treatment
- what to do in an emergency
- by leaflet or poster about the Health and Safety at Work Act and the local Health and Safety Executive's address

**employers must provide free of charge:**

- adequate safety training
- clothing or equipment required to protect you while at work

**as an employee, your responsibilities are:**

- to take reasonable care of yourself and others (including the general public) who may be affected by your work
- to use any equipment provided for you, for its intended purpose and in a proper manner
- not to carry out tasks that you do not know how to do safely
- to let your manager know if you witness anything that is not safe and could place yourself or others at risk
- to co-operate with employers on health and safety matters
- inform the appropriate person in the organisation if you have an accident or witness 'a near miss'.

In effect, both the employer and employee *share* extra responsibilities and any organisation employing more than five people must have a written policy statement of health and safety.

Within care settings, the Act would incorporate infection control, correct lifting techniques, good standards of hygiene, sanitation and cleanliness in food preparation areas, observations and measurements, safe disposal of clinical waste, monitoring for toxic and radioactive contamination, proper heating, lighting and ventilation.

| **Try it out** | Examine the key features of HASAW and select all the points that would particularly apply to you when you are taking routine measurements from a client. Opposite each point give an example of how it would apply. For example:<br>• how to carry out your job safely without risk to yourself and others<br>This would apply to not using mercury-containing equipment that might leak or break, causing a risk of mercury poisoning to both you and the client. |
|---|---|

## COSHH legislation

You should know that COSHH stands for Control of Substances Hazardous to Health as this is helpful and reminds you that the act is concerned with dangerous substances. The key features of this legislation are that employers should:

- complete risk assessments of all hazardous substances used in the workplace
- keep records of risk assessments and review them regularly
- inform employees about any substance hazardous to their health
- provide appropriate training in the use of hazardous substances

- make all efforts to substitute less harmful substances that perform the same tasks.

Hazardous substances may range from correction fluid in offices to disinfectants in cleaning, from drugs used in treatment to radioactive chemicals in care settings and mercury previously in use in clinical thermometers and sphygmomanometers. You can see that mercury-containing equipment is covered by COSHH legislation as well!

## Reporting of Injuries, Diseases and Dangerous Occurrences Regulations 1995 (RIDDOR)

When there is an accident connected with work to either an employee or a member of the public, which involves death or being taken to hospital, then the employer must notify the Health and Safety Executive (HSE) without delay. A completed accident form must follow this within 10 days. Failure to carry out these requirements is a criminal offence and may lead to prosecution. There is a long list of reportable diseases, injuries and dangerous occurrences, but these include:

- acute illness requiring medical treatment where there is reason to believe that this resulted from exposure to a biological agent, its toxins or infected material
- certain poisonings, including mercury
- electrical short circuit or overload causing fire or explosion
- accidental release of any substance which may damage health.

The employer must keep a record of the event, which must include the date and method of reporting, the date, time and place of the event, personal details of those involved and a brief description of the nature of the event or disease.

You can find more details of legislation relating to Health and Safety at Work on www.rmarlowe.freeserve.co.uk/riddor.html and in HSE leaflets.

You will also find that specific details of safe practice have been covered in each section concerned with the physiological monitoring of body systems.

# 3.5 Analysis and accuracy of results

The results of observations and measurements are not very useful if you cannot glean information from them, so you must be able to interpret results carefully and be able to:

- use fractions and decimals to record physiological values
- plot graphs to record body temperature and changes in pulse and respiratory rates, for example
- determine and interpret linear (line) and non-linear graphs, for example changes in pulse and breathing rates and oxygen consumption from spirometer traces
- use formulae, for example to express electrolyte concentrations.

## Using fractions and decimals to record physiological values

Electronic digital displays present information using decimals, so you must be careful to search for the decimal point and record the value accurately. When you are recording values yourself you may find it easier to estimate the distance between two points as a fraction and convert it into a decimal later. Remember that this is an estimation and cannot be accurate to many decimal places. For example, if you estimate that the reading is one-third of the difference between two points on a scale, there is no point in recording 0.333 as your estimation is not to one-thousandth accuracy, so 0.3 will be adequate.

Each figure to the right in order from the decimal point represents 1/10th and so the first figure to the right is 1/10th, the second figure 1/100 (i.e. 1/10 × 1/10), the third figure 1/1000th and so on. Figures to the left of the decimal point are whole numbers, again with a ten-fold difference. The first figure is under 10, the second figure records in multiples of tens, the third figure in multiples of hundreds, the fourth multiples of thousands, the fifth figure multiples of ten thousands and so on.

| Try it out | |
|---|---|
| | The figure 565.75 would be: five hundred and sixty five point seventy five.<br>Say the following figures out loud to yourself:<br>0.6, 56.10, 100.3, 12 999.5<br>*(Answers at the end of the unit.)*<br>You will notice the space between the 12 and the rest of the last number, this signifies that you are in the thousands. One million would be written 1 000 000 and three hundred million 300 000 000. |

When you add or subtract decimals be careful to place the decimal points under one another (unless you are using a calculator, or course). For example, when adding the decimals listed above simply add the numbers in the columns and place the decimal point underneath the others:

| | |
|---|---|
| | 0.6 |
| | 56.10 |
| | 100.3 |
| | 12 999.5 |
| Total | 13 155.50 |

| Try it out | |
|---|---|
| | Using the same four figures (0.6, 56.10, 100.3 and 12 999.5), try adding the three smaller numbers together and subtracting the total from the largest number.<br>*(Answer at the end of the unit.)* |

Fractions are not used as much as decimals to record values as they are more difficult to add and subtract.

| Try it out | |
|---|---|
| | Add $^1/_3$ to $^1/_4$<br>Add 0.33 to 0.25<br>Which was easiest? |

To add fractions you must find the lowest common denominator of the two bottom figures. In the case above it is 12 (both 3 and 4 divide into 12). Then multiply the top figure by the number of times the bottom figure divides into the lowest common denominator. So:

3 goes into 12 four times and 4 × 1 = 4, so $^1/_3$ is the same as $^4/_{12}$

4 goes into 12 three times so 3 × 1 = $^3/_{12}$

When both fractions have been converted to 12ths you can add the top figures, in this case $^7/_{12}$. Even then, this is hard to deal with although you would recognise that

$\frac{6}{12}$ is the same as $\frac{1}{2}$ (dividing upper and lower figures by 6 to cancel down), so $\frac{7}{12}$ is a little over half. Decimals are much easier to cope with.

If you wish to subtract fractions you should proceed in the same way but subtract the top figures. For example, $\frac{1}{3} - \frac{1}{4} = \frac{4}{12} - \frac{3}{12} = \frac{1}{12}$

You may need to convert fractions to decimals.

To convert $\frac{1}{4}$ into a decimal then divide 1.00 (the top figure) by 4 (the lower figure) the answer is 0.25. You can add as many zeros after the decimal point as you need but two are adequate for most tasks.

When converting decimals to fractions, place the figure over the meaning of the decimal placing and cancel down.

| **Try it out** | Convert 0.6 to a fraction: $\frac{6}{10}$ is equal to $\frac{3}{5}$ as both will divide by 2.<br>Now convert 0.8, 1.3 and 0.04 to fractions.<br>(*Answer at the end of the unit.*) |
|---|---|

## Plotting graphs

It is necessary to plot graphs in order to see the trends in two or more groups of figures easily and to see how one set of figures vary with another. One set of figures will be under your control, this is very often time, but there may be other things as well, such as concentration.

The vertical axis is the set of figures over which you had no control, in other words your results, this is known as the independent variable. The horizontal axis is the controlled figures. You must label these axes with their title and units of measurement. One of the most common errors is to mix these up and plot the graph upside down!

You must devise a scale for the two axes by counting the squares available on your graph paper and the extent of your figures. For example if you are plotting blood sugar levels against time and you took blood samples for $2\frac{1}{2}$ hours with 12 centimetre squares available on your paper, you have to find a scale for 150 minutes in 12 cm. Dividing 150 by 12 gives you one square equal to 12.5 minutes, a very awkward scale that will take a long time to plot accurately. However, it has given you a place to start. If you make one square equal to 15 minutes ($\frac{1}{4}$ hour) that will be much easier and the reduction in size of the graph is quite small. You should not choose a scale that makes your graph appear in one small corner of the paper, use the paper to best effect.

You must then repeat the procedure for the vertical scale.

| **Try it out** | If blood sugar levels are ranging from 89mg per 100ml plasma to 149mg per 100ml of plasma, the difference is around 60; suppose you have 20 cm squares available for the vertical axis, then what is the best scale for you to use?<br>Although most graph axes begin at zero, they do not have to do so; in this case you can commence at 70, 80 or even 85mg per 100ml plasma. |
|---|---|

Examples of graphs that commence at a number are shown in Figure 3.55 and these are typical of body temperature charts.

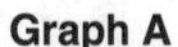

You must indicate the main points on the scale with small marks and numbers and the difference in value between any two adjacent points on the one scale must be the same. The scales for the two or more axes can be different.

Always give your graph a title, for example 'Graph to show how blood glucose levels vary with time'. Next, you must plot the points carefully, finding the places corresponding to the two values on each scale and marking the point at the position they intersect. It is better to plot your points using pencil as it is easy to erase if you make an error. A simple dot or x will suffice to mark the intersection and frequently a small circle is drawn around a point mark so that it can be seen more easily. When your graph is completed satisfactorily, and you are happy with it, you can make your plots more permanent with ink if that is preferred.

If your graph is clearly a straight line but some points are slightly out of place, find the line of 'best fit' which goes through the maximum number of plots. It is acceptable to use a ruler for this. On the other hand, if your graph moves up and down frequently (like a body temperature chart) then join each point up to its neighbour. Some people use a ruler for this, others join the lines freehand. Should your graph be a curve or parabola (U-shaped) you must join the points freehand (in pencil, in case of error) again in 'best fit' mode. Use a writing instrument with a sharp point to do this if you wish to have an accurate graph.

Check that there is a title and labels (with units) to the axes. In some graphs, conditions may change with time; for instance, when exercise starts and ends. This can be indicated below the scale with labelled arrows or a block entitled 'duration of exercise' see graph C in Figure 3.55.

**Graph A**

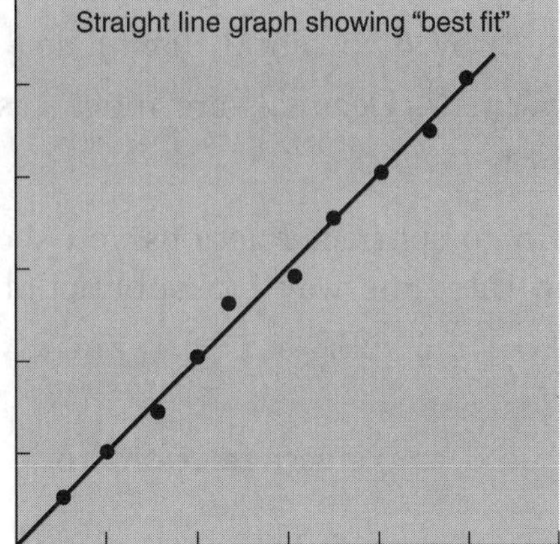


**Graph B**

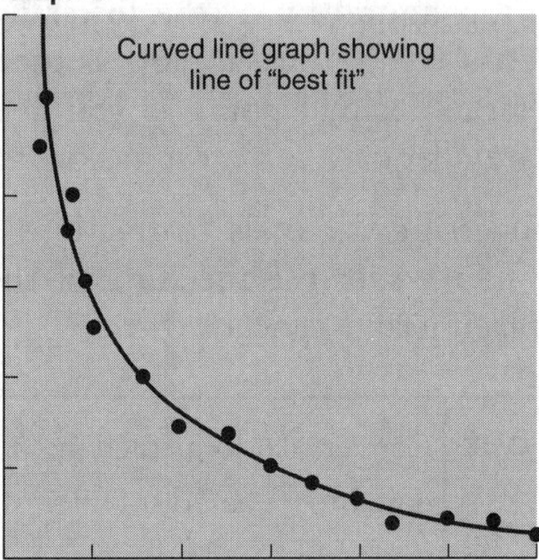


**Graph C**

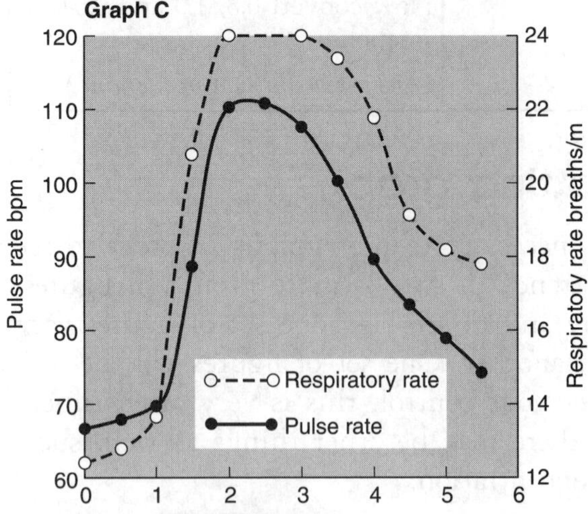


Graph to show pulse and respiratory rate for client C during light exercise

**Figure 3.55 3 types of graphs**

You will notice that graph C displays scales on two vertical axes. Graphs can be used to display two variables against time; the scales are either placed both at one side or on either side of the main graph and the plots or lines indicated with different formats. You have to be very careful to read the right scale for the right value on this type of graph, it is very easy to get muddled up. You can see how the two graphs rise or fall together or when one rises the other falls (known as an inverse relationship) and these relationships are more difficult to observe on separate graphs, see Figure 3.56.

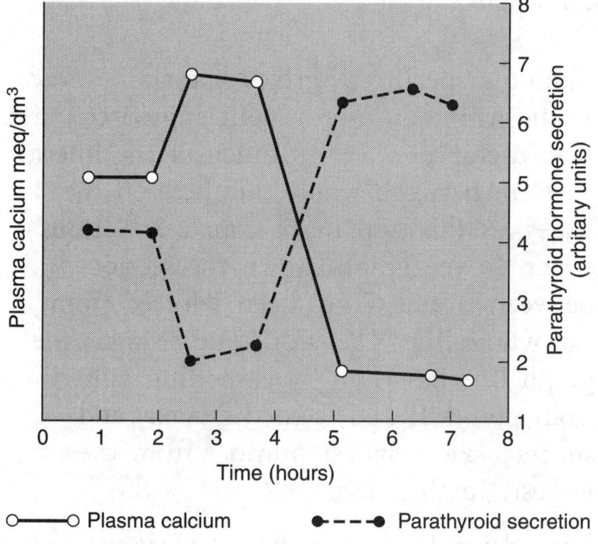


**Figure 3.56 Graph to demonstrate the inverse relationship between plasma calcium and parathyroid hormone**

From this graph it is very clear that when plasma calcium is elevated parathyroid secretion falls, and vice versa, demonstrating an inverse relationship.

When you need to analyse and compare one graph with another you will add text to accompany the graphs. See Figure 3.57 as an example.

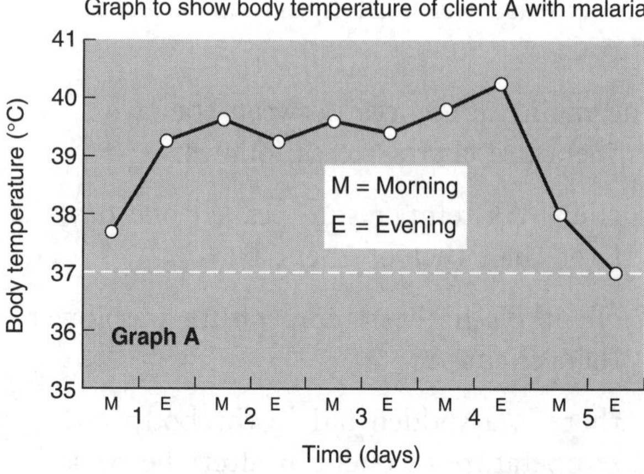


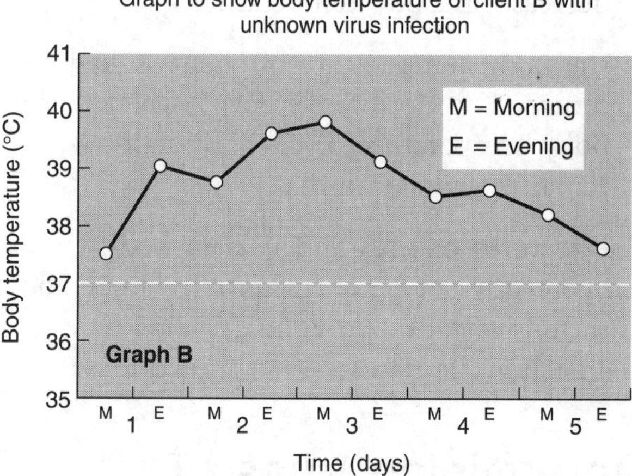


**Figure 3.57 Two graphs to show body temperature of different clients**

*Graph A*, client A: body temperature rose during day 1 and remained between 39.3 and 39.8°C for the next three days. On the evening of day 4 the body temperature peaked at 40.2°C then fell sharply during the night and early morning to 38°C on the morning of day 5 and by that evening the temperature had returned to normal.

*Graph B*, client B: body temperature rose to 39°C during day 1 and continued to climb steadily until it reached a peak of 39.8°C on the morning of day 3. Thereafter the body temperature decreased gradually each day. On the evening of day 5 the body temperature was still lightly elevated at 37.5°C.

The main differences between the two temperature charts are as follows:

- client A's temperature peaked one day later than that of client B
- client B's highest temperature was lower than client A's
- there is a sudden fall in the body temperature of client A after the peak, whereas client B suffered a gradual decrease in body temperature
- the body temperature of client A had returned to normal by day 5 whereas the body temperature of client B still remained above normal.

The features of rises and falls in body temperature can be characteristic of specific infections and can prove useful aids to diagnosing the nature of an infection.

## Determining rates of change

When a variable is plotted against time, it is possible to observe and calculate the rate of change. Clearly, if a graph line rises steeply in a short period of time it means that the variable on the vertical axis (also known as the $y$-axis) has risen so the rate of change is high. Put simply, the steeper the slope of a graph the faster the rate of change. When a graph line is horizontal and parallel to the horizontal (or $x$-axis) the variable has not changed over the period of time.

Examine the graph in Figure 3.58 that shows how insulin secretion after eating increases against time; the rate of change can be calculated from the slope of the graph line.

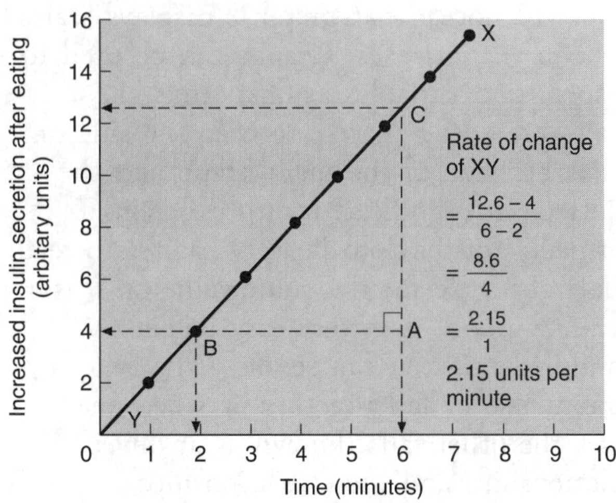


**Figure 3.58 Graph to show insulin secretion increases after eating, at the rate of 2.15 units per minute**

Choose a specific length of the slope to act as the hypotenuse of a right-angled triangle. It is useful to select as much of the line as you can between whole numbers on the scales, as this will make your calculations easier. In the graph shown the section between B and C has been selected from the whole line XY. Work out how far the graph line has risen by extending faint lines from points B and C to the $y$-axis and subtract the smallest number from the largest. In this case: 12.6 – 4 = 8.6.

Extend the lines from B and C downward to intersect the $x$-axis in the same way and subtract as before: 6 – 2 = 4.

We now know that the rate of change of the graph is 8.6 units in 4 minutes, so it is easy to divide 8.6 by 4 to find the rate of insulin secretion after eating, i.e. 2.15 units per minute.

The volume of oxygen consumed when an individual is using an oxygen-filled spirometer with carbon dioxide absorption can be similarly calculated, although the graph is non-linear. As the oxygen is used up, the volume of oxygen declines, producing a downward slope. Draw a sloping line either at the top of the trace, the bottom or in the centre to assume a 'best fit' line again. As you are measuring the **gradient** of the line, the point at which you draw the line is not significant, but all three lines should be parallel.

| **Try it out** | In the spirometer trace, Figure 3.59, find the rate of oxygen consumption.<br>The spirometer has a time trace that indicates minutes, in one minute the trace dropped from A to B so comparing this with the calibration in millilitres you should discover how much oxygen is consumed in one minute. |
|---|---|

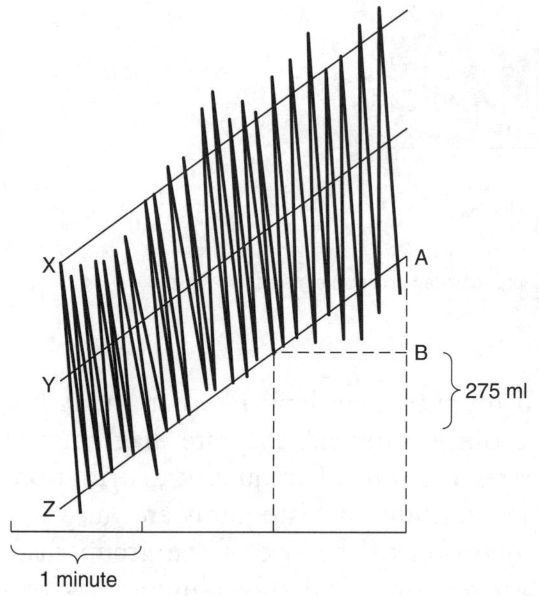


**Figure 3.59 Spirometer trace from subject breathing pure oxygen for 2.5 minutes**

You will have noticed that some of the graphs shown have units on the *y*-axis labelled arbitrary units. This is a useful way of demonstrating fluctuations in a variable without having to handle very small or very large units.

A graph displaying a large number of points that seem unrelated to each other is known as a *scattergram* or *scattergraph*, and in this type of graph the plots are left unconnected (see Figure 3.60).

If you find that the points have a trend then you will have found an inter-relationship or correlation between the two variables that you have been plotting. When there is no distinct trend then the variables are not correlated.

A trend that slopes from left to right upwards is said to have a positive correlation, see Figure 3.60 Graph A. You can see that as height in metres has increased so has the systolic blood pressure. In graph B, no correlation has been identified between insulin secretion and height in metres. When you examine graph C, you can also see a trend but one that slopes downwards from left to right, this is a negative correlation – testosterone secretion has decreased with height in metres.

## Bar charts and histograms

You can also present data in the form of bar charts and histograms. Bar charts are generally used to present discrete data that are separate items. The *y*-axis has a numerical scale but the *x*-axis does not, all the bars have the same width and the frequency is indicated by the height of the bar. See Figure 3.61.

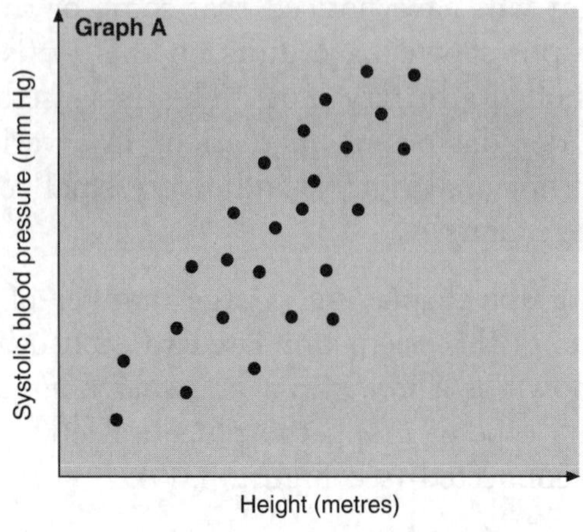


Positive correlation – as height in metres increases so does systolic blood pressure

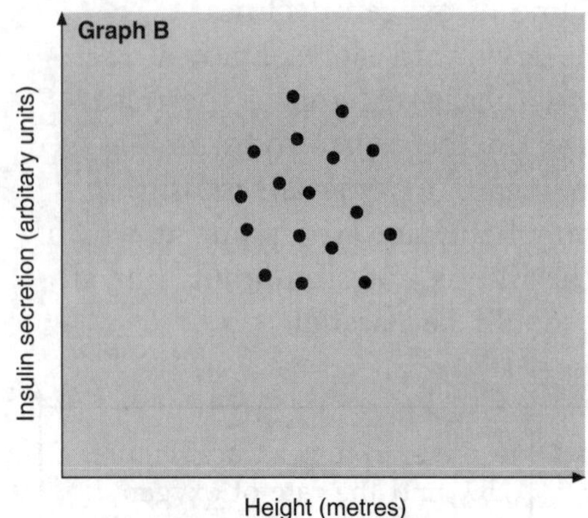


No correlation – insulin secretion is not related to height in metres

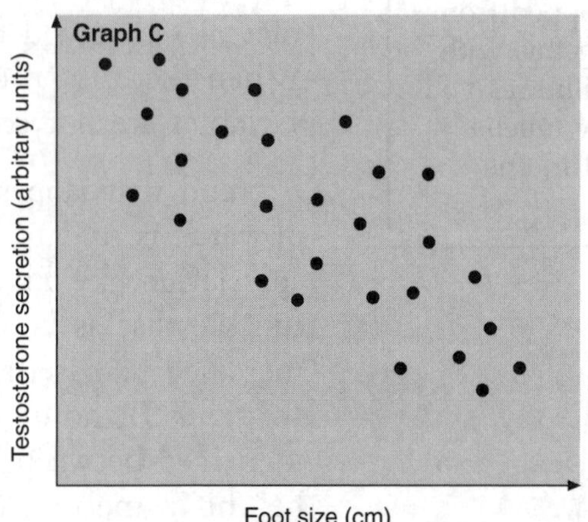


Negative correlation – as foot size increases, testosterone secretion declines

**Note:** The graphs are fictitous to illustrate the concept of correlation in scattergrams

**Figure 3.60 Three scattergrams**

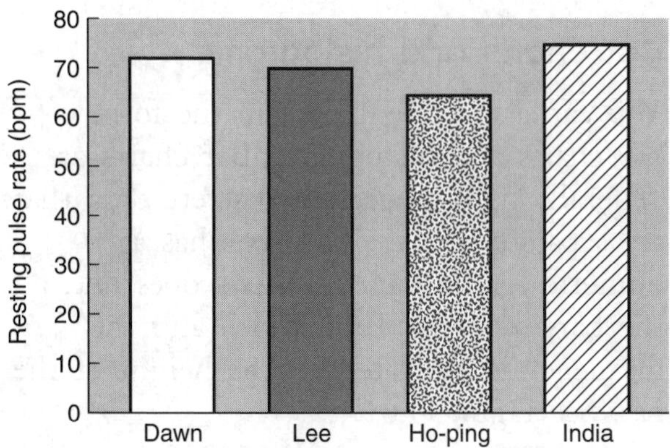


**Figure 3.61 Bar chart to show resting pulse rate for four class members**

Histograms may look like bar charts but are quite different; they are diagrammatic representations of frequency distribution. The columns in histograms are in proportion to the size of the group that they represent and the columns may be different widths. Both $x$ and $y$ axes have numbers and the frequency for a group is proportional to the area of the column. See Figure 3.62.

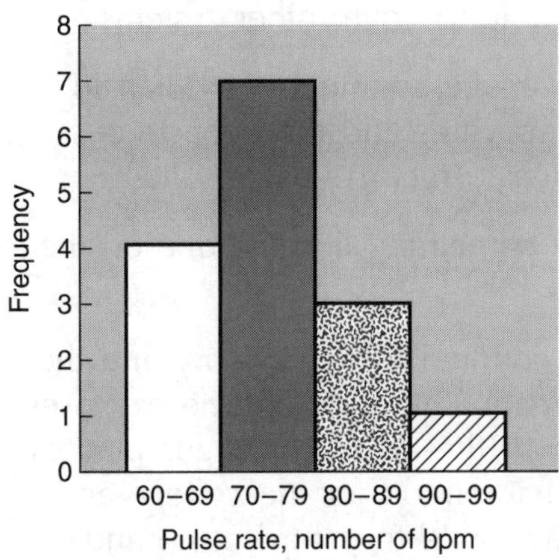


**Figure 3.62 Histogram to show frequency distribution of resting pulse rate in bpm for a group of GNVQ Advanced Health and Social Care students**

## Using formulae

We have already covered using a formula to calculate the concentration of an ion.

Other formulae you might be required to use at some time are:

- changing degrees Fahrenheit into Celsius: subtract 32 and multiply by $^5/_9$
- changing height in feet into metres: height expressed as decimals of feet divided by 3.25
- changing pounds weight into kilograms: divide the weight in pounds by 2.2
- changing volume in gallons into $dm^3$, try this one for yourself! A petrol filling station is a good place to find out if you get stuck.

# Unit 3 Assessment

For this unit you need to demonstrate your understanding of human body systems.

Using non-invasive techniques (this means not puncturing the body surface), you should monitor the physiological status of individuals. You need to measure at least three human body systems and you have to recognise and explain any deviations from the normal range of values. Safe practice should be used with any equipment and you should describe the potential health and safety risks and explain how these can be reduced.

When you have taken your measurements, you will be required to describe the gross structure and function of the three systems and explain how these are inter-related.

Finally, you should describe the homeostatic mechanisms involved in controlling the physiological factors you have measured.

## Routine measurements

Largely, the measurements you will take depend on the equipment you have access to. If you are working in care, then you will probably have modern equipment available for use and a range of clients to test. If you are in school or college, however, you may have a more limited range of equipment and individuals from whom you can take measurements. It is possible to use your peers or family members as 'clients' for your measurements, but you must state clearly who is providing the information.

Most students will be able to monitor heart rate, respiratory rate, peak flow, lung volumes and body temperatures. The body systems involved will be the cardiovascular, respiratory system and skin as part of the (sensory) nervous system. If you are in work, you may be able to cover other systems.

To start with, make a simple diary/plan to record your activities and then construct a chart on which to record your results.

It might look something like the one on the next page.

This student counted the respiratory and the pulse rates 'manually' and kept the exercises the same for all the activities. Angus played competition badminton for the college and the student was able to record pulse and respiratory rates before a crucial match, when Angus was clearly anxious and under stress. At a later date a measurement was taken of pulse and respiration rates, 10 and 30 minutes after lunch.

One of the results tables for this student's portfolio might look something like Figure 3.63.

For body temperature and blood pressure recordings, you might wish to produce a graph similar to a weekly chart for a client in hospital. You could annotate the deviations and explain them in an accompanying piece of text. Peak flow measurements might be added to the temperature/blood pressure chart by recording the values at the bottom or you could construct a separate table. If you use a spirometer, you will have a trace to add to your portfolio; remember that a spirometer trace is usually upside down, for as you inhale the pointer/pen descends and vice versa.

## Safe practice

You will find the health and safety points for each piece of equipment located in the main section dealing with using the equipment. Reread these sections and also remember to ask your tutor for any available manuals.

| Date | Activity | Outcome |
|---|---|---|
| Tuesday, 18th January | Measure Angus's heart rate at rest, during touch toes exercise (ten times) and using the exercise bicycle for ten minutes. Check his health first. Measure body temperature | Measurements were taken every minute and continued until resting rate returned; draw graph to show effects of mild and strenuous exercise on heart rate. |
| Friday, 21th January | Repeat the first activity to confirm results; also take peak flow | Repeated exactly the same, compared charts which were similar |
| Tuesday, 25th January | Angus has the beginning of a cold | Resting pulse was higher and Angus stopped during the bicycle exercise, need to repeat this when cold disappeared, but also explain deviation this time; body temperature also raised; peak flow reduced |
| Friday, 28th January | Repeat activity again, but Angus has a cold | Prepared results chart and graphs; researched physiology and structure of heart |
| Tuesday, 1st February | Repeat activity if Angus fully recovered | Angus still 'chesty', body temperature normal, but peak flow still down, need to repeat when chest clear |
| *And so on, until measurements of heart, respiratory rates, peak flow, spirometry and body temperature records are all complete* | | |

**Activity plan for monitoring Angus McP.'s body systems**

| Date | Results of measurements from Angus McP. a student in my class | | | | | | | | | | | | |
|---|---|---|---|---|---|---|---|---|---|---|---|---|---|
| | Heart (pulse) rate in beats per minute | | | | | | Respiratory rate in breaths per minute | | | | | | |
| | at rest | mild exercise | hard exercise | stress | 10m after food | 30m after food | at rest | mild exercise | hard exercise | stress | 10m after food | 30m after food | notes |
| | | | | | | | | | | | | | |
| | | | | | | | | | | | | | |
| | | | | | | | | | | | | | |
| | | | | | | | | | | | | | |

**Figure 3.63 An example of a results table**

### Interactions of human body systems

You will need to make reference to the interactions of the human body systems. For example:

- the heart delivers and receives blood to and from the lungs via the pulmonary artery and veins
- adrenaline and the sympathetic branch of the nervous system increase the heart rate during exercise, stress and fear
- skin blood capillaries constrict and dilate to assist in cooling/warming of the body
- blood distributes heat around the body
- the respiratory centre in the brain controls inhalation and exhalation by its rhythmic activities.

You will find several more interactions in the text under Body systems.

## Homeostatic mechanisms

Finally, you will need to describe the homeostatic mechanisms which control the physiological factors you have measured; again, you will find this in the relevant section of homeostasis in the chapter related to each body system. In the case of 'Angus', you will need to describe the homeostatic mechanism for heart and respiratory rates and body temperature. You can describe these as text or produce diagrams, as both are acceptable.

To conclude the portfolio, you will make a statement as to the physiological status of the individual you have measured. You might use terms such as:

> *'In excellent cardiovascular and respiratory health and very fit; has no chronic heart and respiratory problems, and has excellent control of body temperature. Is young and healthy at present, but takes no exercise and smokes heavily so may have respiratory and cardiovascular problems with age etc.'*

### For a C grade

In addition to the above you will need to review your monitoring methods to detect possible sources of error.

How accurate were your readings?

Did you take sufficient readings? One or two is not enough.

How accurate was your equipment?

One common error is quoting to several decimal places (usually because you have used a calculator) when the equipment is only accurate to one decimal place. For example, if you are taking temperature readings with an ordinary clinical thermometer, it is very difficult to estimate between two markings on the scale as they are very close together. Look carefully at your equipment scales and record the smallest division you can read accurately; that is the limit of your reading. Digital equipment will provide readings to more decimal places than analogue equipment, and you must read the manufacturer's instructions to find out the limits of accuracy.

When you have shown an appreciation of errors during monitoring, you must indicate whether these errors would have an insignificant effect on your results or make your results fairly unreliable. Clearly, this depends on the type of equipment you are using, your experience in handling the equipment and the sophistication of your equipment: a guide would be that any error of around 5 to 7 per cent can be regarded as insignificant, but when the error is 10 per cent, it is becoming significant. You will not be dealing with very small figures for any measurements.

## Case study – malfunction of homeostatic mechanisms

**Thom is 16 years old and recently he has started to lose weight, drink a lot of water and soft drinks and has had several minor infections. At the moment he is suffering from three rather nasty boils and his mother insisted that he should see the family doctor. The general practitioner gave Thom a thorough medical investigation and asked him for a urine sample that she tested with a glucose strip. She found that Thom's urine was loaded with glucose and diagnosed Diabetes mellitus. Thom was admitted to hospital for further investigations and the diagnosis was correct. He started to have insulin injections and began to feel much improved.**

**Explain how the homeostatic control of blood sugar has gone awry.**

In your explanation, you need to be sure that you use appropriate scientific words and phrases that you will appreciate through reading this and other relevant texts. You will also need to show that you have planned your work and carried out your plan carefully, modifying the plan where you find it appropriate to do so.

You will need to use secondary data to explain how homeostatic mechanisms may malfunction.

You will need to revise the text on control of blood sugar and recognise that in the absence of insulin, glucose (from dietary carbohydrate) cannot enter cells to be used in respiration. If glucose is not being used up inside cells, it will accumulate in the fluids outside cells and eventually, because there is this sugar build-up, any bacteria or other micro-organisms entering through minor wounds will rapidly multiply, causing infections such as boils. A diabetic client needs to control his or her blood sugar well in order to avoid complications like infections.

The urine, being loaded with sugar, attracts water with it due to osmosis and the diabetic client compensates by drinking lots of water. The body cells, unable to use glucose for respiration have to resort to using fats, but this causes the build-up of waste products called ketones. Ketones are harmful in large quantities and the body chemistry starts to go seriously wrong; exhaled breath smells of acetone. Diabetes, if not treated, is life-threatening.

- Use these notes and your text to write up blood glucose homeostatic malfunction.

You can also research Thom's water regulation malfunction as a consequence of his Diabetes. Another opportunity for describing a system malfunction could be during heat stroke, when the body temperature cooling mechanisms fail to switch on and the body needs cooling artificially with damp coverings until the temperature returns to normal.

You will find useful information on the Internet on heatstroke or heat exhaustion: www.thriveonline.com/health/Library/illsymp260.html

You will need to use the data that you collected to show that you know how the body systems are working together to carry out homeostasis. If you have monitored the cardiovascular and respiratory systems, you will be able to describe the control of heart and respiratory rates, particularly with reference to the increases during exercise and stress. You will find the information in the appropriate subject areas, remembering that if you need to take in more oxygen and eliminate the carbon dioxide, both rates will have to increase simultaneously. You can also describe the control of body temperature when heat is produced through exercise and temperature increases.

### For an A grade

You will have to be innovative and committed in your practical work and subsequent analysis. Suggest ways to improve the accuracy of your primary data (i.e. data that you collected yourself). Clearly this will depend on both the equipment you use and on your tenacity.

Do not forget to include every little change that you make to get better results and use your tutor to check out your ideas. When you describe the homeostatic mechanisms, be careful to use appropriate scientific terminology and construct some illustrative flow charts to improve your work. Always include graphics to illustrate your results, line graphs, bar charts, error calculations and so on.

Finally, you should be able to relate the care an individual receives to the malfunction of the homeostatic mechanism. For example, the heatstroke malfunction website will also provide the information on treatment. Wrapping a person in wet or damp sheets will mimic sweating and take heat from the body surface, resulting in the body temperature decreasing. In order to achieve a distinction portfolio, you need to provide reasons for all aspects of your work.

## Test

1 State the definitions of diffusion and osmosis and list the differences between them.

2 Describe the route of a red blood cell passing from the hepatic portal vein to the carotid artery supplying the head.

3 List four functions of the liver.

4 Terry has a tidal volume of 750ml during her workout and a breathing rate of 22 breaths per minute, calculate the volume of oxygen breathed in for a ten-minute period (assume oxygen is 20 per cent of the external air).

5 Define homeostasis.

6 During exercise, Sam's heart rate rises to 120 beats per minute and her stroke volume is 80ml. Calculate her cardiac output.

7 If Sam's heart has the same duration for systole at rest, how long are her ventricles in diastole and filling with blood?

8 If glomerular filtrate is formed at the rate of 125ml per minute and 124ml is reabsorbed, calculate the rate of urine formation. On a very hot day, 124.5ml can be re-absorbed so how much urine will be formed in one hour?

9 List the main ways in which heat is gained and lost by the body.

10 Construct a single graph from the data which follows to show the changes in concentration of glomerular filtrate as the filtrate passes down the nephron.

The first renal tubule extends from 0 to 12mm, the loop of Henlé from 15 to 30mm; second renal tubule from 33 to

| | Osmotic concentration (mOsm/$dm^3$) | |
|---|---|---|
| Distance along nephron tubule (mm) | When the body is short of water | When the body is not short of water |
| 0 | 300 | 300 |
| 3 | 300 | 300 |
| 6 | 301 | 301 |
| 9 | 300 | 300 |
| 12 | 301 | 301 |
| 15 | 328 | 328 |
| 18 | 1000 | 1000 |
| 21 | 1200 | 1200 |
| 24 | 800 | 800 |
| 27 | 180 | 180 |
| 30 | 100 | 100 |
| 33 | 108 | 95 |
| 36 | 122 | 90 |
| 39 | 158 | 85 |
| 42 | 250 | 80 |
| 45 | 300 | 75 |
| 48 | 450 | 73 |
| 51 | 1200 | 70 |

42mm; and the collecting duct from 45 to 51mm. Mark these areas in a suitable place on your graph.

Analyse the graph and explain the results with reference to the function of the nephron.

11 What stimulates the secretion of insulin?

12 The diagram (right) shows a spirometer trace of an individual at rest and during moderate exercise. Find the respiratory rate, the tidal volume and the volume of oxygen consumed in each activity.

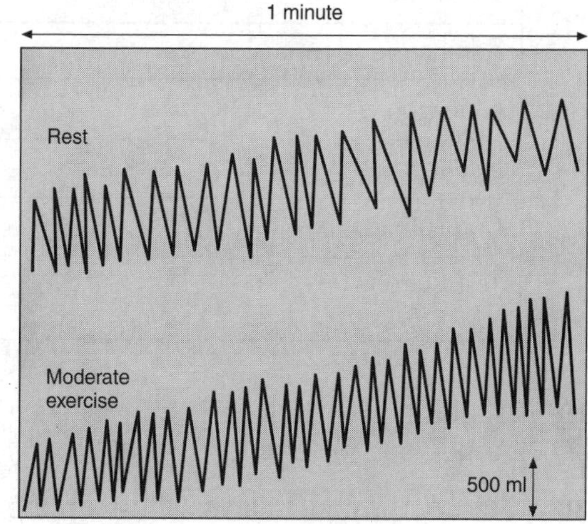


13 What is the difference between a bar chart and a histogram?

14 Why are simple, cheap clinical thermometers being phased out?

15 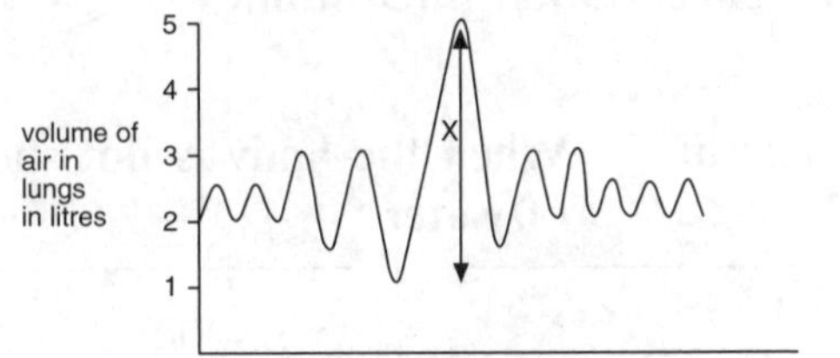


What is represented by the label marked X? Using the same diagram, write another label that represents the tidal volume.

16 Distinguish between aerobic and anaerobic respiration. Where and when does anaerobic respiration occur?

17 Describe the formation of urea. In which body organ is urea produced and how is it eliminated from the body?

18 Complete the following table:

| Name of hormone | Main action of hormone |
|---|---|
| Thyroxine | |
| Adrenaline | |
| Glucagon | |
| Insulin | |
| Cortisol | |
| Testosterone | |

19 Describe how breathing is controlled by the nervous system.

20 Construct a flow chart to illustrate the stages in the digestion of carbohydrate.

## Answers to test

1 Diffusion is the movement of molecules from a region of high concentration to one of low concentration. Osmosis is the movement of water molecules from a region of high concentration to one of low concentration through a partially permeable membrane. Osmosis is only concerned with the movement of water molecules whereas diffusion can occur in gases and liquids. Osmosis takes place through a partially permeable membrane that is usually the cell membrane.

2 Hepatic portal vein, inferior vena cava, right atrium and right ventricle, pulmonary artery, pulmonary vein, left atrium and ventricle, aorta, carotid artery.

3 Liver functions include:

- formation of urea
- storage of glycogen
- production of bile
- main site for heat production
- storage of iron from the diet and old red blood cells
- manufacture of plasma proteins.

4 Terry takes in 750 × 22 ml of air every minute = 16 500ml

In 10 minutes she takes in 165 000 ml of air but only 20 per cent of this is oxygen, so 165 000 × 20/100 = 33 000 ml or 33dm$^3$

5 Homeostasis is the maintenance of a constant internal environment.

6 Sam's cardiac output is 120 × 80ml = 9 600ml per minute or 9.6 dm$^3$ per minute.

7 Sam's cardiac cycle has reduced to 60/120 seconds = 0.5s. As her ventricles will be in systole for the normal period of 0.3s, her ventricles

will be filling and in diastole for only 0.2s.

**8** Urine formation is 125 – 124 = 1 ml per minute, on a hot day this is reduced to 0.5 × 60 = 30ml per hour.

**9** Heat is gained from the external environment and hot food and drink; heat is lost through exhaled air, urine, faeces and the skin. Heat loss from the skin is by conduction, convection, radiation and evaporation of water.

**10**

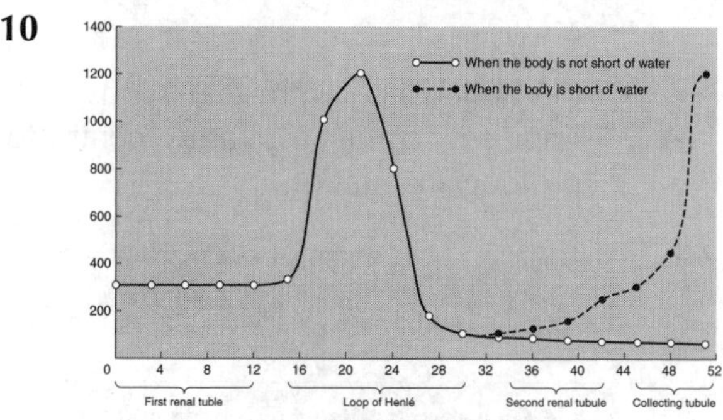


Osmotic concentration refers to the number of solute molecules in comparison to the number of water molecules. When there are few water molecules and many molecules of other types the osmotic concentration is high, conversely many water molecules and few of other types mean that osmotic concentration is low. In the first renal tubule the osmotic concentration is low and unchanging because as many water molecules as other molecules are re-absorbed into the blood. Osmotic concentration in the loop of Henlé soars because this is the area that concentrates sodium ions. The osmotic concentration falls sharply when the filtrate enters the second renal tubule and here the two graph lines separate. This shows that regardless of the body's need for water or not, the process is not specific until the second renal and collecting tubules are entered. When the body needs to conserve water as it is dehydrated, ADH secretion is high and water is re-absorbed in these parts of the nephron producing a highly concentrated urine. When there is no requirement to conserve water, ADH secretion is low and no water is further re-absorbed – making urine dilute.

**11** Insulin secretion occurs when blood glucose rises above a threshold level.

**12** Respiratory rate at rest is 22 breaths per minute, tidal volume is 750ml and oxygen consumption 1 000ml per minute. During moderate activity, the respiratory rate rose to 32 breaths per minute, tidal volume increased to 1 000ml and oxygen consumption was 1 300ml per minute.

**13** A bar chart shows blocks for discrete data and numbers only on the $y$ –axis; histograms show frequency distribution with numbers on both axes. In a histogram the area of the block is proportional to the frequency distribution.

**14** Clinical thermometers contain mercury which is poisonous to body systems if the thermometer breaks or leaks. European legislation and COSHH regulations include the phasing out of mercury-containing equipment.

**15** X represents vital capacity, any small wave at the beginning and end of the graph line represents tidal volume.

**16** Aerobic respiration breaks down glucose and oxygen to provide energy and the waste products are carbon dioxide and water. Anaerobic respiration produces much less energy because it takes place when there is not sufficient oxygen being taken in. The waste product is lactic acid which can only be tolerated for a short period. Anaerobic respiration takes place in muscle cells during strenuous activity.

**17** Urea is formed from the de-amination of amino acids that are surplus to the body's needs. The nitrogen-containing group is broken off and converted into urea. The remainder of the amino acids can be used for energy. Urea is formed in the liver but excreted by the kidneys.

**18** The completed table is as shown:

| **Name of hormone** | **Main action of hormone** |
|---|---|
| Thyroxine | Controls the rate of metabolism in the body and has a significant effect on growth and mental ability. |
| Adrenaline | Prepares the body for flight, fright and fight. Converts glycogen to glucose when blood glucose reserves are low. |
| Glucagon | Also converts glycogen to glucose. |
| Insulin | Converts glucose to glycogen and enables glucose to enter body cells. |
| Cortisol | Anti-inflammatory and helps to control blood glucose. |
| Testosterone | Growth of male sexual organs and glands, responsible for male secondary sexual characteristics. |

**19** The medulla of the brain contains clusters of neurones which represent the respiratory centre; one cluster is responsible for inspiration and the other for expiration. In normal quiet breathing, the inspiratory centre is active for approximately 2 seconds followed by the expiratory centre activity for 3 seconds. Above the medulla in a part of the brain called the pons there are two further centres associated with respiration, these are:

- the pneumotaxic centre, this inhibits the inspiratory centre as the lungs fill with air so allowing expiration to occur
- the apneustic centre that sends impulses to the inspiratory centre to prolong inspiration.

**20**

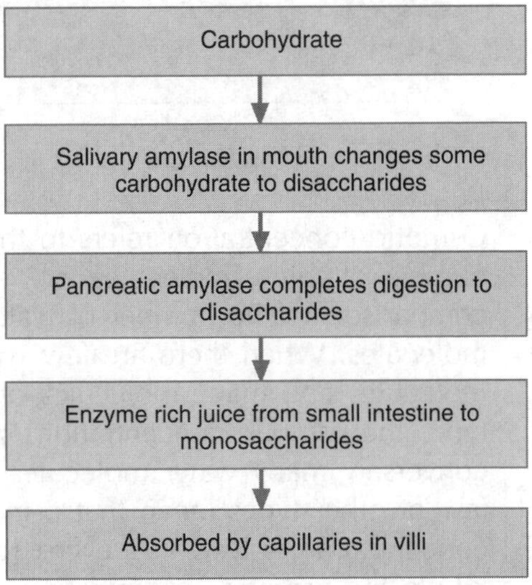

Carbohydrate
↓
Salivary amylase in mouth changes some carbohydrate to disaccharides
↓
Pancreatic amylase completes digestion to disaccharides
↓
Enzyme rich juice from small intestine to monosaccharides
↓
Absorbed by capillaries in villi

## Answers to 'Try it out'

- **Section through chest**, page 136

  A trachea – air passes through to inflate and deflate the chest

  B cartilage rings to prevent trachea collapsing when the head is turned

  C intercostal muscles which contract to raise rib cage upwards and outwards

  D air sacs leading to the alveoli where gaseous exchange takes place

  E pleural space or cavity allows two layers of pleura to move without friction

  F diaphragm sheet of muscle that descends during inhalation to increase the volume of the chest

  G pleura covering the lung, also called visceral pleura enables friction free movement between the lung and the chest wall.

- **Sodium ion concentration**, page 191

  In blood plasma the concentration is 152 meq/dm$^3$ , in intracellular fluid it is 14 meq/dm$^3$, meaning that sodium is not a major intracellular ion

- **Decimal understanding**, page 194

  0.6: zero (or nought) point six

  56.10: fifty six point one (the last zero is not meaningful)

  100.3: one hundred point three

  12 999.5: twelve thousand, nine hundred and ninety nine point five

- **Decimal addition and subtraction**, page 194

| | |
|---|---|
| Add: | 0.6 |
| | 56.10 |
| | 100.3 |
| Total | 157.0 |
| Subtract from | 12 999.5 |
| Answer | 12 842.5 |

- **Converting decimals to fractions**, page 195

  0.8 is $^8/_{10}$ or $^4/_5$

  1.3 is $1^3/_{10}$

  0.04 is $^4/_{100}$ or $^1/_{25}$

## References and recommended further reading

Hinchliff, S., Norman, S., Schober. J., (1998) *Nursing Practice and Health Care*

Gee, G.E. (1994) *Calculations for Health and Social Care,* Hodder and Stoughton

Fullick, A., (1994) *Heinemann Advanced Science: Biology,* Heinemann

Ganong, W.F., (1999) *Review of Medical Physiology,* Appleton and Lange

# Fast Facts

**ADH** Antidiuretic hormone produced from the hypothalamus/posterior pituitary part of the endocrine system to increase water reabsorption in the last part of the renal tubule

**Adrenaline** Hormone produced by the adrenal gland to boost the effects of the sympathetic nervous system

**Aerobic respiration** The release of energy from body cells by the oxidation of glucose

**Alveoli** Thin-walled berry-like swellings that make up most of the lung tissue

**Anaerobic respiration** An inefficient way of obtaining energy from glucose within muscle cells when oxygen is insufficient for the cell needs

**Aortic body** Swelling located close to the aortic arch that contains chemoreceptors monitoring chemical changes in the blood

**Arteriosclerosis** So-called 'hardening of the arteries' when calcium is deposited in the arterial wall, making it more fragile and brittle but harder to the touch

**Atrium** An upper chamber of the heart

**Autonomic system** Part of the nervous system that has two subdivisions called the sympathetic and the parasympathetic

**Bar chart** Graphic representation of discrete data

**Bicuspid valve** The valve that ensures a one-way flow of blood between the left atrium and the left ventricle

**Blood pressure** The force exerted by the blood on the walls of the blood vessels

**Cardiac cycle** The events taking place during one beat of the heart

**Carotid body** Similar to the aortic body, located close to the carotid arteries of the aorta

**Chyme** Paste-like material resulting from the churning of food by the stomach

**CNS** Central nervous system, the brain and spinal cord

**Deamination** The breaking down of surplus amino acids to produce urea

**Diabetes mellitus** An endocrine disorder due to lack of effective insulin that leads to serious disturbance of body metabolism

**Diastole** When the cardiac muscle of atria or ventricles is at rest

**Diuresis** Copious flow of urine

**Electrolyte** Substance that dissociates into ions when dissolved; note that glucose is not an electrolyte

**Enzyme** Biological catalyst capable of breaking down food chemicals in digestion and assisting chemical reactions to occur in the body cells

**Excretion** The elimination of waste products of metabolism from the body

**Feedback** Negative – inhibition of the input by a part of the output or process; positive – further stimulation of the input by a part of the output or process

**Formulae** Mathematical shortcut for determining an unknown value

**Glucagon** A hormone from the pancreas that changes glycogen into glucose

**Heatstroke** A serious failure of thermo-regulation

**Histogram** Graph to show frequency distribution of data

**Homeostasis/homoeostasis** Maintaining the constancy of the internal environment

**Hypothalamus** Part of the brain directly above the pituitary gland that is responsible for many vital processes, including water regulation

**Insulin** Pancreatic hormone that is responsible for lowering blood sugar

**Ion** A charged particle

**Islets of Langerhans** Clusters of endocrine cells within the substance of the pancreas

**Lymph** A milky coloured fluid within the lymphatic system

**Lymphatic vessel** Part of the lymphatic system that contains lymph

**Nerves** Axons and dendrons of neurones wrapped in protective connective tissue

**Neurones** Excitable cells capable of transmitting electrical impulses; sensory or receptor neurones carry impulses from receptors into the CNS; motor or effector neurones carry impulses from the CNS to muscles or glands

**Osmoreceptors** Receptors found in the hypothalamus that detect changes in the osmotic pressure of blood

**Pancreas** Organ that has both a digestive and an endocrine function; located under the stomach and connected to the small intestine via the pancreatic duct

**Parasympathetic nervous system** Part of the autonomic nervous system that is active during resting and non-stressful conditions

**Peak flow** The maximum speed at which air can be forced out of the lungs

**Pituitary gland** Part of the endocrine system that produces many hormones, some of which control other endocrine glands

**Pulse** A shock wave transmitted down the walls of arteries when the ventricles of the heart contract

**Rate of change** Determining how a variable changes in unit time

**Scattergram** Graph to determine whether large numbers of plotted points have correlation

**Semilunar valves** Valves located at the base of both the aorta and the pulmonary artery to ensure a one-way flow of blood through the heart

**Sphygmomanometer** Equipment for recording blood pressure

**Spirometer** Equipment used for measuring lung volumes, breathing rates and oxygen consumption

**Sympathetic nervous system** Part of the autonomic nervous system that is active in fright, flight and fight conditions

**Synapse** A tiny gap between two neurones that is bridged by a transmitter substance to enable the impulse to cross

**Tidal volume** The normal ebb and flow of air into and out of the chest

**Tricuspid valve** The valve ensuring a one-way flow of blood through the heart, located between the right atrium and the right ventricle

**Urea** Metabolic waste product produced by the liver from excess amino acids

**Ureter** Tube carrying urine from the kidney to the bladder

**Urethra** The tube carrying urine from the bladder to the exterior

**Urine** Watery solution of urea and salts produced by the kidneys and eliminated through the bladder and urethra

# Factors affecting human growth and development

Unit 4

**This chapter is organised in four sections. You will learn about:**

- **human development – an overview of physical, social and emotional development.**
- **the development of ability – a review of some key features of personal and skills development throughout life.**
- **factors affecting development – an account of environmental, social and genetic influences which influence individual life chances.**
- **theories of development – an exploration of some of the traditional theories which are used in health and social care contexts to explain influences on human development.**

**Some advice is provided on preparation for a Unit test and some sample test-yourself questions are provided.**

## 4.1 Human development

It is traditional to see our lives as involving certain definite periods of development. Terms like infant, child, adolescent and adult have been used for centuries to classify the age-related status of individuals. During the last century it was common to assume that there was a universal pattern to both physical and social development. During infancy, childhood and adolescence, a person would grow physically and learn the knowledge and skills needed for working life. Adulthood was a time when people would work and/or bring up their own families. Old age was when people would retire. Children would be grown up by the time their parents reached old age.

An American theorist called Havighurst described the developmental tasks of the different life stages (Havighurst, 1972). Some examples of these stages are listed below:

- **Infancy and early childhood**
  Learning to take solid foods
  Learning to walk
  Learning to talk
  Learning bowel and bladder control
  Learning sex differences and sexual modesty.
- **Middle childhood**
  Learning physical skills necessary for ordinary games
  Learning to get along with peers
  Learning an appropriate masculine or feminine role
  Developing basic skills in reading, writing and calculating
  Developing concepts necessary for everyday living
  Developing conscience, morality and a scale of values.
- **Adolescence**
  Achieving new and more mature relations with peers of both sexes

Achieving a masculine or feminine role
Accepting one's physique and using the body effectively
Achieving emotional independence of parents and other adults
Preparing for marriage and family life
Preparing for an economic career.

- **Early adulthood**
  Selecting a mate
  Learning to live with a marriage partner
  Starting a family
  Rearing children
  Managing a home
  Getting started in an occupation.
- **Middle age**
  Assisting teenage children to become responsible and happy adults
  Reaching and maintaining satisfactory performance in one's occupational career
  Relating to one's spouse as a person
  Accepting and adjusting to the physiological changes of middle age
  Adjusting to ageing parents.
- **Later maturity**
  Adjusting to decreasing physical strength
  Adjusting to retirement and reduced income
  Adjusting to the death of one's spouse
  Establishing satisfactory physical living arrangements.

Levinson *et al.* (1978) described the developmental periods in *adulthood* using the categories below:

- 17–22: Early adult transition
- 22–28: Entering the adult world
- 28–33: Age 30 transition
- 37–40: Settling down
- 40–45: Mid-life transition
- 45–50: Middle adulthood
- 50–55: Age 50 transition
- 55–60: Culmination of middle adulthood
- 60 on: Late adult transition and late adulthood.

Levinson *et al.* perceived life as involving definite age-related transitions, where people would have to re-adjust their sense of self and their life goals.

While many people may have life experiences which fit with the tasks described by Havighurst (1972) or the transitions described by Levinson *et al.* (1978), life in the twenty-first century is likely to confront people with a far greater diversity of possibilities, opportunities and problems when it comes to describing periods of development.

Manuel Castells (1996) argues that life has changed so much that the notion of adolescent, adult and later life tasks and transitions is no longer relevant for many people:

> 'Now, organisational, technological and cultural developments characteristic of the new, emerging society are decisively undermining this orderly life cycle without replacing it with an alternative sequence. *I propose the hypothesis that the network society* [the world today] *is characterised by the breaking down of rhythmicity, either biological or social, associated with the notion of a life cycle.*' (Page 446).

Biological, social and economic influences on development are changing because:

- Science is now prolonging life and health for many people – retirement need not be seen as necessary at a set age.
- Reproduction no longer has to start in early adulthood. It is now possible for women to give birth in their 50s!

- People's life plans no longer necessarily focus on a set job role for 'adult' life.
- Retirement can be an optional and even temporary condition that can take place at almost any age.
- Gender, family and reproductive roles are no longer perceived as fixed. One in five women will not have children in their life. A substantial number of people may not marry. Two in every five marriages end in divorce.

We now live in a rapidly changing world where many people can choose their own style of living and plan families, careers and social roles with less and less reference to age. Even so, there are some generalisations about biological, social and emotional development which can be made at the beginning of the new century. These generalised patterns of development may help health and social care workers to understand the needs of people who become clients in the next decade or so.

For the purposes of this book, the following life stages will be used:

- infancy (0–2 years)
- early childhood (2–8 years)
- puberty and adolescence (9–18 years)
- early adulthood (19–45 years)
- middle adulthood (46–65 years)
- later adulthood (65+).

## Physical growth and development

### Infancy (0–2 years)

Every individual has a unique pattern of growth and development. This is because there are so many factors influencing our progress. It would be logical to say that each one us begins from the moment a sperm nucleus from the father joins with the nucleus from the mother's ovum, but the exact time of this process, known as *fertilisation*, is usually unknown. To obtain a more recognisable starting date, doctors will ask a pregnant woman for the starting date of her last menstrual period and add on two weeks. The period when the ovum is available for fertilising by the sperm is halfway between menstruations.

There is, however, a great deal of controversy over when an embryo becomes a human being. This has largely arisen from discussions about abortion. In Britain, the Abortion Act (1967) allowed termination of pregnancy up to the 28th week of gestation; but after lengthy debates in Parliament, the limit was reduced to the 24th week. The debate continues, however, as babies can now survive if born at 24 weeks, owing to the great advances made in modern techniques. Many groups think that the limit should be reduced even further. Some pressure groups (such as Life) and many individuals consider that all abortion is wrong and human life is sacred from the date of fertilisation.

The fertilised ovum, now known as a *zygote*, is one of the larger cells in humans and is just visible to the naked eye. Imagine the smallest dot you can make with a very sharp pencil and this is about the right size. After a short rest period it begins to divide, first into two cells, then four, eight and so on. Quickly the tiny structure becomes a ball of smaller cells – a *morula*. These cells begin to become organised into different areas. Some will be destined to form the new human being, but for a while the majority of the cells are preparing to become its coverings and developing placenta. It is important that these parts are ready to secure the food supply for the developing being as soon as the structure enters the womb, or uterus, of the mother. All the time so far has been spent in travelling down the fallopian tube leading from the ovary into the uterus. At about a week old, the tiny structure, a hollow ball of cells known as a *blastocyst*, arrives in the uterus. The next few days are vital to the embryo. It must bury itself in the *endometrium*, the thickened lining of the mother's uterus and secure a food supply before the mother's next menstruation is due. If this does not happen, the blastocyst will be swept out of the mother's body with the products of menstruation and will die. Once embedded in this way, a process called *implantation*, the tiny embryo releases a hormone into the mother's blood which prevents the next menstruation.

Never again will growth be so rapid. By the third week after fertilisation (week 5 of the pregnancy calculation), the embryo has grown to be 0.5 cm long and has started to develop a brain, eyes, ears and limbs. Some individuals might class the development of the brain as being significant in the date of becoming a human being. There is even a tiny heart pumping blood to the newly-formed placenta to obtain nutrients and oxygen from the mother's blood.

The embryo continues to grow and develop at a fantastic rate until at week 8 all major organs have formed and there is a human-looking face with eyes, ears, nose and mouth. Limbs have formed fingers and toes, and the body length has increased to 3 cm (Figure 4.1). The name changes again – from now until birth it is called a *foetus*.

Growth and development of internal organs continues and the next main stage is at 20 weeks. The mother will begin to feel

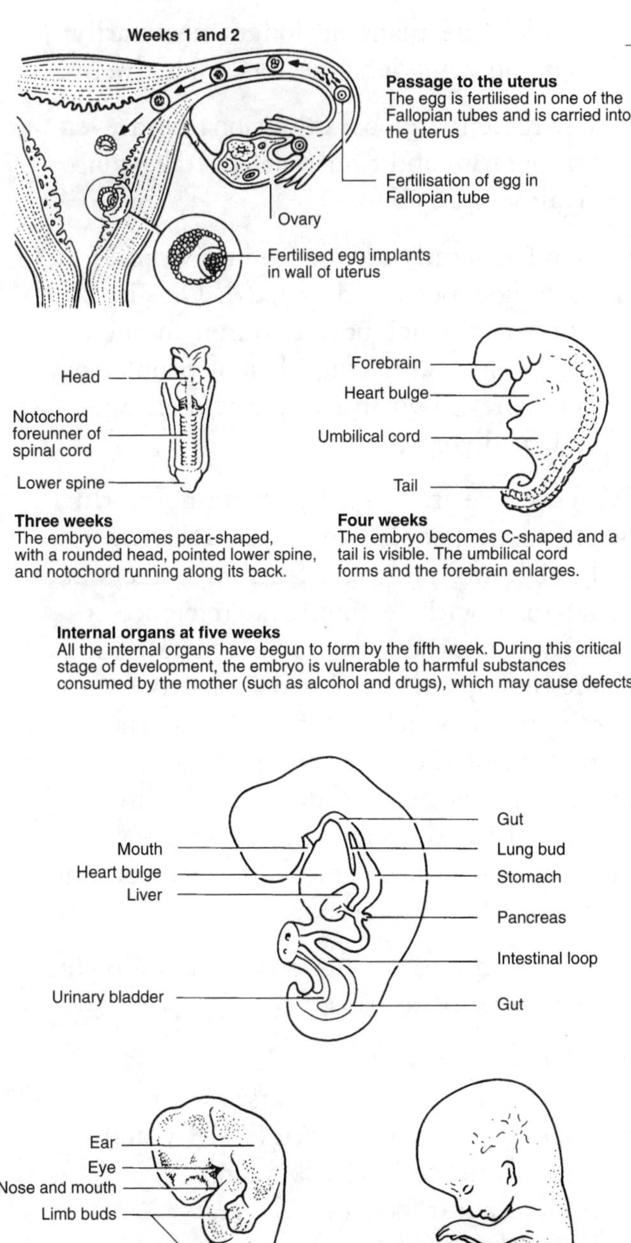


**Figure 4.1 Embryo development**

movements of the foetus, weak at first but getting stronger as the pregnancy progresses. The midwife can hear the heart beats through a trumpet-shaped instrument called a *foetal stethoscope*. The heart beats are very fast and difficult to count without experience.

The foetus is clearly male or female because the external sex organs have developed and the total length is now around 24 cm. The weight of the foetus is close to 0.5 kg already.

**Try it out**

1 Using the table below, draw two graphs to show the changes in length and weight up to birth.

2 Find out the length and weight of a typical 5.5-month foetus.

| Time in months of pregnancy | Length in centimetres | Weight in kilograms |
|---|---|---|
| 1 | 0.35 | Almost none |
| 2 | 3.5 | 0.05 |
| 3 | 8.5 | 0.1 |
| 4 | 15 | 0.2 |
| 5 | 23 | 0.4 |
| 6 | 30 | 0.75 |
| 7 | 38 | 1.5 |
| 8 | 45 | 2.0 |
| 9 | 51 | 3.5 |

As you can see from your graph and the table, at 9 months (40 weeks) the foetus is ready to be born. It is about 50 cm long and weighs around 3.5 kg.

A newborn infant, often called a *neonate*, is a helpless individual and needs the care and protection of parents or others to survive. The nervous system which co-ordinates many bodily functions is immature and needs time to develop. The digestive system is unable to take food that is not in an easily digestible form such as milk. Other body systems, such as the circulatory and respiratory systems, have undergone major changes as a result of birth – the change to air breathing and physical separation from the mother. A few weeks later, the baby's temperature regulating system is able to function properly and fat is deposited beneath the skin as an insulating layer.

## Key principles of development

Although development is a continuous process, it is not an even one affecting all parts of the body equally. However, development always follows the same sequence. The upper part of the body, particularly the head and brain, progresses extremely rapidly, while the lower part of the body, particularly the lower limbs, follows more slowly. This type of development is said to be **cephalo-caudal** and it means 'from head to tail'. Arms and legs, called 'the extremities', develop later than the heart, brain and other organs in the mid-line of the body. So as well as being cephalo-caudal, development is also from the midline to the extremities. The reason for this is not hard to find: most vital organs are controlled by the brain and protected by the trunk. As the baby is

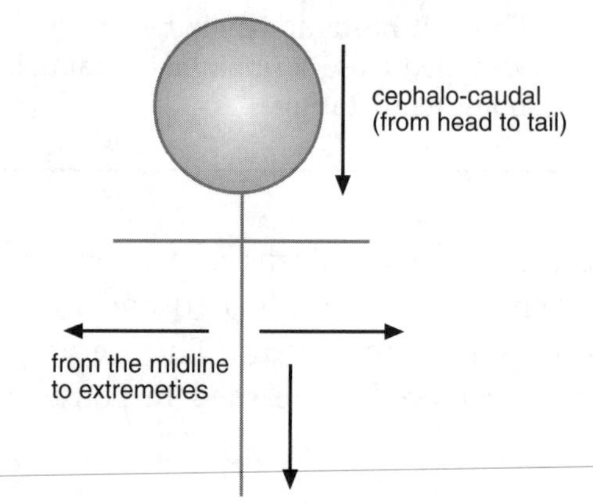


Figure 4.2 The sequence of development

dependent on the mother for nourishment, limbs are not essential to early survival.

### Think it over

Look back at the diagrams showing early development and you will notice the unusual overall shape of the infant's body and the strange proportions of the different parts compared to the whole. For example, measure the length of the whole 8 week-old foetus and then measure the length of the head only. You will find that the head is approximately 50 per cent of the total length, whereas the arms and legs are quite small and weak.

### Think it over

Compare a newly born human to a newly born calf. The mother cow has limited intelligence and wanders about to feed itself on grass. The calf has long well developed limbs to stand almost immediately so that it can follow the mother to feed on her milk, it also has a warm coat to maintain body temperature. The human baby would die if there were no nourishment as it is unable to find the source of milk for itself and cannot follow on its own limbs. It needs to be clothed or wrapped close to mother to maintain body temperature.

For the first three months of a baby's life, movements are unco-ordinated and many *primitive reflexes* are present. These are gradually replaced by learned responses.

## Primitive reflexes

The main reflexes are:

- rooting
- grasp
- moro
- walking.

They are used to test the functioning of the baby's nervous system.

- *Rooting reflex*

The baby turns its head in response to a touch on the cheek. This enables the baby to find the mother's breast and nipple. The suckling reflex occurs when the baby finds the nipple. A finger placed close to the corner of the mouth will cause this sort of response.

- *Grasp reflex*

Any object put into the palm of the baby's hand will be grasped strongly. Often the grasp is so strong that the baby's weight can be supported.

- *Moro, or startle, reflex*

When a baby is startled, its hands and arms are thrown outwards and the legs straightened. The baby often cries and then pulls the arms, hands and fingers inwards as if trying to catch hold of something. This is one of the first reflexes to disappear.

- *Walking reflex*

During the first two months, when a baby is held upright with feet touching the ground, forward movements are made by the legs as if the baby is walking.

| **Try it out** | If you have access to a newborn baby, ask if a doctor or nurse can show you these reflexes. |
|---|---|

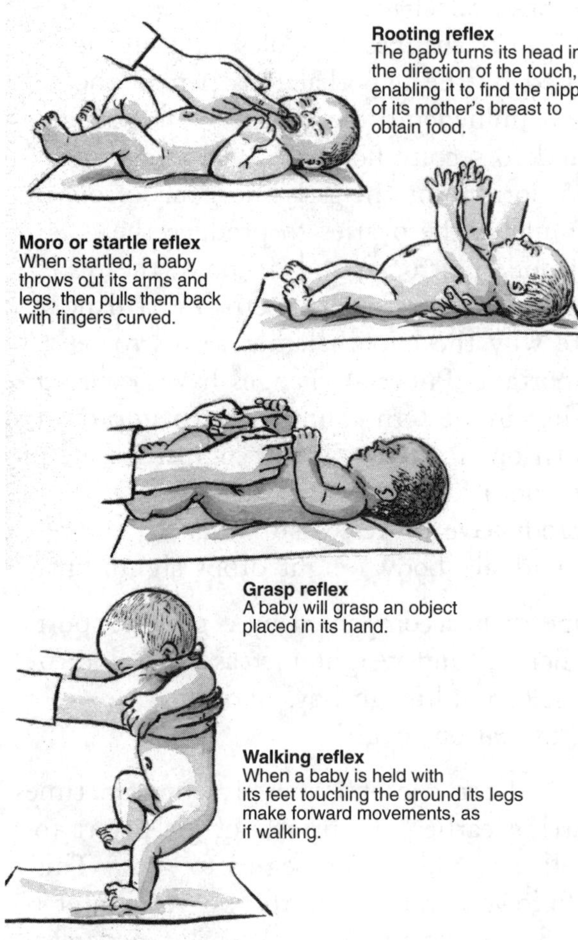


**Figure 4.3 The primitive reflexes of a newborn baby**

## Myelination

Nerve fibres attached to nerve cells gradually acquire a fatty sheath during the first years of life. This is known as *myelination*. Nerve impulses travel a lot faster when they are insulated in this way. Many nerve cells have to 'connect up' with each other and these two processes mean that both muscle and nerve co-ordination slowly increase.

## Early childhood (2–8 years)

During childhood, different parts of the body grow at different rates.

The nervous system, sense organs and head grow very rapidly from birth to 6 years. A 6-year-old's head is 90 per cent of the adult size, and he or she can wear a parent's hat! The reproductive organs remain small and underdeveloped until the onset of puberty (between 11 and 16 years), and then they grow rapidly to reach adult size. General body growth is more steady, reaching adult size at around 18–20 years, but with three 'growth spurts' at 1, 5–7 years, and puberty.

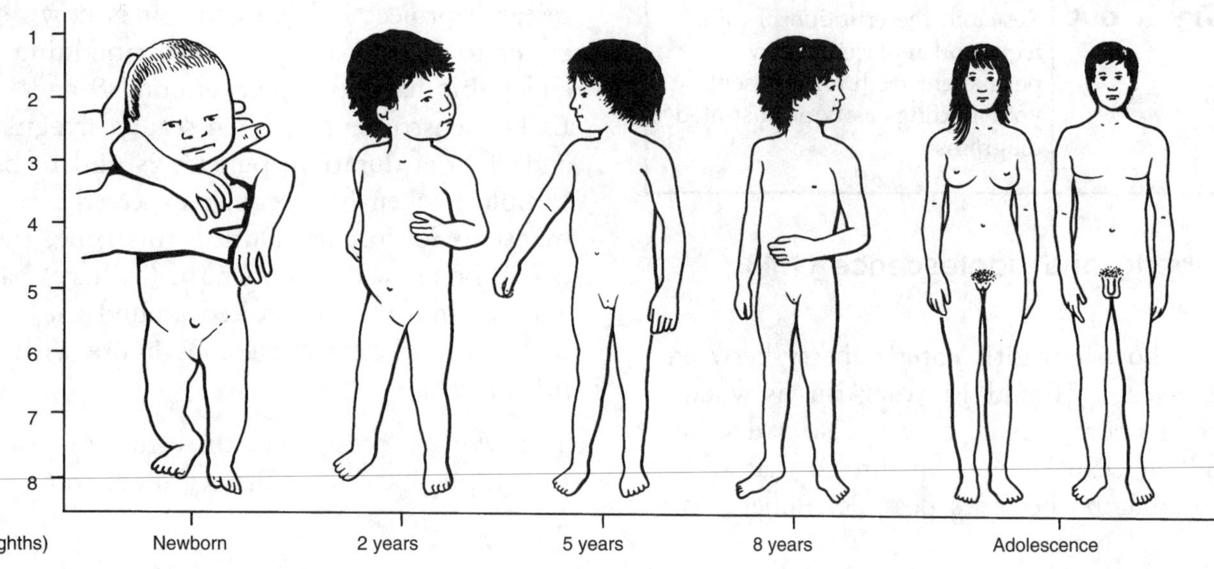


**Figure 4.4 Growth profiles from birth to adolescence**

| **Try it out** | Look at Figure 4.4. Write notes on the changes you can see between birth and 8 years. |
|---|---|

When the skeleton first forms it is made of a flexible material called *cartilage*. This is slowly replaced by bone which is visible on x-rays. Each bone passes through the same sequence of changes of shape as it reaches maturity in a healthy adult. Bone age is, therefore, a useful measure of physical development. Height and weight standards are often associated with age, but are less useful because of the enormous differences which can occur in different individuals.

### Teeth

Babies develop their first set of teeth from the age of 6 months up to 3 years. They are often known as milk teeth, or *deciduous teeth*. From about 6-years-old, these teeth are gradually replaced by the permanent teeth. There are wide variations in dates of both the eruption of milk teeth and their replacement by permanent teeth and, therefore, only average dates can be given.

| **Try it out** | Research the eruption of milk teeth and replacement by permanent teeth and present your findings as two illustrated diagrams. |
|---|---|

### Puberty and adolescence (9–18 years)

Both boys and girls enter puberty between the ages of 10 and 15 years; this is when the secondary sexual characteristics develop and the sexual organs mature so that reproduction becomes possible. Puberty is the physical change which accompanies the emotional changes of adolescence and is caused by the hypothalamus part of the brain influencing the pituitary endocrine gland to secrete hormones known as gonadotrophins. In girls the gonadotrophin stimulates the ovaries to produce the hormone oestrogen and, in boys, the testes produce testosterone. Experts are still not sure why the hypothalamus seems to be important. Pubertal changes have occurred earlier in western countries with improved nutrition. It is also well recognised that, in the condition of anorexia nervosa, reproductive processes fail when an individual's body weight drops significantly.

Puberty is accompanied by a growth spurt in height, and weight increases are due to muscle building in boys and fat accumulation in girls.

Around the age of 10 to 11, but sometimes starting earlier, the breasts of girls start to swell, and pubic hair begins to grow. This is followed around one to two years later by the first menstruation, called the menarche. One hundred years ago the menarche occurred at an average age of 14.8 years; in 1988 it had reduced to 12.5 and a current research project indicates that it is now closer to 10 and 11, with breast budding and pubic hair appearance around 8 and 9. Early menstruation is often scanty, irregular and of brief duration; puberty is said to be complete when full, regular expected menstruation occurs. During this time, the pelvic bones widen, underarm (axillary) hair appears and fat is deposited around the body to produce a curvaceous figure with full breasts.

The whole process takes three to four years to complete and very little growth in height occurs after puberty. Oestrogen is the hormone largely responsible for the physical changes but a second hormone produced during the second half of each menstrual cycle, i.e. progesterone, promotes glandular development of breasts and uterine linings.

Puberty in boys lags behind that of the girls by about two years, so at some time girls can be both taller and heavier than boys; boys eventually overtake girls in height and weight by the end of puberty.

The male penis normally begins to grow bigger around the age of 13 and reaches its full size by 15. The testes in their scrotal sacs also grow rapidly to be followed by pubic, axillary (armpit) and facial hair. Testosterone is responsible for these changes and it stimulates the testes to produce sperm, the prostate glands and seminal vesicles to produce glandular secretions. Some boys can be sexually mature at 14 or even as young as 12 while others have barely started puberty, so there is a wide range of variation in sexual development around these years.

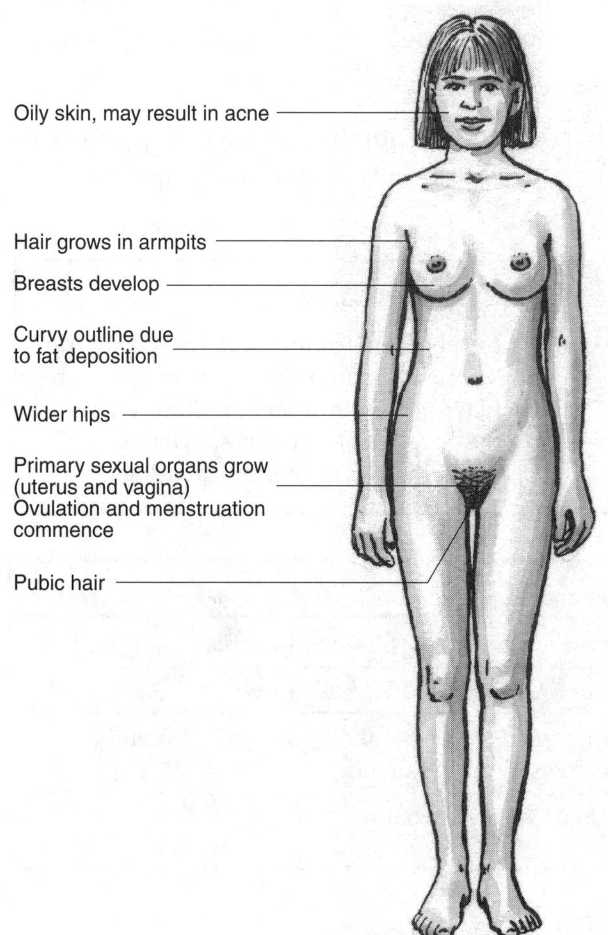


**Figure 4.5 Female body changes at puberty**

There is also a significant increase in the size of the voice box or larynx, so that the vocal cords responsible for voice production not only grow longer but thicker – causing the voice to deepen. Girls' voices also become less shrill over puberty, but this is not so noticeable as the voice change in boys.

Emissions of semen (sperm with accompanying glandular secretions) during sleep are common in adolescent males, the so-called 'wet dreams'.

## Influences on growth

### a) Inherited characteristics

Height and build are thought to be controlled by a number of genes as well as environmental influences. An individual's height, for example, may depend on the proportions of 'tall' and 'short' genes that they have inherited from their parents. Tall parents may have more 'tall' genes than shorter parents and are thus likely, but by no means definitely, to pass on more 'tall' genes to their children. Average height parents are more likely to pass on fairly equal mixtures of 'tall' and 'short' genes. However, during certain types of cell division that precede the production of ova and sperm, there are random exchanges of

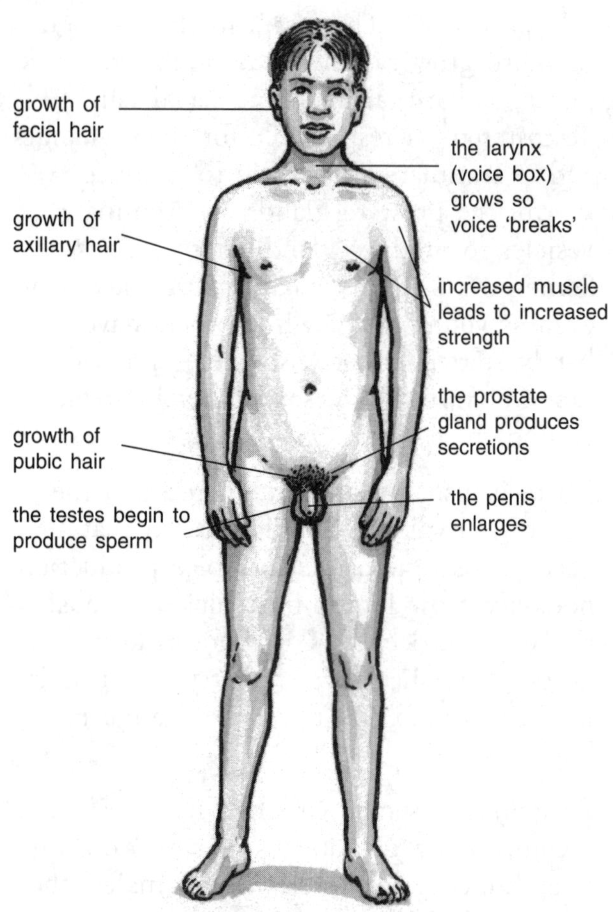


**Figure 4.6 Male body changes at puberty**

genes. It is quite possible for a child of average parents to have a larger 'allocation' of 'tall' or 'short' genes than any brothers or sisters and so to be unusually tall or short.

### b) Health and disease

Clearly, if a mother and her child are in good health there is every opportunity for growth and development to be at the optimum. After weaning, the link between the health of the mother and the health of her children is not so directly tied; however, chronic illness in a mother may mean that she is tired or not fit enough to provide as much stimulation for development as she would otherwise do. Providing that the period of time is not excessively lengthy and alternative care is eventually provided, the child will catch up.

If the child is not healthy, growth tends to be affected as energy supplies may be

> **Think it over**
>
> In the comedy film *Brothers*, Danny de Vito and Arnold Schwarzenneger were playing two brothers at either end of the height and weight spectrum. Unlikely to happen, but possible!

| Male | Female |
|---|---|
| 1 Enlargement of testes and penis | Enlargement of breasts and nipples |
| 2 Pubic, facial, underarm hair growth | Pubic and underarm hair growth |
| 3 Increased muscle and bone size leads to increased strength | Increased fat deposited under skin leads to increased curvy shape |
| 4 Voice deepens (breaks) | Onset of menstruation |

**Table 4.1 Secondary sexual characteristics**

directed elsewhere, for example to combat disease, or to supply muscles for extra work such as in coughing, maintaining balance in deformity, chronic bowel disorders and so on. Any disorder affecting the raw materials required for growth, or hormones concerned with the process of growth, will disturb the process. Some of the conditions which affect growth and development are:

- cystic fibrosis
- endocrine disorders
- diabetes mellitus
- asthma
- coeliac disease
- musculo-skeletal disorders
- gastro-intestinal disorders
- genetic disorders.

**c) Environmental factors**

Children who live in deprived or disadvantaged circumstances may have their growth and development affected by poor home situations, such as inner city high-rise flats with no recreational areas and damp infested interiors. Parents who smoke cigarettes tend to have smaller than average children who do less well at school. Alcoholism in families affects the health and welfare of children, as do any other circumstances that cause anxiety in the home environment. Living close to nuclear establishments has recently been shown to affect children's health, particularly in the incidence of serious diseases such as cancer.

**d) Nutrition and diet**

Malnourishment will affect growth directly, and this could be the influence of too little food or food of the wrong type. A child whose main meals consist of chips or similar foods with inadequate protein, fruit and vegetable content, may appear well-nourished, but lacks essential foods to promote healthy growth and development.

### Think it over

How far do you think genetic influences affect the height and build of people and how far are issues such as diet and lifestyle involved in influencing shape and size?

## Physical development: Adulthood and middle age (19–65)

After puberty, there is little further growth in height but muscle building often continues with increased work and leisure pursuits. Some weight gain is often experienced slowly from the mid-twenties onwards, usually as a result of less strenuous activity and more sedentary work patterns. This is by no means universal and depends very much on the influences dictated by lifestyle.

Between the ages of 45–55, females experience a decline in fertility eventually

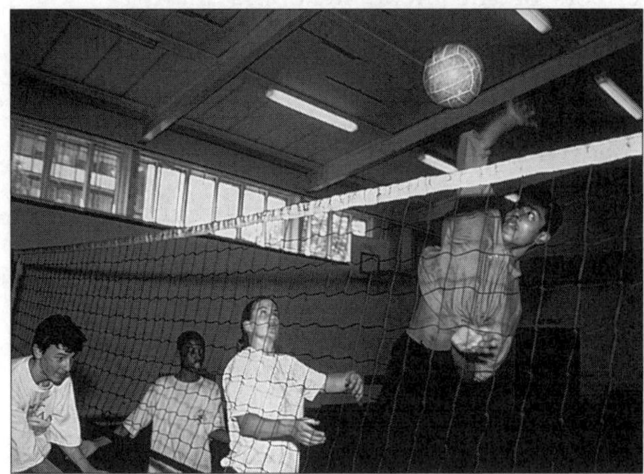

Figure 4.7 Many different factors produce people with different growth patterns

resulting in a complete cessation. This is called the 'menopause'. Menstrual periods become irregular, sometimes scanty and sometimes heavy, and may be accompanied by night sweats and feelings of bloatedness as well as mental and emotional changes such as anxiety, tiredness, confusion and periods of weepiness. The extent of these changes varies tremendously from woman to woman. A few women are able to sail through the menopause symptom-free, whereas others suffer hot flushes and night sweats well into their sixties.

The cause of these effects has been attributed to the lack of viable eggs in the ovary and the high level of pituitary hormones in the bloodstream that are trying to stimulate the ovary into producing the eggs that are no longer there. Many women become less interested in sex after the menopause. As the level of oestrogen in the blood falls, some females suffer a loss of bone density known as *osteoporosis*; their skeletal bones are more brittle and more likely to fracture with falls and injuries. Hormone replacement therapy (HRT) is available to combat the effects of the menopause and many menopausal women accept this regime even though it usually causes monthly withdrawing bleeding similar to menstruation.

Males can experience physical changes in the same way, although of course not the menstrual changes. These form the basis of the so-called 'male menopause' ascribed to a decline in the levels of testosterone.

> **?** At least 20 per cent of men are thought to experience changes due to low testosterone levels as they get older. The figure may even be as high as 50 per cent.

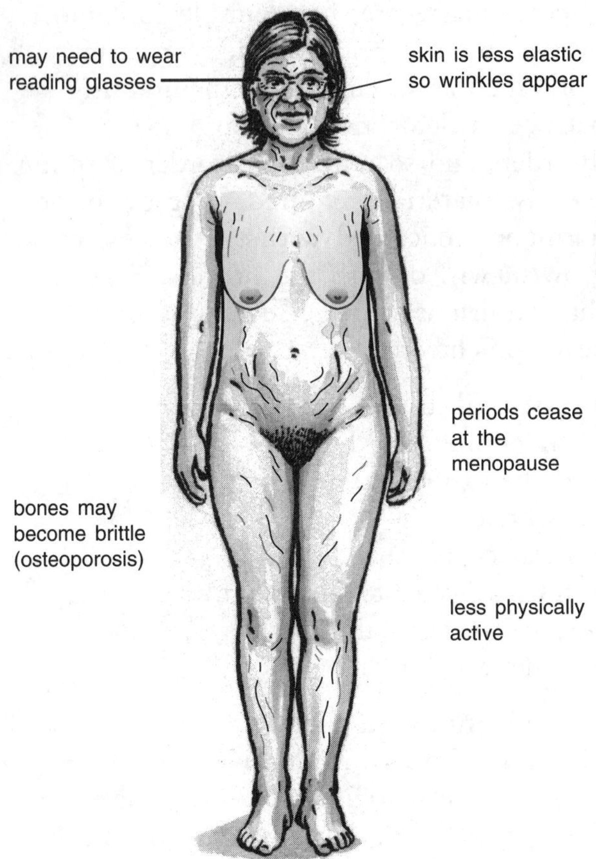


**Figure 4.8 Some physical changes become obvious as people get older**

Men are still able to father children well into their 70s and 80s – assuming the absence of disease and that they were fertile in the first place.

> **?** One in two people over the age of 60 will experience significant hearing loss.

As people get older, they begin to show some wrinkles, greying hair, 'middle age spread', less elastic skin, less muscle firmness and a reduced inclination to be strenuously active. The eyesight begins to change. The focal point for accurate work such as reading gets farther and farther away and reading glasses usually become necessary.

Loss of hair may affect both sexes in the middle years of life, but it is much more common in men. Hair loss in men occurs first from the temples, then the crown of the head, with a gradual widening of the bald area to the sides of the head.

Older people are usually less active than younger people, but often still continue to take in the same amount of food. This usually results in a gradual thickening of the trunk, arms and legs, often called 'middle age spread'. Many people regard this as an inevitable stage in getting older, but generally it is a result of not matching food (and therefore energy) intake with energy output.

### Later adulthood (65+)

Physical and mental changes occur as time passes. Not many people live to be over a hundred years old – the average life span is around 85 years of age in the West.

Sexual activity may decline only a little or a lot, very often depending on the usual life pattern of the individual. Elastic tissue, present in many organs, degenerates with age and this is most readily seen in wrinkled skin. Blood capillaries are more fragile so bruising occurs from relatively small injuries.

The number of nerve cells in the central nervous system steadily decreases from quite a young age and they are irreplaceable. This loss, unnoticed at first, begins to show as one gets older. It results in poorer memory, difficulty in learning new skills quickly and slower reaction times. Senses are less acute, particularly taste, smell and hearing.

The progressive loss of hearing which can come with age is known as *presbyacusis* – sounds are less clear and high tones less audible. It occurs with the degeneration of the sensory hair cells of the cochlea (in the inner ear) and of nerve cells.

The focusing power of the eye weakens with age, beginning at around 45. Often after the age of 65 there is little focusing power left. Large print can usually be seen, but smaller print needs to be held at arm's length, until eventually all focusing is replaced by spectacle lenses (*presbyopia*). Almost everyone over the age of 65 has some degree of cataract, where the lens in the eye has started to become opaque. The condition tends to progress with advancing years and most people have some loss of vision due to cataract formation at around 75 years.

As the body ages it gradually loses its sensitivity to cold, so when body temperature drops an old person may not feel the cold. With age there is a lowered ability to reverse a fall in body temperature, which is why older people are more likely to develop *hypothermia* in cold weather.

Heart, breathing and circulation all become less efficient, causing difficulty with climbing stairs and hills, and with strenuous exercise. A healthy young adult has a blood pressure around 110/75 mm of mercury, but around the age of 60 years this is 130/90 or higher.

Muscle thins and weakens, while joints become less mobile and total height shrinks. Wound healing and resistance to infection decline with age. Functions of organs like the kidneys and the liver slowly decline.

However, there are positive aspects to growing older. Despite the decline of physical systems, a combination of tolerance, wisdom and experience built up over the years enables older people to avoid the mistakes made by younger, inexperienced people.

Healthy older people may have greater emotional control and a more developed understanding of their self-concept than younger people. Socially, older people may have more time to appreciate people and their environment.

## Social and emotional development: an overview

The life story of an individual person will involve the interaction of their genetic structure with the social context and events that make up a person's environment. Human development can also be influenced by the interactive nature of human behaviour and thought. People are not simply moulded into shape by circumstances – people can make choices and interact with their environment in a way which will influence how they adapt to their environment.

This section provides an overview of life stages and describes some of the social issues to which people have to adapt. More specific detail can be found in later sections of this chapter.

## Social and emotional development: infancy (0–2 years)

On average, infants will follow a moving person with their eyes during the first month of life. They will also show an interest in face-like shapes. By two months of age infants may start to smile at human faces and may indicate that they can recognise their mothers. By three months an infant may make sounds and smile when an adult talks. At five months, infants can distinguish between familiar and unfamiliar people. By six months an infant may smile at a mirror image.

It seems as if babies come into world prepared to make relationships and learn about others. Infants try to attract attention, they will smile and make noises to attract adults. It may be the case that infants have an in-built need to make a relationship that will tie or bond them with their carer. The development of a social and emotional bond of love between a carer and infant is one of the key developmental issues during infancy. The nature of 'bonding' was originally emphasised by the theorist, John Bowlby. Bowlby believed that the quality of love between an infant and their carer could have a major effect on the quality of the whole of the rest of a person's life.

### Bowlby's theory of bonding

Bowlby (1953) states, 'What occurs in the earliest months and years of life can have deep and long-lasting effects'.

Bowlby studied mothers and babies in the mid 1940s, just after the end of the Second World War. Bowlby had noticed that some baby animals would make very fixed emotional bonds with their parents. For example, baby ducklings would attach themselves to, and follow, whomever they presumed to be their mother. Wild ducklings will naturally attach themselves to the mother duck. Bowlby had studied

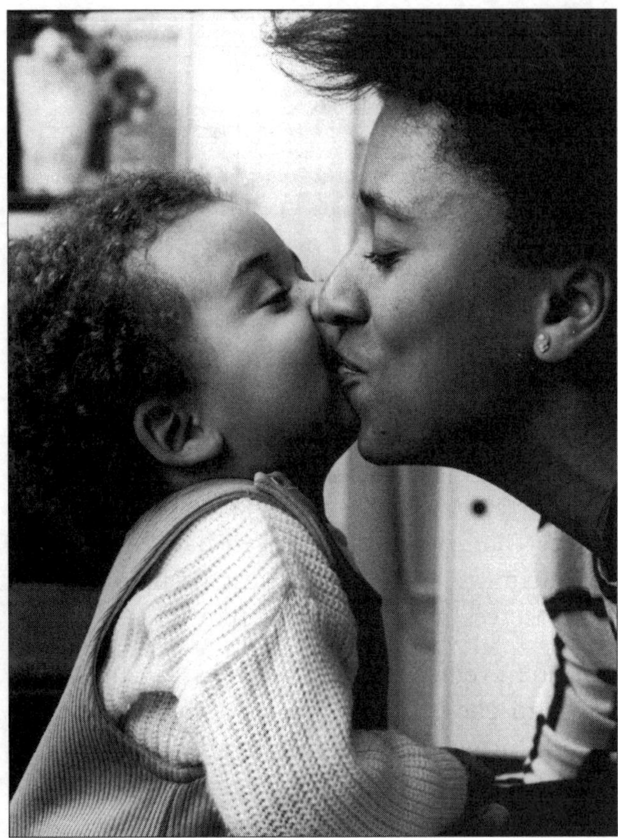

**Figure 4.9 Early bonding is a key developmental issue**

research which showed that ducklings would attach themselves to humans if humans were all that was around during a critical period when the duckling needed to bond.

Bowlby's studies of infants led him to the conclusion that human babies were similar to some types of animal, such as ducks. Bowlby believed that there was a biological need for mothers and babies to be together, and that there was a sensitive or critical period for mothers and babies to form this attachment, which is known as bonding. Bowlby (1953) stated, 'The absolute need of infants and toddlers for the continuous care of their mothers will be borne in on all who read this book.' (Page 18)

If the bond of love between a baby and its mother was broken through separation, Bowlby believed, lasting psychological damage would be done to the child. If a mother left her infant to go to work every day, or just once to go into hospital, there might be a risk of damage. Bowlby believed that children who suffered separation might grow up to be unable to love or show affection. Separated children might not care about other people. Separated children might also fail to learn properly at school, and might be more likely to turn to crime when they grew up.

Some other researchers working outside of the psychodynamic perspective have doubted that babies are really affected so seriously by separation. Michael Rutter (1981) found evidence to suggest that it is the quality of emotional attachment between a carer and the infant that matters. Not being able to make an attachment may damage a child emotionally. But it is the making of a bond of love between the baby and a carer that matters, not whether temporary separations happen.

There is research that suggests that babies can and do make bonds with their fathers and with their brothers, sisters, or other carers. In one study (Schaffer and Emerson, 1964) almost a third of 18-month-old infants had made their main attachment to their fathers. It seems that babies give their love to the person or persons who give them the best quality affection and time.

Alan and Ann Clarke (1976) reviewed a wide range of research. They concluded that children can recover from almost any bad psychological experience provided that later experience makes up for it. It is whole life experience and not just the first years of an infant's life that will decide whether a child grows up to care about other people, or takes to a life of crime. However, although people can recover from separation and poor relationships, it is very important that infants do have a chance to make a loving relationship or bond with carers. The first part of a person's life may set the scene for what will happen next. A lack of love in early life could be a very bad start for a child's emotional development. It would be unwise just to hope that some later quality of life could make up for it.

## Social and emotional development: early childhood (2–8 years)

A child's attachment to parents and carers is just as strong as in infancy, but children no longer need to cling to carers. As children grow older they start to make relationships with other children and learn to become more independent. Young children still depend very much on their carers to look after them, however, and they need safe, secure, emotional ties with their family. Close emotional bonds provide the foundation for exploring relationships with others.

Attachments within a family setting provide a child with opportunities to learn from others. As a child grows he or she will copy what other adults and children do. Children learn attitudes and beliefs by watching the behaviours of parents, brothers, sisters and other relatives toward them. Parents and families create a setting or context in which children learn expected social behaviour. This process of learning social rules is called socialisation.

### Socialisation

Socialisation means to become social – children learn to fit in with and be part of a social group. When children grow up within a family group, they will usually learn a wide range of ideas about how to behave. For instance, at mealtimes, some families will have strict rules that everyone must sit down at the table and it is considered 'rude' if one person starts to eat before the others. Other families may not even have set mealtimes – people may just prepare food for themselves when they feel like it.

In the evenings, some families might sit around the TV together as a social group, while other families might all sit in different rooms doing different activities. Some families are very concerned that people take their outdoor shoes off before coming into the house, and others have no rules about shoes.

Families and similar social groups develop attitudes about what is 'normal' or right to do. Sociologists call these beliefs 'norms'. Each family will have 'norms' that cover how people should behave.

By the age of 2, children usually understand that they are male or female. During the socialisation process, children learn how to act in masculine or feminine ways. Boys may copy the behaviour of other male members of the family, and girls may copy the behaviour of other female members. Sociologists call this learning a gender (male or female) role. Learning a gender role means learning to act as a male or female person.

| **Try it out** | Are, or were, any of the following 'norms' important in your family?<br>• To say 'thank you' or 'thank you for having me' to the head of a household you visited?<br>• To give thanks in prayer before a meal?<br>• To eat hot food with your fingers?<br>• To go to bed at a fixed time – unless there is a special event or festival?<br>• Never to interrupt when an older member of the family is speaking?<br>• That children have set tasks to help adults with the housework?<br>• That male members of the household are responsible for decorating and repairing the house?<br>• That female members of the household are responsible for all the washing and ironing?<br>Make a list of your family's social and behavioural 'norms' and then compare your list with others in your group. |
|---|---|

During childhood, children learn ideas about what is right or wrong. They learn the customs of their culture and family, they learn to play gender and adult roles, and they learn what is expected of them and what they should expect from others. Socialisation teaches children ways of thinking, and these ways of thinking may stay with a person for life.

### Primary socialisation

Not everything that a child learns during first (or primary) socialisation within the family group is learned by copying adults. Children also spend time watching TV, listening to radio and playing computer games. Children will be influenced by the things they see and hear over the media as well as their experiences within the home.

| **Think it over** | Look at the picture of a breakfast scene below. Think carefully – how many influences on the children can you spot? |
|---|---|

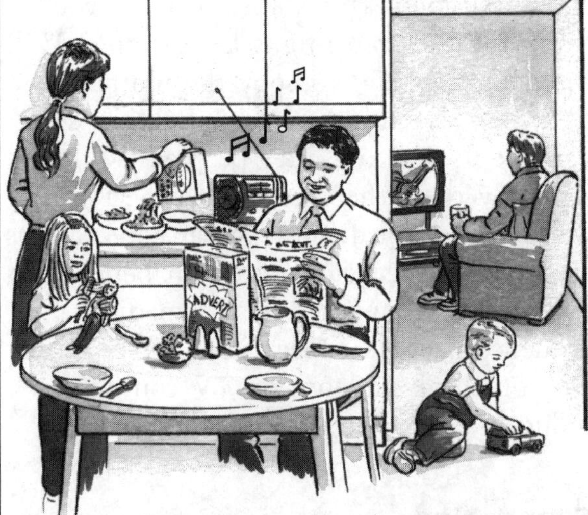


**Figure 4.10 Breakfast time in a family home: how many things to do with socialisation can you spot?**

Did you notice the media influence in this home? The radio sends messages about love and relationships in the songs that are playing. The TV sends messages about news and opinions. The newspaper invites the reader to share its views on current events. Even the cereal packet has an advert encouraging the family to get money and spend it!

Did you notice the gender roles in this home? Who is preparing the children's breakfast, and who is being waited on? What differences are there in the way the two children are playing – what toys have they chosen?

Does playing with dolls or playing with toy cars influence children's expectations in life? Note the length of hair for males and females and their clothes.

Thinking about this scene, what do you think the children might be learning? Will the daughter tend to copy the mother's behaviour as she grows up – will she see her role as 'looking after people'? Will the son copy the father's role and expect to be waited on at mealtimes? What expectations might people develop just from being with each other? How far does the media influence people's expectations of their life? Do you think violence on TV could influence these people in any way?

### Friendships

Young children enjoy playing with others and will often see children that they play with as being their friends. However, 3 and 4 year olds will often show a need or even a preference for being with parents rather than with friends. This is sometimes called 'safe base behaviour' where the child seeks affection and reassurance from parents. By 7 years of age most children will express a preference for playing with others rather than needing the security of being in close contact with carers.

Friendships become increasingly important as children develop independence. Older children will seek friendships based on trust. Friends are special people who are trusted – not just people that are available to play with. Gender role seems to have a major impact on the way older children play. Helen Bee (1994) quotes studies in the USA which suggest that while 5 to 6 year olds will sometimes play in mixed gender groups, it is rare for 7 to 8 year olds to do so. Children of 8 years mainly play with friends of their own gender group. Boys are often less formal and less polite to friends than they are to strangers, but they will often develop networks of relationships which can include quite a wide circle of friends. Helen Bee (1994) suggests that girls often form smaller circles of friends. Close friendships among girls are based on mutual beliefs and a willingness to agree with each other.

> **Think it over**
>
> These observations of social behaviour are based on evidence from ten or more years ago. Is this what you experienced yourself as a child and do these patterns of gender differences still work the same way today?

## Social and emotional development in later childhood (9–18 years)

### Puberty and adolescence

As children grow older they become more independent. Friendship groups become increasingly important and can exert a major influence on behaviour. For a few individuals the norms and beliefs of friends may conflict with the values and norms learned during primary socialisation.

### Secondary socialisation

As children grow older they go to school and learn to read and use computers. The range of influences on them grows larger. However, although children make friends and learn new ideas at school, the main group experience for most children will still be with their family and kinship group.

Children's needs for love and affection and the need to belong to a group will usually be met by the family. If a child is rejected or neglected by the family, he or she will be at risk of developing a low sense of self-worth and poor self-esteem.

During adolescence the importance of the family group begins to change. Between 11 and 15 years of age adolescents become very involved with their own group of friends. Most adolescents have a group of friends, usually people of the same age, who influence what they think and believe. This is the second influential group to which people belong, and it creates a second type of socialisation, that sociologists call secondary socialisation.

After the age of 12 or 13, a person's sense of self-worth is likely to depend more on the reactions of others of the same age than on what parents say. During adolescence it is important to be accepted by and to belong with friends and peers. Adolescents may tend to copy the way other adolescents behave, although they usually retain the values and cultural norms they learned during primary socialisation.

Socialisation does not finish with secondary socialisation. People continue to change and learn to fit in with new groups when they go out to work and when they start their own families.

**Primary socialisation** = first socialisation within a family or care group

**Secondary socialisation** = later socialisation with friends and peer groups

### Think it over

Try to remember when you were 14 or 15 years old. Can you recall what you and others in your class at school thought about the following topics? What sort of beliefs and values did your parents have at that time? Which beliefs are closest to your beliefs now?

1 It is important to get a good job.
2 It is bad and dangerous to use drugs.
3 It is important to go out and have a good time.
4 Wearing the right clothes to look good is a priority.
5 Saving money is a priority.

## Change and transition during adolescence

Adolescence can involve major pressures to change and adapt as young people go through rapid social, emotional and physical development. Sources of pressure may include:

- The need to make new friendships when transferring schools.
- Coping with change within a family group. (Nearly one in four children may expect divorce or the loss of a parent within their family before the age of 16. One in eight children will live with one or more step parents.)
- Coping with academic pressures to succeed and achieve good school results.
- Developing friendship networks and making relationships with 'best friends'.
- Balancing the beliefs and demands of family and the beliefs and values of friendship groups.

- Understanding sexuality and making sexual relationships.
- Coping with the transition from school to work – some adolescents and young adults experience a loss of self-esteem during this transfer.

A historical view of adolescence was that it was a time of 'storm and stress'. Stanley Hall (1904) believed that the biological and social pressures on teenagers inevitably caused an experience of emotional turbulence. This belief may have been reinforced by the 'teenage rebellion' that characterised the 1960s and 1970s in the USA and Europe.

In this period of history many parents had fixed expectations that their children would follow traditional gender, work and family roles, but as the world economy changed, many teenagers adopted lifestyles and beliefs which challenged traditional assumptions. It was possible to ignore the huge changes in technology and society and instead to see these challenges to tradition as a symptom of storm and stress. Recent authors such as Berryman (1991) and Zimbardo et al (1995) question the view that adolescence is generally stressful or necessarily involves conflict with parents. The emerging picture of adolescence over the last 20 years suggests that the majority of people experience a smooth transition and are able to adapt to the changes involved in this period of life without emotional distress.

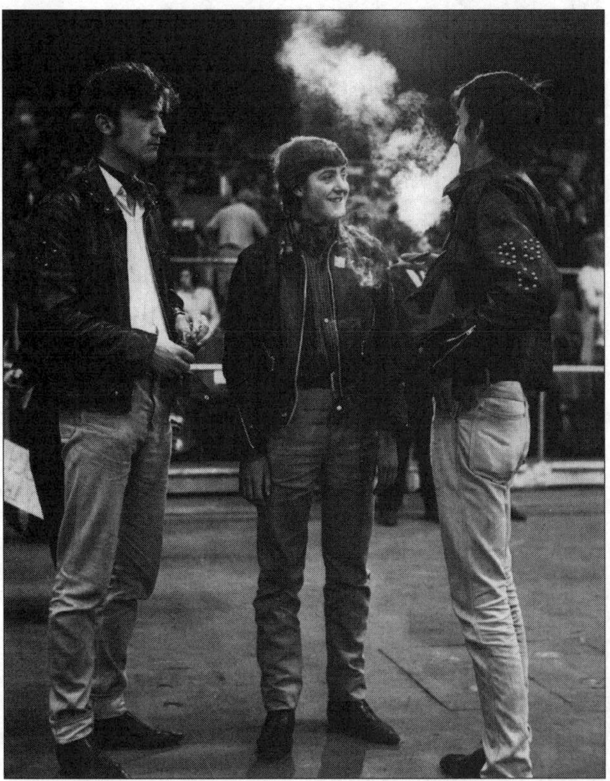

**Figure 4.11 The 1960s were characterised by teenage rebellion**

### Think it over

What areas of change did you experience during puberty?

Thinking of people you know, has change been experienced as a storm of emotional confusion or has it been more of a time of exciting problems to solve?

Toward late adolescence people will begin to think about, plan or take on job responsibilities. Adolescence is a time when many people actively seek new experiences in order to explore the world and develop the skills and knowledge needed for later life. Fifty years ago, the change from adolescent exploration to taking on adult responsibility was often quite obvious. Starting work or leaving home to get married could mean the start of a settled adult lifestyle. Nowadays, many people continue to explore social relationships and are constantly learning new skills and knowledge for most of their adult life. For many people, the transition from adolescent social lifestyles to 'adult social lifestyles' is no longer clearly marked in western culture.

## Social and emotional development in early adulthood (19–45 years)

In Britain people are given the right to vote when they are 18, and 18 years of age is usually taken as the beginning of the social category of adulthood.

Early adulthood is often a time when people continue to develop their network of personal friends. Most young adults establish sexual relationships and partnerships. Marriage and parenthood are important social life events which are often associated with early adulthood. Some adults delay or decide not to have children as they prioritise personal development and careers. The pressure to get paid employment and hold down jobs is also a major social issue for adults.

As in all periods of life, early adulthood involves the need to adapt to social and emotional pressures. The demands of family and career are a source of growing pressure for many young adults. The Henley Centre (1999) published a report called 'The Paradox of Prosperity'. The report

### Think it over

Look at the table below which describes the number of sexual partners that people claim to have had in the previous year. The pattern seems to suggest that as people become older there is an increasing tendency to have just one partner. Is this to do with age, or is it to do with culture, or is it both?

| England | Percentages | | | | | |
|---|---|---|---|---|---|---|
| | 16–19 | 20–24 | 25–34 | 35–44 | 45–54 | All aged 16–54 |
| **Males** | | | | | | |
| None | 48 | 14 | 7 | 8 | 11 | 13 |
| One | 24 | 49 | 78 | 80 | 82 | 71 |
| Two or more | 28 | 38 | 16 | 13 | 8 | 16 |
| All males | 100 | 100 | 100 | 100 | 100 | 100 |
| **Females** | | | | | | |
| None | 30 | 17 | 9 | 10 | 13 | 13 |
| One | 37 | 53 | 81 | 86 | 85 | 76 |
| Two or more | 33 | 30 | 10 | 4 | 2 | 11 |
| All females | 100 | 100 | 100 | 100 | 100 | 100 |

Source: Health Education Monitoring Survey, Office for National Statistics and Health Education Authority

Table 4.2 Number of sexual partners in the previous year: by gender and age, 1998 highlights some of the pressures on adults today.

'Significant factors contributing to family breakdown are the growing pressures of work and the pursuit of material gains. Women, in particular, consider that they have sacrificed the chance of having children or even forming relationships for the sake of their career. Men on the other hand, are more likely to miss out on a home life.' (Page 25.)

One study quoted in the report found that 23.7 per cent of men and 22.2 per cent of women claimed that they had missed their children growing up because of their career choices. A similar percentage reported that they had put 'work before family'. The Henley Centre reports that 37 per cent of people feel that their working hours are increasing and 55 per cent believe that they have been subjected to more pressure at work over the past three years. In addition 59 per cent of people believe they are burdened with excessive time pressure, while 21 per cent claim to be 'very concerned about the amount of free time I have'.

Balancing work and relationships is not the only change or transition which young adults need to adapt to. Adult life can involve a range of transitions and changes which create a need for social and emotional adaptation.

Holmes and Rahe (1967) produced a catalogue of life events to which people frequently have to adapt. Barrie Hopson (1986) states that this general index was found to be consistent across European countries and with the cultures of Japan, Hawaii, central America and Peru. Naturally, the amount of work needed to readjust to a life event differs for each individual. Each person has particular vulnerabilities, strengths and weaknesses. The Holmes-Rahe scale is no more than a general overview, which was originally researched in the USA in the 1960s.

| Life event | Value |
|---|---|
| Death of partner | 100 |
| Divorce | 73 |
| Marital separation | 65 |
| Going to prison | 63 |
| Death of a close family member | 63 |
| Personal injury or illness | 53 |
| Marriage | 50 |
| Being dismissed at work | 47 |
| Marital reconciliation | 45 |
| Retirement | 45 |
| Change in health or family member | 44 |
| Pregnancy | 40 |
| Sexual difficulties | 39 |
| Gaining a new family member | 39 |
| Business or work adjustment | 39 |
| Change in financial state | 38 |
| Death of a close friend | 37 |
| Change to a different line of work | 36 |
| Change in number of arguments with partner | 35 |
| Mortgage larger than one year's net salary | 31 |
| Foreclosure of mortgage or loan | 30 |
| Change in responsibilities at work | 29 |
| Son or daughter leaving home | 29 |
| Trouble with in-laws | 29 |
| Outstanding personal achievement | 28 |
| Partner begins or stops work | 26 |
| Begin or end school | 26 |
| Change in living conditions | 25 |
| Revision of personal habits | 24 |
| Trouble with boss | 23 |
| Change in work hours or conditions | 20 |
| Change in residence | 20 |
| Change in schools | 20 |
| Change in recreation | 19 |
| Change in religious activities | 19 |
| Change in social activities | 18 |
| Mortgage or loan less than one year's net salary | 17 |
| Change in sleeping habits | 16 |
| Change in number of family get-togethers | 15 |
| Change in eating habits | 15 |
| Holiday | 13 |
| Major festival, e.g. Christmas | 12 |
| Minor violations of the law | 11 |

**Table 4.3 The Holmes-Rahe life-event scale**

The value scale suggests that on average the death of a partner involves ten times the change, and perhaps the threat, that being caught for speeding does. Changing to a new school is half as stressful (on average) as a new sibling being added to the family.

The Holmes-Rahe scale may be a useful list of changes and transitions which might happen to adults. But it is important to remember that few people are 'average'. In your own personal life you may rate some issues as far more or less stressful than the scale suggests.

In 1997 the Holmes-Rahe scale was tested out in Nevada (USA) and a new scale suggested. The 15 most stressful life events are listed in Table 4.4.

| | |
|---|---|
| 1 | Death of partner |
| 2 | Divorce |
| 3 | Death of close family member |
| 4 | Marital separation |
| 5 | Fired from work |
| 6 | Major illness or injury |
| 7 | Jail term |
| 8 | Death of close friend |
| 9 | Pregnancy |
| 10 | Major business readjustment |
| 11 | Loan repayment demand |
| 12 | Gain new family member |
| 13 | Marital reconciliation |
| 14 | Change in health of family |
| 15 | Change in financial state |

**Table 4.4 The 15 most stressful life events (1997)**

These tables give some overview of the social issues that adult life requires people to deal with.

## Social and emotional development in middle adulthood (46–65 years)

Early adulthood is particularly associated with starting a career, making relationships and partnerships, and for many people starting a family. 'Middle adulthood' from 46 to 64 years of age is likely to be more associated with maintaining work roles, relationships and meeting family commitments. Early adulthood may focus on developing a lifestyle which has to be developed and maintained as life progresses. The issues identified by Holmes and Rahe (1967) are relevant across the whole of the adult life-span.

One of the distinctions between middle and early adulthood is the increasing significance of having to support parents as well as children. Some 'middle age' adults find that time pressures actually increase as they become older. It can be very difficult to balance the demands of financing their chosen lifestyle, meeting commitments to their own children, commitments to parents, commitments to a partner and/or friends, and commitments to the local community.

Many people feel sandwiched with time pressure. When children leave home some adults may feel that time pressures have been removed. However, other individuals may feel that they have lost part of their social purpose when children no longer need their support.

?

The Henley Centre report 'The Paradox of Prosperity' reports that;

- 82 per cent of the UK population (15 and over) claim to suffer from stress.
- Almost a quarter of the UK population claim to have suffered a stress-related illness in the previous year (1999 research).
- Workplace absenteeism, largely attributed to stress, cost UK businesses £10.2 billion in 1998.

## Social and emotional development in later adulthood (65 years and over)

The age at which men can start to receive the state pension in the UK is 65. In the future this will also become the age at which women can access the state pension (it is still 60 years of age at present). Therefore 65 is seen as a possible age to use as a social definition of being 'elderly'. Most 65 year olds do not see themselves as old however, and some writers distinguish between the 'young-old' (65 to 80) and the later years (80 plus). Many 80 year olds will still reject the term 'old' however!

As with all periods of life there are immense variations in how life is experienced. A person's social class, wealth, health, gender and ethnicity (race) may have far more significance on the type of life they lead than simply how old they are. Key age-related issues include:

- Retirement: the great majority of people over 65 do not undertake paid employment in order to maintain their lifestyle. There is wide variation in the incomes that people live on, ranging from people who are dependent on state benefits through to people who have extensive savings and company pensions.
- Free time: the majority of people over 65 no longer have to care for children, although some may act as carers for relatives or friends. For those who are free of work and care pressures, retirement can represent a time of self-

| Period of life | Life event |
|---|---|
| Infancy | Emotional attachment and bonding |
| Childhood | Adapting to social roles and norms.<br>Learning social skills.<br>Making friends. |
| Puberty | Adapting to own sexuality<br>Developing new friendships<br>Adapting to norms of peers.<br>Developing social skills. |
| Early adulthood | Adapting to demands of work and finance, relationships/family. |
| Middle adulthood | Adapting to change in roles.<br>Coping with unwanted change. |
| Late adulthood | Adapting to reduced stamina and possibly to disability. |

Table 4.5 Adaptation to life events

development when they can indulge interests in hobbies, travel, socialising, and learning for its own sake. For some others, retirement and loss of a care role creates a feeling of uselessness and loneliness.

- The risk of disability: as life progresses, physical impairments may influence mobility, hearing, vision, memory and general performance of daily living activities. Depending on the support available, and on the perceived significance of an impairment, these impairments may create disabilities which restrict the satisfaction an individual achieves from life.
- Financial and social resources: a person's enjoyment of later adulthood may be influenced by the level of financial resources they have; their perceived health including what people believe they can do; and their network of support from community, family and friends. (See section 4.3 for further details of these issues.)

# 4.2 Development of skills and abilities

## Gross and fine motor skills

Motor skills is the term used to describe the ways in which muscles are used and co-ordinated to produce movements and perform tasks. Some actions demand the use of large muscles, such as those found in the trunk and legs. Actions using large muscles, and complete limbs, are called *gross motor skills*. Other actions are much smaller and precise, using small muscles such as those in the fingers. These actions are called *fine motor skills*. All over the world children appear to develop their motor skills more or less in the same order, regardless of the place in which they live. However, children have very different experiences because of their different cultures and, therefore, may not pass through some stages on the same time-scale.

For the purpose of study, we will divide the span of life into significant stages, remembering that these are rather artificial distinctions.

**Think it over**

Think about small children between the ages of two and five that you know well, perhaps members of your family, neighbours or friends. How many of them have cycles or other play equipment?

The availability of activities and equipment may greatly influence the development of fine and gross motor skills. Children who do not have access to equipment may develop more slowly than children who are not disadvantaged. Poverty and deprivation may restrict the development of skills.

### Infancy (0 to 2 years)

- *Gross motor skills in the first six months*

The new-born infant will lie on his or her back with the head turned to one side and if turned over onto the front, the head is similarly turned. There is no support from the infant's muscles if pulled to a sitting position. At one month of age, the infant can lift the head briefly and this movement becomes stronger and lasts longer over the

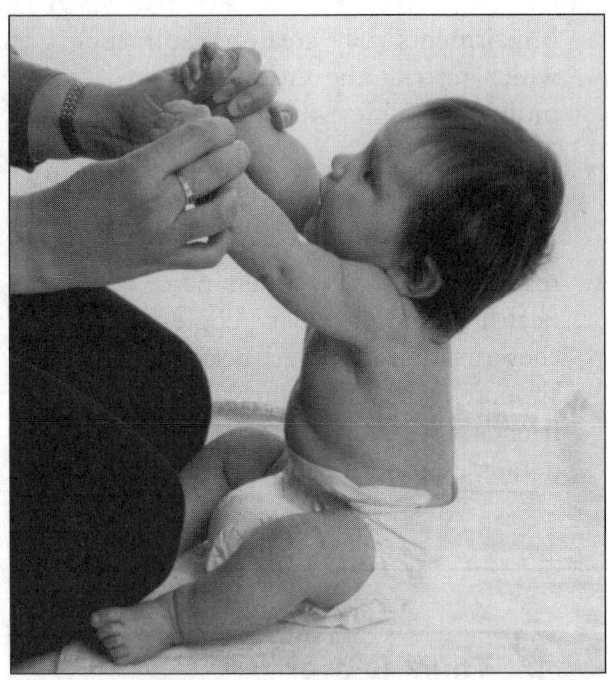

Figure 4.12 This baby shows little head lag while being pulled to a sitting position

succeeding weeks. Arms and legs move but there is no control and no purpose behind the movement. Up to two months, the infant can lift the head briefly in the lying position and can turn from the side to the back. There is still head lag when pulled to sit at this stage.

Towards the three-month stage, the head lies centrally and when the baby is on the front, he or she can support the head and chest on the forearms. Arms and legs are moved energetically and when pulled to sitting there is little or no head lag.

Babies move their heads to watch people or objects and are inquisitive about everything. This is the stage when objects are grasped in the palm of the hand and everything ends up in the mouth! The baby can sit with support for a short period.

- *Fine motor skills in the first six months*

At first, there is very little fine movement, but gradually the baby's eyes are attracted to light and bright objects. The nervous system is not yet sophisticated enough to send precise nervous signals to control tiny muscles. The baby shows more interest in the surroundings and increasingly follows people and objects as they move around. Towards the three month stage, the baby becomes interested first in playing with his or her fingers and later with the feet. Rattles can be held for a short time.

- *Gross motor skills six to nine months*

Gross motor skills are developing fast at this stage. The baby can sit for quite a long time without support, move from front to back and some can even walk around the furniture holding on to things.

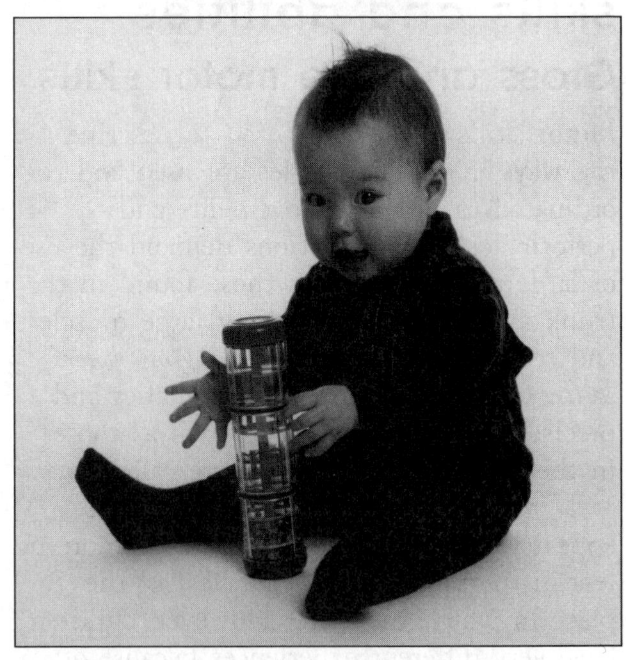

Figure 4.13 The baby can sit alone without support

- *Fine motor skills around six to nine months*

Transferring objects held in one hand to the other becomes part of fine motor play, and if a toy accidentally falls to the ground the baby looks for it. Objects are still mouth-tested and interest is shown in everything. Towards nine months the baby starts to use the thumb and first finger to pick up small objects like crumbs. This is known as the *pincer grasp.*

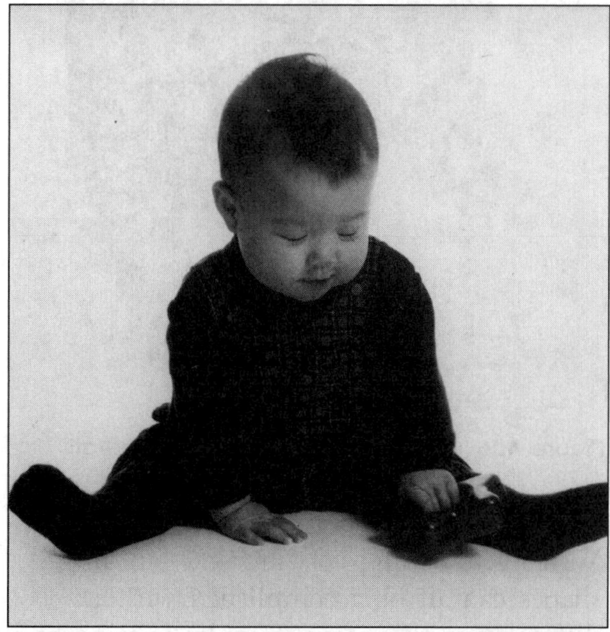

**Figure 4.14 The pincer grip is used to grasp an object**

- *Gross motor skills from nine months to one year*

The baby is usually mobile at this age, either crawling, bottom-shuffling, walking on hands and feet (called bear-walking) or even walking. Furthermore, most babies can even crawl upstairs or onto low furniture.

- *Fine motor skills from nine months to one year*

The pincer grasp is well developed and the art of deliberately throwing things on to the floor is great fun! Pointing to objects and poking at them is interesting and the baby will copy the actions of adults or siblings. The baby can handle food well with fingers and if given a spoon will try to use it in the correct way to feed her or himself.

- *Gross motor skills from twelve to eighteen months*

Rapid progress is made with confident walking, kneeling, crouching, climbing (even stairs can be managed in a forward direction) and carrying things. Infants of this age fall down quite a bit, but rapidly set off again. They do not need furniture or people to climb up on.

- *Fine motor skills from twelve to eighteen months*

The infant can hold a pencil and scribble on paper as well as build a tower of a few blocks. Infants of this age enjoy looking at picture books, but tend to turn several pages together, and are now used to picking up small objects with the pincer grasp.

- *Gross motor skills up to two years*

The infant can run, climb and kick a ball with confidence. Stairs are managed well but with two feet onto each step.

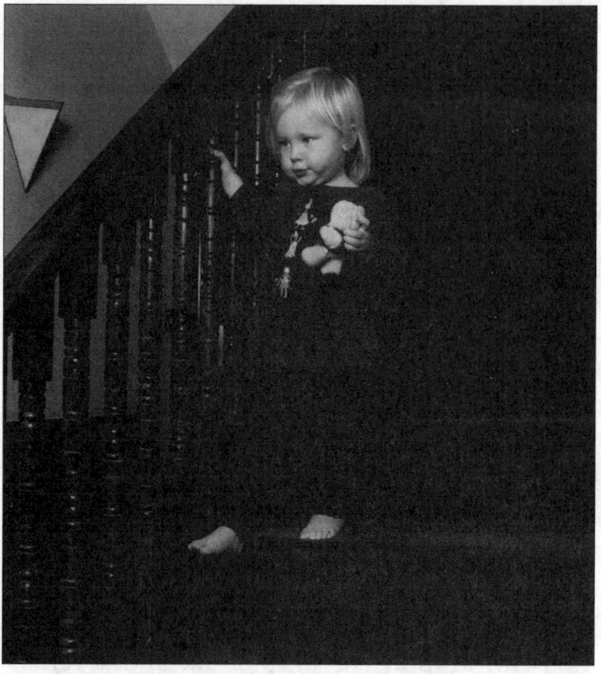

**Figure 4.15 This child can walk downstairs well**

• *Fine motor skills up to two years*
Drawing now becomes more recognisable with lines, dots and even circles forming parts of the picture. The infant concentrates for longer on drawing, painting and building towers of several bricks. Picture book pages are now turned one at a time and stories are greatly enjoyed.

## Early childhood (2 to 8 years)

• *Gross motor skills in the third and fourth years*
Jumping becomes an important part of playing games, together with tiptoeing and standing on one leg. Stairs are managed with one foot on each step although coming down stairs may still be two-footed. Ball play is now important with throwing and catching added to the kicking. Children can manage small tricycles and pedal cars with ease and love to use simple apparatus like swings and climbing frames.

• *Fine motor skills in the third and fourth years*
Pencil and brush control between the thumb and first two fingers mean that drawing and painting become very important activities. Scissors can be used to cut shapes and children of this age begin simple craftwork with paper, card and paste. Beads and cards can be threaded and drawings can show recognisable people, houses and trees.

• *Gross motor skills from five to eight years*
A child in this age range is quite agile with a good balance and can ride a two-wheeled cycle, use gymnastic apparatus at school, skip and can play ball games with good tactics. Moving to music can be important to some children and dancing is often popular. Many children start to learn to swim around the ages of six and seven (usually breast-stroke is first), and gradually add more strokes to their repertoire in the succeeding years.

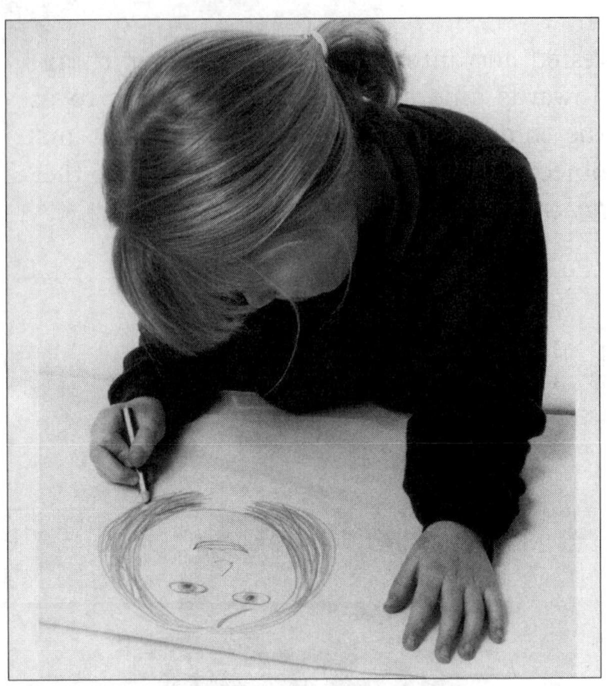

Figure 4.16 Children enjoy drawing in detail

• *Fine motor skills from five to eight years*
Writing, drawing, copying and building shapes can all be accomplished without difficulty at this stage. Simple knitting and stitching can be carried out and the child can thread a large-eyed needle. Many children begin to learn to play a musical instrument at this stage.

## Puberty and adolescence (9 to 18 years)

Most gross and fine motor skills are established by the time a child reaches puberty and the main change lies in the development of muscle strength and strategies if specialisation is involved.

• *Gross motor skills during puberty and adolescence*
Competence comes with practice and a large number of adolescents become excellent swimmers, dancers, gymnasts and footballers; for these are the important training years for a talented youngster. Muscular strength added during adolescence further enhances these abilities.

- *Fine motor skills during puberty and adolescence*

At secondary school, adolescents may learn to type (or word process), play a musical instrument well, sew, knit, cook and use sophisticated technical equipment. Learning to drive is an important goal for most teenagers and it usually provides increasing independence once mastered. Sport of all types is important and using racquets for tennis, badminton or squash produces strong flexible wrist and finger movements.

## Early adulthood (19 to 45 years)

Many new skills are learned in this period that could have developed earlier, but the added strength of full maturity and often an increasing income assist in the introduction of new activities which are often to do with sport and leisure. Skiing, snow-boarding, sailing and golf are pastimes pursued with vigour, strength and increasing maturity. There is often a combination of gross and fine motor skills used in many adult sports.

> **Think it over**
>
> Make a list of the activities that young adults take up which further develop their gross and fine motor skills.

## Middle adulthood (46 to 65 years)

On the whole, exciting, physical sports tend to wind down during this stage of adult life. Golf is popular well into later life and large numbers of older adults use their gross motor skills in gardening and walking. Fingers may start to become less nimble, although crafts such as sewing and knitting may go on until late adulthood. Generally, poor eyesight is the factor that causes these activities to reduce, particularly sewing.

## Later adulthood (65+ years)

We have mentioned some activities that tend to persist into the sixties and seventies, but many older people suffer from arthritis and stiffened joints so that their fingers become less mobile.

> **Think it over**
>
> You may see an older person in a supermarket or other shop taking a long time to get small coins from his or her purse or pocket. Many small items could get dropped on the floor and the person might complain that they are becoming clumsy. Arthritis and eyesight are factors that influence the ability to handle small objects.

It is important to realise that the old saying:

'You can't teach an old dog new tricks'

should be taken with a good pinch of salt. You can teach an old dog new tricks, but it takes longer!

Carers must be patient when working with older adults. The temptation to take over is very strong, but every time this happens they are one step nearer to helplessness.

> **Think it over**
>
> *Use it or lose it.* This is a good thing to remember when working with older people in a care setting. When you observe an older person struggling to walk to the toilet or get money from a purse, be patient.

Do not assume that older people cannot help themselves; many aged people manage very well and still continue gardening, walking or perhaps knitting until they are very old. Dancing is a good exercise that can help with both balance and movement.

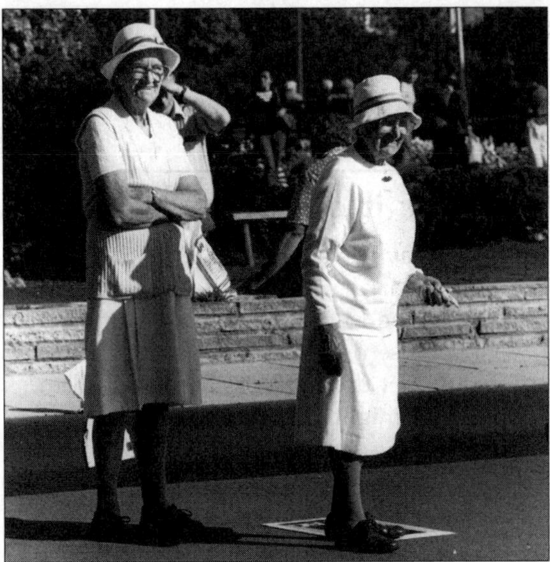

**Figure 4.17 Many older people still enjoy life to the full**

## Intellectual ability

Intellectual ability focuses on the mental skills people use to interpret and make sense of the world. The development of thinking skills is usually referred to as cognitive development.

### Cognitive development

Cognitive development covers the development of knowledge, perception and thinking. Over the past 40 years the study of cognitive development has been dominated by the work of Jean Piaget (1896–1980) and his colleagues. The study of 'object permanence' and 'conservation' refer to aspects of Piaget's theory of development. Piaget originally developed his theories of cognitive development by observing and questioning young children. When his own children, Jacqueline, Laurent and Lucienne were born, Piaget was able to illustrate his theory by observing their actions.

Piaget's theory of cognitive development specifies that children progress through four stages:

1 the sensorimotor stage – learning to use senses and muscles (birth–$1^1/_2$ or 2 years)
2 the pre-operations stage, or pre-logical stage (2–7 years)
3 the concrete operations stage, or limited logic stage (7–11 years)
4 the formal operations stage – formal logic/adult reasoning (from 11 years).

Piaget believed that the four stages were caused by an in-built pattern of development that all humans went through. This idea and the linking of the stages to age-groups are now disputed. There is some agreement that Piaget's theory may describe some of the processes by which thinking skills develop.

### 1 Sensorimotor stage

Throughout life we have to learn to adapt to the circumstances and puzzles that we come across. This process starts soon after birth.

To begin with, a baby will rely on in-built behaviours for sucking, crawling and watching. But babies are active learners. Being able to suck is biologically necessary so that the baby can get milk from its mother's breast. The baby will adapt this behaviour to explore the wider range of objects by sucking toys, fingers, clothes, and so on. If the baby is bottle-fed, he or she will be able to transfer this sucking response to the teat on the end of the feeding bottle. Learning to respond to a new situation, using previous knowledge is called *assimilation*. The baby can assimilate the bottle into his or her knowledge of feeding. Later when the infant has to learn to drink from a cup, he or she will have to learn a whole new set of skills that will change the knowledge of feeding. This idea of changed internal knowledge is called *accommodation*. People learn to cope with life using a mixture, or balance, of assimilation and accommodation as their internal knowledge changes.

During the sensorimotor stage, the infant is slowly adapting to the world by developing his or her own motor actions. At first, the infant learns to co-ordinate tongue and lip movements to feed. By 3 months of age, an infant might start to reach for things and grasp things to suck. By 9 months, the infant might crawl towards an object that could be grasped. In all these actions the child is slowly building a knowledge of how to cope with the environment.

## Spatial awareness

Young infants do not have adult eyesight. Their brains and nervous systems are still developing and their eyes are smaller in proportion to their bodies. They are effectively short-sighted, able to see close detail better than more distant objects. Piaget's observations convinced him that infants were unable to make sense of what they saw. If a 6-month-old child was reaching for a rattle and the rattle was covered with a cloth, then the child would act as if the object had now ceased to exist. It was as if the object had been absorbed into the cloth!

Piaget believed that young infants would have great difficulty making sense of objects and that they were unable to use mental images of objects in order to remember them.

Infants will also have great difficulty in making sense of objects. If a feeding bottle is presented the wrong way round, the young infant will be unlikely to make sense of it. The infant may not see a bottle as we would – they will see an unusual shape.

### Think it over

The world for the infant might be a very strange place. If we close our eyes we will be able to use our memory for spaces, 'our spatial awareness', to walk around a room with our eyes shut. According to Piaget, young infants have no memory of visual objects when they close their eyes. If they can't see an object, it no longer exists.

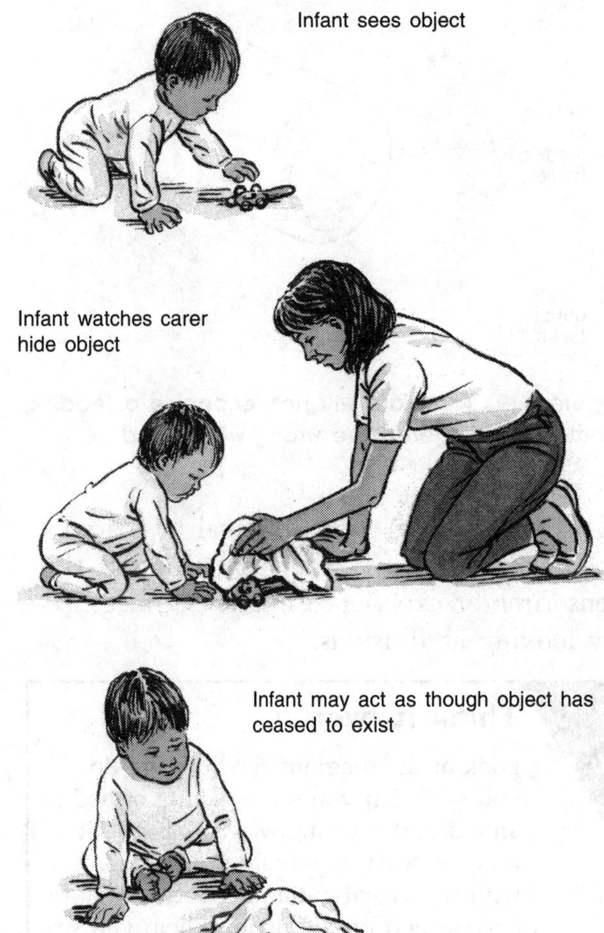


**Figure 4.18** The sensorimotor stage

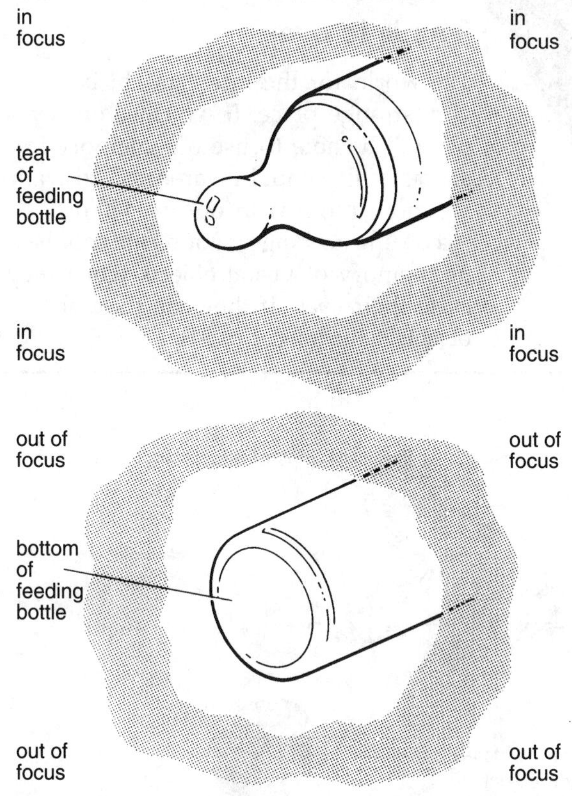


**Figure 4.19 An infant will not recognise a feeding bottle if it is offered the wrong way round**

As adults, we have a vast visual or spatial memory for objects – but something of the sensorimotor experience might be imagined by looking at illusions.

### Think it over

Look at the diagram above. What do you see? Can you see a picture of both an old and a young woman? If not, it may be because you are not familiar with the visual patterns involved. Try to get a friend or colleague to help you see both images.

Piaget guessed that the young infant may be unfamiliar with almost everything that surrounds him or her. An infant would be unable to interpret what objects like feeding bottles were, or even to know that their own body ended and that there was an outside world.

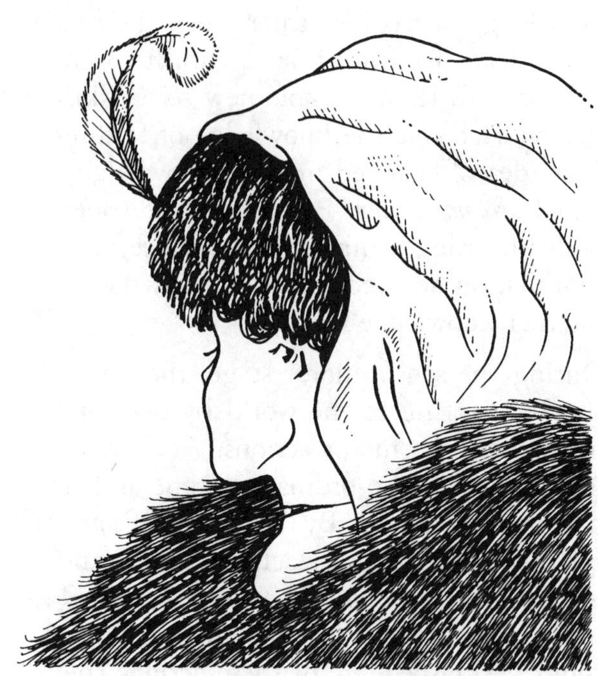

Toward the end of the sensorimotor period, children would begin to internalise picture memories in their minds. Piaget noticed this in his daughter, Jacqueline, at 14 months of age. Jacqueline had seen an 18-month-old child stamping his feet and having a temper tantrum. The next day, Jacqueline imitated this behaviour. Jacqueline must have been able to picture the behaviour in her mind in order to copy it later.

At the end of the sensorimotor period, children are regarded as being able to remember images and to make sense of objects that they see.

### Object permanence

The sensorimotor period ends when the child can understand that objects have a permanent existence. The child knows that objects still exist even if he or she is not looking at them.

At the end of the sensorimotor period, children will know that their father and

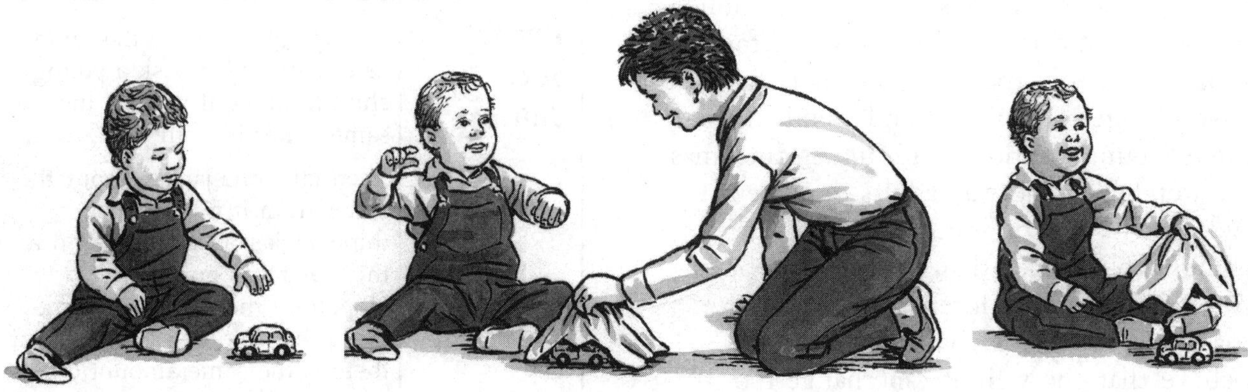

**Figure 4.20 Understanding the concept of object permanence (around 18 months)**

mother still exist even if they are not to be seen. If the child loses a toy he or she will start to search for it, because it can be pictured and because the child has learnt how objects work. If an object can't be seen, it will have gone somewhere – not just 'gone'.

The end of the sensorimotor period is also a time when the child is beginning to use one- and two-word utterances to recognise and describe things. Piaget believed that language was a powerful tool that a child could use to help organise his or her knowledge of the world.

## 2 Pre-operational stage

Pre-operational means pre-logical. During this stage Piaget believed that children could not operate in a logical or rational way. Between 2 and 4 years of age, children were pre-conceptual – they could use words and communicate with adults, but they might not really understand what they were saying. For example, a 2-year-old might use the word 'cat' to mean any animal that he or she sees, and might not really have the same idea of cat that an adult has. By 5 years of age a child might name objects correctly, but still not understand the logic behind things that he or she says. Pre-operational children don't always understand how *meaning* works in language.

The classic demonstration of pre-logical thinking involves studies of children's thinking about number, mass and volume. Pre-operational children do not *conserve* these qualities. Conservation means that you know that a line of 10 buttons has the same number of buttons as a pile of 10 buttons. A young child might say there were more buttons in the line than in the pile, 'because it's longer'. The child is not conserving number. The child appears to not understand that 10 buttons in one place is the same as 10 somewhere else. The child can count to 10, but not understand what he or she is doing.

### Conservation experiments

| **Try it out: Weight** | Show a 5-year-old child a pair of weighing scales and get the child to make two balls of plasticine that weigh exactly the same.<br><br>Check that the child agrees that the two balls are equal in weight (mass). Then roll one ball out into a sausage shape. Ask the child if he or she thinks the two balls will still weigh the same. |
|---|---|

A 5-year-old might answer 'no' – the long one will weigh more now! This statement is illogical. If only the shape and not the mass have changed, then it should weigh the same. Young children don't understand mass (or weight) in the way adults do. Their judgements can be influenced by the way things look, rather than by the concept of 'weight'. Young children may not *conserve* mass – if the shape changes, they may believe that the weight can change too.

| **Try it out: Number** | Set out ten buttons in each of two lines. Ask a child to count the lines. Ask if there are the same number of buttons in one line as in the other. The child will agree that they are equal, there are ten buttons in each line. Now take one button away from one line, but space them so that the two lines still look the same length.<br>Ask the child if there are more buttons in one line than the other. |
|---|---|

A 5-year-old might tell you that there are the same number. So nine buttons is the same as 10 buttons if the lines still look the same! The child is not conserving number. Once again, as in the experiment on weight, children's judgement seems to be dominated by the way things look. The child's attention is centred on visual appearance rather than logical understanding of the way number works.

Try the volume experiment (above right). The child will probably say there is more water in the tall jar! The child is not conserving volume. If the two amounts of water were the same in the beginning, how can there now be more water in the taller jar? Where would this extra water have come from? The child is making a judgement centred on appearance rather than logic.

| **Try it out: Volume** | Fill two glass jars to the same level with water. Ask a young child to judge if there is the same water in both jars.<br>Then take one jar and pour the water from it into a taller, thinner glass cylinder. Ask if all the water has gone in. Hopefully the child will agree that it has. Now ask the child if there is the same amount of water in the first jar and the tall jar. |
|---|---|

### Egocentricity

The pre-operational child is not only pre-logical, but according to Piaget, the child is also unable to imagine other people's perceptions. In a now famous experiment, Piaget showed 4–6-year-old children a model of three mountains. Piaget moved a little doll around the model and asked the children to guess what the little doll could see. Piaget gave the children photographs which showed different views of the mountain. The children had to pick out the photograph that would show what the doll saw. Children were also invited to try using boxes to show the outline of the mountains that the doll could see.

The young children couldn't cope with this problem. They chose pictures which showed what *they* could see of the model mountains. Piaget concluded that children could not understand other people's perspectives. Children were centred on their own way of seeing things – they were *egocentric*. Egocentric means believing that everyone will see or feel the same as you do. To understand that other people can see things from a different view, a child would need to de-centre his or her thoughts. Piaget believed that pre-operational children could not think flexibly enough to imagine the experiences of other people.

The pre-operational period is a time when children begin to develop an understanding of their world but where thinking is limited. A 3-year-old child has the spatial ability to remember how to find his or her way round a room or house, but cannot explain what he or she does. A 4-year-old cannot copy simple diagrams that he or she is shown. A child's drawings of people may suggest that he or she doesn't really conceptualise how people's bodies are made up of arms, hands, fingers, and so on.

Observations of play might suggest that Piaget's view of egocentric thought is correct. Young children might speak with other children when they play, but they do not always seem to listen to others or watch others for their reactions. Piaget believed that emotional and social development were strongly influenced by cognition. The child's ability to reason and use concepts would lead the development of social skills and emotional development. Children might learn to de-centre and understand others' viewpoints when they could use concepts and make mental operations that would free them from being dominated by the way things look. This freedom from egocentricity and the ability to think logically come with the development of concrete operations.

### 3 Concrete operations stage

Children in the concrete operations stage can think logically provided the issues are 'down to earth' or concrete. Children can solve logical puzzles provided they can see examples of the problem that they are working with. The concrete stage implies an ability to think things through and 'reverse ideas'. Very young children have problems with verbal puzzles like, 'If Kelly is Mark's sister, who is Kelly's brother?' At the concrete stage, children can work out the logic of the relationship – Mark must be Kelly's brother if she is his sister. They can explore relationships in their minds. In terms of spatial ability, 7–11-year-old children are likely to be able to imagine objects as they would look from various directions. Drawing ability suggests that mental images are much more complex and complete.

Children in the 'concrete' stage still cannot cope with abstract thought or with formulating theories and hypotheses to explain the world. Although children may be able to imagine objects from different viewpoints, they may still not be able to explain their ideas using language. If a problem becomes too abstract, then it will prove difficult for a child in the concrete period. For example, if you ask a question like 'Samira is taller than Corrine, but Samira is smaller than Lesley, so who is the tallest?', an 8-year-old child may not be able to cope. An 8-year-old child may not be able to imagine all this information in a way that will enable him or her to answer the question. If 8-year-olds can see Samira, Corrine and Lesley, then they will be able to point to the tallest.

Children of 8–11 years may tend to concentrate on collecting facts about topics that interest them. But their real understanding may still be limited compared to older children and adolescents.

### 4 Formal operations stage

When children and adolescents develop formal logical operations they have the ability to use their imagination to go beyond the limitations of everyday reality. Formal operations enable an adolescent or adult to see new possibilities in everything. Piaget stressed the ability of children to use formal deductive logic and scientific method in their thought. With formal logic, an adult can develop hypotheses about the puzzles that life sets. The adult with formal operations can reason as to why a car won't start. Adults can check their hypotheses out. Perhaps the car won't start because there is an electrical fault. Perhaps the fuel isn't getting into the engine. Is the air getting in as it's supposed to? Each hypothesis can be tested in turn until the problem is solved.

## Hypothetical constructs and abstract thinking

The adolescent or adult with abstract concepts and formal logic is free of the 'here and now'. They can predict the future and live in a world of possibilities.

So that's me – fine, but I want to be different!
So how do I change? What's the plan – new clothes, go to the gym?

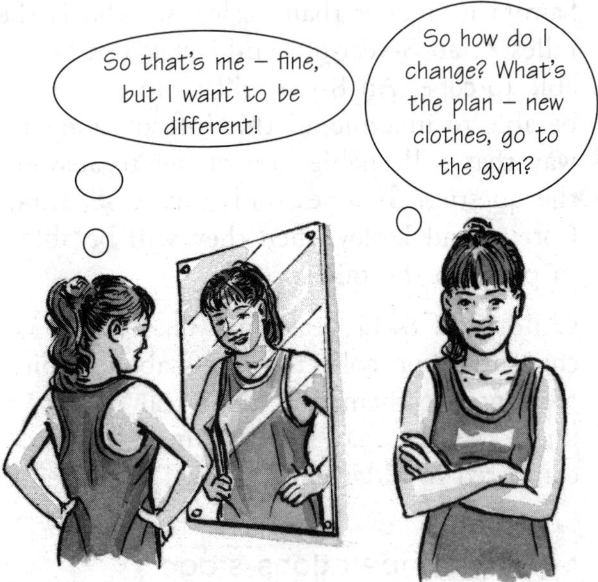

... but adolescents see themselves differently

Although Piaget originally emphasised logic; the ability to 'invent the future' may be the real issue of interest for many adolescents. For example, an 8-year-old will understand how mirrors work and even understand that people can dress differently, change the way they look, and so on. The 8-year-old is likely to accept that the way they look is just 'how it is', and is very unlikely to start planning for a change of future image. With hypothetical constructs an adolescent can plan to change his or her appearance and future.

Many adolescents will have theories or concepts about the way people in their social group should look. In order to make

### Think it over

Hypothetical constructs and abstract thinking may play an important part in care work. Each person that a carer works with will have a range of social, emotional, intellectual and physical needs. People's needs are not always 'concrete'. People don't usually just need a bus pass, a walking aid, or food and shelter. Understanding the emotional needs of a bereaved person will require a carer to understand abstract concepts like denial and acceptance. Understanding the social and emotional needs of an adolescent might involve understanding relationships and self-concept. All these concepts are abstract. It is easy to see how the breakdown of relationship can cause pain, or the success of a relationship can cause joy, but the word 'relationship' is abstract. We can see the effects of relationships but we can't see relationships as if they were concrete objects.

Being able to build interpretations or construct hypotheses about emotional needs may be an important skill in care work.

relationships, it will be important to present themselves in the right way, to be seen as being attractive. Adolescents and adults may spend time planning their image. Body-building, diets, new clothes, new jewellery, new hairstyles might be chosen to create the desired appearance. People build or construct an idea of the person they want to be. Because they have the mental power to think through various possibilities, they are able to re-design the way they look.

## Was Piaget's view of cognitive development the whole story?

Over the past 25 years a range of research has built up which suggests that human development is not as straightforward as Piaget's theory of stages suggest.

### Object permanence

Berryman *et al.* (1991) quote research by Bower (1982), which suggests that 8-month-old infants have begun to understand that objects have a permanent existence. Bower monitored the heart beat of infants who were watching an object. A screen was then moved across so that the infant couldn't see the object for a short while. When the screen was removed, sometimes the object was still there and sometimes it had gone. Infants appeared to be more surprised when the object had disappeared. This should not happen if 8-month-old infants have no notion of object permanence.

Bower suggests that infants can begin to understand that their mothers are permanent from the age of five months. Infants begin to understand that their mothers move and exist separately from other events. Berryman *et al.* (1991) state: 'It seems that Piaget may well have underestimated the perceptual capabilities of the infant, and that some sensorimotor developments take place at an earlier age than he suggested'.

### Conservation

The reason why children got 'logical' tasks wrong may not be that they are completely illogical or egocentric. Part of the reason why children got the tasks wrong may be that they did not fully understand the instructions they were given. Another reason may be that Piaget was right and that young children do centre on perception. They judge things by the way they look. Even so, this may not mean that they have no understanding of conservation.

Jerome Bruner (1974) quotes a study by Nair which used the water and jars problem. This time the experiment used language and ideas that would be familiar to the child. The adult experimenter started with the two full, clear plastic tanks and got children to agree that there was the same water in each.

The adult then floated a small plastic duck on one tank of water, explaining that this was now the duck's water.

Children could now cope with the change. Many children would now say that the two amounts of water were the same because the duck kept his water.

Children may be able to make logical judgements if the problems are made simple and put in language that they can understand. Bruner believed that in the original jars problem, young children may have centred their attention on the way the jars looked. Young children might have understood that water stayed the same, but

Yes, the water is the same amount
All the duck's water went in, so there is still the same amount

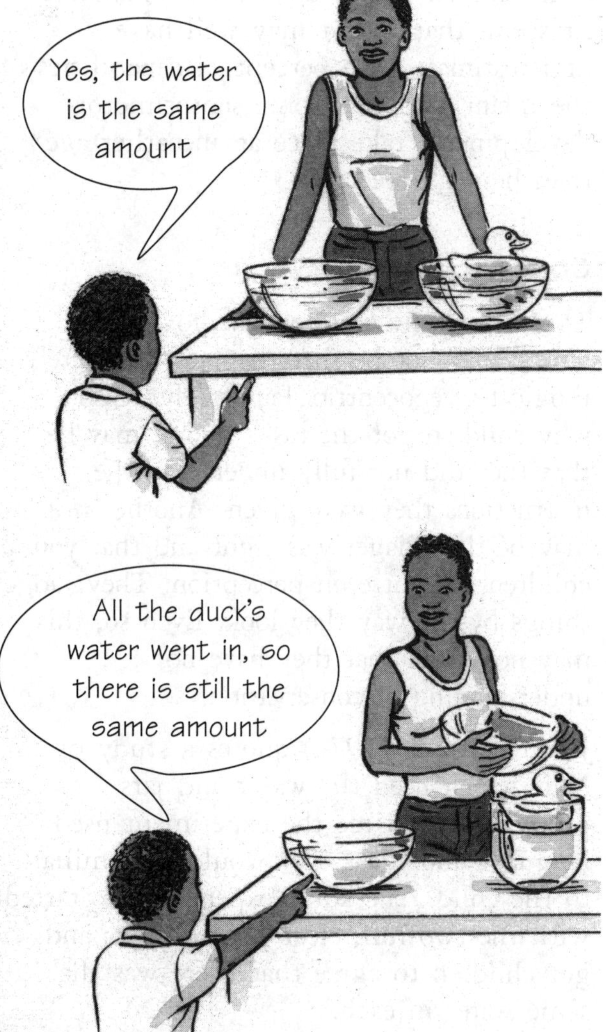

Figure 4.21 Pre-operational children can be logical

Which line has more counters?

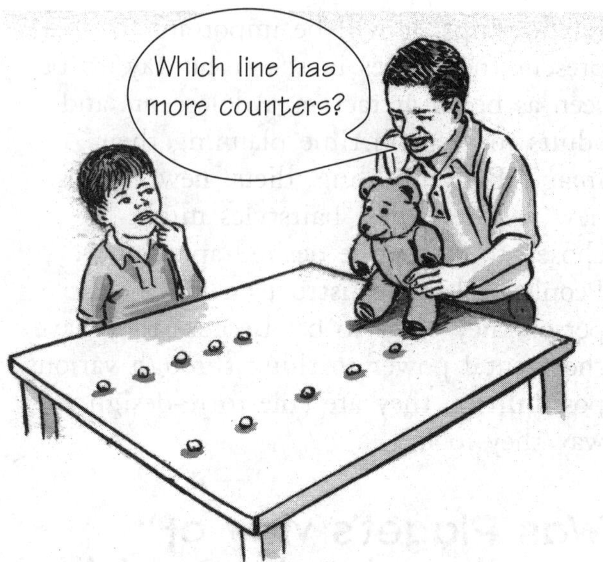

they became confused because their picture (or iconic) memory suggested that height should make volume bigger.

McGarrigle and Donaldson (1975) repeated the counters task. This time a 'naughty teddy' would make one line longer. Children of 5 and 6 were now more able to understand that there were still the same number of counters. In a play-type setting, children may not be so fixed on the 'look' of a line, and may be able to use their developing knowledge of conservation.

It is clear that very young children take time to understand how to use concepts and that 4–7-year-olds can easily make illogical judgements. It is likely that children do develop an understanding of the logic in language at between 4 and 7 years. Piaget may have underestimated children's thinking ability.

Just because children get a problem wrong, it does not necessarily mean that they have no idea of the issues involved.

### Egocentricity

Piaget believed that young children were unable to de-centre their perception from the way things looked, to be able to understand logical relationships. Pre-operational children were supposed to be egocentric to the point where they could not imagine that anyone could see or experience things differently from themselves. Paul Harris (1989) reports that children as young as 3 years of age do understand others' perspectives and do try to comfort others even though they are not themselves distressed. Nicky Hayes and Sue Orrell (1993) quote research from Barke (1975) who found that 4-year-old children could choose a view that a *Sesame Street* character could see – and from different positions. Hayes also quotes research from Hughes (1975) who found that young children were able to hide a doll from another doll using partitions. The children could imagine who would see things at different angles.

Why did children fail at the 'three mountains' task if nowadays children seem to be able to understand others' perspectives? One possibility is that the task may have been too formal and too complicated for young children. In Piaget's experiment, children had to work out which photos went with perspectives, or work with complicated systems of boxes. In the studies reported by Hayes and Orrell, children were playing with characters that they understood in 'safe', informal settings. Children may not always display their full potential for reasoning in formal test settings.

Piaget's belief that pre-operational children are completely egocentric may not be safe. Modern research does not confirm his original findings.

### Hypothetical constructs and abstract thinking

David Cohen (1981) is scathing in his criticism of Piaget's focus on logic:

> 'Furthermore, outside the domain of science, there are realms like art, music and literature which, while not illogical, hardly involve the kind of narrow logic that Piaget harped on. Perhaps even higher education – outside certain disciplines such as philosophy and mathematics – does not require that deep skill in formal logical thinking.' (Page 185.)

Cohen quotes research by Watson and Johnson-Laird (1972) which suggests that at that time 92 per cent of London undergraduates did not use formal operations or hypothetical thinking to solve what was a logical problem. The majority of the population may not use formal logic as Piaget originally suggested that they would. Later in his career, Piaget claimed that it was the ability to use formal logic which developed at perhaps 11 or 12 years of age. He acknowledged that many individuals might never actually use that ability. Even so, the finding that many university students may not think in a generally logical and scientific way does throw doubt on the importance of formal operations as a general developmental stage. Segall *et al.* (1990) report a number of cross-cultural studies which may suggest that formal operational logic is dependent on education and training rather than being some natural capability that simply unfolds in humans.

Cohen (1981) devotes a chapter to his critique of Piaget's theory entitled 'cross-cultural flaws'. Within the chapter, he

#### Think it over

Piaget's experiments with conservation of volume, mass and number do often work in the way that he originally discovered. If you work or live with children you may be able to try them out. The story of cognitive development will not be a simple story showing that Piaget's ideas are absolutely correct in discovering the nature of the human mind, or that his theories are hopelessly wrong. Understanding of human nature grows and develops as time moves on. Piaget's observations and theories may still be useful in helping us to remember the limitations of children's understanding.

In summary, it may be that Piaget's four stages underestimate the capabilities of young children and overestimate the capabilities of the average adolescent and adult.

raises a range of difficulties and paradoxes which have occurred when Piaget's theories are tested outside of European and North American cultures. Cohen reports that one piece of work in Algeria suggested that 7-year-olds could conserve volume, 8-year-olds could not, but once again 10-year-olds could – a 'zig-zag' pattern. It may be that cultural systems of meaning can influence children's judgement and that even conservation can be strongly influenced by cultural beliefs and norms.

## The influence of inherited and environmental factors on cognitive development

Piaget believed that cognitive development was due to an *interaction* between environmental learning and genetic influences. He understood that genetic influences and environmental influences combined to create a new system, on which development depended.

The system which enables a person to learn and understand involves the regulation of knowledge through *assimilation* and *accommodation*. For example, consider the experience of learning to swim. Learning to float to begin with is not easy – you have to get the feeling of how it works. Once you've got the idea, then it's easy. This learning comes in a kind of automatic way. You may not be able to remember how you did it. Piaget thought that learning to float was 'regulated' by an automatic correcting and 'fine tuning' action. He called this *autonomous regulation* – you gradually get the 'feel' of how to do something.

If you are going to swim, you will have to experiment with arm and body movements. At first you may get it wrong and take in mouthfuls of water. Eventually you may get the actions right. You learn by activity or by what Piaget called *active regulation* – trial and error type of learning.

A lot of skills, such as listening or non-verbal communication, are learned by active trial and error and fine tuning of our behaviour. We do not learn them by thinking about them but through practice.

If you want to be a really good swimmer and enter swimming competitions, you will

This feels fine
I've got the idea
Turn faster, keep head down, keep breathing rhythm
COACH
"Streamline your body more"

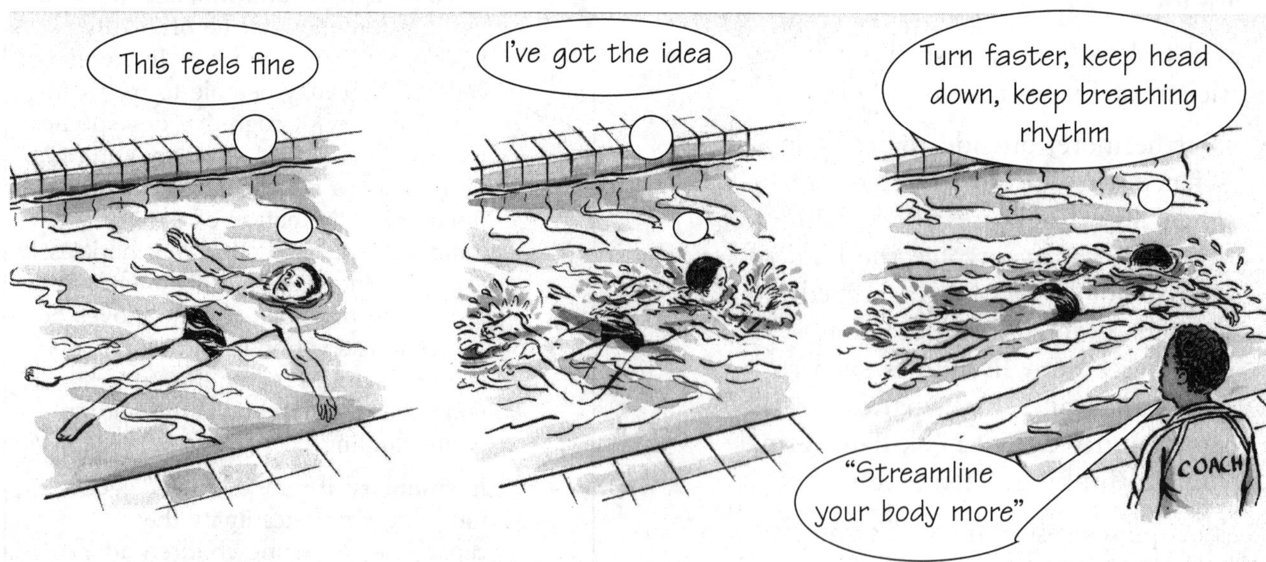

**Figure 4.22 The ability to use concepts can help in the improvement of skills**

probably need *conscious regulation* of your learning. This is where you do work out and conceptualise what you are doing. You will need to work out a training routine, you will need the right diet, you may need to improve the way you turn your body and use arms and legs to swim. To get it right you may need to get your mind involved. The same applies to learning to listen, to communicate with people in social care, or to reassure people who are upset. Basic skills might be developed naturally or unconsciously, but advanced skills require the ability to analyse or to evaluate what you are doing using concepts.

Piaget believed that people often started to learn from practical action. Skills could be dramatically improved by learning to use concepts to analyse action, and then autonomous, active and conscious regulation systems could be used together. With the ability to use concepts, mature learners can imagine a situation or skill that they want to improve. Imagination may even help competitive swimmers to improve their skills.

It may be that children do learn skills by learning practised actions and only later being able to conceptualise them. Some adults may be able to learn by using concepts before they try practical activities.

### Think it over

Think of a skill that you have. Did you learn it through practical work? Could you improve it by analysing and evaluating it?

## Intellectual development during adulthood and later life

Many adults will need to continue to develop their mental skills. Adults who work in professional jobs may develop special mental skills where they control and monitor their own thought processes. This ability is sometimes called *metacognition*. Many adults will specialise in particular styles or areas of mental reasoning.

Zimbardo (1992) suggests that adulthood may involve learning to cope with continual uncertainties, inconsistencies and contradictions. Logic alone may not be sufficient to cope with life. Skilled judgement and flexible thinking are needed. Some psychologists have gone on to call this adult stage of advanced thinking a *post-formal stage* – adding a fifth stage to Piaget's theory. As people grow older, happiness may depend on thinking skills that many cultures have referred to as wisdom.

## Intelligence and individual difficulties

The way that children develop thinking and reasoning skills is described by theories of cognitive development. The concept of intelligence is used to describe the quality of thinking that people display. Psychologists have tried to measure individual performance of intellectual tasks since the time of Francis Galton (1822–1911). Galton is often seen as the person who founded the study of individual differences. Galton measured a range of human differences such as height and weight and sensory abilities over a four-year period from 1886 to 1890. He introduced the notion of the normal distribution curve to explain how people varied in characteristics such as height, weight and intellectual ability.

## The normal distribution curve

The normal distribution curve describes what happens when a random process is at work. For example, imagine what happens if you knock a packet of washing powder over. As the grains fall from the box on to the floor the majority of grains will stay directly underneath the packet. Some will spread out to the sides and just a few will roll away to the edges of the heap.

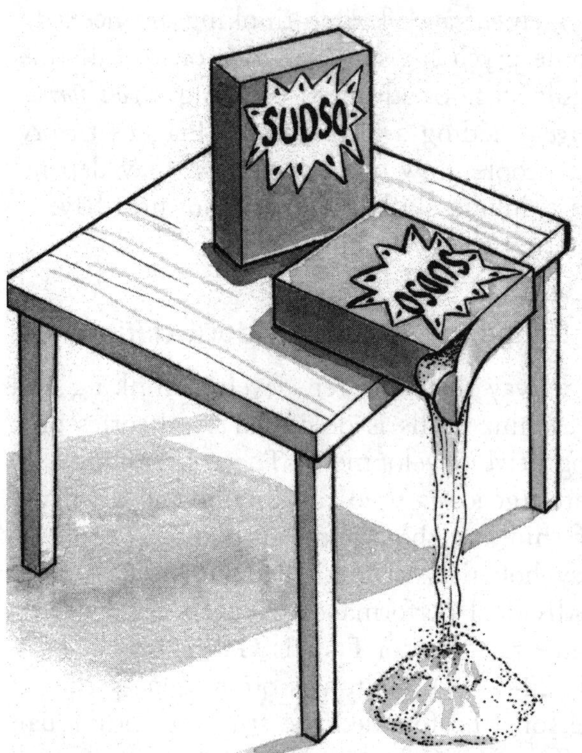


**Figure 4.23 Soap powder falling on the floor will create a normal distribution**

The grains react with each other and gravity in a random way – causing a heap which fits the pattern of a normal distribution curve. Galton and many psychologists who followed his initial ideas believed that intelligence must be normally distributed. This means that the majority of people develop an average ability. Only a few people develop very limited levels of ability and only a few people develop very high levels of ability.

## What is intellectual ability?

At the beginning of the last century, researchers began to design tests of human ability to measure intelligence. These tests were designed to provide an intelligence quotient or I.Q. score. A person's amount or 'quotient' of intelligence is measured against the normal distribution or 'bell curve'. Typically a scoring system might use a scale system like the one in Figure 4.24.

So, in this system, if you score less than 70 I.Q. points this would mean you are unusually low in intelligence. 100 points is average. Above 130 points means unusually high intelligence. 140 would be exceptional, with scores above this achieving genius status.

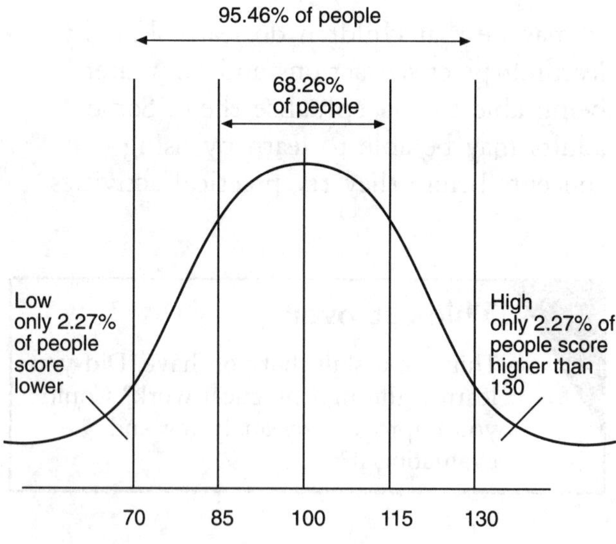


**Figure 4.24 The 'bell curve' describes the mathematics of a random process**

?

Not all I.Q. tests use the same scoring system: there are tests which are graded differently from the scale above which can make it easier to get a high score. If a person says they have an I.Q. of 148, they may have taken a test with a different standard deviation than 15 points. Their 'real' score may only be 130!

Intelligence is measured by testing people's ability to solve puzzles or to use their knowledge to answer questions. Some tests are done by having a lengthy interview where the questions are asked, and other tests are done by completing a series of test papers in an exam-like setting. Some I.Q. tests have measured a wide range of abilities. For example, the Wechsler Adult Intelligence Scale (1955) measured eleven areas (see box below).

**The Wechsler Adult Intelligence Scale** (1955) measured:

- Comprehension (understanding issues described in language)
- Arithmetic (number work)
- Similarities (spotting the common issues between concepts)
- Digit span (memory for strings of numbers)
- Vocabulary (knowledge of words)
- Digit symbol (translating numbers into a code)
- Picture completion (spotting what is missing in a diagram)
- Block design (making patterns with coloured wooden blocks)
- Picture arrangement (putting pictures into the correct sequence)
- Object assembly (solving jigsaw puzzles).

But what is intelligence? Although everyone seems to assess themselves in terms of this concept there is no real agreement as to what it is! Guildford analysed intelligence tests as long ago as 1956 and concluded that different tests measure quite separate abilities. Your ability to spot what is missing in a picture may be quite separate from your ability to know the meanings of long words in the Wechsler test described above. Some psychologists believe that intelligence is the ability to use abstract thinking and make logical arguments. Others see intelligence as being a person's ability to adapt to their environment. The confusion about intelligence has been around for many years. One famous view is that, 'Intelligence is whatever intelligence tests test'!

Recent work on intelligence stresses the existence of different types of mental ability. Robert Sternberg (1986) stresses the importance of practical intelligence. Some people can work out complex mathematical problems: so they have abstract mental ability, but they can't work out how to cross the road safely. Sternberg would argue that the ability to cope with practical problems is a form of intelligence which is often ignored by academics. Howard Gardner (1984) argued that there are seven types of intelligence and that it is important to talk about 'intelligences' rather than believing in some single quality of ability. Gardner's seven types of intelligence are listed below:

- Linguistic
- Mathematical
- Visual/spatial
- Musical
- Bodily-kinesthetic
- Intra-personal
- Interpersonal.

### Think it over

How do you rate your own intellectual abilities on Gardner's seven areas? Look at the pie chart below to help you.

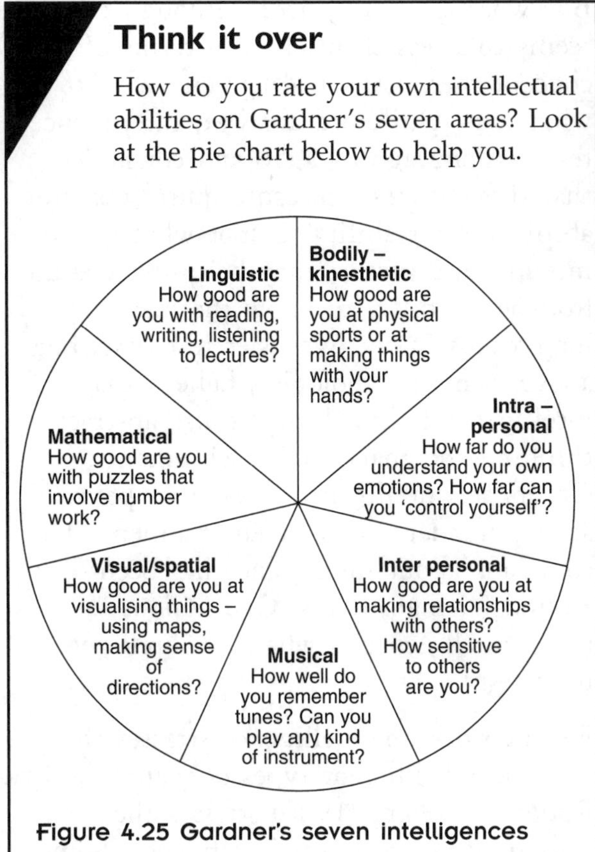


**Figure 4.25 Gardner's seven intelligences**

Gardner (1984) believed that intra-personal intelligence (the ability to understand your own emotional feelings) was a highly important factor enabling people to be successful in life. This idea was developed by Daniel Goleman (1996), who developed the term *emotional intelligence* from Gardner's idea of inter and intra-personal intelligence. Emotional intelligence is the ability to understand and use your own feelings to help cope with issues in life. For example, a person with low emotional intelligence might feel bored with having to write a piece of work. The feeling might dominate their mind and stop them from working, because they have no choice but to do what their feelings tell them. A person with high emotional intelligence might be able to mentally adjust their own feelings – in order to allow themselves to concentrate. People with a high emotional intelligence can make themselves work if they decide they really want to.

Goleman (1996) quotes five areas that emotional intelligence covers:

1 Knowing one's own emotions – self-awareness and understanding of emotion

2 Managing emotions – being able to influence your own feelings

3 Motivating oneself – making emotions work for you and not against you

4 Recognising emotions in others – sensitivity to others

5 Handling relationships – being responsive to other people and understanding their emotions.

### Think it over

How good are you at the five areas above? How important is emotional intelligence – is it more or less important than reasoning skills in your life at present?

Are you born with your intelligence or can you learn these abilities? For much of the last century people argued about genetic and environmental influences. Experts in genetics generally agree that both environment and genetics interact. This means that while people may be born with differences, the environment can and does have a major influence on how these differences work out. Everyone can develop their intelligences and their emotional intelligence if they have the opportunity. (See the next section for further details.)

## Life-span development of intellectual ability

Traditional measures of intellectual ability (I.Q. tests) measure a mixture of abilities, and they have been used for much of the last century. In general, studies suggest that: *intelligence is strongly influenced by learning and experience*. Education can have a major impact on the development of intelligence. Michael Howe (1997) reviews a range of studies of adopted children, schooling and educational courses designed to change ability and motivation. He concluded: 'Intelligence is not at all unchangeable. It can be increased, and very substantially. Doing that on a large scale takes resources, of course, but the task can be done. The enormous gains that would follow would almost certainly outweigh the costs.' (Page 63)

## Intelligence test results are not fixed for life

As children grow and as people become older their results on tests can vary. Studies as long ago as 1941 demonstrated how

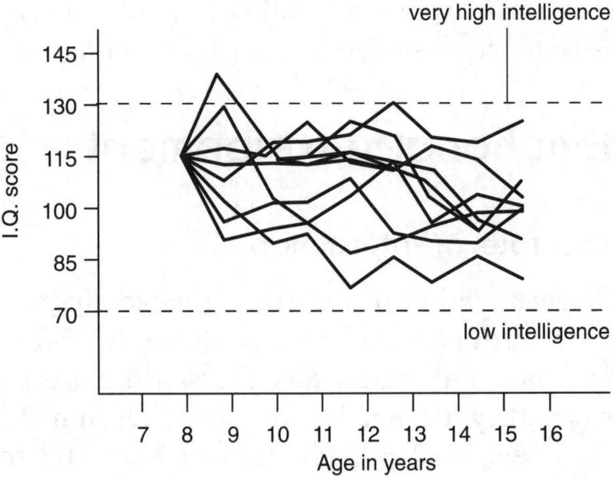


**Figure 4.26 A graph of I.Q. scores from 8 children who all scored the same at age 8 (quoted in Deerborn and Rothney's Harvard growth studies 1941)**

children's intelligence can vary on a year-by-year basis as their unique genetic growth pattern interacts with different life circumstances and events.

## Measures of intelligence do not always predict career success

Intelligence test results are related to (or correlated) with social class. In other words, in the past, some people had better opportunities for career success and learning because of the family they were born into. In the past, studies show that social class had a general influence on the career and earnings that people might expect (I.Q. results also loosely relate to achievement and wealth). Daniel Goleman (1996) argues that intelligence test results fail to explain why some people are successful and others with similar abilities are not. Michael Howe (1997) also concludes that I.Q. results are not very useful for predicting individual achievements in the future.

## Some abilities may change more than others as people get older

There is evidence to suggest that abilities such as general knowledge and language do not start to decline until old age in most people. A psychologist called Catell used the term **crystallised intelligence** to describe past learning and language ability. The abilities have become hardened or crystallised. Abilities such as thinking speed and deductive reasoning are called **fluid intelligence**. These abilities seem to decline from middle adulthood onwards in many people. Younger people (adolescents and young adults) also perform more effectively on tests of memory than most older people.

In the 1940s, psychologists in the USA tried to understand the effects of ageing on intelligence by testing people of different ages. They discovered that 20 year olds did best on the tests and then people seemed to get worse as age groups got older. This led to the idea that intelligence disappears with age! It is not true that intelligence peaks at 20 or 25 years of age. The reason that older groups did less well was probably that they had had less education and less of a chance to develop their ability in the first place. Schaie (1983) studied real people as they grew older and found that many individuals increased their intelligence in their 20s and 30s, with little evidence of any general loss of intelligence during adulthood.

### Use it or lose it?

A critical issue which may contribute to the loss of ability with age is that mental skills may need to be exercised if they are to be kept. Denny (1982) argues that skills which are not used will decline or waste away faster than skills which are exercised. Perhaps the loss of ability which some older people experience with respect to number work and logical problem solving may be due to not using these skills. 'Crystallised' language skills show less decline because they are exercised more.

It is possible to speculate that retirement may influence some people to give up intensive reasoning or problem-solving work. Where this happens, intellectual ability may decline more rapidly than would otherwise happen.

> **Think it over**
>
> Think of older people that you know or have met. What opportunities did they have to exercise their mental abilities? Do you think some people might give up on mental activity in later life?

### Does wisdom increase?

Intra and inter-personal intelligence (emotional intelligence) may continue to develop in many people as they make relationships during early and middle adulthood. Some people may continue to develop emotional intelligence well into later life. The development of these skills may in part be behind the belief held in many cultures that older people increase in wisdom.

Kitchener and Brenner (1990) explain that older adults often develop an ability to make skilled reflective judgements when dealing with complex non-routine problems. This may be an ability which takes experience and time to develop. This ability is 'not associated with the young' (page 226) and may also in part be what is associated with the idea of 'wisdom'.

Perhaps many older people substitute reflective thinking skills for the more rapid reasoning skills tested by traditional I.Q. tests. One view of ageing is that speed of thinking declines but wisdom increases. Age in itself may not be as important as the differences – between individuals and the lives that people lead – in predicting a person's level of intellectual functioning.

## Emotional development

### The role of interaction

Piaget's studies of infants suggested that they are unaware of an outside world and may not understand that the world exists when they are not looking at it. During the pre-operational period, children were said to be egocentric – incapable of imagining different thoughts and feelings or viewpoints from their own. Only as development progressed to logical thought were children seen as able to free themselves and de-centre their imagination.

Paul Harris' study of children and emotion (1989) casts doubt on these assumptions. As already mentioned, babies seem capable of recognising voices and emotional tone at seven months of age (Walker-Andrews, 1986). Harris quotes cross-cultural studies by Paul Elkman *et al.*, which suggest that there are set facial expressions for happiness, distress or anger. There is much evidence in Paul Harris' 1989 review that babies can recognise these basic, perhaps universal, emotional expressions. Emotional development may not be dependent on cognitive development as Piaget's stages suggest. Instead, children may come to imagine and understand others' feelings and reactions long before they can conceptualise or describe these issues with language. David Cohen (1981) claims that Piaget mainly studied babies' motor reflexes and movements, and that he may have gained a different view of early life if he had only studied facial expression.

Can infants respond to adult emotional expression? Paul Harris' review of research suggests they can. A study by Mary Klinnert (1984) involved children aged one and one-and-a-half years being shown new toys. The mothers of the infants would smile or look worried when certain toys were presented. If the mothers looked fearful their infants would tend to return to them and stay close by them.

Harris states, 'By 12 months, we can conclude that infants not only react within a social dialogue in an appropriate manner to an emotional expression, they are also guided by an adult's emotion in their behaviour toward objects or events in the environment'.

A study by Sorce *et al.* (1985) explored how a mother's expression would influence her baby's confidence to crawl across a 'visual cliff'. A visual cliff looks like a drop, but a strong sheet of glass is used to make sure a baby cannot come to any harm. Usually babies will not crawl across what looks like a serious drop. This may be an in-built survival reaction. The cliff was adjusted to look like a slight drop – so that the baby would be uncertain whether to cross or not.

Sorce *et al.* found that most babies crossed the visual cliff if their mothers smiled, but none of the babies crossed if their mothers looked fearful. Harris concludes that infants' exploratory behaviour is influenced by adult emotional reactions. 'The evidence described so far shows that quite early in the first year of life, babies adjust their social behaviour to the emotion expressed by their caretaker'.

## Egocentricity

Harris (1989) describes a range of research which demonstrates that 2-year-old children can recognise distress in others and will often seek to comfort them. There are instances of children under 2 years of age trying to comfort a parent who has hurt his or her foot. Although individual children vary enormously, in general, 'Young children begin to try to alleviate distress in another person; they comfort their parents and siblings at home, and later they comfort other children in the nursery school, particularly if they are hurt'.

Research by Stewart and Marvin (1984) suggests that 3 and 4-year-old children who comfort younger brothers and sisters were good at taking the emotional perspective of their brothers or sisters. So a 3-year-old who is not upset by his or her mother leaving the room can provide comfort to a younger child who is upset. Harris claims that young children actively try to alter the emotional state that others are in. Children are not just imitating or copying behaviours that they have seen. If younger children were egocentric, they would not be able to understand the emotional needs of their brothers and sisters. This research on emotional development casts doubt on the idea that young children cannot de-centre and see others' viewpoints.

Research by Dennie Wolf *et al.* (1984) documents how children use their imagination about other people. Wolf explored how children play with dolls. At around one and a half years of age, children just pretend to look after their dolls. They might pretend to feed, wash or put them to bed. Between two and two and a half years children begin to imagine dolls as talking, and as having desires and emotions. Between three and a half and four years, children can imagine their dolls as characters who make plans and interact with other characters. Harris believes that young children can and do imagine emotional states and can guess how real life events might lead to emotional reactions in others.

It seems that children have powerful imaginations and that they can understand the reactions and needs of others. In many ways this contradicts the picture of child development put forward by Piaget. It would appear that children do have difficulty in using concepts to describe or 'own' their own emotions, however. A 3-year-old child may feel jealousy at the arrival of a new baby sister. He or she may want to help with the baby, but may also say such things as, 'the baby should be cut up and thrown away'. These mixed emotions are clearly demonstrated by children but Harris noted that they could only start to explain such complex feelings from the age of 10 onwards. Conceptual awareness – the ability to use language to explain complex emotions – may need to wait for the developments outlined by Piaget.

### Showing emotion

The way children and adults display their feelings may have a great deal to do with the social roles, norms and values that children learn. Harris (1989) quotes cross-cultural studies which suggest that people can be trained to suppress the expression of emotion, or to develop and exaggerate emotions of happiness, distress or anger. How they learn to express their emotions may depend on the social and cultural context in which they find themselves.

### Self-awareness

Two-year-old children appear to be able to recognise and respond to emotions in other people. It may be that they learn to understand human relationships and the individual expression of emotion as a result of social experience. George Mead (1934) believed that self-awareness developed from children's ability to imitate adult behaviour and to imagine characters. When children play, they can copy actions that they have seen. They do not need to fully understand – they just do the action. For example, a young child might pretend to be a dog, just because the child had watched the family's pet dog.

By 4 or 5 years of age, children might start to act out adult behaviour patterns. Again, children do not really need to understand adult behaviour, they just copy what they think they see. In this way, children can start to copy, or assimilate, adult roles. For

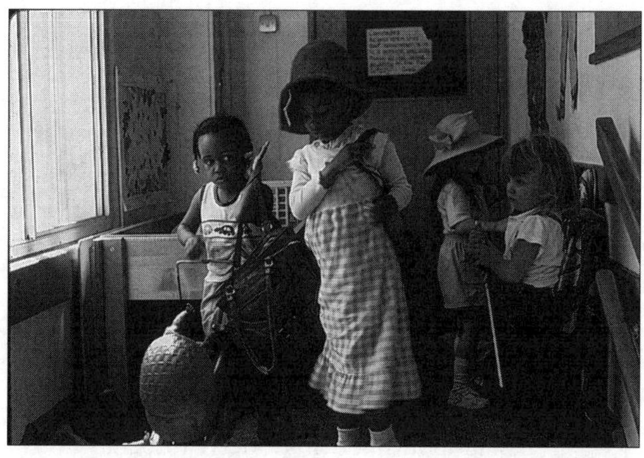

Figure 4.27 Young children will imitate adult behaviour

example children might imagine that they are working together in a kitchen, cooking something for some imaginary children. As they play, they may copy behaviour that they have seen adults perform.

As well as imitating adults, children will imitate things they have seen on TV. This might involve dramatic scenes like rescuing people, nursing people in hospital and, of course, car chases and fights. When children play, they are using imagination to create characters and to take on the roles of other people.

Mead believed that children might start to create a character for themselves – they would start to invent a 'me'. This idea of a 'me' comes about because children can understand social roles and put themselves in the place of other people.

> **Think it over**
>
> Have you ever watched young children inventing characters or talking to imaginary people? Have you seen the influence of TV or of family roles in what they do? Can you see what children may be imitating?

As children develop self-awareness, their idea of a 'me' will be strongly influenced by the culture in which they grow up. 'Culture' includes the beliefs, norms and values that a specific group of people develop. Children will grow up with varying norms and values depending on their social context.

## Self-concept

Children will come to be socialised into the beliefs, values and norms of their initial family or care-giving group. Later, children will be influenced by the beliefs, values and norms of the friends with whom they mix and play. Children adopt others' values and norms in order to be accepted into social groups. They will need to understand the rules of games or sports that they wish to play. In order to be liked and to be popular, they have to show that they fit in with others. Mead (1934) believed that children come to learn general social rules and values at this stage. They might be able to imagine 'generalised others' or general social demands which they need to live up to.

Mead believed children might learn to display emotion as expected within the social roles and cultural context in which they live. They do not simply do what others teach them to do, however. They internalise values that are built into a sense of self. This sense of self determines what they actually do.

These roles may become part of the child's self-concept and social identity. This sense of self will guide the individual to exaggerate, suppress or even substitute

That's me!
Self-awareness
I can picture myself playing with others.
Imagining self through play
I belong with this family.
Self is influenced by being in a family group
I belong with these people. I am like them.
Self-concept is influenced by groups of friends during adolescence
I am ...
1 ...
2 ...
3 ...
Full adult self-concept helps people to be successful in work and love

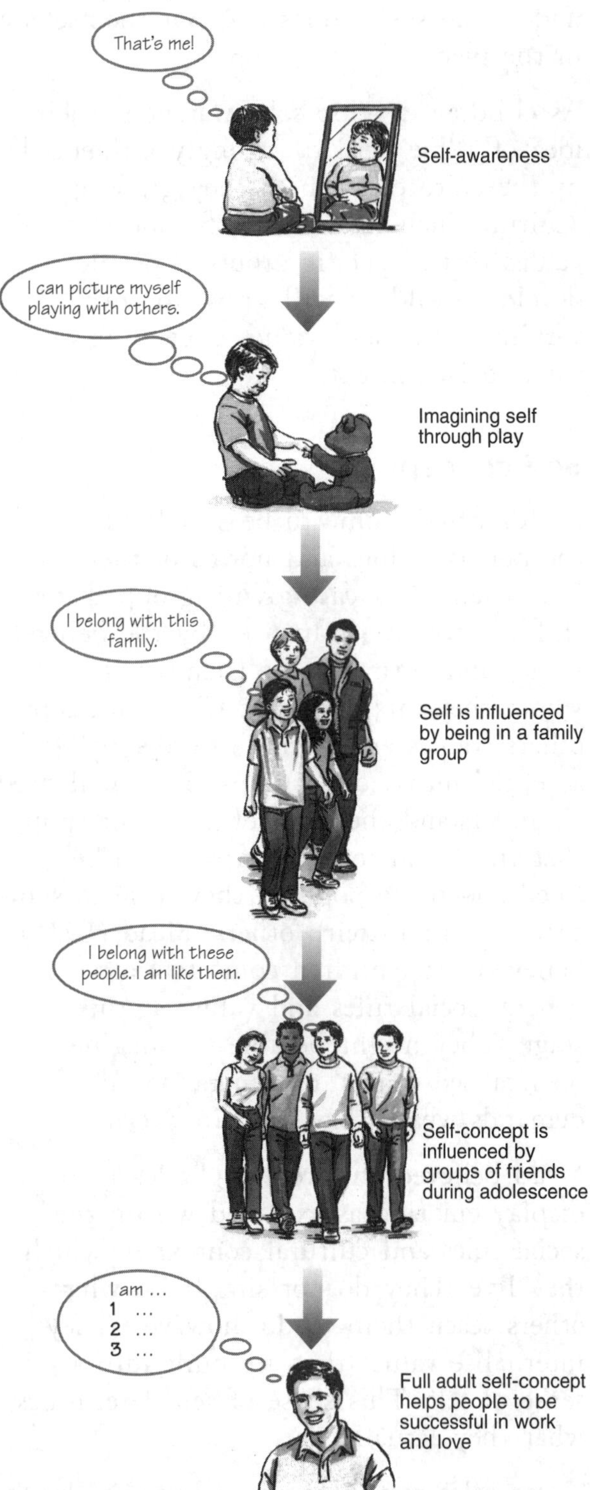

**Figure 4.28 The development of self-concept begins with self-awareness**

> **Think it over**
>
> A boy might imagine himself as a person who is tough and doesn't cry if he gets hurt. By adopting this gender role he may conform to the beliefs of other boys he mixes with.
>
> Gender role might require this particular boy to suppress the emotion of distress at being wounded and to even display the emotion of being pleased. A girl living in the same neighbourhood may need to behave slightly differently in order to fit in with her friends.

emotional expression. In some social classes and geographical areas, boys may learn to exaggerate feelings of anger and aggression in order to achieve social status. In another social class group, boys may learn to express anger in terms of clever verbal behaviour with little hint of emotion. Some girls may learn to suppress feelings of distress in order to look 'in control'.

It is tempting just to say that society does this to people – that people develop the emotions for which society trains them. Mead's theory provides an explanation of how social influences work on an individual. It is the idea of a self, a 'me' that explains how social values influence individual behaviour.

During adolescence this sense of self becomes of central importance. Erik Erikson (1963) believed that biological pressures to become independent would force adolescents into a crisis which could only be successfully resolved if the individual developed a conscious sense of self or purpose. He wrote, 'In the social jungle of human existence, there is no feeling of being alive without a sense of ego identity'. (Page 240.) Other theorists have regarded the development of self-concept or identity as more gradual, and less centred on biological maturation. A clear sense of self may lead a person to feel worthwhile and to have a sense of purpose. A sense of self might provide a person with the confidence to cope with changes in life.

The development of a secure sense of self may be needed in order to:

- make effective social and sexual relationships with others
- cope with work roles where we have to make independent decisions
- cope with complex interpersonal situations where 'emotional intelligence' (Goleman 1996) is needed in order to use appropriate skills such as assertion
- cope with our own internal or intrapersonal feelings in order to enable us to motivate ourselves
- develop self-confidence and self-efficiency in social or work settings.

General factors which will influence the development of self-concept include those outlined in Figure 4.29.

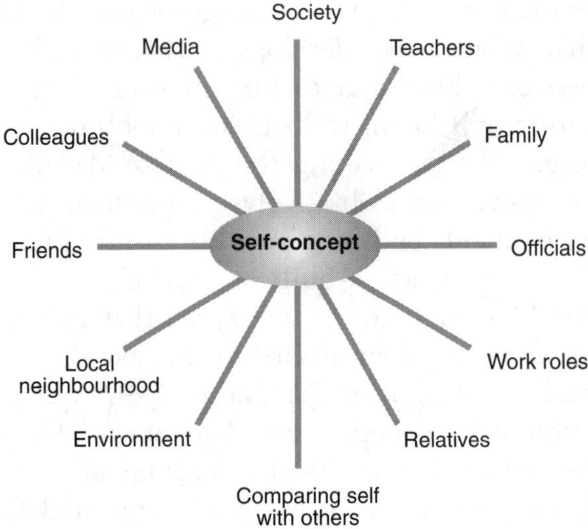


**Figure 4.29 Influences on self-concept**

> **Think it over**
>
> Examine the list of influences in Figure 4.29. How have each of these issues influenced your own sense of who you are? What are the most important influences on your life?

The differences in expression of self-concept between the various age groups might be summarised as in Figure 4.30.

| Age | Expression of self-concept |
|---|---|
| Young children | Self-concept limited to a few descriptions, for example, boy or girl, size, some skills |
| Older children | Self-concept can be described in a range of 'factual categories', such as hair colour, name, details or address, etc. |
| Adolescents | Self-concept starts to be explained in terms of chosen beliefs, likes, dislikes, relationships with others |
| Adults | Many adults may be able to explain the quality of their lives and their personality in greater depth and detail than when they were adolescents |
| Older adults | Some older adults may have more self-knowledge than during early adult life. Some people may show 'wisdom' in the way they explain their self-concept |

**Figure 4.30 Differences in self-concept between different age groups**

| Age | Stage of development |
|---|---|
| $1^1/_2$–2 years | Self-awareness develops – children may start to recognise themselves in a mirror |
| $2^1/_2$ years | Children can say whether they are a boy or a girl |
| 3–5 years | When asked to say what they are like, children can describe themselves in terms of categories, such as big or small, tall or short, light or heavy |
| 5–8 years | If you ask children who they are, they can often describe themselves in detail. Children will tell you their hair colour, eye colour, about their families and to which schools they belong |
| 8–10 years | Children start to show a general sense of 'self-worth', such as describing how happy they are in general, how good life is for them, what is good about their family life, school and friends |
| 10–12 years | Children start to analyse how they compare with others. When asked about their life, children may explain without prompting how they compare with others. For example: 'I'm not as good as Zoe at running, but I'm better than Ali.' |
| 12–16 years | Adolescents may develop a sense of self in terms of beliefs and belonging to groups – being a vegetarian, believing in God, believing certain things are right or wrong |
| 16–25 years | People may develop an adult self-concept that helps them to feel confident in a work role and in social and sexual relationships |
| 25 onwards | People's sense of self will be influenced by the things that happen in their lives. Some people may change their self-concept a great deal as they grow older |
| 65 onwards | In later life it is important to be able to keep a clear sense of self. People may become withdrawn and depressed, without a clear self-concept |

**Figure 4.31 The development of self-concept**

An overview of the developmental stages of self-concept might be summarised as in Figure 4.31.

## Language skills

### Pre-language

On average, children do not usually start to use words until they are about 12 months old, and they start to use two words together at about 18 months of age. The first 18 months of life are referred to as 'infancy', which originally meant 'incapable of speech'. Language abilities develop gradually and infants may be able to use words to name experiences. However, infancy is still considered as a 'pre-language' stage of development.

Babies can make crying sounds from birth. During the first two months of life, they will tend to cry if they are upset or in pain. From about the third month of life, they make 'cooing' sounds if they are content and happy. The range of sounds that babies make develops gradually, and between about four to nine months of age babies will begin to 'babble'. Babbling might involve making sounds like 'dadada' or 'mamamama'. It involves experimenting with sounds and it is possible to interpret this stage as an in-built or 'innate' developmental stage. It may be that babies are building their ability to use sounds ready for language. Zimbardo (1992) quotes research from Petitto and Marentette. These two researchers analysed recordings of hearing-impaired infants who were cared for by hearing-impaired parents. It seems that hearing-impaired infants go through a stage of babbling with hand movements in response to the sign language used by carers. Petitto and Marentette believe that 'babbling' is not confined to learning to make sounds, but that it is a stage for learning to use language, whether that language is spoken or sign language. The pre-language stage of babbling may have something to do with organising an infant's abilities ready for language.

Infants listen to a wide range of sounds that might be used in language. It seems that they start to focus on the sounds that a particular language uses by eight months of age. It may be that infants 'lock' on to a particular range of sounds and then lose the ability to distinguish the fine detail of sounds used in other languages.

Zimbardo (1992) quotes research from Janet Werker, who studied the ability of children and adults to hear the different sounds (or phonemes) used in English and in Hindi. Infants under eight months could hear all differences, regardless of whether they were exposed to English or Hindi as their language. After eight months this ability seemed to be lost. Only Hindi-speaking children could hear and distinguish the fine detail of sounds in their language. 'Thus, infants start with sensitivities to sounds that they lose if these contrasts are not used in their language.' (Zimbardo [1992], page 155.)

The first 12 months of life, therefore, are a time when infants may begin to build their ability to make signs or sounds ready for language. But it is quite wrong to suppose that, because the young infant does not use language, adults and infants do not communicate during this time.

Infants pay particular attention to faces. Studies in the 1950s suggested that babies tend to smile at human faces. Robert Fantz (1961) found that babies between one and 15 weeks of age would spend longer looking at diagrams that looked like human faces than at other patterns. Julia Berryman *et al.* (1991) quotes studies which suggest that babies start to recognise faces at between the sixth and ninth weeks of life. It is likely that babies are born with a readiness to smile at human faces. As learning develops, an infant may be able to pick out his or her own mother's face and respond to expressions.

Research by Arlene Walker-Andrews (1986) suggests that seven-month-old babies can recognise happy or angry voice tones. The babies were shown two films side by side, one film showing a face with a happy expression, and one film showing a face with an angry expression. The babies then heard an angry voice or a happy voice. The infants looked more at the happy face when they could hear the happy voice and more at the angry face when the angry voice was played.

Infants communicate with gaze and with facial expressions and sounds. Adults seem to have a set way of communicating with infants. They often talk more slowly and in a higher pitched voice when talking to infants. Adults may also use exaggerated facial expressions and sounds. This type of communication is called 'baby-talk'. A father might use slow, gentle sounds to comfort an infant, 'There...there...all...go...to...sleep...now'. And higher rising sounds catch the baby's attention, 'Hello, what's this...what's this then...look at this.' Research by Anne Fernald (quoted in Zimbardo, 1992) suggests that parents use baby-talk in many different cultures. Babies appear to respond to the baby-talk style even if it is in a language they are not used to.

Parent/infant games like 'peek-a-boo' may also help infants to learn the idea of social

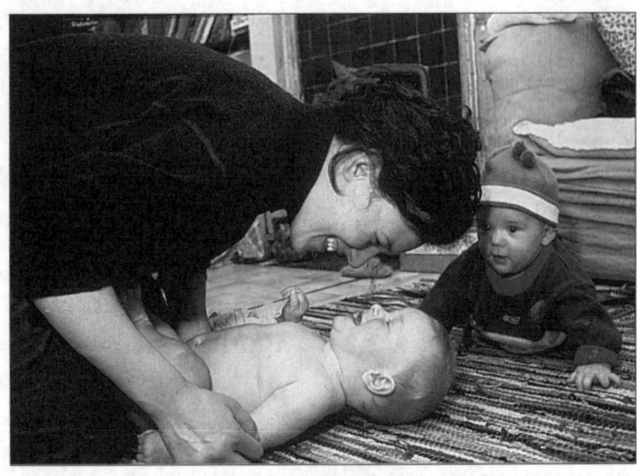

Figure 4.32 Babies and young children learn to communicate with their primary carers at a young age

relationships and turn-taking in communication.

Children may begin to produce their first words between 9 and 16 months of age. Richard Gross (1992) states the average age for first words as 12 months.

The rate at which children learn to use words will depend on their social context and their cognitive development. Social interaction with brothers, sisters or other carers may help a child to speak. Piaget (1896–1980) believed that cognitive development had to reach the necessary stage before language would develop. He believed that thought processes lead the development of language. Another famous theorist, Lev Vygotsky (1894–1934), believed that language development was motivated by the experience of communicating with others. Vygotsky believed that social interaction, or social relationships, provided the basis for both the development of thinking and the development of language ability. A child might want a toy that he or she cannot reach. The child's father might point at the toy and say, 'Is this what you want?' The child might then copy the idea of pointing. The child learns to point because of his or her social experience.

Later the child will be able to use language in order to meet his or her social needs, as well as using ideas like pointing.

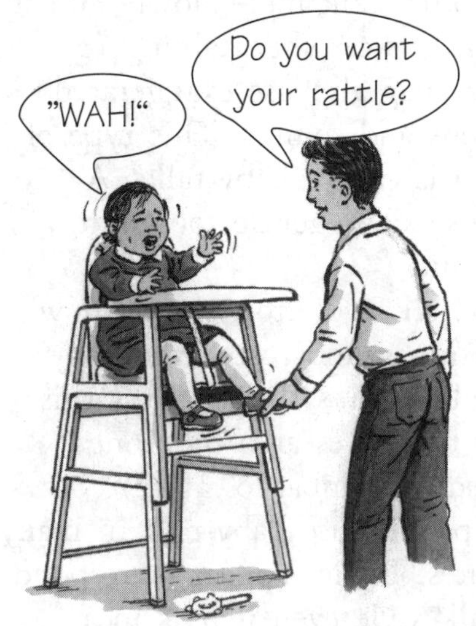


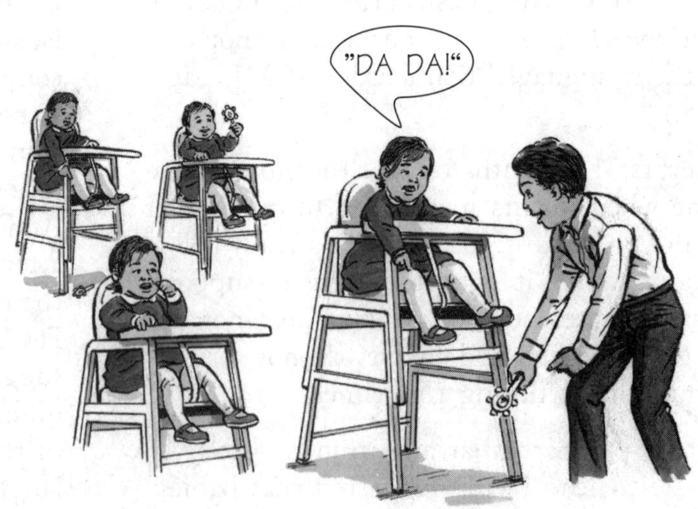


Figure 4.33 Social interaction influences learning

### Think it over

If you live or work with young children, what can you do to help them develop language?

If social relationships are important, then an infant's development may be supported with high quality play and interaction. Speaking to the child and playing with the child using lots of clear facial expression and gesture may be useful.

Whatever the balance between social and cognitive explanations for language, young children are astonishingly good at learning words. Between the ages of one and a half and six years, children may develop a 14,000–word vocabulary. This works out as almost one word for each hour that the child is awake (Zimbardo, 1992).

To begin with children will use a single word: the 'One word stage' (Gross 1992). They may use a single word to name an experience or an object which they have seen, such as 'dadda', which can be used to mean, 'Look, I can see my father (daddy), or 'I want daddy to come here', or 'Where is daddy?' A carer may be able to tell what the child means because of the setting or context in which the word is used, or the way that the child says it.

## Language: developing words

Language development involves a gradual shift from babbling to the proper use of words, and so children will often continue to use nonsense sounds as well as single words during the 'One word stage'. These nonsense words are sometimes called 'jargon'. The single words that a child uses are usually linked to objects with which the child is in frequent contact.

Between about 18 months and two and a half years of age, children begin to communicate with two-word phrases. They might make up phrases like:

| | |
|---|---|
| 'Want drink' | meaning 'I want a drink'. |
| 'Nicky sleep' | meaning 'Nicky wants to go to sleep'. |
| 'Cat goed' | meaning 'The cat has gone out'. |

Brown (1973) described these short phrases as a kind of telegraphic speech. The child is sending a message as if by telegram where words have to be cut down to a minimum. The young child does not know many words and seems to concentrate on sending a message in the most 'economical' way.

Brown (1973) describes the development of language in terms of five stages:

1 Telegraphic two-word statements.

2 The beginning of grammar. (Grammar means the way in which language is structured or used. During Brown's second stage the child might start to structure what he or she says, for example 'I want drink', 'The cat goed'.)

3 Asking questions, such as 'What that?', 'Where is cat?', 'When we see doggy?'.

4 The use of sentences with more than one clause, for example 'The cat come in and the doggy come in'.

5 Sentences used in an adult way.

As children learn to ask questions and make sentences they appear to follow their own rules of grammar. For example, they will invent their own ideas of plurals. 'Gooses' sounds like a logical way of describing more than one goose. As adults, we know that the word for more than one goose is 'geese' – but young children may not accept this idea.

*Carer*: 'Where have you been today?'
*Child*: 'We went to feed the **gooses**.'
*Carer*: What did you feed the **geese** with?'
*Child*: 'Can't know.'
*Carer*: 'Did you enjoy it?'
*Child*: 'Yes the **geeses** splashed!'

The young child still puts an 's' on the end of geese as this fits his or her idea of grammar.

Gross (1992) quotes research by Braine (1971) and Tizard *et al.* (1972) which suggests that trying to teach young children grammar has little effect. Instead, there is evidence that trying to correct children's speech might actually slow their development of vocabulary. It appears that children may 'learn grammatical rules despite their parents.' (Gross, 1992, page 784.) Research by Slobin suggests that parents pay little attention to grammatical correctness, 'and even if they did, it would have little effect.' (Page 784.)

Although children appear to establish adult grammar and a reasonable vocabulary of words by the age of 5 or 6 years, Berryman *et al.* (1991) caution that children between 5 and 10 years of age still have trouble interpreting the meaning of complex sentences. Berryman *et al.* quote a study by Carol Chomsky, where children were shown a blindfolded doll and asked, 'Is the doll hard to see or easy to see?' Young children said 'that the doll was hard to see, because it was blindfolded.' The younger children appear to have interpreted the sentence to mean that the doll was doing the seeing. Berryman *et al.* provide further evidence that 5 to 6-year-olds have difficulty in understanding complex sentences and state : 'It is misleading, then, to think of language development as something which is more or less over by the time a child is about four or five. Important language learning continues throughout much of childhood.' (Page 101.)

Although adolescents and adults may have advanced language competence, changing demands in employment or social life may mean that communication skills have to be constantly refined and developed. Adults may continually improve their social skills and their ability to listen to and understand others' viewpoints. Vocabulary for technical terms is constantly changing. Language learning may never 'finish' until an individual dies.

### The influence of inherited and environmental factors on language

In 1957, Burrhus F. Skinner put forward the idea that children learn language because of the influence of the environment. Skinner believed that parents would provide more attention and pleasurable reactions when an infant made 'correct' sounds or utterances. In this way a child would gradually learn to speak and use language. The child would respond to the smiles and approval of carers. By trial and error, a child could work out how to communicate with others. The child would repeat verbal behaviour that was rewarded (or reinforced) and drop sounds or speech that did not work in terms of getting a pleasurable response.

Very few people now believe that this completely explains how language is learned. Children learn language with very little teaching (one word per hour between one and a half and 6 years). Children do not respond to being taught grammar. Children in totally different cultures across the world seem to pick up the complexities of language development at the same age. This points to the possibility that children may have an in-built ability to learn language.

Noam Chomsky argued that children are born with a 'language acquisition device'. This means that humans have an in-built mechanism to help them recognise language and speak languages. Chomsky believed that children simply need to hear language in order to begin to develop language. The language acquisition device would enable them to understand the 'deep structure' which all languages follow. Individual languages use different sounds and have special rules of grammar. Chomsky called these individual rules a surface structure. All languages have the same underlying rules or structures and these deep structures are something that babies are born to recognise.

Professor Steven Pinker (1994) has gone further than Chomsky and claimed that the human ability to use language is not only inherited, but that language was produced as a result of evolutionary pressures. According to Pinker, language ability will be built into each person's genetic code. The language acquisition device is genetic and has come about because good communication skills would have given our ancestors increased advantages in terms of reproduction and survival.

Pinker claims that most successful species develop special abilities. Hawks can see a mouse move from great distances. Bats can navigate by using sonar and sound waves. Many species of birds migrate across whole continents without losing their way. Pinker's idea is that language is a special ability which has enabled the human species to become so successful. Because it is so important and valuable to human survival, language has evolved as part of the human nature (our brains may be pre-wired to develop language). This genetic potential might be similar to the potential that enables birds to fly. Flight is a special ability that birds are born with. Language is perhaps our 'special act'.

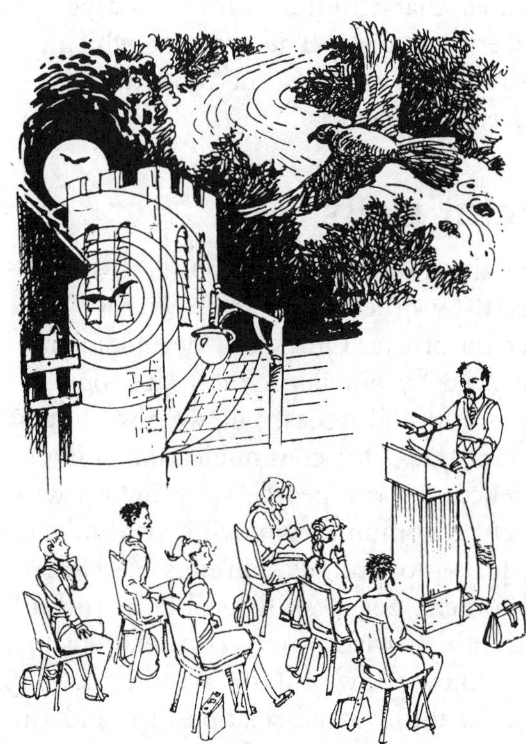

**Figure 4.34 Language is a special ability developed by our species**

Whether language developed because of evolution or not, there is now a widespread expectation that a genetic basis for human language ability will be discovered. Professor Myrna Gopnik claims to have evidence for a genetic component for language. Her studies focus on a language disorder which 'runs in' families and which reduces individuals to learning language by rules, rather than quickly and easily. Gopnik may have evidence of the existence of a genetic failure in the human language acquisition device, evidence that would suggest a genetic component to language (report in *Times Higher Educational Supplement*, 7 April 1995).

If the broad theories of Chomsky, Pinker and Gopnik are correct, it would suggest that the underlying ability to learn language is influenced by an in-built or genetic factor. The actual sounds, words and grammar that children learn will depend on their environment. The speed at which children learn will also be influenced by their environment.

## Social skills

From the moment we are born we are affected by other people and we have an effect on others. Our social development is influenced by our family and later our friends and colleagues, but we also influence other people. Our communication skills are influenced by the people we grow up with, but our communication skills also influence the quality of the relationships we have with others. Social skills enable us to build relationships with others, but relationships also influence how our social skills develop. Understanding social relationships and the skills which develop and maintain these relationships involves understanding an interactive process.

### Relationship skills

> **Think it over**
>
> Think about all the conversations and interactions you have had with other people so far today. How did you learn to 'get on' with others? Are some people better at making friendships and relationships than others? What makes people popular or good at relationships?

In the same way that people 'naturally' develop language skills, some people seem to develop social skills of communicating and making relationships with others. But even if we do not have an in-built tendency to communicate and make relationships, people also have to learn how to 'get on with others'.

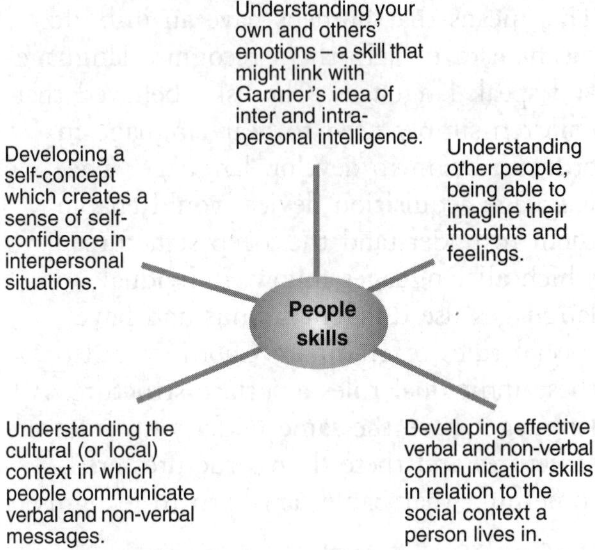


**Figure 4.35 Making good relationships with others depends on people skills**

These skills are learned by:

1 Experiencing other people's conversational skills and the reinforcement or lack of reinforcement of your own responses (see the section on reinforcement on page 318). Some social skills may be learned through trial and error.

2 Watching other people and copying their actions. Play provides an opportunity to experiment and practise social skills.

3 Building a cognitive and emotional understanding of other people using thinking and emotional skills. People interpret the behaviour of other people using concepts and theories which they learn. Unit 2 provides a detailed analysis of the communication skills needed to be effective in relationships.

## The importance of relationships

Relationships create the social context in which children grow and learn. Relationships are also vital in order to protect individuals from stress. Stress can damage our health and development.

Mildred Blaxter (1990) published the results of a national survey into health and lifestyles. She reported that, 'self-perceived stress was strongly associated with poorer health of every kind' (page 104). She notes, 'Social loss or social isolation are particular forms of stress which have been shown to be particularly dangerous to health. "Life events" such as widowhood or other bereavement, divorce, job changes, unemployment, migration, even moving from one home to another, are all associated with increased risk of morbidity (disease) or mortality (death).' (Page 103.) One key factor, which appears to be vital in protecting people from the effects of stress, is having close social support networks. Friends, family, partners and community links, all seem to act as a buffer against stress. Michael Argyle (1987) writes, 'Many studies have found that distress is caused by stress. This effect is, however, greatly reduced or minimised if there are supportive relationships. This is known as "buffering".' (Page 25).

So friends and supportive relationships may protect an individual against stress. They may be vital to maintain self-esteem and, perhaps, self-concept or identity when these are threatened. Relationships may be critical when our sense of self is threatened. According to Argyle, a key issue is the quality of support.

Argyle noted that both males and females found conversations with females to be 'pleasanter, more intimate – to involve more self-disclosure' and to be more 'meaningful' than conversations with men, when this was researched in the early 1980s. This may be an interesting and important aspect of gender role socialisation.

Blaxter (1990) reported that, 'Family relationships and close bonds have been shown to be strongly protective, perhaps through effects on self-esteem and feelings of control. Certainly, the relationship between social networks and health has been found to be so strong that it can be used predictively in relation to mortality.' So it seems that people with poor social support may be at more risk of dying from an illness than those with closer relationships. Argyle quotes a study of 7000 people in California during the 1970s (Berkman and Syme, 1979). Those with supportive social networks had a much lower death rate even after initial health, health practices, obesity, smoking, drinking and social class had been taken into account. In terms of support, marriage produced the strongest protection, with friends and relatives then offering more protection than belonging to churches or other organisations.

But how do relationships make a difference to a person's physical health? Argyle (1987) writes,

> 'One way in which stress is bad for health is that it impairs the immune system, the natural defence against disease. Social support could restore the immune system, by its power to replace negative emotions like anxiety and depression, and their accompanying bodily states, by positive emotions. A second way in which relationships may affect health is through the adoption of better health practices. Those who have good relationships are able to cope with

stress by seeking help and social support. Those without are more likely to use other means of coping, like smoking and drinking.' (Page 184.)

Blaxter's study (1990) provides evidence that there is a positive relationship between marriage, or living with a partner, as compared to being single. This relationship was particularly significant for men and, indeed, older men. For men especially, living alone was associated with more illness and poorer psychological and social well-being. The number of social roles a person had (roles like parent, worker, regular worshipper) also related to measures of good health. Although these general findings from a survey cannot be used to make predictions for individual health and happiness, it does appear that partners, friends, family and community social links help protect people from stress. People with close supportive relationships may have useful resources to fall back on when they encounter life-event threats. Socially isolated people may lack a buffer to protect themselves against the anxiety, strain and threat that change may cause.

If you were about to bring a new baby into the world you would want to make sure the child enjoyed most of the positive things listed in Figure 4.36.

Social skills cover the way we communicate with and get on with other people. We will copy the cultural views of our friends and family. We will judge our appearance in terms of the people we mix with. We may take on a male or female gender role because of the influences of friends, family and the local community.

Our friends, family, relatives, teachers and community are similarly influenced by:

- the local environment
- their education and developmental maturity
- their cultural background and gender roles
- the wider influences in western culture, including newspapers, TV, radio, the Internet, computer games and so on.

It is possible to think of these influences working at different levels, like the circles in Figure 4.37.

| **Try it out** | Using the circles shown in Figure 4.37, think of the names of 3 people who have influenced you. Write down what effect their influence has had on your development.<br><br>Can you think of examples of the ways the media have influenced how you think about yourself? |
|---|---|

## Developing a sense of self-confidence

The social learning theory of Albert Bandura emphasises the power of the environment to influence the way people think and behave. Bandura stressed the fact that people imitate and copy other people. We adopt roles and social behaviours because of the outcomes that we expect for ourselves. If being polite and friendly helps us to get accepted into a particular group, and we want to belong to that group, then we may try to imitate the polite and friendly behaviours that we have seen others act out. Social learning theory complements the interactionist theory of George Mead – we learn to imagine and copy the reactions that will lead to pleasant outcomes for us.

| Good relationships can produce: | Poor relationships can produce: |
| --- | --- |
| *Infancy*<br>Secure attachment between the infant and parents<br>A rich learning environment<br>A safe, loving environment which meets a child's emotional needs | A failure to make a secure or safe emotional attachment between parents and the child<br>Neglect, rejection of the child |
| *Early childhood*<br>A secure home from which to develop slowly<br>Parents who can cope with the stressful behaviour of young children<br>Friendships with other children | A stressful home situation<br>Neglect or rejection of the child<br>Inconsistent attempts to control a child<br>Parents who become angry or depressed because of the child<br>Isolation from other children |
| *Later childhood*<br>Membership of a family or care group<br>Socialisation into a culture<br>Friendships with others at school<br>Increasing independence from parents<br>A feeling of being confident and liked by other people<br>A feeling of being good at things | Stress and change if parents fight each other or separate<br>No clear feeling of belonging with a group or culture<br>Limited friendships<br>Feelings of not being liked by others<br>Feelings of not being good at anything or not as good as others |
| *Adolescence*<br>Independence but still with the support of the family<br>A network of friends, a sense of belonging with a group of friends<br>A culture shared by friends<br>A positive environment that has opportunities for the future | Conflict and fighting with parents and family<br>Few friends, feeling depressed and rejected<br>No feeling of belonging with other people<br>No clear sense of who you are<br>The feeling that life is not worth much |
| *Adulthood*<br>A network of friends and family who help and support you<br>A secure, loving, sexual relationship<br>Good relationships with work colleagues<br>The ability to balance time pressures between work, partner and other family relationships<br>A feeling of being secure and safe, with other people to help you | Feelings of isolation, loneliness, rejection and no feeling of belonging with friends<br>No support<br>Changing relationships<br>No social protection from stress<br>Low self-esteem |
| *Old age*<br>A network of family, friends and partner to provide emotional support<br>Control of own life<br>A sense of purpose | Few friends, no social support<br>No social protection from stress<br>Isolation<br>No sense of purpose |

**Figure 4.36 The effects of personal relationships at different stages of a person's life**

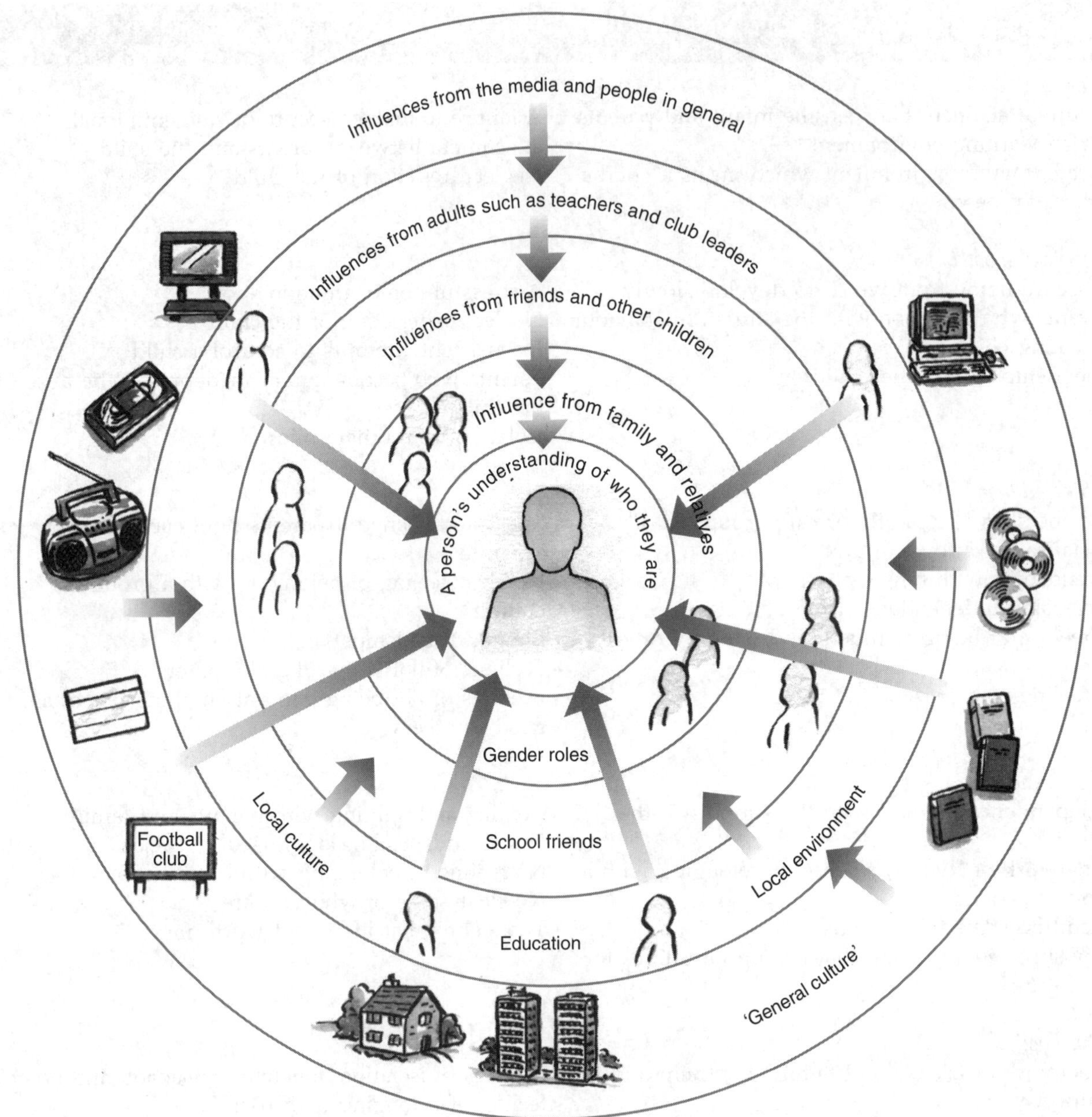


Figure 4.37 Circles of influence

Bandura's 1989 theory of self-efficacy may help to illustrate how social learning influences us. Albert Bandura uses the term self-efficacy to cover a person's ability to understand his or her capabilities, motivation, thought patterns and emotional reactions. Self-efficacy is how you estimate your abilities – what you believe about yourself. Self-efficacy is learned from past experiences, watching and thinking about what happens to others, copying others and from the feedback we get from other people. High self-efficacy means believing you will succeed at a task. Low self-efficacy means believing you will fail.

Once a person believes he or she is good at something, this belief will provide motivation to keep building on success. Of course, the opposite is also true. If you believe you are no good, then you will probably withdraw from the activity and avoid it.

### Think it over

How would you advise someone to develop conversational and relationship skills? What happens if you join a group but other people are not interested in talking to you?

## Case study: Ashra's Story

Ashra is 16 years old; she has just started on a new course. Starting a new course means mixing with new people. When Ashra first met her new colleagues she thought, 'Oh, these aren't my kind of people, how will I get on with them?'.

Ashra had always been popular at school and could usually encourage others to talk to her. On the first day of the course she found the courage to talk to two students who knew each other but who she had never met before. Ashra was delighted when both students responded in a warm and friendly way. Not only was she making friends but she thought to herself, 'I am good at getting people to talk to me and getting them to like me. I guess that I have good social skills'. This idea of being good creates a special feeling for Ashra, she starts to imagine that she is clever and 'good with people'. Ashra starts to think that she will be good at conversation work with the whole group.

Because Ashra thinks that she is good at conversation she feels confident to talk to all the new people in the group. Because Ashra is confident she succeeds in getting all the other students to see her as a leader. Ashra becomes very popular.

Ashra's success with people grows out of her belief that she is good at relationship skills. High self-efficacy means having an accurate belief that you are good at something. If you have this belief it may help you to develop your skills and become even better.

Self-efficacy could become a general feature of an individual's personality. It is learned from experience where an individual interacts with teachers, tests and social roles.

Some people may learn to think of themselves as capable individuals, who will be able to cope with the puzzles and problems that life holds. Others may fail to develop this view of themselves. Some people may go through life without believing they can influence what happens to them. These people may experience their lives as a series of events which just 'happen to them'. An evaluation of self as a capable decision-maker may be needed before individuals can be assertive and before they can take responsibility for their own lives.

## Play

Any activity that is not obviously focused on achieving some social goals such as money, food or prestige, is called play. Play is most commonly associated with young children, but 'play' behaviour takes place across the life-span, so why do people of all ages spend time on play activities? One answer is that play meets the different needs that people have.

- **Play meets physical needs**

In the past, theorists pointed out that play behaviour was a way of using up energy. We are not designed to rest continuously: people (particularly children) have a physical need for activity and exercise. Physical games meet this need. Play also provides time out from stressful activity. Some games and activities help people to relax. Exercise and relaxation are important for a balanced life.

- **Play meets emotional needs**

A psychodynamic (or Freudian) explanation of play is that it helps people to cope with emotional tensions. Acting out a role, such as a child pretending to be a teacher, may provide the child with a sense of power and control. The adult playing computer games may also be meeting a need for emotional tension release or a sense of control which is missing in real life.

- **Play enables people to learn**

When infants play with toys they are developing their motor skills and their understanding of objects. Young children will play out actions that they see adults perform – perhaps setting a table for dinner or pressing the buttons on a music system. Play may help children to make mental sense of or 'represent' the outside world in the child's imagination.

Older children may act out roles that they see adults perform. Taking on a role may help a child to imitate and learn the social skills and behaviour they will need as they grow older. Adolescents and adults continue to develop practical and social skills as they engage in role-play or with electronic games. Retirement may provide an opportunity for new learning and much of this new learning may be linked to enjoyable recreational activity.

- **Play can create a social context for development**

Vygotsky believed that we mainly learn and adapt in order to meet social needs. We need to be able to interact with our family; we need to belong with work colleagues. Play between a child and his or her family will create a social context where social skills can develop. Older children, adolescents and adults will 'play' or undertake leisure activities with friends. 'Play' can provide a social setting for the development of social communication and interaction skills.

## Types of play

The word 'play' can cover many different types of activity. Children's play mainly involves exploring, practising, social learning and pretending (see Figure 4.38).

## The development of play

When they are aged less than two years of age, children tend to play alone. At around two years of age, children may play side by side with other children, although they may still concentrate on their own activity. Children may start to share activities with other children at about three years of age. By four or five years of age, children may

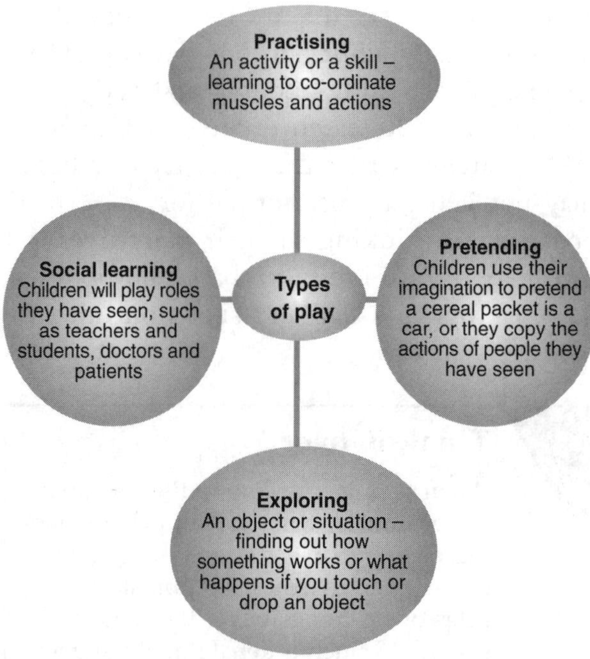


**Figure 4.38 Children's play can involve several different types of activity**

play in small groups and follow activities or games with simple rules.

By seven years of age, most children develop same-sex friendship groups. Children may often prefer being with their friends rather than doing other activities. By 10 years of age, friendship groups often share similar attitudes and values. Friendship groups start to have an influence on children's beliefs and behaviour during childhood.

## The development of morality and moral judgement

Children's beliefs about what is right and wrong are strongly influenced by the beliefs of the people they live with and mix with. The way children talk about what is right and wrong is influenced by their level of intellectual development. Kolberg (1976) published his ideas about how children and adults might progress through six different stages of moral thinking. These stages are outlined below:

1 **Punishment and obedience** Things are wrong if you get told off or punished for doing them. You should do what you are told because adults have power.

2 **Individualism and fairness** You should do things that make you feel good or get praised, and avoid things that get punished. It is important to be fair to everyone. For example, 'If I help you, you have to help me!'. 'If I get pushed in a queue, then I have the right to push other people!' There is a simple belief that everyone should be treated in exactly the same way. For example, if everyone gets the same food, this must be fair. Children at this stage will find it hard to work out that 'the same food' is not fair because it will discriminate against some people and not others. If everyone is given meat, this will be good for some people, but not for vegetarians!

3 **Relationships** As children grow older, relationships with others become important and children begin to think about the way they are seen by others. At this stage, children start to think about 'good' behaviour as behaviour that pleases others. Being good is about meeting other people's expectations of you. Ideas of loyalty, trust and respect come into children's thoughts and feelings. For example, a child might think 'I can trust my friend to keep a secret because they are a "good person".'

4 **Law and order** Adolescents and adults start to think in terms of a 'whole society'. Rules and laws are seen as important as they enable people to get on with each other. Being good is not only about relationships with friends and

family, but also about relationships with people in general.

5 **Rights and principles** Some adolescents and adults develop an understanding of what is right or wrong in terms of social principles and values. Laws are valid and must be obeyed because of social consequences or the principles of justice which should govern society. Laws can be changed depending on the needs of society.

6 **Ethical philosophy** Adults that reach this stage will believe in a system of ethical reasoning. The individual will follow a system of values and principles which can be used to justify and guide action. Laws and regulations are judged in relation to the individual's own system of reasoning, and individuals take personal responsibility for their own actions.

These levels of moral judgement are strongly influenced by the level of cognitive development and education that an individual has received. The first two stages rely on pre-logical or pre-operational thinking. Stages three and four are associated with concrete logical thinking. Stages five and six require formal logical thought. Many adults do not develop clear systems of reasoning about moral and ethical issues. Research quoted by Cohen (1981) suggests that the majority of adults may not generally use formal (or operational) thinking in their daily lives. The majority of adults probably do not develop to stages five and six as outlined in Kolberg's theory.

### Think it over

When people you know discuss equal opportunities, what sort of debate takes place? Do people concentrate on what can happen to you if you break the rules or on things being the same for everyone? Such a debate might suggest that moral thinking is at levels one or two. Do people discuss equal opportunities in terms of relationships or the need for a just society? This might put the debate at Kolberg's levels three or four. If people discuss the relativity of value systems or the ethical context of equal opportunities then this would be a discussion at levels five or six.

In real life, much adult debate might focus on levels two to four. Why do you think this is?

# 4.3 Factors affecting development

## Genetics and their interaction with the environment

### What are genetics?

Steve Jones (1993) explains that genetics is a language, 'a set of inherited instructions passed from generation to generation'. (Page xii.) Jones argues that genes are like the words in a language. The way genes are arranged can be seen as the rules for language – a grammar. Genetics also has a literature, 'the thousands of instructions needed to make a human being'.

Genes contain the information or 'the instructions' needed to make living organisms. At a molecular level this information is held in DNA (deoxyribonucleic acid). Each cell nucleus in a living person contains this genetic material.

Scientists are working very hard to understand this language system. By April

2000 the human genome project had worked out how the genes of one human chromosome work. It is expected that scientists may map and understand how the entire genetic sequence works by 2003. Understanding the genetic code will create a vast new range of medical treatments. Drugs which can even be made for individual patients will be possible.

Will this new knowledge enable us to re-design or even create people? The opinion of experts is a definitive 'No!' What we are unravelling is the language of the instruction system that creates human biology. We are on the threshold of understanding the human *genotype*, the underlying pattern for making people. An individual human being is called a *phenotype*. This distinction in terminology is important because people are not simply 'caused' by underlying genetic instructions. As Nicky Hayes (1995) says, 'The genotype doesn't determine the phenotype, although it may point us in certain directions rather than others.' (Page 140.)

Professors Rose, Lewontin and Kamin (1984) state, 'Genotype and environment interact in a way that makes the organism unpredictable from a knowledge of some average of effects of genotype and environment taken separately.' (Page 269.) Jones (1993) puts it very straightforwardly, 'Genetics has almost nothing to say about what makes people more than just machines driven by biology, about what makes us human.' (Page xi.)

Every individual person is a unique creation made from the inseparable and intertwined influences of genetic instructions and experience. To be alive, you will have had to have a code (genetics) to guide the construction of your body. That body could not have been built if there were no materials and no environment to build it in. Some individuals may have a genetic design or potential to grow tall, but they will not achieve this potential if they do not have enough protein in their diet as a child. The environmental and genetic influences interact. An individual, a phenotype, is the result of an interactive process, not just an example of an underlying genotype or genetic pattern.

## Some very powerful genetic influences

We have known for many years that particular conditions result from genetic influences. Genes are carried on chromosomes. Usually a person has 23 pairs of chromosomes in each cell nucleus. These pairs are made up of one set of chromosomes from the mother and one set from the father. It is possible for a person to be born with three 'number 21' chromosomes, instead of two. Where this happens, the three-chromosome pattern causes 'Down's syndrome.' A person with Down's syndrome may have a learning disability and may have a physical appearance which includes a rounded face and shorter height. The extra genetic material on the additional chromosome clearly has a strong influence on the individual's development.

Richards (1993) identifies Huntingdon's disease and hereditary ovarian and breast cancer as two areas of disease which are linked to a *dominant genetic pattern*. This means that it only requires one parent to have the genetic pattern for children to inherit the illness. Other inherited diseases like beta thalassaemia and cystic fibrosis may only be passed on if both parents carry the genetic pattern responsible for these illnesses (a *recessive pattern*). Increasing knowledge has enabled tests to be designed to show whether a person is carrying one of these genetic patterns. These patterns could lead their children to develop an illness later in life. Counselling can be offered to people who are found to carry the genes for these illnesses, to enable carriers to plan their lives and avoid passing the genes on to children.

## Genetic influences and environmental factors

Dominant genes and chromosome abnormalities may have dramatic influences on individuals. Most genetic influences are likely to be more complex.

A rare disease which is caused when two carriers produce a baby is phenylketonuria or PKU. People with PKU cannot process phenylalanine, a substance found in most diets. So in the past, babies with PKU became poisoned. They did not develop intellectually and were likely to die from their genetic defect. Nothing can be done to change the genetic make-up of people with PKU. But nowadays most babies have no problem with the illness. At birth, they are tested for PKU and a special diet can be given if the test is positive. The special diet means that the genetic inability to process phenylalanine has no effect. So people with PKU grow up to be healthy and intelligent. PKU is caused by genetics, but is made harmless by the right environment.

> **Think it over**
>
> Are genetic or environmental influences most important when thinking about PKU? The answer may be that it is a mistake to try to separate genetic and environmental influences. In some senses, PKU is 100 per cent genetic and 100 per cent environmental.

Jones (1993) provides a range of examples which work like PKU. Anencephaly and spina bifida are disorders which cause the spinal cord to develop incorrectly. They also appear to 'run in families'. It is now known that poor diet may sometimes influence how genes work. Vitamin supplements during later pregnancy can reduce the risk of the genes causing the illness.

Jones argues:

> 'Even lung cancer has a genetic component. It is, as everyone knows, most common among smokers however, smokers … who are unfortunate enough to inherit a gene for susceptibility are far more likely to contract cancer than are those who do not. If everybody smoked, lung cancer would be a genetic disease.' (Pages 230–1.)

He then goes further and speculates:

> 'Most people know that smoking causes cancer and that a fatty diet may lead to heart disease. Certain genes predispose their carriers to the harmful effects of smoke or fat; and some individuals may be able to drink, smoke or eat lard with impunity. Perhaps it will become possible to choose the vices best fitted to ourselves.' (Page 234.)

Findings at the Patterson Institute for Cancer Research in Manchester (1995) suggest that about one person in ten inherits a general susceptibility to cancer.

Jones' point is that genetics interact with their surroundings. Some genetic diseases only happen if a person also catches a virus to trigger the disease response. Some cancers are genetic but come into operation because of diet. Some genes may cause cancer if triggered by chemicals or radioactive substances. Jones quotes the case of people

I'm 80 and fit as a fiddle!
I've had 2 heart attacks. I don't smoke and I exercise regularly

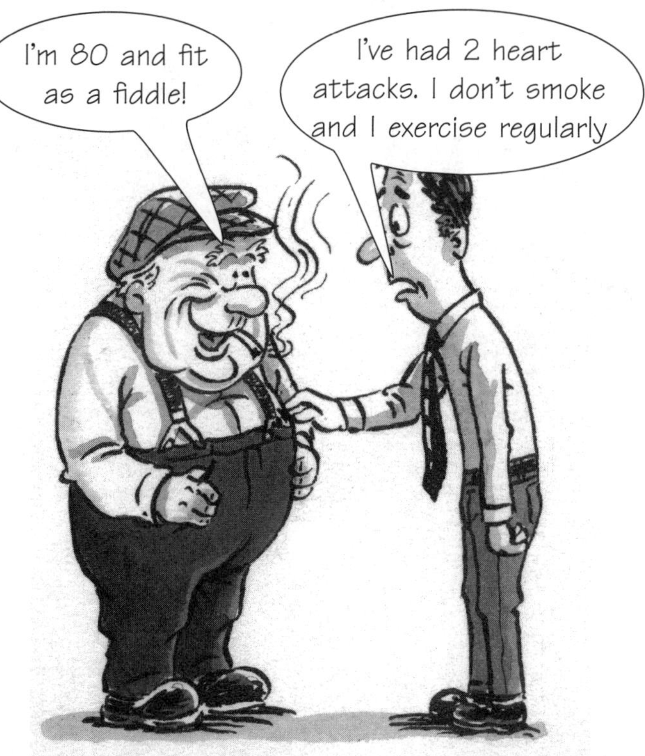

**Figure 4.39 Are genetic or environmental influences at work here?**

who live on the island of Nauru in the Pacific. They used to eat fish and vegetables, but now that they have greatly increased their consumption of sugar and fat (a western diet), eight out ten adults have diabetes – a susceptibility that didn't matter until they started to eat a western diet.

> **Think it over**
>
> Is diabetes on the island of Nauru caused by environment or genetics?

One of the reasons for studying the human genetic code is to find answers to the puzzles of genetically inherited disease. There may be ways in which environmental influences, drugs, vitamins and so on, can influence the effects of our genetic code. The environment may often be able to 'un-cause' the consequences of our original genetic plans.

## How the environment can modify genetic influences

If genetics and environment are inseparable when understanding disease, then what of studies of personality and ability? Plomin (1989) reviews research on the heritability of personality and intellectual factors. Personality traits and intelligence test results provide measures which can be studied in relation to potential inheritance. This area is highly controversial, but Plomin claims evidence that traits like extroversion and ability are influenced by genetic inheritance. Plomin also finds evidence that genetic influences are inseparably linked to environmental influences. It is not simply that intelligence or personality is passed from parents to children.

There is evidence that the environment has a potential to modify genetic influences. Plomin (1989) writes, 'As the pendulum swings from environmentalism, it is important that the pendulum be caught mid-swing before its momentum carries it to biological determinism. Behavioural genetic research clearly demonstrates that both nature and nurture are important in human development.' (Page 110.)

> **Think it over**
>
> Imagine a man in his forties. He goes to his doctor with complaints of being short of breath, sometimes feeling dizzy, and being generally unfit and unwell. The doctor discovers high blood pressure. If the doctor knew a little more about the person he or she could diagnose the situation as follows:
>
> 'Well as I see it, you are an unemployed member of social class 5 (lower class). Your social habits involve excessive drinking, smoking, lack of exercise, and a poor high-fat, high-sugar

diet. Your life situation provides you with little chance of changing your ways. Your family won't really support you to change your lifestyle – you are poor. Frankly you have little chance of recovery – expect to die!'

Or alternatively the doctor could have said:

'Well, tests of your genetic pattern suggest that you are at risk of developing heart disease. Some people are lucky, but I'm afraid you've inherited a tendency to heart disease – nothing I can do about that, it was all fixed before you were born – expect to die!'

Hopefully there are no doctors who would behave as in these two examples. The advice actually given would be more like:

'You have a history of heart disease in your family and it seems that you are not doing the right things to help yourself. I can't help you with money, jobs or family, but there are some things that we could do – would you take up an exercise programme if you had someone to help you? Would you follow a diet? Would you give up smoking? Can you find a sense of purpose that would make these things possible? You aren't guaranteed to live a long life if you can do these things – but at least you can try!'

The first two reactions are deterministic. The make-believe doctor is interpreting the social or the genetic pressures on an individual as fixing (or determining) what will happen. Social influences do affect people – statistics provide evidence of this. Genetic influences do affect people. But what happens to a person depends on the interplay of these factors. They also depend on the reaction of the individual. There are different levels of explanation that can be used for any area of human behaviour.

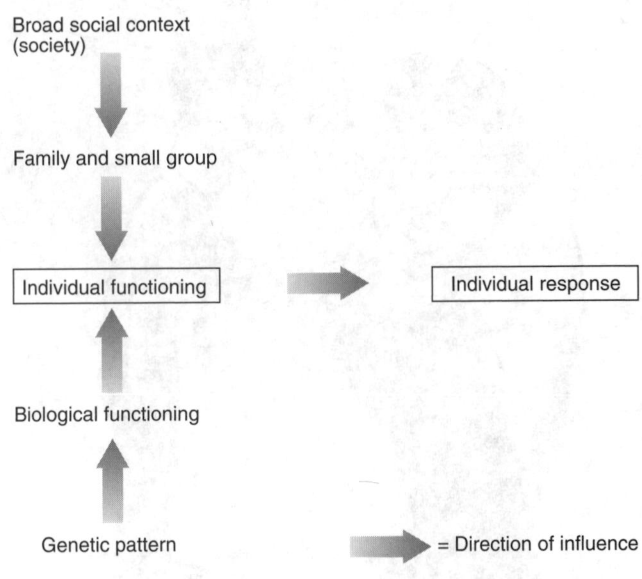


**Figure 4.40 Different levels of explanation for behaviour**

Society, belief systems, wealth, and social roles, all have a strong influence on the way families and friendship groups behave. Individuals are socialised to behave in terms of the norms and values that they learn in these groups. Genetics also influence our biological nature. Aspects of ability, temperament and susceptibility to disease will also influence how we react. The influences of biology and social groups have been interacting in us since our birth.

## Determinism

There is broad agreement amongst the majority of authors in the fields of psychology and biology that human ability, personality and susceptibility to disease result from the interaction of genetic and social influences. There are individuals who insist that human nature is the result of social influences and that genetics either do not exist or have very little influence. This view is sometimes described as *social determinism* – the idea that everything about a person is fixed by his or her social circumstances. Historically, this view has been associated with the philosopher John Locke (1632–1704). Locke believed that a newborn baby was a 'blank slate' for the environment to write on. Any baby could become anything depending on the way he or she was brought up.

More recently, Karl Marx's analysis of social influences was used as a basis for a similar argument. People became what their class membership made them. Some extreme views derived from Marxism suggested that individual people were no more than representatives of particular groups. Group influences controlled or moulded what you were. So a white, middle-aged male would have to think differently from a young working-class male. A black, middle-class woman would think the way her race and class made her think. If you could control social influences, then you could control all human behaviour.

The opposite view is *genetic* or *biological determinism*. This view says that people are born to become what their inheritance dictates that they should become. There is a long history to this viewpoint in European culture. Originally a religious leader, John Calvin (1509–1564) taught that people were pre-determined to achieve salvation or not. Calvin saw human nature as fundamentally corrupt and wicked. The philosopher, Thomas Hobbes (1588–1679) took up this theme in accepting that human nature inevitably led people to be destructive. People had to be controlled in order to keep their inborn tendencies in check.

## Popular views of biological determinism

At the time of the philosopher René Descartes (1596–1650), Europeans seem to have understood children as being made up from what was in their two parents. Whatever came out in a child must have in some way existed in the parents. If a child was attractive, clever or wicked, those qualities must have come from the parents. Steve Jones (1993) explains how later people believed that qualities ran 'in the blood'. In the 1800s, Europeans literally believed that it was the blood that created the abilities and personalities of children. This is the reason for terms like 'royal blood' and 'blood lines' and 'blood relatives'.

The popular understanding was that when two people had a baby, the baby would be half one parent and half the other – because of the mixing of the blood!

So can you see which half of the baby is me and which half is you?

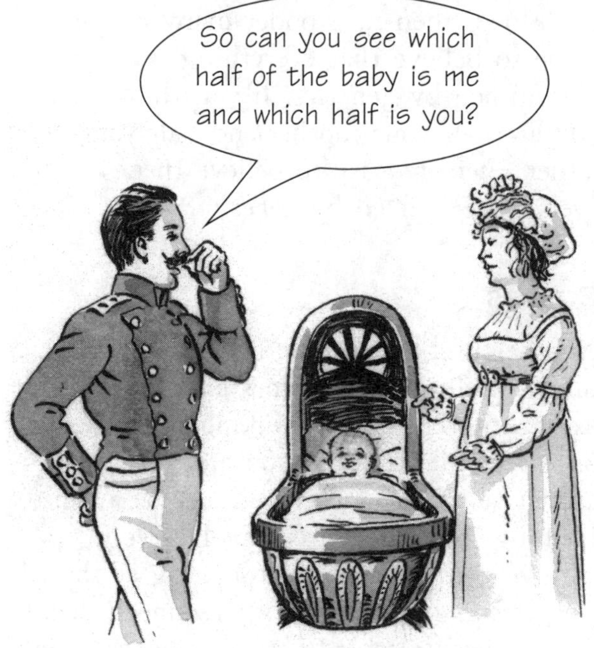

**People used to believe that a baby was made up of half one parent and half another**

Since the time of Gregor Mendel (1822–84), biologists have come to understand that genetics do not work this way. A baby is not a simple continuation of the features of his or her parents. Even the idea of dominant and recessive genes does not explain the full complexity of genetic inheritance. It may be more appropriate to think of a child as a unique outcome of the interaction of his or her mother and father's genetic patterns.

Richards (1993) provides evidence that many people still think of inheritance in terms of the old Victorian idea. Some people appear to believe that if one of your parents had cancer then you will get it. If neither had cancer then you must be all right! This kind of thinking is very inaccurate and does not fit recent understandings of the complex way in which genetic material may work.

If people still believe the old Victorian ideas and just substitute the word 'genes' for 'blood' then no wonder many people come to believe that everything is determined by genetics. If you think that you are half your mother and half your father, then it's easy to believe that everything is fixed by genes.

### Causes

Another problem people may have with understanding genes comes back to levels of explanation. Western thinking often focuses on discussing *causes*. If you are clever, attractive or wicked, there must be a cause. Looking for causes often involves very simple ideas. Rather than looking at the way things interact and interconnect, people often concentrate on ever more general ideas of cause. So a person can say, 'When I think, my thoughts are caused by all sorts of electrical messages in my brain. These messages are caused by chemical reactions; the chemical reactions are caused by the biochemistry of my genes. Therefore, everything I think goes back to my genes.' Equally a person can say, 'When I think, I am thinking in patterns that I have learned. I have learned to think the way I do because of my social experiences. My social experiences have been caused by society. Therefore, everything I think is caused by society.'

Both these arguments are inaccurate – they only pick up some of the issues and ignore the complexity of human experience.

#### Think it over

The word 'cause' can lead people to some very strange conclusions. Imagine asking three people where they went for their holiday last year and why they chose that destination.

The first person says, 'Spain. Society and the social construction of holidays made me do it.'

The second person answers, 'Spain. It was the biochemical reactions in my head that made me do it – biochemical reactions which have their origin in evolution since the beginnings of the world'.

The third person says, 'Spain. I went there because I thought I would enjoy it!'

You would probably see the first two people as 'not fully functioning human beings' or to put it more bluntly, 'weird'. Reducing everything to distant and abstract causes can lead to explanations at the wrong level.

It would be hard to enjoy a social life (and probably hard to have one) if you didn't think in terms of individual and personal systems of meaning. Without an individual

Society makes me think the way I do
Biology controls my thought
I think for myself

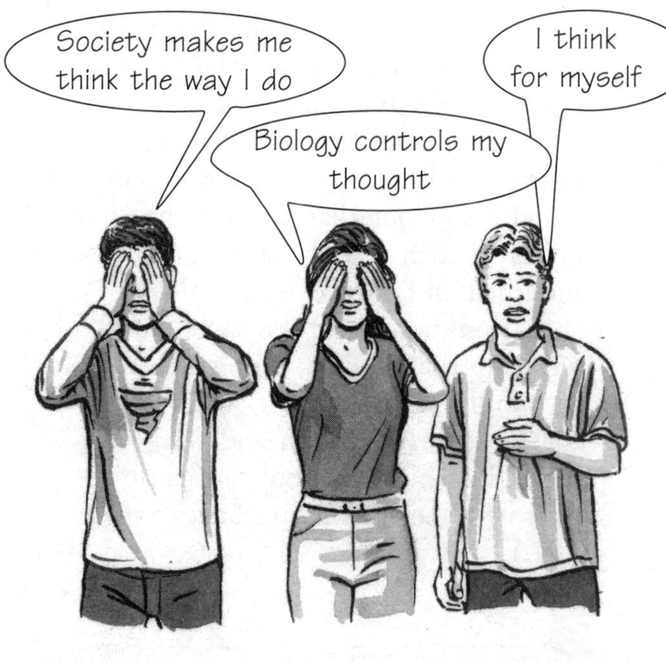

**Figure 4.41** It is inaccurate to think that our lives are determined either by society or by genetics

level of explanation, how do you understand the skill of interpersonal communication?

All the levels of explanation have a part to play in care work and in understanding human need. It is important not to allow the word 'cause' to twist thinking into reducing everything to biochemistry. It may be equally important not to allow the idea of cause to persuade us to explain everything away in terms of 'society'.

## The politics of determinism

To say that everything is fixed by genes, or that everything is fixed by society, gives a nice simple explanation. Each is also an explanation with political consequences. If a person who visits the doctor is given the explanation he or she has a 'genetic weakness', the doctor might conclude the conversation by saying, 'we can't do anything – so go away and die quietly.' The idea of things being fixed can be used to avoid responsibility.

What's the point in spending money on cancer treatment and research, if the possibility of whether people develop cancer or not is fixed? Politically, it could be argued that tax cuts are better than spending money on people with heart disease and cancer – some people can be seen as 'no hopers' if you believe in simple genetic determinism.

Social determinism also leads to theories about political power. Once again, the individual need not matter. Individual problems can only be put right if a particular kind of government takes control. Issues about health immediately become issues about political power and who should be in control of world economic issues.

The situation becomes even more extreme if areas like wealth, intelligence, personality and crime are seen as genetically determined. It could then be possible to claim that the poor are poor because they are inferior, that crime can't be tackled socially, that education is wasted on some groups in society, and so on. Genetic determinists might be able to argue for the abolition of free health and education – they could use the argument that 'It's wasted on people who are "no hopers"'. A genetic determinist could argue, 'If people have it in them to lead prosperous, healthy, worthwhile lives, then they will. If people haven't got it in them, then why should taxpayers waste money on them?'

Professors Rose, Lewontin and Kamin (1984) state:

> 'Over the past decade and a half we have watched with concern the rising tide of biological determinist writing, with its increasingly grandiose claims to be able to locate the causes of the inequalities of status, wealth and power between classes, genders and races in Western society in a reductionist

[everything reduces or goes back to genetics] theory of human nature.' (Page ix.)

Rose *et al.* devote a whole chapter to the politics of biological determinism. Nicky Hayes (1995) reviews some of the theories of genetic determinism and states:

'These people are not purveying scientific theory, but ideology. It is a political perspective with very direct political implications: it legitimises the inequalities of society by arguing that these arise from inherited differences; and negates attempts to create a better society by implying that they are doomed to failure from the start.' (Page 132.)

## The interaction of nature and nurture

The debate about inherited and environmental influences is sometimes referred to as the *Nature* (inherited influences) *versus Nurture* (environmental influences) debate. This is a poetic way of putting the issues that may go back to Shakespeare. Shakespeare created the character Caliban in his play *The Tempest*. Caliban is described as a person 'upon whose nature nurture could never stick'. This means that he was fixed by inheritance. The nature/nurture debate was going on long before genes or chromosomes were discovered.

Rose *et al.* conclude,

'The contrast between biological and cultural determinism is a manifestation of the nature– nurture controversy that has plagued biology, psychology and sociology since the early part of the nineteenth century. Either nature plays a determining role in producing the similarity and differences among human beings, or it does not, in which case, what is left but nurture? We reject this dichotomy. We do assert that we cannot think of any significant human social behaviour that is built into our genes in such a way that it cannot be modified and shaped by social conditioning...yet at the same time, we deny that human beings are born as tabulae rasae [blank slate], which they evidently are not, and that individual human beings are simple mirrors of social circumstances.' (Page 267.)

" WELL, I KNOW HEART DISEASE RUNS IN OUR FAMILY – IF IT'S IN YOUR GENES, IT'LL GET YOU – THAT'S WHAT I SAY! "
SUGAR
BEER
CRISPS
HI FAT SNACK

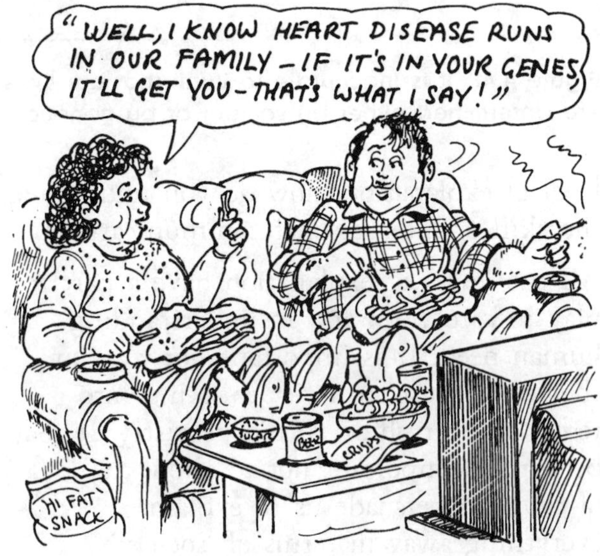

**Figure 4.42 The nature–nurture debate will continue to run and run**

Can criminal behaviour be influenced by genes? Professor Patrick Bateson, writing in *The Independent* (18 February, 1995) commented on articles claiming that biological make-up might hold the key to criminal behaviour, or that unemployment might be the cause. He said, 'The sad thing was the determinism that accompanied the media coverage of the claims. It was obvious that, in certain quarters, the dreadful old nature–nurture debate was rampant once again'. Later, he states, 'By degrees, both sides in the nature–nurture dispute have come to appreciate that behavioural development cannot be treated as though it were wholly under the control of the genes or wholly influenced by the environment.'

It is possible to look at issues like temperament, language learning and the in-built reactions of babies and say that these are all genetic, and so, therefore, a certain proportion of language or personality is genetic. Bateson argues that this is wrong. To explain why, Bateson uses the example of baking a cake. A cake is more than the ingredients that go into it. A cake is the result of a process. When a cake is mixed and later baked, the butter, sugar, eggs, flour, milk, raisins and water all alter. The taste of the cake and the texture of the cake is different from the taste of the cake mixture. Bateson argues that human development is a process. The contribution of environment and the contribution of genetics is impossible to separate:

> 'You would not expect to recognise each ingredient and each action involved in cooking as a separate component in the finished cake... The development of individuals is an interplay between them and their environment. Individuals choose and change the conditions to which they are exposed; then they are themselves changed by those conditions to which they are exposed.'

Rose *et al*. (1984) also use this cake metaphor.

The question as to how much human development is due to environment and how much is due to genetics could be answered by saying that it's a bit of both. But even this answer is wrong. The influence of both nature and nurture is an influence on a process. Development is a process. Jones (1993) states:

> 'An attribute such as intelligence is often seen as a cake which can be sliced into so much "gene" and so much "environment". In fact the two are so closely blended that trying to separate them is more like trying to unbake the cake. Failure to understand this simple biological fact leads to confusion and worse.' (Page 227.)

Human beings are infinitely more complex than mixing and baking a cake. The cake stays baked – it becomes a finished product. Humans are never finished. Human learning and change continue until an individual dies. Although the cake metaphor is limited, it does provide a way of understanding why it is unwise to separate the influences of nature and nurture.

Professor of genetics Steve Jones (1993) summarises the nature–nurture debate with the following paragraph:

> 'Most modern geneticists find queries about the relative importance of nature and nurture in controlling the normal range of human behaviour dull, for two reasons. First, they scarcely understand the inheritance of complex characters (those like height, weight or behaviour which are measured rather than counted) even in simple creatures like flies or mice, and even when studying traits like size or weight which are easy to define. Second, and more important, geneticists know that the perpetual interrogation – nature or nurture? – is largely meaningless. Its only answer is usually that there is no valid question.' (Page 226.)

So how much of the flavour of your cake is due to flour and water, and how much is due to baking?
What a leading question! Perhaps if I say a bit of both he'll go away

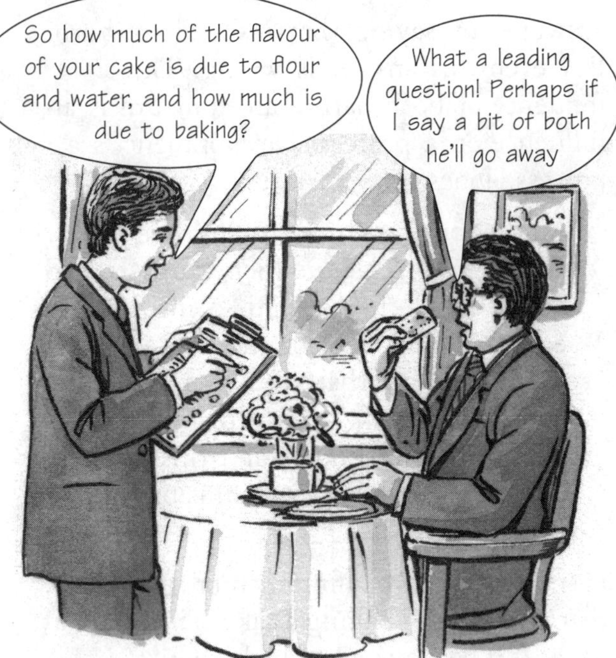

**Figure 4.43 A cake is more than the ingredients that go into it: it is the result of a process**

A conclusion would appear to be that nature and nurture cannot be usefully abstracted from the process of development, but that nature and nurture form a process of interaction which progresses across the life-span of any organism. Environment may completely override genetic influences, as in PKU, or genetic influences may sometimes have powerful effects, depending on the environment with which they interact.

## Socio-economic factors which influence development

Human development is an interaction of genetic and environmental influences, but the environment can be very different for different individuals. Some children grow up in an environment which offers lots of opportunity for them to lead a fit, healthy and successful life. But some children are born into an environment that offers them less chance of leading a healthy and fulfilled life. The term 'social exclusion' is used to identify people who are seriously disadvantaged in terms of opportunities for social and economic development.

The government set up the Social Exclusion Unit in December 1997 to explore ways of improving opportunity and reducing social exclusion. This group produced a report in 1999 called 'Opportunity for All – Tackling Poverty and Social Exclusion'. In this report the government states:

> 'Our aim is to end the injustice which holds people back and prevents them from making the most of themselves. That means making sure that all children, whatever their background and wherever they live, get a first class education, giving them the tools they will need to succeed in the adult world. And it means making sure that children can live and play in clean, safe environments, and that the community in which they live is thriving and supportive. Put simply, our goal is to end child poverty in 20 years.'
>
> From 'Opportunity for All' document (page 1)

The government says its goal is 'that everyone should have the opportunity to achieve their potential. But too many people are denied that opportunity. It is wrong and economically inefficient to waste the talents of even one single person'.

The 'Opportunity for All' paper also states that:

- The number of people living in households with low incomes has more than doubled since the late 1970s.
- One in three children live in households that receive below half the national average income.

- Nearly one in five working-age households has no one in work.
- The poorest communities have much more unemployment, poor housing, vandalism and crime than richer areas.

The report goes on to say that the problems which prevent people from making the most of their lives are as follows:

- *Lack of opportunities to work.* Work is the most important route out of low income. However, the consequences of being unemployed are more far reaching than simple lack of money. Unemployment can contribute to ill health and can deny future employment opportunities.
- *Lack of opportunities to acquire education and skills.* Adults who are without basic skills are substantially more likely to spend long periods out of work.
- *Childhood deprivation.* This is linked with problems of low income, poor health, poor housing and unsafe environments.
- *Disrupted families.* The evidence shows that children in one-parent families are particularly likely to suffer the effects of persistently low household incomes. Stresses within families can lead to exclusion and, in extreme cases, to homelessness.
- *Barriers to older people living active, fulfilling and healthy lives.* Too many older people have low incomes, a lack of independence and poor health. Lack of access to good-quality services is a key barrier to social inclusion.
- *Inequalities in health.* Health can be affected by low income and a range of socio-economic factors, such as access to good-quality health services and shops selling good-quality food at affordable prices.
- *Poor housing.* This directly diminishes people's quality of life and leads to a range of physical and mental problems. It can also cause difficulties for children trying to do their homework.
- *Poor neighbourhoods.* The most deprived areas suffer from a combination of poor housing, high rates of crime,

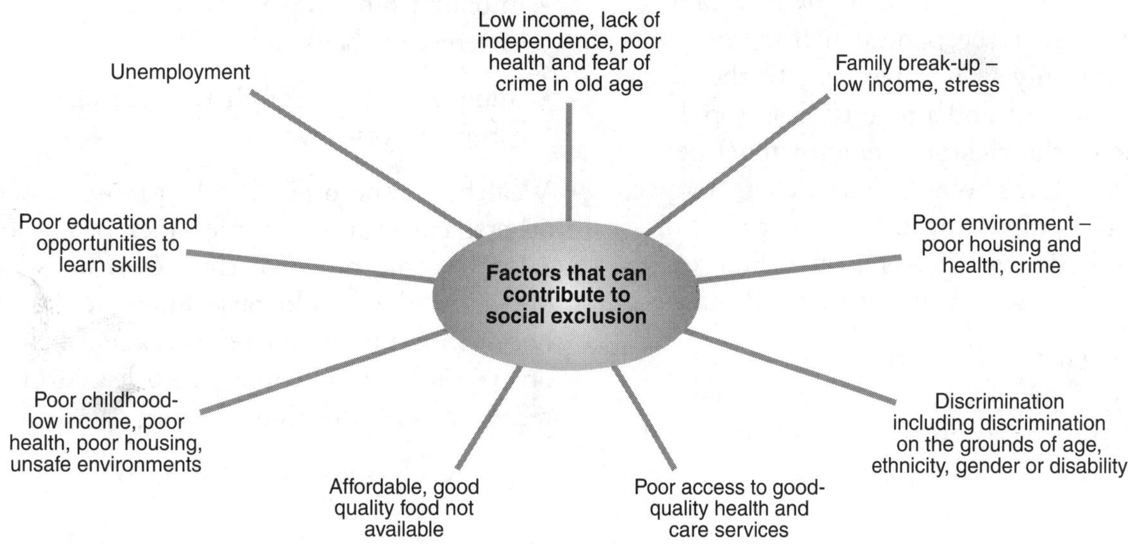


**Figure 4.44 Factors that can contribute to social exclusion**

unemployment, poor health and family disruption.

- *Fear of crime.* Crime and fear can effectively exclude people within their own communities, especially older people.
- *Disadvantaged groups.* Some people experience disadvantage or discrimination, for example, on the grounds of age, ethnicity, gender or disability. This makes them particularly vulnerable to social exclusion.

## The effects of wealth and income

The economic resources possessed by an individual or family make a major difference to the quality of life a person leads. Economic resources include wealth and income. *Wealth* includes:

- savings, in banks or building societies
- the value of your home if you own it
- shares, life assurance and pension rights
- any other property that belongs to you.

Wealth is not shared out evenly in the UK. Figures for 1996 reported in *Social Trends 2000* show that the poorest half of the population only own 7 per cent of the country's wealth and property. The top 1 per cent of the richest people own 19 per cent of the UK's wealth. The richest 10 per cent of the population own 52 per cent of the wealth. If wealth was a cake, Figure 4.45 shows how it would be shared out.

*Income* is what really matters to the vast majority of people, your weekly income enables you to pay for your home, and feed and clothe yourself. Income mainly comes from:

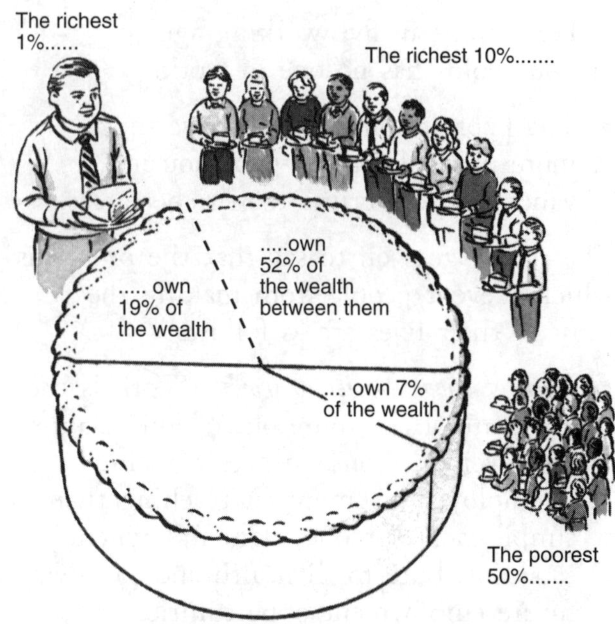


**Figure 4.45 The UK wealth cake (based on 1996 figures reported in Social Trends 2000)**

- wages you are paid
- profits from your business if you are self-employed
- benefits paid by the government
- money from invested wealth, such as interest on bank accounts or bonds
- money raised through the sale of property you own.

Wealth, on the other hand, might matter to others. For example, some older people have a low income but own their own house; if necessary, they could raise money on their home through special remortgage schemes or even sell up and move into leased or rented accommodation.

> ? *Social Trends 2000* reports that: 'In 1997–98, over 50% of households reported having less than £1,500 in savings, with 30% reporting no savings at all. In particular, 71% of single parent households and 41% of single adult households had no savings.' (Page 97.)

## Low income

The DSS paper 'Opportunity for All' (1999) reports that more people live on low incomes than in the past. 'The proportions of people living in households with relatively low incomes more than doubled between the end of the 1970s and the beginning of the 1990s. One of the main reasons for this increase in numbers of people with low incomes has been the growth of numbers of working-age households where no one is working. The proportion of working-age households where no one is working has doubled since the end of the 1970s. The most disturbing aspect of this growth in worklessness is the number of people trapped on benefits for long periods of time. Just under three million working-age people have been claiming income replacement benefits for more than two years'. (Chapter 2, pages 1 and 2.)

*Social Trends 2000* reports that 18 per cent of the population lived in households with low income during 1997 to 1998 (low income is defined as less than 60 per cent of average income). *Social Trends 2000* reports that, 'Children are disproportionately present in low income households: in 1997–98 there were 3.2 million children living in such households in Great Britain. Two out of five of these children were living with one parent only, and more than half were living in households where no one was in paid work'. (Page 93.)

'Opportunity for All' (1999) reports that 'nearly one in five households with children has no working adult [a figure which is] significantly higher than all other European countries'.

Living in a low-income household might have an impact on the development of a child in a number of ways (see Figure 4.46).

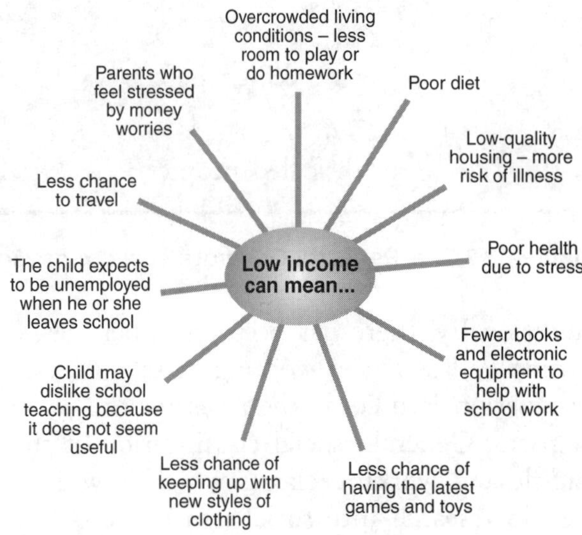


**Figure 4.46 A child's development will be influenced adversely by living in a low-income household**

## Social class and health

It would be very unusual for wealth and power to be distributed evenly in any society. The concept of social stratification is used to divide society into different layers (or strata) of wealth and power. In the UK, these layers or social strata are usually referred to in terms of the class system.

| | Social class | Examples of occupation in each class |
|---|---|---|
| Middle class | *Class 1*<br>Professional people | Doctor, lawyer, accountant, architect |
| | *Class 2*<br>Managerial and technical people | Manager, teacher, librarian, farmer, airline pilot |
| | *Class 3A (non-manual)*<br>Clerical and minor supervisory people | Sales representative, office worker, policeman |
| Working class | *Class 3B (manual)*<br>Skilled people | Electrician, tailor, cook, butcher, bricklayer |
| | *Class 4*<br>Semi-skilled people | Farm worker, postman, packer, bus conductor |
| | *Class 5*<br>Unskilled people | Porter, labourer, window cleaner, messenger, cleaner |

**Figure 4.47 The Registrar-General's social classification**

Traditionally, there has been an upper class, a middle class and a working class. Occupation is used as the basis for the Registrar-General's social classification of the middle and working classes which is widely used in research into social issues (see Figure 4.47).

The occupations given as examples for each class are chosen because they are linked to more than a level of income. They are ranked according to the general standing of the occupations within the community, which means that people in these occupations have a particular place or status in society and the behaviour and lifestyle associated with it.

This is illustrated by the way that Class 3 is divided into two, with 'non-manual' placed above 'manual' in the ranking of occupations. Although a skilled manual worker's income may be higher than that of a clerk, he or she is still regarded as being in the working class. Non-manual (or 'white collar') workers are seen as tending towards the middle class and are expected to have many of the values and norms of behaviour associated with middle-class culture.

The class system is being revised and a new class system is expected to be used in the 2001 census. For information, the new social classification structure is outlined in Table 4.6.

Research on the impact of social class on health has used the old '6 group' classification system described above. In 1998, Sir Donald Acheson published an 'Independent inquiry into inequalities in health', a report which had been commissioned by the government. This report provides dramatic evidence not only of differences between the health of people in different class groups, but that if anything these differences have become more extreme since the 1970s.

| | |
|---|---|
| **1.1** | Employers and managers in larger organisations, for example company directors. |
| **1.2** | Higher professionals, for example doctors, solicitors, teachers. |
| **2** | Lower managerial and professional occupations, for example nurses, journalists. |
| **3** | Intermediate occupations, for example clerks, secretaries. |
| **4** | Small employers and own account workers, for example taxi drivers, painters and decorators. |
| **5** | Lower supervisory, craft and related occupations, for example plumbers, train drivers. |
| **6** | Semi-routine occupations, for example shop assistants, hairdressers. |
| **7** | Routine occupations, for example cleaners, refuse collectors. |

*Those who are long-term unemployed form a final, eighth group.*

**Table 4.6 Social classifications expected to be used in the 2001 census**

People in the lower social classes are more likely to die before the age of 65 than are people in the higher social classes. The table is copied from Acheson (1998, page 13). This table shows that health may be improving in England and Wales, but that it may be improving more for the higher social economic groups than it is for the lower socio-economic groups.

The Acheson report details how disease, accidents and suicide affect people in the different social classes. Table 4.9 shows the 'death rates' or mortality rates for men aged 20–64. Most of the data suggests that health is improving, but more for the higher groups than the lower groups. Suicide rates for lower-class men have actually become much worse since the early 1970s!

### Think it over

Why is there nearly five times the rate of lung cancer in social class V than in class 1? Why nearly three times the amount of heart disease? Why over three and a half times the suicide rate and four times the accident rate between these classes? What might be the reasons for these figures?

| | *Women* (35–64) | | | *Men* (35–64) | | |
|---|---|---|---|---|---|---|
| | 1976–81 | 1981–85 | 1986–92 | 1976–81 | 1981–85 | 1986–92 |
| **All causes** | | | | | | |
| I/II | 338 | 344 | 270 | 621 | 539 | 455 |
| IIIN | 371 | 387 | 305 | 860 | 658 | 484 |
| IIIM | 467 | 396 | 356 | 802 | 691 | 624 |
| IV/V | 508 | 445 | 418 | 951 | 824 | 764 |
| *Ratio IV and V against I and II* | 1.50 | 1.29 | 1.55 | 1.53 | 1.53 | 1.68 |

**Table 4.7 Death before the age of 65 by social class (Acheson report, 1998)**

## All causes

rates per 100,000

| *Social class* | *Year* 1970–72 | 1979–83 | 1991–93 |
|---|---|---|---|
| I – Professional | 500 | 373 | 280 |
| II – Managerial & Technical | 526 | 425 | 300 |
| III(N) – Skilled (non-manual) | 637 | 522 | 426 |
| III(M) – Skilled (manual) | 683 | 580 | 493 |
| IV – Partly skilled | 721 | 639 | 492 |
| V – Unskilled | 897 | 910 | 806 |
| England and Wales | 624 | 549 | 419 |

## Lung cancer

rates per 100,000

| *Social class* | *Year* 1970–72 | 1979–83 | 1991–93 |
|---|---|---|---|
| I – Professional | 41 | 26 | 17 |
| II – Managerial & Technical | 52 | 39 | 24 |
| III(N) – Skilled (non-manual) | 63 | 47 | 34 |
| III(M) – Skilled (manual) | 90 | 72 | 54 |
| IV – Partly skilled | 93 | 76 | 52 |
| V – Unskilled | 109 | 108 | 82 |
| England and Wales | 73 | 60 | 39 |

## Coronary heart disease

rates per 100,000

| *Social class* | *Year* 1970–72 | 1979–83 | 1991–93 |
|---|---|---|---|
| I – Professional | 195 | 144 | 81 |
| II – Managerial & Technical | 197 | 168 | 92 |
| III(N) – Skilled (non-manual) | 245 | 208 | 136 |
| III(M) – Skilled (manual) | 232 | 218 | 159 |
| IV – Partly skilled | 232 | 227 | 156 |
| V – Unskilled | 243 | 287 | 235 |
| England and Wales | 209 | 201 | 127 |

## Stroke

rates per 100,000

| *Social class* | *Year* 1970–72 | 1979–83 | 1991–93 |
|---|---|---|---|
| I – Professional | 35 | 20 | 14 |
| II – Managerial & Technical | 37 | 23 | 13 |
| III(N) – Skilled (non-manual) | 41 | 28 | 19 |
| III(M) – Skilled (manual) | 45 | 34 | 24 |
| IV – Partly skilled | 46 | 37 | 25 |
| V – Unskilled | 59 | 55 | 45 |
| England and Wales | 40 | 30 | 20 |

## Accidents, poisoning, violence

rates per 100,000

| *Social class* | *Year* 1970–72 | 1979–83 | 1991–93 |
|---|---|---|---|
| I – Professional | 23 | 17 | 13 |
| II – Managerial & Technical | 25 | 20 | 13 |
| III(N) – Skilled (non-manual) | 25 | 21 | 17 |
| III(M) – Skilled (manual) | 34 | 27 | 24 |
| IV – Partly skilled | 39 | 35 | 24 |
| V – Unskilled | 67 | 63 | 52 |
| England and Wales | 34 | 28 | 22 |

## Suicide and undetermined injury

rates per 100,000

| *Social class* | *Year* 1970–72 | 1979–83 | 1991–93 |
|---|---|---|---|
| I – Professional | 16 | 16 | 13 |
| II – Managerial & Technical | 13 | 15 | 14 |
| III(N) – Skilled (non-manual) | 17 | 18 | 20 |
| III(M) – Skilled (manual) | 12 | 16 | 21 |
| IV – Partly skilled | 18 | 23 | 23 |
| V – Unskilled | 32 | 44 | 47 |
| England and Wales | 15 | 20 | 22 |

Table 4.8 Death rates for men aged 20–64 (Acheson report, 1998)

Argyle (1987) states, 'The lower social classes are affected by most illness more often, take more days off from work, and die a little sooner because of them [the illnesses]. This is partly due to inequalities in the conditions of life – smaller homes, less heating, larger families, less good food, and so on.' (Page 189.) Argyle goes on to argue that middle-class people also make more use of preventative health services such as antenatal clinics, vaccination programmes and cervical screening, than do working-class people. 'Doctors spend more time with middle-class patients and there is evidence that National Health Service expenditure on middle-class people is 40 per cent higher than on those in Classes 4 and 5 – because Classes 1 and 2 know how to make better use of the system.' (Page 190.) Argyle suggests that middle-class people may have responded to health education campaigns more effectively than working-class people in the past. In particular, there is evidence that middle-class people smoked less, were slimmer and took more exercise than working-class people in the past.

A study by Mildred Blaxter (1990) finds a very strong relationship between low income and disease, disability, illness and poor psychological and social (psycho-social) health. But it seems that it is poverty which is associated with ill-health, rather than the case that health gets better the richer you are! Her studies show that there might be just slightly more illness and disease for the very rich than for the more moderately well-off. Money itself does not seem to create health; but a lack of money may be strongly associated with disease and illness. Blaxter writes, 'The apparently strong association of social class and health is primarily an association of income and health.' (Page 72.) Blaxter's study found that self-perceived stress was strongly associated with poorer health of every kind, but, 'It is notable that the relationship was particularly strong for men in manual classes, at all ages.' (Page 104.)

## Poverty and nutrition

The Acheson report (1998) refers to 'food poverty' and notes that people in low socio-economic groups 'spend more on foods richer in energy and high in fat and sugar, which are cheaper per unit of energy than foods rich in protective nutrients, such as fruit and vegetables'. (Page 65.) 'People on low incomes eat less healthily partly because of cost, rather than lack of concern or information. Therefore increased availability of affordable 'healthy' food should lead to improved nutrition in the least well off'. (Page 66.) The Acheson report (1998) notes evidence of the following among people in low socio-economic groups:

- they tend to eat more processed foods containing high levels of salt, thus increasing the risk of cardiovascular disease
- there is more obesity in low socio-economic groups than in higher groups – increasing the risk of ill-health
- babies born to mothers in low socio-economic groups are more likely to have reduced birth weights than higher groups. Low birth weight is linked with the risk of cardiovascular disease in later life
- women in lower socio-economic groups are less likely to breast feed their babies. Breast feeding helps to protect infants from infection.

People who are poor will find it harder to travel to supermarkets and cannot stock-up on cheaper food or take advantage of 'special offers'. The Acheson report notes that 'healthy food' often costs more than processed food which contains higher amounts of sugar and salt. Poverty may push people to choose an unhealthy diet, because it can be harder and more expensive to choose a healthy one.

### Smoking

Smoking was estimated to cause 30,000 deaths from lung cancer and 16,000 deaths from other cancers in 1995. The Acheson report points out that there are major class differences in this behaviour. The report states that only 2 per cent of men and 16 per cent of women in professional occupations smoke, whereas 41 per cent of men and 36 per cent of women in unskilled occupations smoke. The report notes that people in the lower socio-economic groups find it harder to give up smoking.

Poverty may remove many of the small daily satisfactions of life, such as buying small presents for friends, going out and giving yourself treats. Poverty or low income may also provide a source of stress for individuals. This stress may be linked to the self-esteem and identity of people who may not be able to keep up with the consumer values which are promoted by advertising and which are a big part of contemporary society. If you have lost the consumer race, you may be inclined to evaluate yourself as a loser. This alone could create stress.

When a person feels stressed, anything which promotes an easing of tension will be very desirable. A study by NCH Action for Children (1994) found that, 'two-thirds of children interviewed said they smoked to "escape" their problems, while one in three said they drank, and one in six took (illegal) drugs.' Sarah Hirsh of the anti-smoking charity, Quit, is quoted as follows in *The Independent* 9 March 1994: 'As smoking rates increased in line with poverty, it was not surprising that women found it more difficult to stop. Women who are in the lower social groups may be stuck at home with no luxuries. Many tell us on the helpline that smoking is all they have got.'

Oakley (1989) quoted in Nettleton (1995) 'found that smoking was significantly inversely related to income, housing tenure, access to a car, telephone ownership and central heating.' (Page 54.) In other words, the poorer women were, the more they were likely to smoke. Nettleton theorises that poor health 'choices' like smoking may enable people to cope with poverty. 'Thus whilst affecting women's physical health, smoking may facilitate their mental well-being.' (Page 54.)

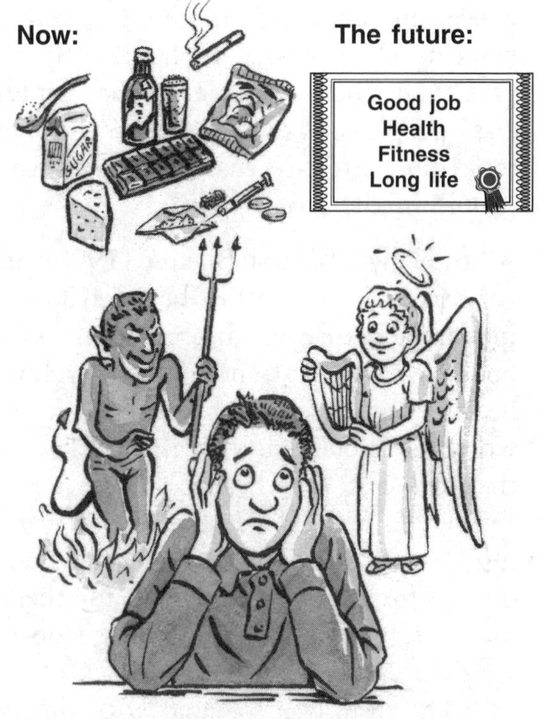


Figure 4.48 It is not always easy to make the 'right' choices

People who are poor and/or stressed may find it harder to trade a long-term future for tempting and stress-relieving treats that can be enjoyed in the present.

> **Think it over**
>
> What 'treats' do you and your family allow yourselves? What might be the effect if poverty prevented you from having these treats?

## Access to health services

Private health care may sometimes provide a faster service than the NHS. Certain drugs and treatments may be available to private patients, but may be limited to NHS patients. Some voluntary groups campaign against the 'postcode lottery' where some people do get access to the latest treatments but people living in other areas do not. For example, the drug beta-interferon has been proven to slow the progress of multiple sclerosis but only three per cent of NHS patients in the UK are prescribed it.

The Acheson report 1998 identifies an 'inverse law' which appears to exist in some aspects of care and preventative medicine. The 'inverse law' means that communities with the greatest need receive the lowest level of service whilst those with the lowest need receive the highest level of resources.

In the field of access to prevention services the Acheson report states:

> 'Communities most at risk of ill health tend to experience the least satisfactory access to the full range of preventative services, the so called "inverse prevention law". Prevention services include cancer screening programmes, health promotion and immunisation. While differences are most noticeable amongst socio-economic groups it is likely that, for example amongst Bangladeshi women, additional inequalities in access are experienced. Lack of access to women practitioners can be a deterrent to Asian women taking up an invitation for cervical screening. Local studies have shown that access to female practitioners is poorest in areas with high concentrations of Asian residents and that practices with a female doctor or nurse are more likely to reach the cervical cytology targets set out in the GP contract. Sub-regional and small area analysis illustrate this inequality for areas such as Liverpool and Birmingham where, using nine indicators of primary care services, the most deprived areas tended to be the least well served. Within London, health promotion claims by GPs are highest in the least deprived and lowest in the most deprived areas.'

With respect to medical services, the Acheson report states:

> 'Since mortality from coronary heart disease in South Asians is 40 per cent higher than the general population, intervention rates for large Asian communities might be expected to be higher than average. The evidence shows the opposite after adjusting for socio-economic and geographical factors. Similarly, rates for coronary artery bypass grafts and coronary angioplasty are not generally higher in areas with the greatest need.
>
> 'An "inverse care law" is still evident in relation to the distribution of medical and nursing staff in relation to need. A number of studies have also shown that deprived areas suffer increasing difficulty in recruiting GPs.

This situation has been exacerbated – especially in inner London – by the poor quality of primary care premises, large numbers of single-handed GPs, GPs approaching retirement and practices without training status. This inequity extends beyond that of GPs to other primary care staff including practice nurses, health visitors and district nurses.' (Page 116.)

Further details of the differences between social class areas and the provision of health care during the 1990s can be found in Unit 5. While there is evidence of inequality in the provision of health services the Acheson report notes that reliable research into the details of this issue is limited.

## Housing

People in the professional classes often feel sufficiently confident about their future and their ability to take on a mortgage to buy their own home. People in the higher social classes can choose where and how they would like to live.

People in the unskilled social categories tend to have less choice sometimes, forcing people to rent property in more densely populated housing areas. *Social Trends 2000* states: 'Among the economically active, nine out of ten household heads in the professional, and employer and manager groups were owner-occupiers in 1998–99, compared with half of those in the unskilled manual group.'

Wealth and income will affect the lifestyle that people enjoy with respect to housing. Wealthier people will often live in more

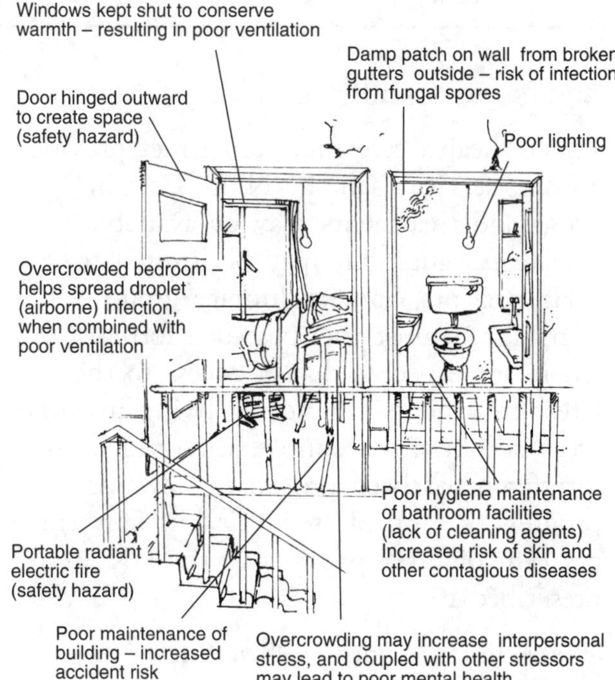


**Figure 4.50 Poor housing may contribute to a wide range of hazards to health and social well-being**

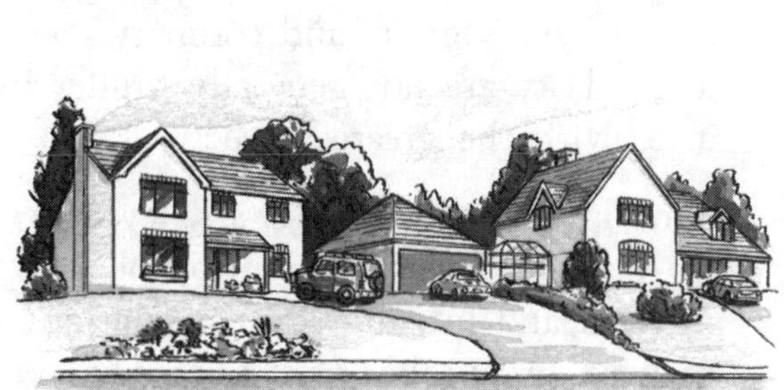

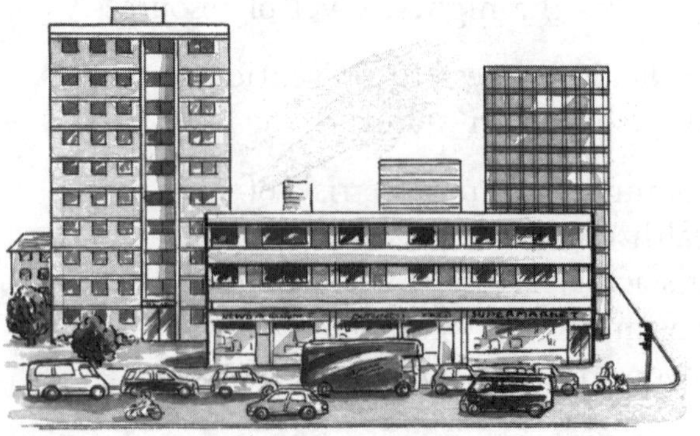

**Figure 4.49 Your home can have a great impact on your health and well-being**

spacious, and less stressful conditions than people on low incomes.

According to the Acheson report, 'Poor quality housing is associated with poor health. Dampness is associated with increased prevalence of allergic and inflammatory lung diseases, such as asthma'. Almost half of all accidents to children are associated with architectural features in and around the home. Households in disadvantaged circumstances are likely to be the worst affected by such accidents.' (Page 52.)

Older properties are often less insulated than modern properties. Many older people on low incomes worry about the cost of heating in their homes. Older poorly maintained homes are likely to cost more to heat than recently built properties. Many people in temporary accommodation or cheap rented accommodation may also live in poorly maintained housing, which may have consequences for their health.

For some people who live on a low income in high-density housing the following problems may create stress:

- noise from neighbours
- more chance of being woken up at night
- stress from neighbours' behaviour
- nearby busy roads where traffic fumes create pollution
- overcrowded rooms and facilities (waiting to get in the bathroom, etc.)
- more risk of becoming a victim of crime
- poor car parking and travel facilities.

?

The British Crime Survey (1997) which covers a two year period, found that only 3.9% of households in rural areas were burgled compared with 6.3% of households in urban areas and 10.3% of households in inner-city areas! (Source, *Social Trends 2000*.)

The Rowntree Report (1995) drew attention to the fact that some neighbourhoods were particularly stressful to live in, because of high levels of poverty, unemployment, crime and vandalism.

The Social Exclusion Unit Paper 'Opportunity for All' (1999) explains that some communities are 'trapped outside mainstream society.' The problems faced by deprived communities include:

- unemployment
- lack of educational opportunities
- high crime
- poor health
- poor services.

Growing up and living in the most deprived neighbourhoods may greatly restrict an individual's chance of developing their full intellectual, social or emotional potential. The problems of poor facilities and crime may stop employers from starting businesses. Poor facilities and crime may be linked to unemployment. Unemployment may contribute to poor facilities because people have little money to spend. Growing up in a neighbourhood with widespread unemployment, crime and poor facilities may do little to motivate children to achieve a good education. If people do not achieve a good standard of education they may find it harder to get jobs. The problems 'feed off' each other, creating housing estates and areas which are stressful to live in. The neighbourhood in which children live therefore may have a major impact on a person's life chances of growing up to lead a fulfilled life.

## How problems are concentrated in poor communities

### Unemployment

The 'Opportunity for All' paper notes that 'unemployment rates are twice as high in the 44 most deprived local authority districts compared with the rest of England.' Inner cities often have extreme concentrations of joblessness, perhaps because inner city residents do not have the education and skills needed for the jobs that are available. The report also notes that race discrimination is likely to be a factor in creating unemployment in many communities.

### Crime

The 'Opportunity for All' paper notes that 40 per cent of all crime may happen in just 10 per cent of areas in England. 'The most deprived local authority districts in England experience poor housing, vandalism and dereliction two or three times higher than the rest of England'.

### Poor services

The 'Opportunity for All' paper notes that 'Of 20 unpopular local authority estates in England surveyed in 1994, none had a supermarket or a range of shops, and no more than five had a post office, a GP/clinic, a launderette or a chemist.' Poor communities tend to have:

- a poor range of shops
- above average cost for food and essentials (one study found that food in small shops can cost 60 per cent more than in supermarkets)
- poor public transport
- poor access to information technology and even telephones
- poor access to financial services.

(Points adapted from 'Opportunity for All,')

The disadvantages found in some housing estates and communities mean that life is both more stressful and shorter than for people in wealthier areas. The 'Opportunity for All' paper quotes a study which suggests that mortality (death) rates are 30 per cent higher in the most deprived local authority districts in England as compared with the rest of the country.

### Education

Education levels in the poorest communities are lower than for the country generally. The government regards the improvement of primary and secondary school achievements as a major priority, in order to equip people with the skills needed to achieve jobs and careers.

The Acheson Report (1998) notes that schools in deprived neighbourhoods are likely to suffer more problems than schools in more affluent areas. 'Schools in disadvantaged areas are likely to be restricted in space and have the environment degraded by litter, graffiti, and acts of vandalism. This contributes to more stressful working conditions for staff and pupils. Children coming to school hungry or stressed as a result of their social and economic environment will be unable to take full advantage of learning opportunities. Stress, depression and social exclusion may reduce parents' capacity to participate in their children's education.' (Page 38–39.)

Education has a link with health in that low levels of educational achievement are associated with poor health in adult life (Acheson, 1998.) This link may be caused by the fact that poverty causes both poor educational achievement and poor health.

Social class is a major factor which influences access to higher education. In 1998–99, 31 per cent of people under the age of 21 were undertaking a higher education course at university or college. But 72 per cent of young people from the professional classes were taking a higher education course compared with only 13 per cent of children from an unskilled background. (Source: *Social Trends 2000*.) *Social Trends* notes :

> 'Young people (aged 21 and under) from the partly skilled and unskilled socio-economic groups are particularly under-represented in higher education in Great Britain. The participation rate for the unskilled group more than doubled, from 6% in 1991/92 to 13% in 1998/99. However, their participation rate is still only a fraction of that for the children of professional families. This, in part, reflects lower achievements at A-level and equivalent for these groups.'

It is likely that the combined effects of poor resources, low expectations and the need to earn money often influence young people from low income families to give education a low priority. The government is now trying to introduce new initiatives such as 'Connexions' and Educational Maintenance Allowances to encourage young people from low-income families to achieve A-levels and access to higher education. In the past there were strong environmental influences which tended to exclude people from a working class background from the higher levels of educational achievement.

**Think it over**

Why do you think young people from an unskilled background are less likely to take a higher education course? In the longer term, what effects could higher education have on young people's life prospects?

## Local and global environmental influences

Social, emotional, intellectual and even physical development are strongly influenced by socio-economic status and the local neighbourhood culture and expectations which people experience. Broader influences such as pollution and stressful living conditions also affect the health of individuals.

The Acheson Report (1998) quotes a report which estimates the damage that air pollution causes:

> 'Air pollution in urban areas, in the form of particulate matter, is responsible for bringing forward 8,100 deaths a year and bringing forward or creating an additional 10,500 hospital admissions for respiratory disease a year. In addition, in both urban and rural areas in the summer months, ozone is responsible for bringing forward 12,500 deaths and bringing forward or creating an additional 9,900 hospital admissions for respiratory disease.' (Page 58.)

The Acheson report repeats the Department of Health's view that air pollution does cause ill health and premature death.

## Causes of air pollution

Air pollution has been a problem in cities for many years. In the 1950s and early 1960s, London in particular used to suffer from smog – a thick fog mixed with soot and sulphur dioxide from coal smoke. Many homes and industries burned coal for heat or power. The Clean Air Acts and new electric and gas heating systems solved that problem, and smog disappeared. Since the 1970s the number of cars and other vehicles on the roads have been steadily increasing. There are fears that a new kind of invisible, or chemical, smog is affecting people's health.

Vehicle exhausts produce a range of pollutants including carbon monoxide, nitrogen oxides, volatile organic compounds and particulates. During periods of high pressure (or anticyclonic) weather, the air in cities may become relatively still. Sunlight reacts with exhaust gases to produce ground-level ozone. Ozone protects the planet when it is part of the ozone layer high up in the atmosphere. At ground level, however, it creates breathing problems for people with asthma or other respiratory illnesses. The World Health Organisation suggest a safe limit of 50 parts of ozone per billion parts of air. This limit is now often broken in cities during spells of warm, still, sunny weather.

Data reported in *Social Trends* make it clear that motorised traffic is now the major source of air pollution, particularly in urban areas of the United Kingdom. The good news is that levels of air pollution are falling, but levels may not be falling fast enough to meet the health needs of people in urban settings.

> 'The Department of the Environment, Transport and the Regions funds three national automated networks to monitor air pollution: one based in rural areas, one in urban areas and one monitoring levels of hydrocarbons. These give hourly measurements of five main pollutants: ozone, sulphur dioxide, nitrogen oxides, carbon monoxide and particulate matter (PM10) at various locations around the country. Between 1971 and 1997 emissions of PM10 fell by about three-fifths and sulphur dioxide fell by nearly three-quarters. The fall in sulphur dioxide emissions was primarily due to the reduction in the use of coal by power stations. The EC Large Combustion Plants Directive requires the United Kingdom to reduce emissions of sulphur dioxide by 60 per cent from large combustion plants by 2003, taking 1980 as the baseline. Emissions of carbon monoxide peaked in 1973 at 9 million tonnes and then fell by two-fifths by 1997. The decline in carbon monoxide, and also nitrogen oxide, emissions is attributed in part to the introduction of catalytic converters on petrol cars and the small increase in the use of diesel cars. In 1997 road transport accounted for three-quarters of all carbon monoxide emissions and almost half of nitrogen oxide emissions in the United Kingdom.'
>
> *Social Trends 2000* (Page 187.)

PM10 or particulate matter are very tiny soot-like particles which are too small to see. They may tend to collect in buildings, especially buildings which are close to busy roads. People living in polluted air may breathe in millions of these particles which may become stuck in their lungs. Within the lungs, particulate matter may trigger an inflammatory reaction.

Particulates may collect in buildinngs
Oxides of nitrogen
Volatile organic compounds
Carbon monoxide
Ozone develops at ground level

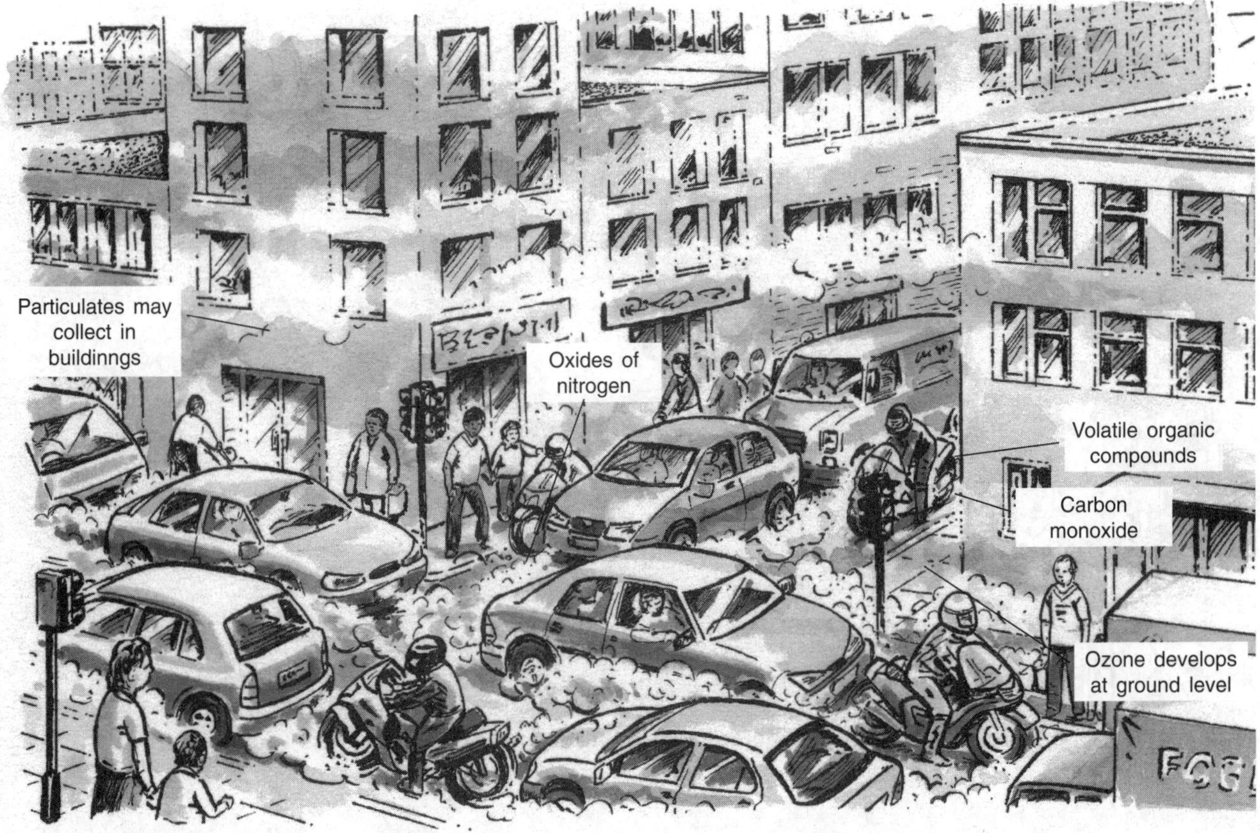

**Figure 4.51 There are many sources of pollution in urban areas and on busy roads**

The government has proposed a new form of vehicle tax for cars to help encourage people to buy cars which create less air pollution. From 2001 there will be four tax bands which rate new cars on how much carbon dioxide they produce. Diesel cars will pay slightly more than petrol cars in a given tax band, because in general they produce more particulate pollution even though they produce less carbon dioxide.

## General sources of pollution

Air pollution may be the major pollution hazard which affects the health of people in the UK as well as contributing to 'global warming'. Not all air pollution comes from traffic. Domestic fuel consumption, from such appliances as gas fires and gas central heating boilers, contribute to air pollution as do factories and power stations. Land and water pollution can also cause problems for some localities. Figure 4.52 shows some general sources of pollution.

## Noise pollution

Noise appears to be a growing problem which may create stress and ultimately ill-health for some people. Environmental health officers received six times the complaints about noise from homes in 1996–97 than were made in 1981. Noise can prevent people from sleeping or resting and may create a feeling of being 'out of control' or unable to influence a person's environment or domestic setting. The Noise Act 1996 enables local authorities to

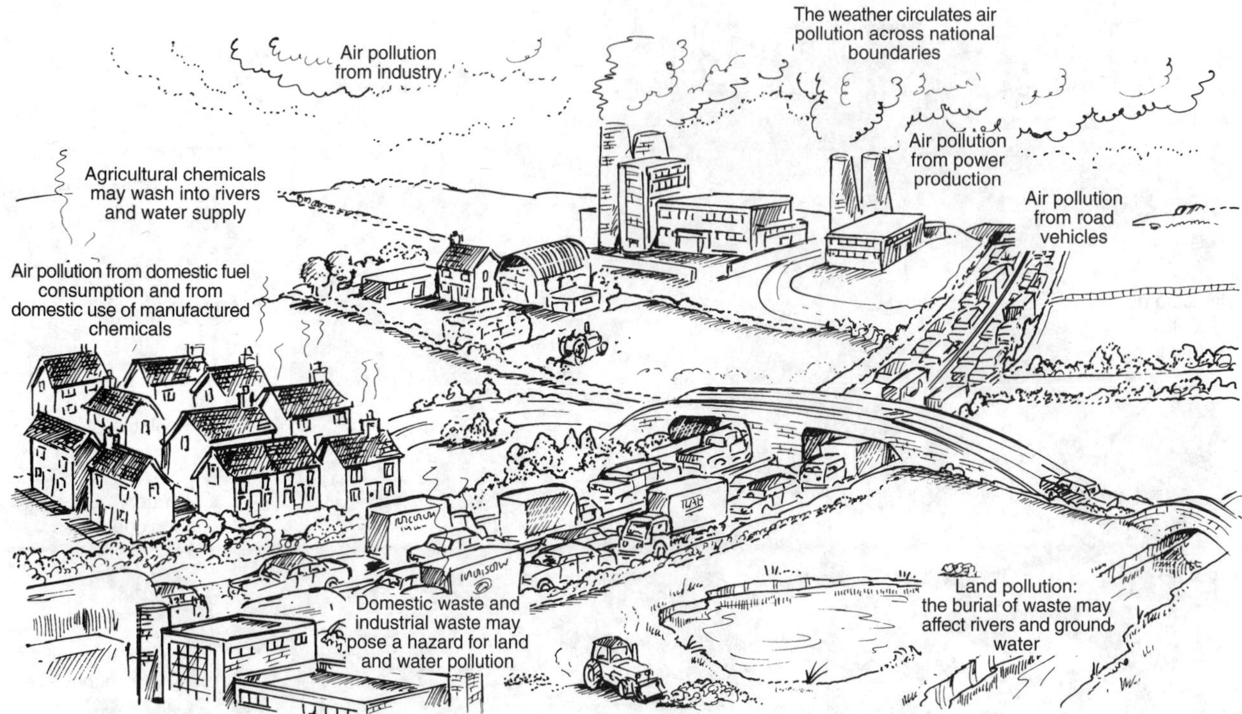


Figure 4.52 There are many different sources of pollution

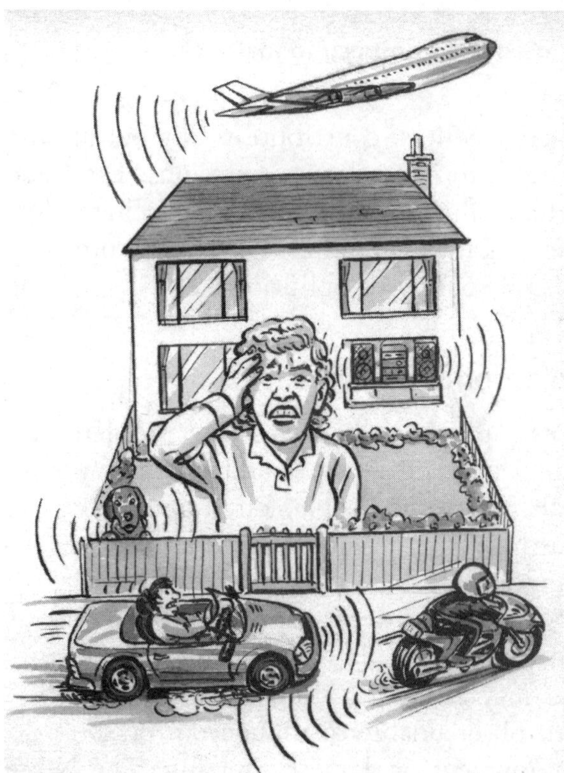

Figure 4.53 Noise is a form of pollution which can create stress

confiscate equipment where people interfere with the rights of others by making excessive noise.

## The interrelation of genetic, socio-economic and environmental factors

We have seen how genetic influences cannot be separated from environmental influences. Diet and pollution, stress levels and lifestyle influence foetal development. Throughout life people will be influenced by the social and economic contexts in which they find themselves. Wealth and income are likely to influence diet, housing, the type of neighbourhood lived in and the quality of education that a person receives. Environment will not determine what happens any more than genetics will. But different levels of influence interact to create a context that we develop in. Figure 4.54

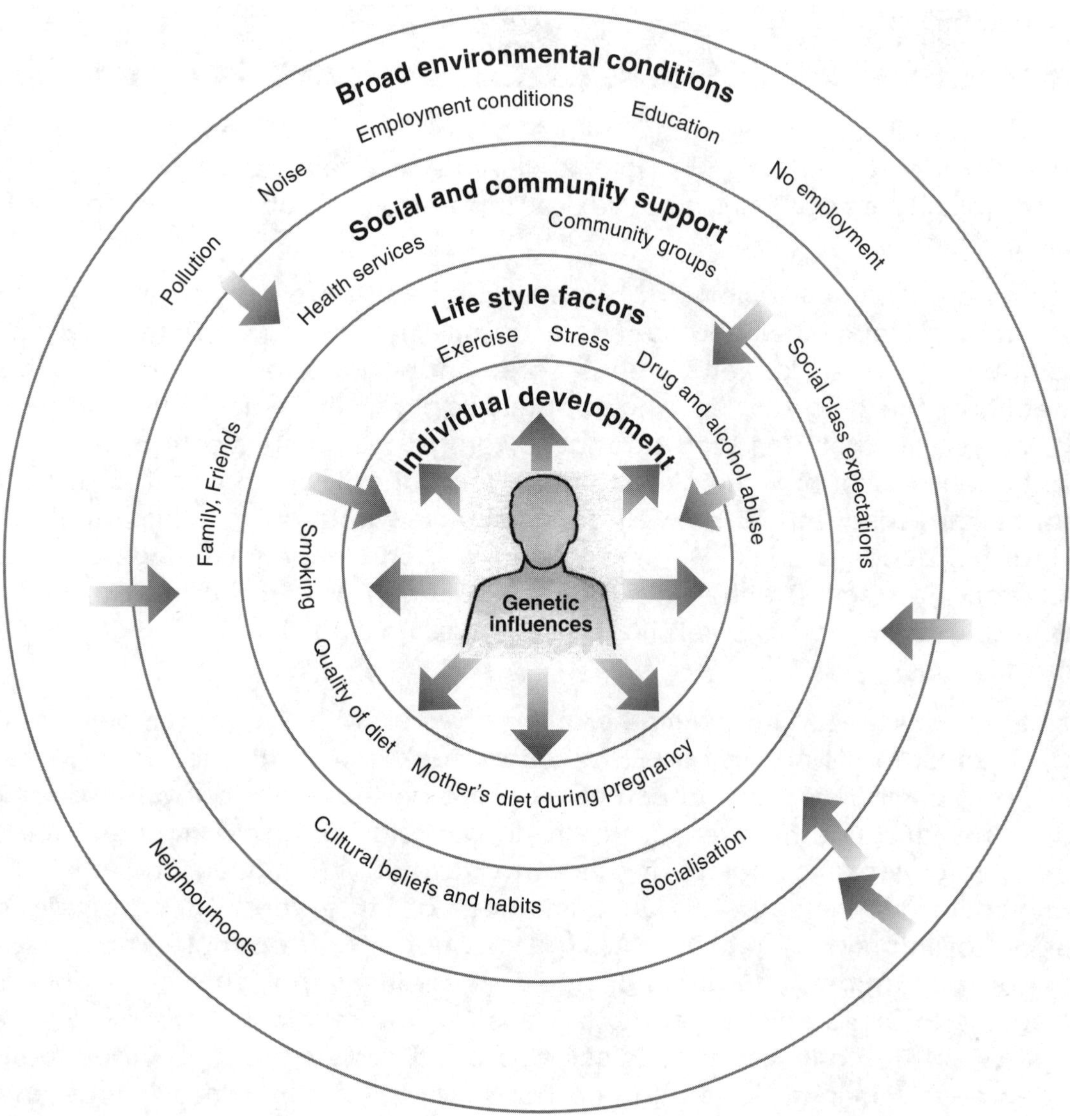


**Figure 4.54 Different levels of influence on development**

explains some of the levels of influence which will affect individual development.

Two children could start off in a similar environment and with similar genetic patterns but life events could lead to very different outcomes. The term 'life chances' is used to describe the way our environment may create more chances for some people than others, i.e. people born to professional parents are likely to have more chances of obtaining a good job and having good health throughout their lives than are children born to low income parents. But although 'chances' are not even, remember that many people from low income backgrounds do lead happy and fulfilled lives and some people from professional families may experience poor health, stress and lack of fulfilment. There is an element of chance which will come into every life. Human life is not fully determined or fixed either by genetics or by social context.

# Case study: Jack and Maxwell

Jack and Maxwell are brothers and both share a genetic tendency to become dependent on alcohol. They are born to parents who rent accommodation in a deprived housing estate. Jack and Maxwell's parents split up and Jack goes to live with his mother.

Maxwell's story: Maxwell remains at home and his father re-marries. Maxwell does not get on with his stepmother and spends a lot of time playing with the children on the estate where he lives. Maxwell's friends hate school and are impressed by the status and wealth of the drug dealers who supply people in the neighbourhood. By the age of eleven Maxwell has tried a range of drugs, including alcohol. His concentration at school is impaired through lack of motivation and the effects of substances he has tried. As Maxwell grows older he frequently drinks alcohol and finds that he 'needs a drink'. By seventeen he spends many evenings drinking and cannot manage to cope either with further education or with the idea of getting a job. By early adulthood Maxwell has few friends, no qualifications and serious health problems.

Jack's story: Jack goes with his mother and grows up with his grandmother who takes a close interest in his development. At school Jack mixes with friends who are interested in computers. Jack does not play out on the street but often goes to a friend of the family in the evening where he can play on the computer. Jack is able to join in on a weekend project at school to develop information and communication technology skills. Jack imagines a future where he can make a career out of information technology. He does not mix with people who drink alcohol or take drugs. At 16 years of age Jack believes that drinking is unhealthy and decides to avoid alcohol (partly because of the religious views of his grandparents). By early adulthood Jack has good 'A' levels and decides to study for a degree. He is in good health and has a range of supportive friends and relatives and believes he has few problems.

### Questions

1 What is the balance of genetic, environmental and 'chance' influences in these two stories?

2 If you were to imagine more complex stories, how could you weave the issues in Figure 4.54 into a story?

3 How have the issues in Figure 4.54 influenced you so far in your life?

# 4.4 Theories of human development

## Stages of development

It is easy to see life as a series of stages which people pass through. Babies look and behave very differently from young children, but adolescents are very different from children. Infancy, childhood, adolescence, adulthood and old age can be seen as different stages in life.

In past centuries Europeans often saw the human life-span as being like the four seasons of the year. Infancy and childhood were like spring, full of new beginnings and new possibilities. Adolescence and early adulthood were like summer – the most exciting and best time of the year. Adulthood was autumn, a time of harvest and fulfilment. Old age was winter – a time of decline and death! Shakespeare saw the male life cycle as having seven stages. He runs through them in a famous speech in his play *As You Like It*, Act 2: scene 7.

1 Infancy

2 The school boy

3 The lover

4 The soldier (or warrior)

5 The justice (or judge)

6 The shrunken, impaired older man

7 Last of all, 'second childishness and mere oblivion'

These theories of life stages were picked up by Charlotte Buhler (originally in 1933). According to her theory, biological stages of development create a basis for understanding our lives. There are five stages of biological development as listed below:

- 0–15 years — Progressive growth but no reproduction ability.
- 15–25 years — Progressive growth but with the onset of reproduction ability.
- 25–45 or 50 years — Stationary growth with reproduction ability.
- 45–50–65–70 years — Beginning decline with loss of reproduction ability in women.
- 65–70–death — Biological decline.

Buhler's view of life can be seen as a trajectory. A shell fired from a gun has a trajectory. If it is fired in the air it will curve upwards, along and then downwards. Life can be seen as a pattern where the biological forces of growth and decline interact to create an inevitable physical pattern of development.

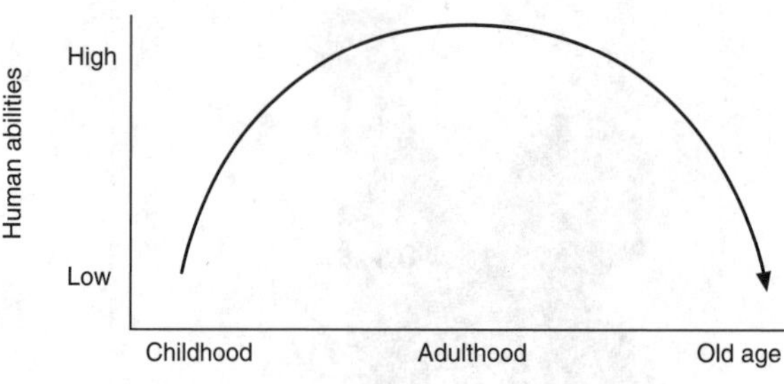


**Figure 4.55 The trajectory view of life**

Buhler believed that biology provided the framework for psychological development. The five biological stages gave rise to people's understanding of themselves. People would begin to form life goals and ambitions between 15 and 25. They would attempt to achieve these goals between 25 and 45. Between 45 and 65 people would assess their success. After 65, people would experience a sense of fulfilment, or of resignation to fate or of failure. In this perspective, life can be understood in terms of a biological clock which is ticking away, your ambitions and views change as your body changes!

Arnold Gesell also worked within the perspective of biologically determined development. Gesell introduced the notion that human development could be measured in terms of biological maturation. Maturation is the genetically programmed 'unfolding' of abilities and behaviour. Gesell's main work was carried out from the 1930s to 1950s and he is responsible for mapping out the milestones of development in physical, language, adaptive, personal and social skills. This became known as normative development or measurement. Any child who did not meet the milestone development map became labelled as 'abnormal'. Nowadays, this is thought to be inappropriate by many people, particularly those working in the field of learning disability. The measurement was a comparison between children in age bands, not linked to any external criteria. He devised his scale of normative measurement by observing and filming thousands of children over the years using building blocks, bells and wooden cups. This is why you may come across phrases such as 'can build a tower of six or more blocks at the age of 2 years'. Today, normative measurement is used to indicate general trends in development rather than to distinguish which child is 'normal' and which 'abnormal'. Gesell's work was biased towards physical or motor development.

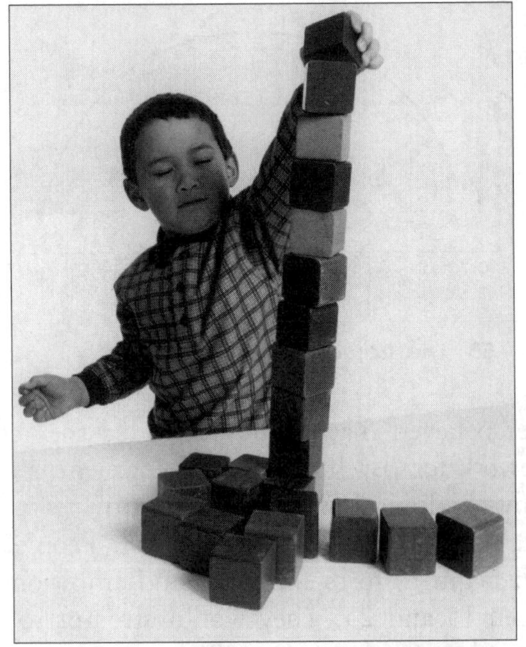

**Figure 4.56 Building a tower of blocks is part of Gesell's scale of normative measurement**

Gesell's study of language development was based almost entirely on counting the words in a child's vocabulary, as well as the phrases used and the different types of sentences. Although Gesell's work is still used today it is interpreted differently, we no longer label children solely based on normative measurements.

Buhler's and Gesell's views are rarely used without criticism, but the idea that biology determines people's lives is still quite common. Many people still ignore the interaction of social and environmental factors with genetic maturational effects or argue that they are of limited significance. (See page 284 in this unit for further details of 'biological or genetic determinism'.) People who believe in 'genetic determinism' are likely to understand life in terms of fixed patterns of growth and decline.

## Early experience: Freud and Erikson

Sigmund Freud (1856–1939) developed a stage theory of human development, but Freud emphasised the interaction of biological drives with the social environment. Freud's theory emphasises the power of early experience to influence the adult personality.

Freud's theories are usually called psychodynamic theories. 'Psycho' means mind or spirit and 'dynamic' means energy or the expression of energy. Freud believed that people were born with a dynamic 'life energy' or 'libido' which initially motivates a baby to feed and grow and later motivates sexual reproduction. Freud's theory explains that people are born with biological instincts in much the same way that animals such as dogs or cats are. Our instincts exist in the unconscious mind – we do not usually understand our unconscious. As we grow we have to learn to control our 'instincts' in order to be accepted and fit in with other people. Society is only possible if people can 'control themselves'. If everybody just did what ever they felt like, life would be short and violent and civilisation would not be possible. Because people have to learn to control their unconscious drives (or instincts) children go through stages of psychosexual development. These stages result in the development of a mature mind which contains the mechanisms that control adult personality and behaviour.

## Freud's stages of psychosexual development

- **The Oral stage:** Drive energy motivates the infant to feed, activities involving lips, sucking, biting, create pleasure for the baby.
  Weaning represents a difficult stage which may influence the future personality of the child.
- **The Anal stage:** Young children have to learn to control their muscles and in particular the control of the anal muscles. Toilet training represents the first time a child has to control their own body in order to meet the demands of society. The child's experiences during toilet training may influence later development.
- **The Phallic stage:** Freud shocked Europeans a century ago by insisting that children had sexual feelings towards their parents. Freud believed that girls were sexually attracted to their fathers and boys were sexually attracted to their mother. These attractions are called the Electra and Oedipus complexes: named after characters in ancient Greek mythology who experienced these attractions. As children develop they have to give up the opposite sex parent as a 'love object' and learn to identify with the same sex parent. Children's experience of 'letting go' of their love may have permanent effects on their later personality.
- **Latency:** After the age of 5 or 6, most children have resolved the Electra and Oedipus complexes (Freud believed that this was usually stronger and more definite in boys, i.e. girls often continue with a sexual attachment to their father!). Children are not yet biologically ready to reproduce so their sexuality is latent or waiting to express itself.
- **Genital:** With the onset of puberty adolescents become fully sexual and 'life drive' is focused on sexual activity.

### Think it over

Freud's theories are often hard to accept in a society which is 'out of touch' with nature, but have you ever watched animals such as kittens develop? Young kittens focus all their energy on getting milk from the mother cat – life energy seems almost visible. As kittens grow to young cats they will sometimes attempt to mate with parents! Freud's theories were based on the idea that people are animals – but animals that have to adapt their behaviour to the needs of society. Perhaps we adapt so far, that we forget or even deny our inner 'animal' drives?

## Freud's mental mechanisms

Freud believed that we are born with an *id*. The 'id' is part of our unconscious mind that is hidden from conscious understanding. The 'id' is like a dynamo that generates mental energy. This energy motivates human action and behaviour.

When a young child learns to control their own body during toilet training the ego develops. The 'ego' is a mental system which contains personal learning about physical and social reality. The 'ego' has the job of deciding how to channel drive energy from the unconscious into behaviour which will produce satisfactory outcomes in the real world. The 'ego' is both unconscious (unknown to self) and conscious (a person can understand some of their own actions and motivation).

The super ego develops from the ego when the child gives up their opposite-sex parent as a 'love object'. The 'super ego' contains the social and moral values of the parent that has been 'lost' as a potential partner.

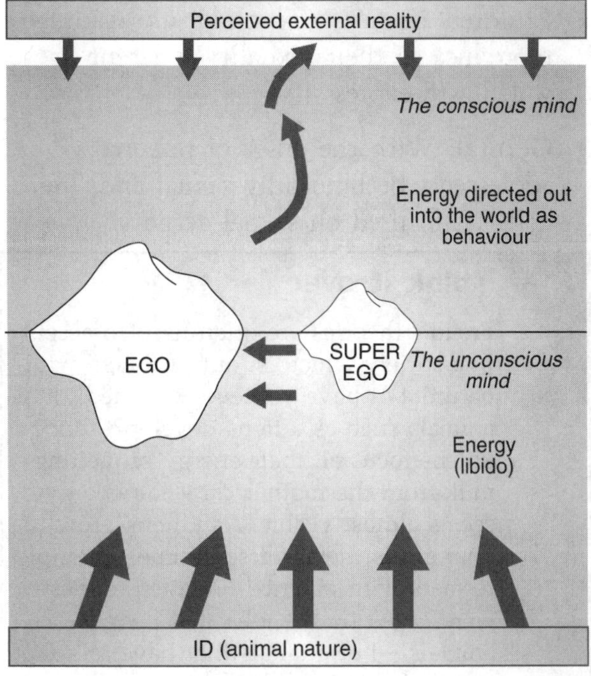


Figure 4.57 Freudian mental mechanisms

Throughout adult life a person has to find a way to release drive energy that is compatible with the demands of society and with the demands of the super ego. Sometimes people may feel sandwiched between the demands of their biology and social pressures. Typically, today's world often creates pressure to 'achieve a good career' and please parental values by 'doing well'. For some people, the desire to enjoy their sexuality and perhaps have children may conflict with the pressure to achieve. The way people cope with these pressures will be strongly influenced by childhood experiences in the Oral, Anal and Phallic stages according to Freudian theory.

## Erikson's stages of development

Erik Erikson (1902–1994) based his theory on Freud's psychodynamic ideas. Erikson's first three stages of development are similar to Freud's and are developed from Freud's theory. The major difference between Freud's and Erikson's theory is that Erikson believed that people continue to develop and change throughout life. Freud only explained how early experience might influence adult life. Erikson believed that the events of adolescence and beyond were equally important to understanding people's personality and behaviour.

Erikson originally stated that there were eight periods of developmental crisis that an individual would have to pass through in life. These crises were linked to an unfolding maturational process and would be common to people of all cultures because they were 'psychosexual' in origin rather than linked to issues of lifestyle or culture. How an individual succeeded or failed in adapting to each crisis would influence how their sense of self and personality developed. The early stages of development provide a foundation for later development. Each stage is described in terms of the positive or the negative outcomes that may happen following the developmental stage. Many people achieve an in-between outcome.

Erikson's eight life stages:

1 *Basic* trust versus *mistrust*

2 *Self-control* versus *shame and doubt*

3 *Initiative* versus *guilt*

4 *Competence* versus *inferiority*

5 *Identity* versus *role confusion*

6 *Intimacy* versus *isolation*

7 *Generativity* versus *stagnation*

8 *Ego-integrity* versus *despair*

The explanation for these stages is as follows:

- **Basic trust versus mistrust (1)**
*Birth to $1^1/_2$ years.* Infants have to learn a sense of basic trust or learn to mistrust the world. If children receive good quality care this may help them to develop personalities which include a sense of hope and safety. If not, they may develop a personality dominated by a sense of insecurity and anxiety.

- **Self-control versus shame and doubt (2)**
*$1^1/_2$ to 3 years.* Children have to develop a sense of self-control or a sense of shame and doubt may predominate. They may develop a sense of willpower and control over their own bodies. If this sense of self-control does not develop, then children may feel that they cannot control events.

- **Initiative versus guilt (3)**
*3 to 7 years.* Children have to develop a sense of initiative which will provide a sense of purpose in life. A sense of guilt may otherwise dominate the individual's personality and lead to a feeling of lack of self-worth.

- **Competence versus inferiority (4)**
*Perhaps 6 to 15 years.* The individual has to develop a sense of competence, or risk the personality being dominated by feelings of inferiority and failure.

- **Identity versus role confusion (5)**
*Perhaps 13 to 21 years.* Adolescents or young adults need to develop a sense of personal identity or risk a sense of role confusion, with a fragmented or unclear sense of self.

- **Intimacy versus isolation (6)**
*Perhaps 18 to 30 years.* Young adults have to develop a capability for intimacy, love and the ability to share and commit their feelings to others. The alternative personality outcome is isolation and an inability to make close, meaningful friendships.

- **Generativity versus stagnation (7)**
*Perhaps 30s to 60s or 70s.* Mature adults have to develop a sense of being generative, leading to concern for others and concern for the future well-being of others. The alternative is to become inward-looking and self-indulgent.

- **Ego-integrity versus despair (8)**
*Later life.* Older adults have to develop a sense of wholeness or integrity within their understanding of themselves. This might lead to a sense of meaning to life or even to what could be called 'wisdom'. The alternative is a lack of meaning in life and a sense of despair.

Both Freud's and Erikson's views of human development are based on the notion that human biology creates a 'life trajectory' where stages of crises are inevitable. Both Freud and Erikson accept that individual social experiences will interact with biology to create an individual personality. The psychodynamic view of development emphasises the importance of individual experience and the interaction of biological stages and the environment. The relationship between children and parents is seen as a key influence on the development of personality. Personal development is understood in terms of definable stages.

The idea that human development fits eight stages (or five stages) of coping with crises or change does not make intuitive sense to everyone. While there may be some important ideas about emotional development in psychodynamic theory, some authors claim that the theories are both too rigid to provide a full understanding of development. Many people fail to identify with the idea of developmental crises. Many people seem to experience change as a smooth sequence of gradual adjustment. Psychodynamic theory provides an interesting way of interpreting past life experience – but it is possible to question whether people in the future will experience the biological pressures that Erikson originally identified in the middle of the last century. Castells (1997) argues that science now gives people not only the power to live longer, but also the power to delay reproduction and the effects of ageing. Sexuality can be decoupled from reproduction so that sexual behaviour becomes a form of recreational pastime rather than linked to a biological time clock for reproduction! As technology gives people the power to intervene in their own biological nature, notions of biologically controlled stages of development may become increasingly dated, at least with respect to adult life.

### Think it over

Thinking back over your own life, did you experience times of crisis linked to issues like competence or inferiority in your own school life?

Do you think that your life will involve change through periods of crisis or more gradual and gentle change?

## Cognitive stage theories: Piaget

While Freud and Erikson seek to explain emotional development, Piaget (1896–1980) developed a stage theory of cognitive or intellectual development. Piaget's stages are:

- the Sensorimeter Stage – birth to $1^1/_2$ or 2 years
- the Preoperational Stage – $1^1/_2$ or 2 years to 6 or 7 years
- the Concrete Operational Stage – 6 or 7 to 11 or 12 years
- the Formal Operational Stage – 11 or 12 onwards.

Piaget believed that children progressed through a series of qualitatively different stages. During these stages children think in different ways. To begin with infants can only think in terms of memories of sensory experiences and motor or muscle movements. Language in the preoperational stage enables a child to represent or interpret the world using concepts. Before six or seven years of age these concepts are not used in a logical way. During the concrete operations period children can think using mental operations, such as being able to understand the 'logic' in the way numbers work or the way weight and volume work. Finally, adolescents develop the ability to use deductive logical reasoning to solve problems.

Despite some argument about the nature of Piaget's stages most theorists accept that children do develop their thinking ability as they grow older. Adults may go beyond 'formal operations' and develop a deeper, more intuitive ability to make skilled judgements in their field of work.

Piaget's theory relies on the idea of an unfolding maturational process that gives children and adolescents new mental powers at different stages. Maturation is influenced by an unfolding genetic pattern – but the way this pattern works is also influenced by the environment. Children have to have an interesting and stimulating setting to encourage them to develop and use their powers. Piaget never believed that children might develop independently of their experience! Biology interacts with teaching and learning to create new skills and abilities.

Some key assumptions in Piaget's theory are that:

- Infants, children and adults actively seek to understand the world that they live in. People build mental representations or theories of the world in their minds because it is human nature to do so.
- Children learn through experience. Teachers can only help with or facilitate learning by helping to create useful experiences. Teachers and parents do not directly implant learning into children minds.
- As children grow older they develop increasingly complex ways of interpreting the world.
- Developing theories about the world involves processes called *assimilation* (taking things in), *accommodation* (changing ideas and theories when new information is discovered), and *equilibration* (creating a balance between theory and experience in order to make sense of the world).

A simple explanation of Piaget's theory of learning might be based on a young child's experience of animals. Perhaps a child goes to a park and sees ducks for the first time. The child has already seen pictures of animals in books and has seen other animals in real life. The child will take or assimilate the idea of 'ducks' as a new category of animal. As the child experiences more examples of ducks, the child will need to adapt their idea of what ducks can look like – this is called 'accommodation'. The child will now have a balanced theory of what ducks are and will be able to identify them effectively.

As the child grows older the child will lose their equilibration on this idea when they have to make sense of the idea that ducks are birds and not animals! Life involves constant development and changing of ideas.

In Piaget's theory, learning is a process which is constantly working to enable people to cope with or 'adapt' to their environment. Teachers should never try 'to put ideas into children'. Teachers are most successful when they create useful experiences which stimulate children to make sense, or make new sense, of their experience. Learning and knowledge are controlled by the individual who needs the learning. Piaget's theory sees learning as a very independent and individual activity.

Children cannot learn skills before they are maturationally ready. Trying to teach abstract theories (such as psychodynamics) to five year olds would never work, no matter what teaching skills a person had.

First experience of ducks
Ducks are brown ducks are animals too!
Mental act of assimilating experience into knowledge of animals
Experience of looking
Second experience of ducks
That duck is white
Mental act of accommodating (changing ideas about ducks)
Equilibration
Ducks look like and can be many different colours – I can identify ducks when I see them

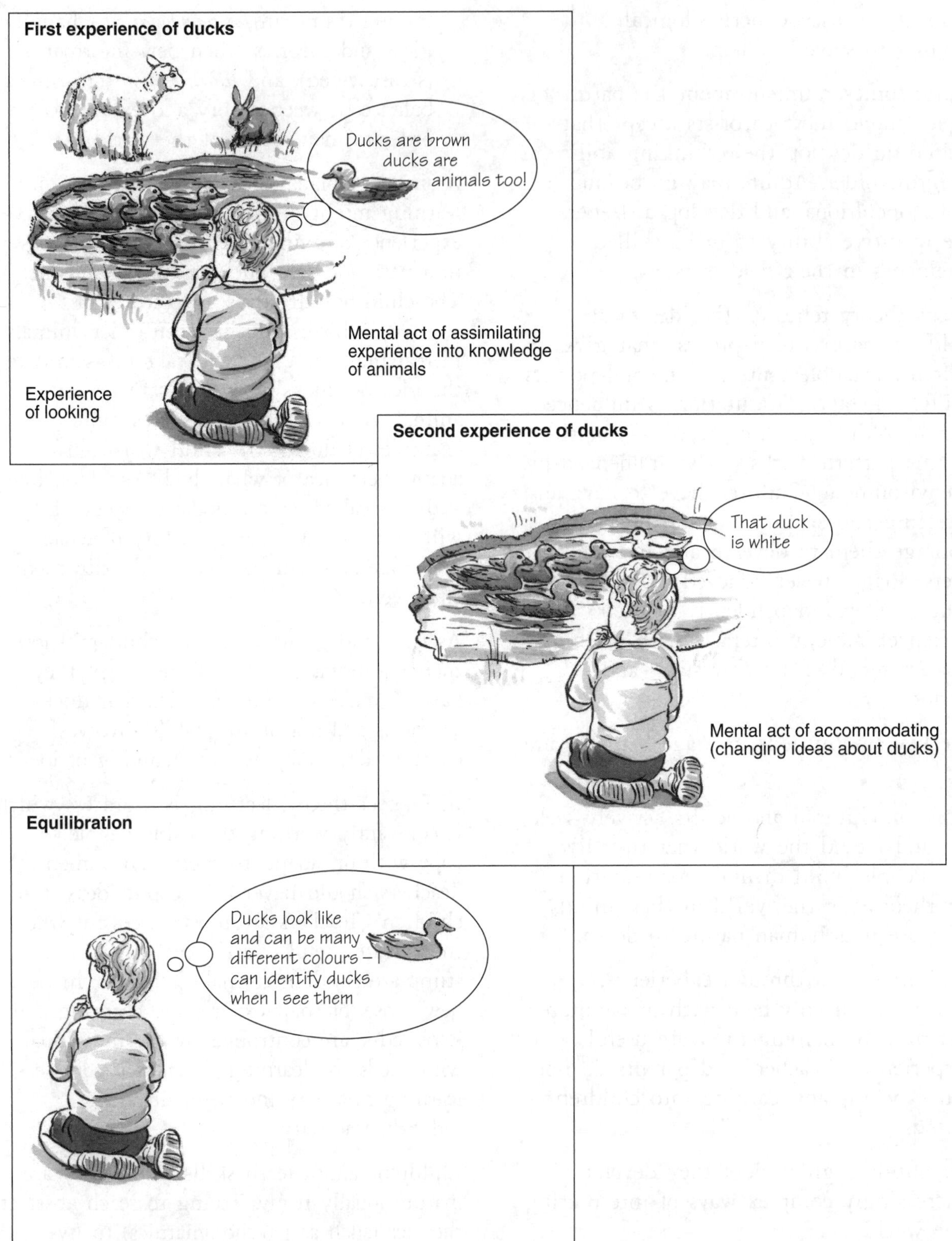

**Figure 4.58** Developing ideas about the world involves assimilation, accommodation and equilibration

### The limitations of Piaget's theory

Researchers have found problems with Piaget's idea of stages. It does seem that young children are more able than Piaget thought, and that adolescents and adults may be less able – or at least may make less use of formal logic than his theory implied. Recent research also suggests that Piaget's stages may not work in the simple and straightforward way a process of maturation might imply. Children can 'conserve' and behave logically if problems are described in language which they can easily follow. It may be that stages provide a neat and easy way to think about development but the real picture is much more complicated.

## Theories of development which do not use stages

Some theorists believe that learning is the main force which controls human development. People are seen as being immensely adaptable: they will adapt to the environment and life experiences they encounter.

The Russian physiologist, Ivan Pavlov (1849–1936) and the American psychologist, Burrhus F. Skinner (1904–1990), both worked in the first half of the last century to develop theories of learning. Both Pavlov and Skinner believed that the environment controlled behaviour. They thought that the way people developed skills and abilities was entirely due to the influence of the environment. There were no general stages of development because people are simply conditioned to learn and develop.

### Conditioning

In 1906, Pavlov published his work on conditioned learning in dogs. Pavlov had intended to study digestion in dogs, but his work ran into difficulties because his animals anticipated that their food was due to arrive. Pavlov became interested in how the dogs learned to anticipate food. Pavlov was able to demonstrate that the dogs would salivate (or dribble) when ever they heard a noise, such as a bell being rang, if the noise always happened just before the food arrived. The dogs had learned to 'connect' or associate the sound of the bell with the presentation of food. It was as if the bell replaced the food: the dogs' mouths began to water to the sound of the bell. The dogs associated sounds with food. This learning by association was called conditioning.

'Conditioned learning' is not really such a big discovery. Oscar Wilde (a famous author of the time) is reported to have said, 'Doesn't every intelligent dog owner know that.' In the first half of the last century many people believed that learning by association (conditioning) represented the discovery of the basic mechanism whereby learning took place. It was easy to assume that all learning and perhaps all intellectual and emotional development were due to learning by association.

### Skinner's theories of conditioning

Skinner argued that learning is caused by the consequences of our actions. This means that people learn to associate actions with the pleasure or discomfort that follows from action. For example, if a child puts some yoghurt in his or her mouth and it tastes nice, the child will associate the yoghurt with pleasure. In future the child will repeat the

# Case study: Reinforcement at work

Amita is an infant who is eating while sitting in a highchair. Amita accidentally drops the spoon with which she is eating. Amita reacts with surprise that the spoon has gone. Her mother picks the spoon up and gives it back to Amita, smiling and making eye contact as she does so. This makes Amita feel good. Amita's mother goes back to her own dinner and stops looking at Amita. By accident Amita drops the spoon again. Once again her mother gives Amita attention and the spoon is returned. Once again Amita feels good. Half a minute later Amita drops the spoon on purpose – dropping the spoon has become reinforced. The consequences or outcomes of dropping the spoon feel nice because it is followed by attention.

action of eating yoghurt. On the other hand, if the yoghurt does not taste good he or she may avoid it in future. We learn from our experiences in the world.

Behaviour that operates on the environment to create pleasant outcomes is likely to strengthen or reinforce the occurrence of that behaviour. Behaviour operates on the world and so Skinner used the word 'operants' to describe behaviours which create learned outcomes. The term *operant conditioning* is used to describe learning through the consequences of action.

The terminology of conditioned learning:

- **Classical conditioning** (Pavlovian conditioning): learning to make association between different events.
- **Operant conditioning** (Skinnerian conditioning): learning to repeat actions which have a reinforcing or strengthening outcome. In other words, people learn to repeat actions which have previously felt good or are associated with 'feeling better'.

## Reinforcement

Skinner believed that learning could be explained using the idea of reinforcement. Reinforcement means 'to make stronger'. For example, reinforced concrete is stronger than ordinary concrete; when a military base is reinforced, it becomes stronger. A reinforcer is anything that makes a behaviour stronger.

### Think it over

Look at the case study above. Without understanding reinforcement Amita's parents might say that the child is being naughty, or that she is playing a game. Stressed parents could even take the food away – to stop her being naughty! Skinner would have argued that 'naughtiness' was an adult misunderstanding. What is happening is that Amita's behaviour of dropping the spoon is being 'reinforced' by her mother. Her mother is teaching her to drop the spoon although she does not realise what she is doing. Reinforcement is happening because Amita is getting a 'nice feeling' each time she drops the spoon and her mother gives it back.

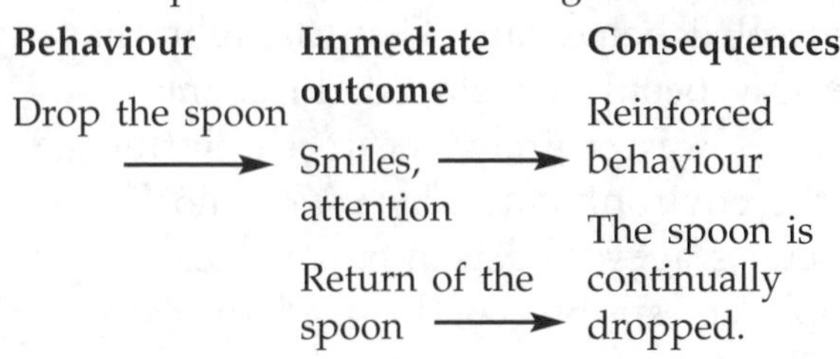


Figure 4.59 How reinforcement works

## Case study: Sarina and Jodie

***Sarina***

Sarina walks to school each morning with friends. Her friends enjoy talking to her and are always pleased to see her. At school Sarina is quite good at completing her work; teachers often praise her and write positive comments on her work. Sometimes other people will say things like, 'Ask Sarina to help, she's very clever'. Sarina looks forward to school and likes to work hard in class.

***Jodie***

Jodie travels to school alone. At school she is picked on by some older girls who try to steal her pocket money. Jodie is a little slower than the other girls in her class and is sometimes 'told-off' for not putting things away in time or not completing her work. Because Jodie gets bullied she is not 'popular' and does not get a lot of social attention from the other children.

***Question***

How will conditioning theory predict the future for these two children?

### How conditioned learning influences behaviour and development

Some habits may be directly learned by classical conditioning, while many of our interests and achievements in life may have been influenced by operant conditioning or reinforcement. Pleasant and unpleasant experiences may affect our social, emotional and intellectual development.

Look at the case study above and compare the two stories.

The case study above shows that Sarina gets a lot of positive reinforcement for mixing with others and for working with teachers and for doing school work. Mixing with others feels enjoyable and doing work feels enjoyable; therefore these behaviours are reinforced and will get stronger. Sarina is likely to try harder and work longer than some others because of reinforcement.

Jodie does not get much reinforcement from mixing with others or trying to do her work. Because Jodie is bullied she finds school 'punishing'. Punishment is the opposite of reinforcement and it will block Jodie's social behaviour and development. Teachers do not reinforce Jodie's attempts to study and so she is likely to withdraw from academic work. Punishment can stop behaviours in the same way that reinforcement can increase behaviour. Jodie may experience a process such as that described by 'learned helplessness' in Chapter 2.

Jodie's social, intellectual and emotional development may be blocked by her learning experiences whereas Sarina's development is reinforced. Sarina may go on to become very happy and successful in adult life because of the learning experiences she receives. Jodie may find it hard to get on with others and may be less successful. Theories of conditioned learning may offer an explanation of Jodie's lack of success.

It is very important to remember that life experiences cause conditioning. Most conditioning happens without anyone planning or intending it. Reinforcement and punishment frequently take place in educational and social care settings. They happen whether or not anyone intended reinforcement or punishment to happen.

The concepts of conditioning and reinforcement offer some useful tools for understanding the ways in which life experience can influence human development. However, they may not explain the whole complexity of human experience.

### 'Imitation learning' (Bandura)

Albert Bandura (born 1925) argues that conditioning only partly explains what is happening when people learn. He argues that people also learn from what they see and hear and that people often imitate or copy others without external reinforcement or conditioned association taking place.

Bandura was able to demonstrate that children will copy the behaviour that they see in adults in a famous experiment carried out in 1963. Children who saw adults behaving aggressively towards a 'bobo doll' were much more likely to get aggressive toward the doll when they had a chance to play with it than were children who saw more usual behaviour. This experiment confirmed that we are not just influenced by reinforcement, we are also influenced by what we see in the media and what happens to other people. Bandura argues that people will model themselves on other people who appear to be being rewarded or 'reinforced'. People copy or model themselves on people they associate as being like themselves, but who seem successful.

**Think it over**

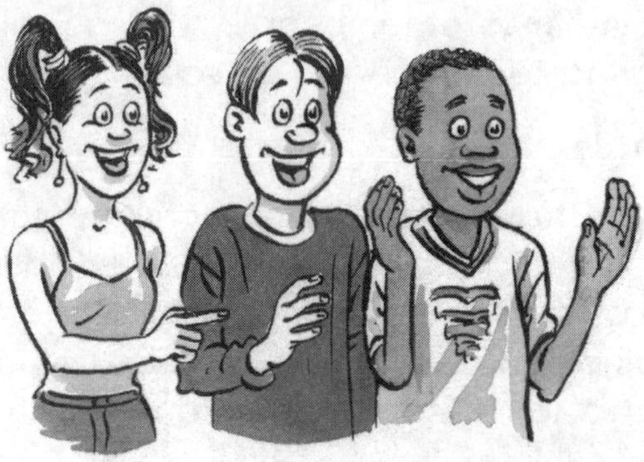

If people imitate what they see others rewarded for, how might the following life experiences influence a person?

- Seeing an elder brother or sister praised for school achievement.
- Seeing a friend being praised and looked up to because of violent behaviour.
- Seeing a neighbour do well from gambling with shares on the internet.
- Seeing a person gain respect and being 'looked-up to' because they deal in drugs.
- Seeing a person being praised and thanked for caring for a relative.

Learning undoubtedly influences human development, and conditioning and imitation learning almost certainly go a long way to explain how neighbourhoods and local environments influence people at an individual level. Theorists like Skinner believed that learning theory could explain the whole of a person's development. Skinner even went so far as to argue that language was learned entirely through reinforcement. Personality and ability were also explained in terms of environmental influences. Nowadays few people would accept such an extreme view. Individual biological differences and maturational processes almost certainly interact with learning to cause people to develop as they do. Learning theories are useful in helping to explain individual differences in development, but they may not be sufficient on their own to explain human development.

### Humanistic theories

Psychodynamic and learning theories represent two major 'schools of thought in psychology'.

Another perspective which deserves mentioning is the humanistic view of human nature. Abraham Maslow's theory is briefly mentioned here because it is central to understanding human need, particularly in a caring context. Maslow's hierarchy of need is another non-stage interpretation of influences on development. Abraham Maslow (1908–70) believed that humans have an inbuilt framework of needs. We have a range of deficit needs which have to be met before we can truly develop to meet our full potential. This means that we have:

- Physiological needs – for food, warmth, shelter, sex, etc.
- Safety needs – to feel physically and emotionally free from threat
- A need to belong – a need for social inclusion and attachment to others
- Self-esteem needs – a need for respect and to develop a secure sense of self/self-concept.

If any of these needs are not met then an individual will invest time and energy in trying to meet these needs rather than in progressing to the higher levels of development.

In an ideal world everyone would have their physical, safety and belonging needs met from birth. Everyone would grow up in a safe, secure, loving network of carers. The task of childhood and adolescence would be to develop a secure sense of self-esteem. Once self-esteem is established, adulthood could focus on the full development of a person's potential. Full development would include in-depth intellectual and artistic skills. In a perfect world each person would be 'free' to self-actualise. Self-actualisation means 'becoming everything one is capable of becoming'. People who achieve self-actualisation might have special qualities including:

- a more accurate perception of reality
- greater acceptance of self and others
- greater self-knowledge
- greater involvement with major projects in life
- greater independence
- creativity
- spiritual and artistic abilities.

People who self-actualise achieve a high degree of satisfaction from life.

Maslow believed that only a few people have the chance to achieve self-actualisation in North American or European culture. The majority of people spend most of their life struggling with deficit needs, feeling stressed and worrying about issues such as money or about self-esteem.

The Paradox of Prosperity (1999), a paper prepared for the Salvation Army by the Henley Centre, argues that although material prosperity is increasing in western

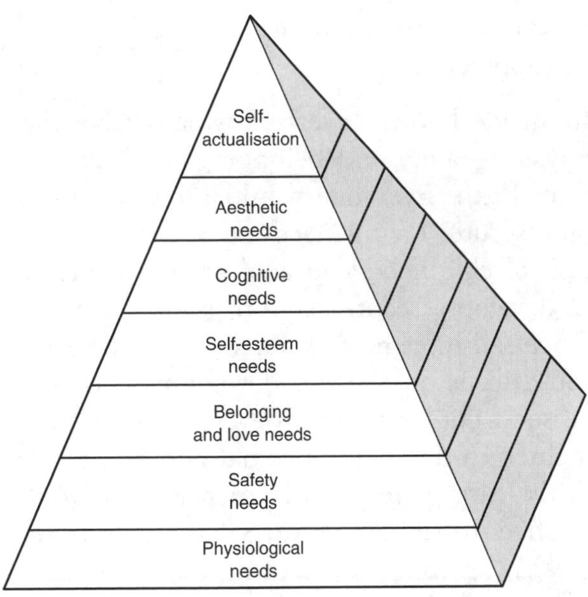


**Figure 4.60 Maslow's hierarchy of needs (based on Maslow, 1954)**

society, the chances of a fulfilling life are decreasing. By 2010 more people will experience life stress, fewer people will find satisfying relationships, few people will feel secure and 'safe' and fewer people will be able to meet the conditions for self-actualisation.

Maslow's theory offers a simple overview of balanced developmental needs and appropriate goals for living. His views may be useful in informing our understanding of quality of life.

## The importance of social context – Vygotsky

All the theories of development and learning reviewed in this section so far focus on the individual child and adult, seeking to explain development in terms of maturation, the impact of the environment, internal mental theories or some combination of these influences. Lev Vygotsky (1896–1934) proposed a theory which emphasises the importance of a child's social context in influencing development. Vygotsky believed that thinking, memory and perception were strongly influenced by the culture in which a child lives. A child's understanding of the world develops from the child's interaction with other people as well as with 'the environment'.

### Constructivism

Constructivism is a perspective which explains human development and human behaviour in terms of the way an individual builds an interpretation of the world. Put very simply, the way a person learns to think about and conceptualise an experience will influence how they behave and react.

> **Think it over**
>
> Imagine you were attacked by a person with a large stick while you were walking and that you were hurt and bruised as a result.
>
> Now imagine you were accidentally hit by an opponent while playing hockey and that you were hurt and bruised as a result.
>
> In both these experiences the pain and injury might be identical, but your feelings and reactions would probably be very different. The way a person makes sense of their experience makes a huge difference to what they feel and think. Constructivism emphasises that it is not what happens in a person's life that matters as much as the way people come to interpret and build their understanding of events.

Piaget is sometimes regarded as a constructivist because his theories emphasise the way children build their own mental interpretations of the world. Vygotsky also studied the way children built an understanding of life. Vygotsky's theories are different from Piaget in that Vygotsky believed that internal thinking and understanding were developed through social activities such as play and conversation. The way parents and teachers interact with a child would strongly influence the nature and speed of a child's development. Piaget believed in an underlying process of maturation which would result in stages of thinking skills development. Vygotsky believed that action and interaction with others would determine development – not some underlying biological process. Vygotsky's theories can be referred to as being 'social constructivist' because of his emphasis on social interaction as being the major influence on the way a child builds their understanding of the world.

Vygotsky's view of development leads to some important conclusions about development:

- the culture and socialisation a child experiences will greatly influence the nature and level of skills that he or she will eventually develop
- the quality of parental communication and teaching that a child experiences will greatly influence the skills that they develop
- the quality of conversation, play and instruction a child receives will influence how their language and intellectual skills develop.

Vygotsky offers two important concepts to help explain how children learn, these are '**Internalisation**' and the '**Zone of Proximal Development**'.

## Internalisation

Vygotsky believed that successful cognitive development depended on a child being able to build an internal 'understanding' of activities and skills. Internalisation might follow a process such as in the example below:

> A mother tries to encourage her son to complete a jigsaw puzzle. The mother explains how jigsaw puzzles work and demonstrates how to search for correct pieces and put them together. At this stage the child is socially involved with play and communication but the child does not understand how to do a jigsaw puzzle. The child will then attempt to find pieces of the puzzle, the mother will help him and repeat ideas to encourage him. The child may begin to talk out loud to help him make sense of his actions. The child is beginning to learn but has not yet internalised the skill of solving jigsaw puzzles. Finally, after lots of help, guidance and encouragement the child can work on the puzzle independently. He will be excited and will say how good he is at puzzles! At this stage the child has learned how to solve the puzzle – the child has internalised the external guidance and concepts his mother provided.

If you were teaching a child to read you might ask him or her to read out loud. Reading out loud helps a child to practise skills, but 'Vygotskyans' might question whether the child was internalising anything. In other words is the child really learning when he or she reads out loud? 'Vygotskyans' might ask the child to explain the story they had read. By asking the child to explain, the teacher or parent is creating a social learning situation which requires the child to internalise ideas and concepts which might otherwise only be repeated without understanding. Teachers who follow Vygotsky's views are likely to try to encourage a high level of cognitive performance from children – they will want children to internalise and understand rather than simply 'do' things.

**Think it over**

Compare the ideas on internalisation of a jigsaw puzzle with the ideas on Piaget's theory of accommodation, assimilation and equilibration. Consider how Piaget's theory assumes children develop their own theories and might even develop on their own, whereas Vygotsky argues that teaching and communication with others is vital for the development of skills and knowledge.

### The Zone of Proximal Development

Vygotsky not only believed that skilled teaching and parenting were important in influencing development, he also introduced a theory to guide cognitive development. Very simply this theory is that teachers and parents should try to understand the level of thinking a child was working from and then try to move the child on to a deeper level, but always staying within what was possible for a child to understand. The zone of proximal development is the range that a child's thinking and understanding might realistically be developed in a given subject area.

An example of the zone of proximal development might relate to a child's understanding of the concept of fairness. A father might be talking to his seven-year-old daughter. The daughter might say that fairness is when 'everyone gets the same' e.g. when she and her younger sister each get the same size slice of apple pie to eat. The father may have a much more complex understanding of equal opportunities based on ethical reasoning. The father will not be able to explain ethical philosophy to a seven year old, because such theories cannot be assimilated or linked with the child's current understanding (this means that they lie outside the child's zone of proximal development). The father could try to move his daughter's thinking on by mentioning that the younger sister does not like apples – so just giving everyone the same food isn't really fair. Fairness is not having exactly the same treatment – it's having an 'equal feeling at the end'; so the younger sister has to have something different for things to work out fairly. In this example the father is trying to encourage the daughter to develop a deeper understanding of equality and fairness working within issues that the daughter can understand. This is working within the zone of proximal development.

Vygotsky's theories provide a useful additional perspective to understanding development which focuses on the nature and quality of language and concept development. The way parents and teachers guide children may be very significant in influencing cognitive development. Other learning theories fail to explore the importance of communication and concept development in the way that Vygotsky's theories do.

## An overview of the theories

A diagrammatic overview is set out in Figure 4.61.

Freud/Erikson: early experiences influence adult life

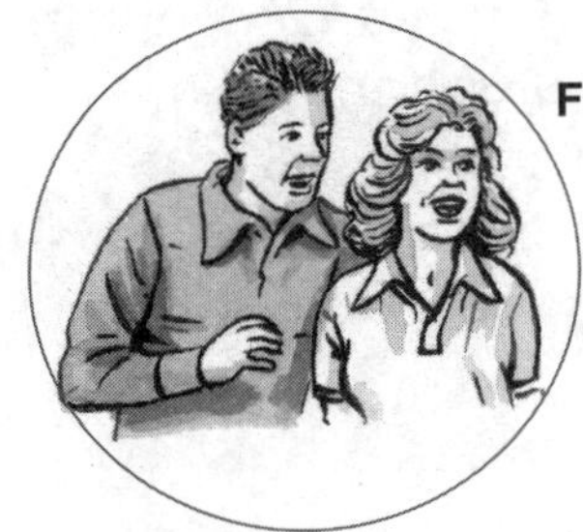

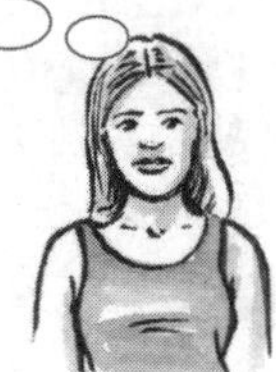

Mental mechanisms are influenced and created by developmental crises

Piaget: children progress through stages of cognitive development

Child matures in stages
Adults may facilitate or help but children build their own systems of thinking

I can work it out

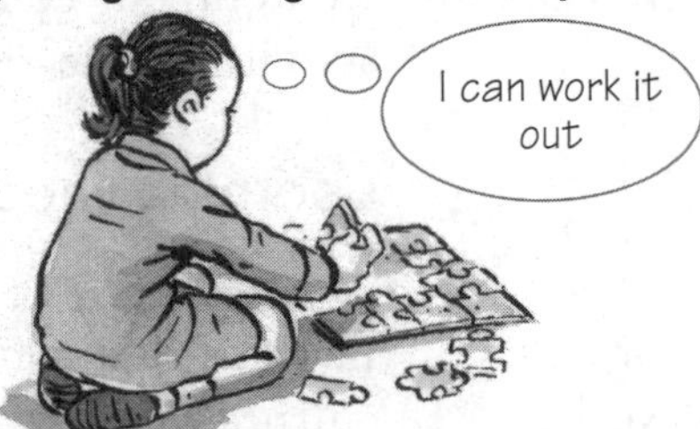

Skinner and Bandura: children are conditioned to learn from their experiences

Reinforcement or punishment moulds our behaviour

Learning by imitation:Bandura

I like this. I'll keep doing it
That's good!
I can copy that

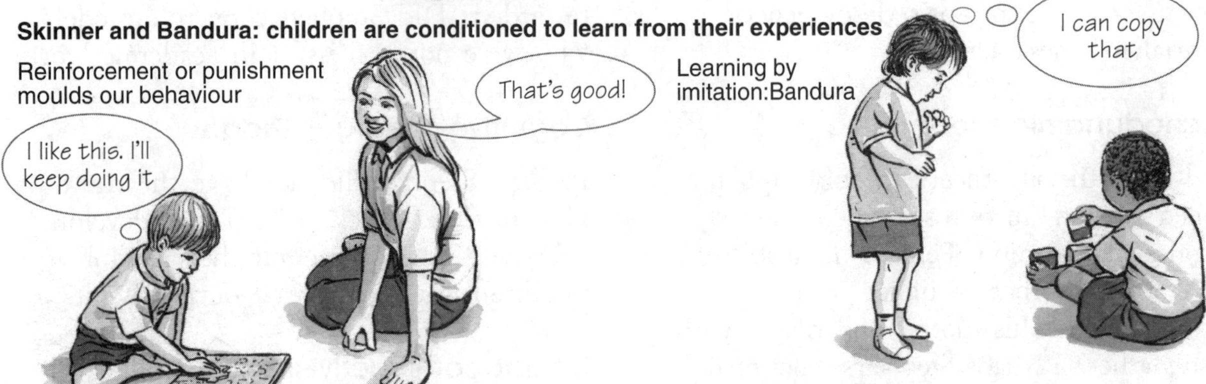

Vygotsky: social context is all important (social constructivism)

I'll help them internalise their understanding

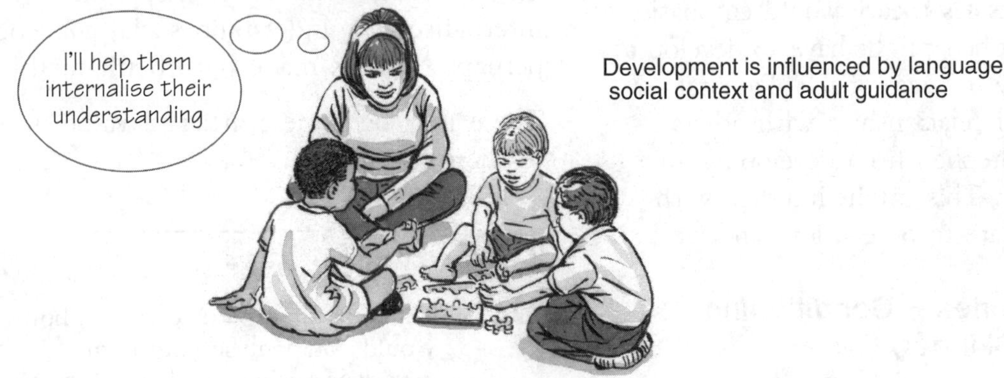

Development is influenced by language, social context and adult guidance

**Figure 4.61** Overview of theorists

# Case study: Stephen

**Stephen is now 20 years old. Stephen appeared to enjoy a healthy and happy childhood but he never did very well at junior school. When Stephen was 12 years old his mother and father got divorced and his mother remarried. Stephen did not get on well with his new stepfather. Stephen stayed at school until he was 18 but never did very well in his exams. He went to work for a DIY store as his first job but found that he couldn't get on with the other staff. Stephen left his job because of arguments with his employers.**

The different theories of development explain issues in Stephen's life in different ways.

### Genetic determinism

Theories which emphasise genetic maturation would probably explain poor academic performance and poor social skills in terms of a lack of aptitude or genetic potential for these activities.

### Psychodynamic theory

Freud and Erikson's theories would explain Stephen's action in terms of unconscious struggles in the mind. Perhaps his inability to get on with others is linked to his relationship with his mother and rivalry with his stepfather? Perhaps Stephen's emotional development and achievement at school has been disturbed because of tensions between his parents. Erikson's theory would emphasise the struggle Stephen might have to develop a working identity or sense of self. Parental conflict and poor relationships with others might prevent Stephen from developing an effective identity. This might interfere with his ability to relate to others, love and work?

### Learning theories – Conditioning (Pavlov and Skinner)

Perhaps Stephen did not get sufficient reinforcement to motivate him to be successful in school work? Did Stephen's environment condition him to avoid certain activities or learn to give up some tasks?

### Learning theories – Imitation (Bandura)

Perhaps Stephen did not grow up in a culture where success in academic work was rewarded? Did Stephen copy role models who were not successful in academic work?

### Cognitive theory – Piaget

Perhaps Stephen did not have the right kind of experiences to help him develop effective 'internal' mental theories during his intellectual and social development?

### Social constructivism – Vygotsky

Perhaps Stephen's parents and teachers were not sufficiently skilled to help him internalise and understand social concepts – perhaps this has made it difficult for him?

There may be some truth and value in all of these theories.

### Think it over

Thinking about your own life, how would you analyse your own experience using the theories in this section? Can you find some value or relevance in each theory?

# Unit 4 Assessment

Unit 4 will be assessed through an external test. To prepare for this you need to be able to explain how a wide range of factors influence human development. You might consider the factors which influence adolescence and life-long adult development. You might prepare some case studies of individuals which map out:

- the way individuals have developed and changed
- the physical development patterns that individuals may experience
- the cognitive, social and emotional changes that individuals may experience
- the interaction of genetic, social, economic and wider environmental influences on human development
- the theories and perspectives which try to explain human development.

## For an E grade

To pass the unit and achieve an E grade you will need to be able to:

1 describe patterns of physical growth and development

2 describe the development of gross and fine motor skills, intellectual ability, emotional development (including self-concept and self-confidence), language and social development such as the development of communication and relationship skills, play, and moral judgement.

3 describe how genetic, socio-economic and other environmental factors may influence development

4 describe some of the main theories of development.

## For a C grade

To achieve a C grade you will need a deeper understanding of how the issues above might interrelate. You need to be able to use theory in order to contrast the development of different individuals. Use Figure 4.54 and the stories of Jack and Maxwell, page 308, to help you think about comparing the development of the individuals.

You will also need to be able to explain how socio-economic issues will influence the development of 'skills' such as language, self-efficacy, moral judgement and so on.

You will need to understand a range of theories presented in this unit well enough to analyse how development may be affected by the context that a person grows up in and the life events that they experience.

You should discuss case studies and life histories and use different areas of theory to analyse and explain what might be happening. One of the best ways of revising for a test is to spend time thinking and discussing how ideas and theories might work. Trying to memorise some facts may help toward an E grade but you will need to practise applying theory to real life if you are aiming for a higher grade.

## For an A grade

At A grade you not only need to be able to explain life histories using the theory in this unit, but you will also need to provide detailed evaluation of how various factors may interact to influence development. When you read a case study it is always possible to think of different interpretations of the person's context and events (see the case study of Stephen, page 326). The skill required at A grade is not finding the 'right answer' but the skill of justifying a chosen answer which could realistically 'fit the facts'.

At A grade you should provide an evaluation of case study material which discusses the relative importance of different factors in influencing development. You should try to 'justify' or explain why your ideas are good.

Once again the best way to develop evaluative skills will be to practise evaluation by discussing and arguing issues through with others. Just having a good memory will not be enough to achieve this level.

At this level you should also have thought through how social policy, social and health care, and science could help to improve people's quality of life and therefore human development. You should have ideas for creating a healthier environment, reducing social exclusion, ideas for protecting people from potential negative consequences of their genetics and promoting opportunities for people to fulfil their intellectual, social and emotional potential. In this way you may be able to explain how 'the effects of factors [which affect development] may be enhanced or minimised'.

Finally, you should reflect on how different theories of human development might influence the interpretation of the development of an individual. Different theories pick out or emphasise the importance of factors such as early experience, learning, social context, genetics and so on. At A grade you should be able to discuss these theories and use them to evaluate the relative importance of different factors.

Use the unit test which follows to practise for the external assessment.

## Test

Read the case study below and then answer the questions which follow.

### Case study 1: Jason

Jason is 18 years old and will soon be taking exams which will influence his future career. He would like to continue to study although he does not know what he might want to study or what career he could progress to. He is not sure if he can afford to go to university and thinks that it might be better to get a job. He has spent time with careers advisers but still feels 'confused' about his future.

Jason grew up and lives in a high density housing estate on the outskirts of a major city. His father divorced his mother when he was eight and Jason's mother re-married and he now lives with her and his stepfather. Jason was very upset by these changes but has since come to accept the new family which he is part of.

Jason has several periods of difficulty at school. He was an only child and found it difficult to mix with other children when he first started school. He found it difficult to learn to read and was well behind other children in his reading ability by the age of 10. He enjoyed physical activities but he developed chronic asthma which limited his ability to play physical games such as football.

Over the last four years Jason's school work has improved and he was able to get good grades at GCSE. Jason says that he used to hate school because he was 'picked on' by other pupils due to his asthma. He says that work is more interesting now and he finds it easier to do homework.

### *Questions*

1 Describe the major changes in personal relationships that might be expected to have occurred as Jason passed through the life stages of infancy, early childhood, childhood and adolescence.

2 The psychodynamic perspective emphasises the importance of early experience in influencing personality. Explain some key stages which this perspective would predict Jason to have experienced.

3 Jason developed asthma which prevented him from being successful at physical activities. Why might some children in a given locality develop asthma but others do not?

4 Jason found it difficult to read and developed his reading abilities more slowly than other children in his class. Think of four different explanations which might account for differences in learning performance as children develop.

5 Jason lives in a crowded housing estate. If this estate also had a high general unemployment and crime rate, how might this environment be expected to influence Jason's education and career prospects?.

6 Jason now finds it easier to do homework and enjoys school more than earlier in his life. Give one good explanation as to why this change may have come about and link your idea to theories of 'skills development'.

Read the case study below and then answer the questions which follow.

## Case study 2: Jessie

Jessie is 84 years old, her husband died six years ago. She has osteoarthritis which affects her fingers, hands and back. This arthritis causes pain when Jessie attempts to undertake daily living activities. Jessie becomes breathless when she tries to walk or do any heavy work. This breathlessness is due to cardiovascular problems.

Jessie pays for regular home care support because she has difficulty with housework and with collecting shopping. She is also a little forgetful and worries about making mistakes when she tries to pay bills. Jessie sometimes appears to be depressed when her carer visits. She has limited social contact as her friends find it difficult to visit her due to their own health problems. Jessie's son emigrated over 30 years ago and although he keeps in contact he rarely visits. Jessie's daughter lives over 60 miles away and connot provide regular social support.

### *Questions*

1 Jessie is facing a range of emotional threats. List two possible risks to emotional well-being that she may experience.

2 The psychodynamic theorist, Eric Erikson, believed that late adulthood involved a particular life crisis. Briefly describe the eighth crisis which older people may expect to experience within this theoretical perspective.

3 The psychodynamic perspective is just one way of understanding human development. Contrast this perspective with two alternative views that could be used to explain Jessie's situation.

4 Jessie is finding it increasingly difficult to cope with daily living activities. When she tries to pay bills or do housework things often go wrong. Behaviourists would see this as a punishing experience. How will punishment influence Jessie's behaviour?

5 Jessie sometimes appears depressed. Explain some of the factors which might contribute her depression and justify why these factors are relevant.

6 If social care services took over Jessie's daily life routine, what dangers might this cause?

7 All care workers would agree with the value statement that it is morally wrong to abuse others. How would you try to explain this value to:

a a six-year-old child
b a mature and intellectually able adult?

What key intellectual differences would you expect to find between these two people?

8 Smoking is generally accepted to be very dangerous for health. Some young people take up smoking and others do not. Using your knowledge of social development and learning theories, justify two explanations which might account for this difference.

9 Social class appears to be a major factor in influencing people's educational attainment, health and even length of life. Explain what is meant by social class classifications.

10 List three secondary characteristics that feature in a female during puberty.

11 Describe the symptoms that could be alleviated by hormone replacement therapy.

12 Which endocrine glands secrete the following:

a oestrogen
b testosterone.

13 Gesell devised a map of milestones of development. What is the technical term for this map?

14 Place the following motor skills into gross and fine categories:

- Stands without support
- Builds a tower of six or more cubes
- Catch a ball
- Run up and down stairs one foot at a time
- Uses a pincer grasp to pick up fine objects
- Holds rattle without dropping it
- Rolls from front to back.

## Answers

*Case study 1*

1 During infancy Jason would be expected to bond with his parents. In early childhood he would develop associations with other children founded on the 'safe base' of parental relationships. In later childhood Jason would be expected to become increasingly independent of his parents and develop friendships with other children. During adolescence Jason might have developed close friendships with 'peers' as well as with groups of peers. Jason might be expected to explore sexual relationships and partnerships during adolescence.

2 The psychodynamic perspective would identify the following three stages as influencing Jason's development:

Oral – infants learn to trust or mistrust the world.

Anal – children learn to control themselves to meet social pressures.

Phallic – children have to resolve a crisis about relationships (or love) in relation to parents, a sense of initiative or guilt may follow.

Erikson also identified later stages of:

**Learning to be competent**. A sense of competence and confidence may develop, or at the other extreme a child may be left with feelings of inferiority or failure.

**Identity crisis**. Adolescents and young adults need to develop a sense of personal identity or else fail to develop a secure sense of self.

3 • Different individuals may have different levels of tolerance to conditions which cause asthma. Some children may develop a high level of immunity to

asthma, others may not. Genetic differences may influence the way people develop illnesses and impairment.

- Different individuals may be exposed to different levels of pollution or other environmental factors which may make a health problem more serious.

**4** Possible explanations include:

**a** Individual children have individual patterns of development. Jason's personal pattern of environment-genetic interaction may have resulted in him appearing to be 'behind' but to then 'catch up'.

**4** Possible explanations include:

**a** Individual children have individual patterns of development. Jason's personal pattern of environment-genetic interaction may have resulted in him appearing to be 'behind' but to then 'catch up'.

**b** Individuals have different intelligences – individuals prefer to learn in different ways. Perhaps teaching has changed to a style which helps Jason to learn or perhaps he has found a way to learn using his preferred styles. This creates the appearance of catching up.

**c** Emotional needs – Jason found it hard to settle with other children, his own relationships may have been stressed when his father divorced his mother. Stress at home may have caused problems with learning.

**d** Jason says he was 'picked on'. Stress within the school may have created a barrier to learning.

**e** The social context Jason lived in may not have provided motivation to learn. Perhaps Jason has developed a new motivation to do with the 'new' family or perhaps new friends.

**f** Jason may have missed classes due to physical ill health.

**5** Living in a high stress environment might result in low motivation to work at school because of:

**a** A lack of role models, i.e. people who had succeeded through study.

**b** Poor opportunities for homework and study, perhaps due to overcrowding or noise.

**c** Poor health because of overcrowding, noise, pollution. Poor health may interrupt school work.

**d** Reduced self-efficacy due to past experiences of failure.

**e** The development of low expectations for achievement in relation to socialisation, and learning in relation to others' expectations.

**f** The lack of social support with learning (Vygotsky's theory that social support is essential for learning).

**6** **a** Jason's social contact may have altered – perhaps he gets help and support with homework, encouraging learning (Vygotsky's theory).

**b** Perhaps experiences of success create an increase in self-efficacy (Albert Bandura's theory).

**c** Perhaps teaching has changed and Jason is able to use his abilities more effectively than previously (Gardner's theory of multiple intelligences).

**d** Perhaps Jason's environment includes reinforcement for learning and school work (Skinner's theory of learning).

*Case Study 2*

1 Risks may include:

- A loss of competence or ability to manage daily living activities (a threat to belonging).
- A belief that life is 'ending' (physical threat).
- A feeling of being powerless or out of control due to inability to manage daily living tasks (threat to emotional safety).
- A feeling of being taken over by others who have to look after her (threat to emotional safety)
- A feeling of being rejected – relatives and friends don't visit (a threat to belonging).
- A feeling of being devalued or worthless (a threat to self-esteem).

2 Erikson's eighth crisis is a stage of struggle to maintain ego-integrity versus being overwhelmed by despair. Ego-integrity involves maintaining a sense of self-esteem and purpose for most people. Ego-integrity and despair are extremes, many people will achieve a view of 'self' that is somewhere in between these two definite outcomes. People who do despair may become depressed. People who maintain a sense of self-esteem may have a positive outlook on their life.

3 Other perspectives include:

- Biological determinism – Jessie's life trajectory inevitably results in decline and loss.
- Behaviourism – Jessie's environment no longer provides reinforcing or rewarding experiences. Her environment is punishing, causing her to withdraw from attempts to control daily living activities.
- Cognitive – Jessie may have difficulty making sense of the changes which are impacting on her. She may lack the social support necessary to help her to make sense of her experiences.
- Humanistic – Jessie's self-esteem and other emotional needs are unmet. She is unable to live an emotionally fulfilling life without social support.

4 Punishment causes people to stop repeating a behaviour, but punishment does not guide people to make alternative responses. If all of Jessie's attempts to cope with housework and bills are punished she will 'give-up' and withdraw. Seligman sees punishment as a route to learning to become helpless.

5
- Failure to cope and loss of control may result in 'punishing' experiences leading to withdrawal and depression (Seligman's theory of learned helplessness).
- Socialisation may lead to a loss of self-esteem (self concept theory and Maslow's theory of human need).
- Inactivity may reduce physical health (activity and exercise help to maintain health).
- Jessie may be in a stage of emotional crisis – despair and depression may result (Erikson's theory).
- Jessie may be unable to cope with transition (Hopson's theory or other theories relevant to coping with change).

6 If other people take control it might encourage Jessie to withdraw. Other people taking control may reduce Jessie's self-esteem and sense of purpose. She may become depressed if she loses a sense of self-worth due to no longer making decisions about her own life.

7 You might emphasise ideas like fairness when working with a six-year-old or

saying, 'How would you like it if it happened to you?' Explaining values to the adult might involve reference to social needs – what kind of society do you want to live in, or reference to rights and principles on a more philosophical level. Piaget's or Kolberg's theories are relevant to this answer.

The key difference is that intellectually advanced adults are able to think in a more complex way. Young children will have only a narrow pre-operational or concrete logical way of making sense of moral judgements. Explanations that work for adults may not be understood by six-year-olds.

**8**
- Some individuals may smoke because their initial experiences are physically reinforced. Some individuals may be genetically disposed to addiction. Some individuals may find smoking less habit forming than others due to their biological nature.
- Some individuals may smoke because of social reinforcement. If a person mixes with others who expect or reward this behaviour then they may develop the habit. Mixing with people who reject smoking may help to prevent the development of this habit.
- The presence or absence of adverts and other media messages may have different levels of influence on people depending on their local culture, socialisation and self-concept.

**9** Social class is measured by the Registrar-General's Social Class Classification System. This system classifies occupations according to their social status. For many years, a six category system was used to measure social class, with Social Classes 1, 2, 3a, 3b, 4 and 5. This system was replaced by an eight category system in 1998. Both systems attempt to assess the status of occupations – but the recent system also takes issues such as job security, pension entitlement and control of workload into account. Status is partly – but not completely – influenced by incomes and benefits associated with occupations.

**10** Growth of primary sexual organs, onset of menstruation, development of axilliary and pubic hair.

**11** Hot flushes/night sweats, osteoporosis, depression, heavy menstruation, weepiness, anxiety.

**12** Oestrogen – ovary; testosterone – testes.

**13** Normative measurement.

**14**
- Stands without support – gross
- Builds a tower of six or more cubes – fine
- Catches a ball – fine
- Runs up and down stairs one foot at a time – gross
- Uses a pincer grasp to pick up fine objects – fine
- Holds rattle without dropping it – fine
- Rolls from front to back – gross

# References and recommended further reading


Acheson, D. (1998) *Independent inquiry into inequalities in health* HMSO

Argyle, M. (1987) *The Psychology of Happiness* Methuen

Bandura, A. (1989) 'Perceived self-efficacy in the exercise of personal agency' in *The Psychologist* 2 (10) 411–24

Berryman, J. *et al.*, (1991) *Developmental psychology and you* BPS books and Routledge

Bee, H. *Lifespan development* Harper Collins

Berkman, L. F. and Syme, S. L. (1979) Social networks, lost resistance and mortality *American Journal of Epidemiology,* 109

Black, D., *et al.* (1980) 'The Black Report' in Townsend, P., *et al.* (1988) *Inequalities in health* Penguin

Blaxter, M. (1990) *Health and lifestyles* Routledge

Bowlby, J. (1953) *Child care and the growth of love* Penguin

Bowlby, J. (1969) *Attachment and loss* Vol. 1, Hogarth Press

Brown, R. (1973) *A first language: The early stages* Harvard University Press

Bruner, J. (1974) *Beyond the information given* George Allen & Unwin

Buhler, C. (1933) *Der menschinche lebenslauf als psychologiches problem* Hirsel. Printed in German

Castells, M. (1996) *The rise of the network society* Blackwell

Catell, R. B. (1963) 'Theory of fluid and crystallised intelligence: A critical experiment' *Journal of Educational Psychology* 54

Clarke, A.M. and Clarke, A.D.B. (eds) (1976) *Early experience: myth and evidence* Open Books

Cohen, D., (1981) *Piaget : Critique and Reassessment* Croom Helm

Dearborn and Rothney (1941) *Predicting the child's development* (Harvard Growth Studies) Sci-Art Publishers, USA

Denny, N. W. (1982) 'Ageing and cognitive changes', in B. Wolman (ed.) *Handbook of Developmental Psychology* Prentice Hall

Erikson, E. (1963) *Childhood and society* Norton

Fantz, R. (1961) 'The origin of form perception' in *Scientific American* 204, 1097–104

Gardner, H. (1984) *Frames of mind* Basic Books

Goleman, D. (1996) *Emotional intelligence* Bloomsbury

Gordon, D. and Forest, R. (1995) *People and Places 2: Social and economic distinctions in England* School for Advanced Urban Studies, University of Bristol

Gross, R. (1992) *Psychology* (2nd edition) Hodder & Stoughton

Guildford, J. P. (1956) 'Structure and intellect' *Psychol. Bulletin* Vol 53, p267–93

Hall, S. (1904) *Adolescence* Appleton

Harris, P. (1989) *Children and emotion* Basil Blackwell

Havinghurst, R. J. (1972) *Devlopmental tasks and education* (3nd edition) David McKay

Hayes, N. and Orrell, S. (1993) *Psychology: an introduction* (2nd edition) Longman

Hayes, N. (1995) *Psychology in Perspective* Macmillan

Henley Centre (1999) *The paradox of prosperity* Salvation Army/Henley Centre

Holmes, T.H. and Rahe, R.H. (1967) 'The social readjustment rating scale' in *Journal of Psychosomatic research* 11, 213–18.

Hopson, B. (1986) 'Transition: Understanding and managing personal change' in Herbert, M. (ed) (1986) *Psychology for social workers* The British Psychological Society and Macmillan

Howe, M. (1997) *IQ in question* Sage

Jones, S. (1993) *The language of the genes* Flamingo/HarperCollins

Kitchener, K. S. and Brenner, H. G. (1990), in Sternberg, R. (ed.) (1990) *Wisdom* Cambridge University Press

Klinnert, M. (1984) 'The regulation of infant behaviour by maternal facial expression' in *Infant behaviour and development* 7, 447–65.

Kolberg, L. (1976) 'Moral stages and moralization: The cognitive-developmental approach' in Lickona, T. (ed.) *Moral development and behaviour* Holt

Levinson, D. J. *et al.* (1978) *The seasons of a man's life* A. A. Knopf

McGarrigle, J. and Donaldson, M. (1975) 'Conservation accidents' in *Cognition* 3, 341–50

Mead, G.H. (1934) *Mind, self and society* (ed. Morris, C.) University of Chicago Press

Millar, E. (1977) *Abnormal ageing* John Wiley

Pinker, S. (1995) *Language instinct* Penguin

Plomin (1989) 'Environment and genes' in *American psychologist* 44 (2) 105–11

Richards, M.P.M. (1993) 'The new genetics: Some issues for social scientists' in *Sociology of health and illness* 15 (5)

Rose, S., Lewontin, R.C. and Kamin, L.J. (1984) *Not in our genes* Penguin

Rutter, M. (1981) *Maternal deprivation reassessed* (2nd edition) Penguin

Schaffer, H.R. and Emerson, P.E. (1964) 'The development of social attainments in infancy' in *Monographs of social research in child development* 29 (94)

Schaie, K. W. (ed.) (1983) *Longitudinal studies of adult pshycholigcal development* Guildford Press

Segall *et al.* (1990) Human *Behaviour in global [erspective* Pergamon Press

Skinner, B.F. (1957) *Verbal behaviour* Appleton Century- Crofts

Social Exclusion Unit (1999) *Opportunity for all* HMSO

*Social Trends* Vol 30 (2000) HMSO

Sorce, J.F. Emde, R.N., Campos, J.J. and Klinnert, M.D. (1985) 'Maternal emotional signalling' in *Developmental psychology* 21, 195–200

Sternberg, R. (ed.) (1990) *Wisdom* Cambridge University Press

Sternberg, R.and Wagner, R. (eds.) (1986) *Practical intelligence* Cambridge University Press

Stewart, R.B. and Marvin, R.S. (1984) 'Sibling relations' in *Child development* 55, 1322–32

Stopford, V. (1987) *Understanding disability* Edward Arnold

Walker-Andrews, A. (1986) 'Intermodel perception of expressive behaviours: Relation of eye and voice?' in *Developmental psychology* 22, 373–7

Watson, P. and Johnson-Laird, N.J. (1972) *Psychology of reasoning: structure and content* Batsford

Wolf, D., Rygh, J. and Altshuler, J. (1984) 'Agency and experience: Actions and states in play narratives' in Brehterton, I. (ed.) (1984), *Symbolic play* Academic Press

Zimbardo, P.G. *et al.* (1992) *Psychology and life* HarperCollins

Zimbardo, P. *et al.* (1995) *Psychology: A European text* HarperCollins

## Fast Facts

**Accommodation** A process which happens when existing knowledge is changed to fit with new learning.

**Adolescence** Usually understood as the period between 13 and 18 when full adult responsibility is not required but when people are more independent than children.

**Assimilation** Changing our understanding of an issue in the light of new knowledge.

**Asthma** A rapidly increasing long-term (chronic) illness which now affects over 2 million people in the UK and causes over 1600 deaths a year.

**Axillary hair** Hair in the armpits.

**Babbling** A stage infants go through before they can use language. The infant makes sounds which may later help him or her to use words.

**Baby talk** Adults use a high-pitched voice and slow down their speech when talking to infants. Adults may also use exaggerated facial expressions. Baby talk may help to keep an infant's attention.

**Belonging** A feeling of identifying with a particular group of people. Feeling safe and supported by a particular group.

**Bereavement and loss** A process of transition or coping with change following a loss. Loss of a loved person is usually called bereavement. But the process may be similar in any loss, such as loss of a limb. The process may involve phases of shock, searching, using defences, anger and guilt, before final reconstruction of identity is possible.

**Bonding** Making an emotional attachment to a person. Babies usually make an attachment to carers during the first year of life.

**Buffering** To absorb shock and protect people. Relationships often protect people by absorbing the shocks that life might deliver.

**Cancer** The uncontrolled growth of abnormal body cells. Malignant cancer will disrupt normal body functions. In 1991, 25 per cent of all deaths in the UK were caused by cancer. One in four people might be expected to die from cancer, and one in three might develop cancer in their lifetime.

**Cephalo-caudal** From head to tail.

**Circulatory disease** Disease of the heart and blood circulatory system. It was the cause of 46 per cent of all deaths in the UK in 1991. It is the major cause of death in the UK.

**Classical conditioning** Learning to associate two responses – the simplest type of learning.

**Cognition** A term which covers the mental processes involved in understanding and knowing.

**Concepts** Linguistic (language) terms used to classify, predict and explain physical and social reality. They are probably dependent on experience of events, usefulness in terms of simplifying experience and ability to be shared with others.

**Concrete operations** The third stage of intellectual development in Piaget's theory. At this stage, individuals can solve logical problems provided they can see or sense the objects with which they are working. At this stage, children cannot cope with abstract problems.

**Conservation** The ability to understand the logical principles involved in the way number, volume, mass and objects work.

**Construction** Construction means to build or develop. Beliefs about self and others are often built or 'constructed' from our experience within a social context.

**Constructivism** A perspective which emphasises that people invent or build their own understanding of what is real. Different people may come to see and think about the world in different ways.

**Constructs** Individual concepts which don't have to be shareable. Constructs are private ways of evaluating ourselves, others and things. They can be used in patterns to create pre-emptive, constellatory or propositional evaluations.

**Culture** The collection of values, norms, customs and behaviours that make a group distinct from other groups. Cultures have their own system of values which may be linked to religious beliefs. The culture we are raised in may be one of the biggest influences in our lives.

**Crystallised intelligence** Intelligence which relies on past learning and memory for previous problem-solving.

**De-centring** The ability to use concepts and mental processes to free judgement from the way things look.

**Dementia** A term which covers a range of illnesses involving the degeneration (or wasting) of the brain. Dementia is not part of normal ageing. Most very old people show no sign of dementing illness.

**Depression** Used as a clinical term, depression indicates a loss of social and emotional functioning. One in five people may be expected to experience clinical depression at some stage of their lives.

**Determinism** The view that human behaviour is determined or caused either by the environment (social determinism) or by genetics (biological determinism).

**Differential growth rates** The nervous system grows rapidly in the first few years of life, the reproductive organs hardly grow until puberty, while general bodily growth occurs fairly steadily throughout childhood.

**Disability** The loss of ability. Ability is socially constructed, i.e. it depends on the perceptions of social groups.

**Dysfunction** The loss or impairment of a function, something not working so as to fulfil its function.

**Egocentricity** An inability to understand that other people's perceptions or feelings could be different from your own. Piaget believed that pre-operational children were egocentric. More recent evidence casts some doubt on this theory.

**Embryo** The first eight weeks of infant (human) development.

**Emotional development** A focus on the feelings that individuals may have in association with expected relationship patterns in their culture.

**Emotional intelligence** The ability to understand and use own emotions to achieve personal goals rather than being controlled by emotions.

**Emotional maturity** The development of a stable self-concept, or identity, which enables an individual to become independent and take responsibility for his or her own actions.

**Environment** The surroundings that a person or people function in. Environment includes air quality, water quality, landscape, housing, noise, physical and social context – everything that affects people.

**Equilibration** Achieving a balance between our experience and our ability to explain the world to ourselves.

**Fertilisation** The point in time when a sperm nucleus from the father joins with an egg nucleus from the mother. This can begin the process which will lead to new life.

**Foetus** The name given to the developing life within the mother's womb from week 8 to week 40 (birth).

**Fluid intelligence** Intelligence which is used to adapt and solve problems.

**Formal operations** The fourth and final stage in Piaget's theory of intellectual development. People with formal logical operations can solve abstract problems.

**Genetic code** A set of instructions passed from one generation to another for building a living organism.

**Grammar** The rules for organising or using a language.

**Group** A collection of individuals who are seen as being linked by common characteristics such as appearance, interests or behaviour.

**Health** The World Health Organisation's definition of health is, 'A state of complete physical, mental and social well-being, and not the absence of disease or infirmity.'

**Holmes–Rahe scale** A scale of life events which may put pressure on individuals to make a social readjustment. The scale was researched in the USA in the 1960s by Holmes and Rahe. The scale may be a useful starting point for cataloguing life-event threats.

**Humanistic theory** A perspective on human personality and behaviour which regards personality as resulting from an individual's system of thinking and feeling.

**Hypothalamus** Part of the brain that has certain functions including controlling many of the pituitary gland hormone secretions.

**Hypothesis** A theory or idea which can be tested out in practice.

**Hypothetical constructs** Theoretical ideas which can be helpful when trying to solve abstract problems. Part of intelligent adult problem-solving.

**Identity** Put simply, a person's identity is how she understands herself and makes sense of her life in relation to other people and society.

**Impairment** Damage to, or loss of, a physical function of the body.

**Income** Money that an individual or household gets from work, from investments and other sources. Income is usually thought of as income per week or income per month. For statistical purposes, income per year may be recorded.

**Independence** Being able to function without being dependent on others. Adolescence is seen as a time of growing independence in Western culture.

**Infancy** A term used to cover the first 18 months of life.

**Intelligence** A term used to classify differences, human cognitive ability. People may differ in cognitive abilities, but intelligence is not clearly defined.

**Internalisation** Vygotsky's term for building an understanding through social experiences.

**Language acquisition device** Noam Chomsky theorised that people had an in-built ability to learn, think and communicate using language. The language acquisition device enabled children to understand the deep structure which all languages follow.

**Life chances** The view that people are born with different advantages or disadvantages with respect to wealth and health. Some people have a better chance of being socialised into healthy habits than others. Some people will experience less stress than others. Some people may be exposed to poorer housing and poorer diets than others from birth.

**Life crises** Eight developmental stages which influence personality in Erikson's theory of personality.

**Lifestyle choice** The view that people are free to choose their way of life. For example, people may be free to choose a healthy diet, a healthy balance of rest and exercise, healthy habits such as only moderate drinking of alcohol and not smoking.

**Maternal deprivation** Bowlby's theory that children would become emotionally damaged if separated from their mother during a critical period of their early life.

**Media** All the methods of mass transmission of information within society. It includes television, radio and newspapers.

**Menarche** The onset of menstruation.

**Menopause** The end of the fertility period.

**Mental illness** A loose term, used to cover social and emotional disability. Categories include schizophrenia, affective or emotional illness (psychosis), depression and anxiety. Sometimes the term is also used to include dementia.

**Metacognition** Understanding or knowledge of your own knowledge.

**Motor development** How muscles co-ordinate and pull together to enable more and more complicated movements to occur.

**Nature–nurture debate** A debate that has gone on for hundreds of years as to whether inheritance (nature) or environment (nurture) are most important in making people what they are. A modern view claims nature and nurture cannot be meaningfully separated.

**Neonate** A newly born baby.

**Norms** Patterns of behaviour that are expected to be followed by the members of a particular group. Different groups have their own sets of norms to which members are expected to conform. Society as a whole has norms which all are expected to follow, and some of which are backed by legal sanctions.

**Notochord** Forerunner of the spinal chord.

**Object permanence** The understanding that objects exist whether they can be seen or not. Piaget theorised that infants would develop object permanence only at the end of the sensorimotor period.

**Oestrogen** Hormone produced by the ovary (and placenta) that is mainly responsible for secondary sexual characteristics in a female.

**Operant conditioning** Learning to repeat a response because that because that response has been 'reinforced'.

**Peer group** A group of people who share common characteristics or circumstances, and feel themselves to be like one another. We are all members of peer groups, and may join several different peer groups during our lives. Peer groups are an agent of socialisation. We learn our role, and the norms and values of the group, as we become a member.

**Pituitary gland** A small endocrine gland that lies in the mid-line under the hypothalamus; it secretes many hormones including those that stimulate the primary sexual organs.

**Power** A relationship where one person is able to influence or control aspects of the life of another. Power is an aspect of many social relationships. It may be exerted through coercion or authority, or through a combination of the two.

**Practical intelligence** The ability to cope with, and succeed in life. Intellectual abilities which are not measured by language or mathematical tests.

**Pre-conceptual** A period when children can communicate, but do not necessarily understand the meaning of the terms they use.

**Pre-operational** The second stage of Piaget's theory of intellectual development. Pre-operational children are understood as being pre-logical. They cannot reason logically.

**Presbyopia** Long sight that develops from mid-forties onwards in most people.

**Primary socialisation** The socialisation that takes place during early childhood. The language, values and norms of the society the child has been born into are acquired. Through primary socialisation in the family the child learns how to be an accepted member of the group. (See also **Socialisation**.)

**Primitive reflexes** Reflexes which are present in the newborn, but disappear after a few months to be replaced by learned responses.

**Psychodynamic** A perspective on human personality and behaviour which emphasises the importance of early learning.

**Puberty** The physical changes of adolescence.

**Pubic hair** The hair that grows on the lower abdomen between the legs.

**Registrar-General's social classification** A method of stratifying the population along the lines of class. Occupational groups are used as the basis for deciding class membership, and there are five class groups in the scale.

**Regulation** The monitoring and control system. In Piaget's theory the development of knowledge is regulated by a balance of assimilation and accommodation. Autonomous, active and conscious regulation systems may explain how skills are learned and developed.

**Reinforcement** Anything which makes a behaviour stronger, anything which causes behaviour to be repeated because of conditioned learning.

**Role** The behaviour adopted by individuals when they are interacting in social situations. People learn their roles through the socialisation process, and may play many different roles during their lives.

**Self-concept** The use of many concepts to describe, understand and perhaps predict what we are like. Understanding of self.

**Self-confidence** An individual's confidence in his or her own ability to achieve something or cope with a situation. Self-confidence may influence and be influenced by self-esteem.

**Self-efficacy** An individual's ability to understand and perhaps predict his or her own abilities in relation to any tasks or challenge. High self-efficacy involves the belief that you will succeed at a given task. Self-efficacy may become a general feature of a person's identity.

**Self-esteem** How well or badly a person feels about himself or herself. High self-esteem may help a person to feel happy and confident. Low self-esteem may lead to depression and unhappiness.

**Sensorimotor** The first stage in Piaget's theory of intellectual development. Infants learn to co-ordinate their muscle movements in relation to things that they sense.

**Sexual maturity** A stage of physical development that results in the ability of males and females to reproduce.

**Smog** A fog mixed with soot and sulphur dioxide from coal smoke. Smog affected cities in the UK in the 1950s and early 1960s. Chemical or invisible smog may create a serious air pollution problem nowadays. This new air pollution problem is caused by motor vehicles.

**Social class** The status given to different types of occupation or work. Comparisons of social class are used to help understand social differences.

**Social construct** A feature of society about which people share a common understanding. Ideas like 'housewife', 'crime' and 'health' are examples of social constructs. Social constructs have no concrete existence, but they are such an integral part of social interaction that they may seem as though they have.

**Social constructivism** The view that social context influences or even determines the way individuals learn to think about and understand the world.

**Social context** The setting for group and social influences or individual learning.

**Social development** A focus on the way groups may influence relationship patterns within a culture.

**Social exclusion** Being excluded from opportunity – people with fewer life chances to become economically prosperous than the majority of people.

**Social learning theory** A perspective on human personality and behaviour which emphasises the importance of the environment and the ability of individuals to learn from, and copy, the behaviour of others.

**Social networks** Where people are linked to each other like the links in a net. Social networks may provide help and support during times of need.

**Social support networks** Partners, friends, family and relatives, membership of community groups which provide a source of support for own self-esteem. Support may often be provided in the context of conversation which permits self-disclosure (talking about oneself).

**Socialisation** The process by which we learn the norms, values and behaviour that makes us a member of a particular group. We learn the roles that we are expected to play as a group member.

**Spatial awareness** The ability to make sense and respond appropriately to objects in space.

**Status** A measure of the rank and prestige of a person or a group of people. Status helps to define how people are treated by others, and how they see themselves. Status is linked to role, and different roles in a group have different levels of status attached to them.

**Teenage rebellion** A belief that adolescents necessarily reject the norms of older generations. Many modern authors claim that there is little evidence for rebellion as a life cycle stage – it may have been a feature of the 1960s and 1970s.

**Telegraphic speech** A kind of early speech where a child sends a message using only a few words, for example 'Cat goed' meaning 'The cat has gone away'.

**Testosterone** Hormone produced from the male testis that is responsible for the secondary sexual characteristics in a male.

**Threat** Something which is understood as a danger to physical, social or emotional well-being.

**Transition** Periods of major changes in life such as starting work, having children or retiring.

**Values** Beliefs about what is good and bad, right and wrong, worthless or worth striving for. Group values help to explain and define group norms of behaviour.

**Wealth** The value of the property owned by a person. Wealth includes the value of houses, cars, savings and any other personal possessions.

**Zone of proximal development** The range of explanation that is likely to be understood and lead to new learning for an individual. Explanations lie outside this 'zone' when they are too easy and no new learning takes place or when they are too difficult so that an individual cannot understand and learn.

**Zygote** Alternative technical name for the fertilised egg.

# Health, social care & early years services

Unit 5

**It is important that all workers in the health, social care and early years services understand how these services have developed, how they are structured and how they are funded. This information has an impact on their jobs. This chapter is organised in six sections.**

**You will learn about:**

- **the origins and development of health, social care and early years services – including demographic influences**
- **national and local provision of services**
- **informal carers**
- **the funding of services**
- **the effects of government policies on services**
- **access to services.**

## 5.1 Origins and development of services

### Origins of health, social care and early years services prior to 1948

In the mid-1300s an epidemic raged through Europe, reaching England in 1348 and Scotland a year later. What we think of as 'the plague' killed one in three people in England and had a devastating effect on society and the economy. This sudden and drastic reduction in the number of working people encouraged labourers to leave their former masters and to sell their services to the highest bidders. This was viewed as a threat to the established social order and resulted in the introduction of the **Poor Laws**, the first of which came into being in 1389. The Poor Law set a legal **maximum** wage and made it illegal for labourers to leave the manor to which they belonged.

However, the Poor Laws did not prevent the numbers of travelling and homeless people from increasing during the next two centuries. The population also rose rapidly, so adding to the number of homeless people. At this time the monasteries provided some food and shelter to the sick and poor. But following the dissolution (closure) of the monasteries in the 1540s, laws allowing parishes to collect money in order to provide food and shelter were introduced. This 'relief' was provided to those who were old, sick or disabled and to needy children. Able-bodied poor people could also apply for relief but had to work to earn it.

The Poor Laws of the 1500s, which allowed parishes to collect money in order to provide food and shelter, were the start of today's council tax system.

A new comprehensive Poor Law, replacing all the previous ones, was introduced in 1601, stating that each parish should look after their own poor and unemployed. Needy people were categorised into one of three groups: the 'impotent' (helpless) poor; the able-bodied poor; and 'rogues' and 'vagabonds'. Each group was treated in different ways. The impotent poor, (the old, sick, crippled and children) were considered as deserving relief, with children being 'apprenticed' at the parish's expense. The able-bodied who could not find work were admitted to the 'workhouse' and given tasks to do, for which they received very poor rates of pay, until they could find employment. Rogues and vagabonds, who begged, scrounged and stole, were flogged and sent to the 'house of correction' (prison). Persistent offenders were hanged. Often whole families would be committed to the workhouse, including infants and children.

The population had increased again by the end of the 1700s and there were food shortages, caused by war and bad harvests. Many people in work found themselves living below the poverty line. Parishes therefore began to supplement the wages of low-paid workers (similar to today's Income Support).

By 1830 there was growing concern about the cost of parish relief, which had risen from £1.7 million in 1776 to £7 million in 1831. Boards of Guardians were appointed to oversee the expenditure of the new poor law unions and infirmaries (hospitals). At this time the poor were considered to be responsible for their own poverty i.e. that there was work available if only they were not too lazy to look for it, or that they could have avoided poverty in some way. The workhouses were now intended to be a deterrent and very quickly became viewed with hatred and horror, although their policies were not intentionally meant to be cruel.

Huge changes in society resulted from the Industrial Revolution (1760–1840), replacing a mainly rural agricultural society with an urban industrial society. There was a mass movement of people from the countryside to the towns and cities, which created public health problems. The 1848 Act for Promoting Public Health was the result of national and local pressure to improve the condition of the urban environment and to improve the health of the nation. Health-related services, including water supplies, sanitation, food and hygiene inspection, pollution control and, later, housing and community health, were developed. In 1861 workhouses became part of the public hospital system, providing eighty-one per cent of all hospital beds in England and Wales. The rest were provided by voluntary hospitals.

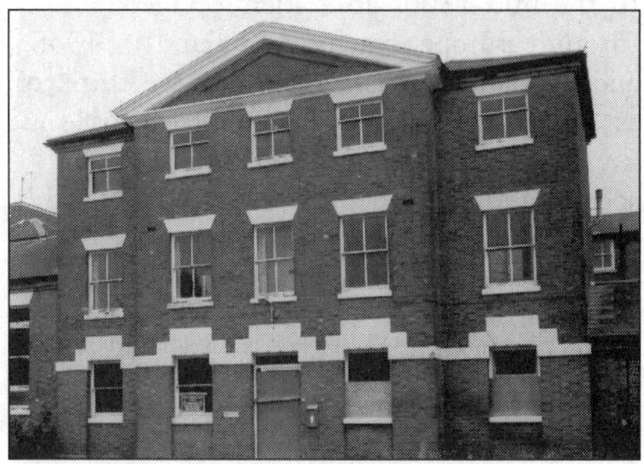

Many old workhouses were used as hospitals, like St Edmund's, Northampton.

> **Think it over**
>
> There are many workhouse buildings still in existence today. Find out if there are any in your area. What are they now used for?

In the late 1800s there was an outcry against the conditions of the sick wards in the workhouses, which led to the appointment of the first medical officer to the Poor Law Board. Public opinion began to change in respect of the sick and it was felt that the deterrent poor law policy should not apply to them. Poor Law Unions were encouraged to establish separate asylums (hospitals), which would care for the sick, insane and infirm.

It was only in the 1860s that there were the beginnings of social justice for children. The introduction of legislation was prompted by the high mortality rate and waste of children's lives and by the obvious misery and exploitation of the poor. In 1868 the Poor Law Amendment Act enabled the Boards of Guardians to prosecute parents who wilfully neglected their children, so causing them to need poor law care. But it was not until the end of the 1800s that the first Act for the prevention of cruelty to children was passed.

By 1900 it was generally viewed that children should be removed from the workhouses and that the Boards of Guardians should provide accommodation for children in 'cottage homes, by the hire of scattered homes, by boarding out and emigration'.

From 1870 onwards various Liberal governments introduced reforms that began to chip away at the old Poor Law. The new initiatives provided the basis for the **Welfare State** system and the notion of state intervention began to be accepted.

However, health services were fragmented and uncoordinated, some were provided by local authorities and others by voluntary organisations. Sometimes there were overlaps and sometimes gaps in the provision of services, which the poorest groups could not afford to access. A National Insurance scheme was introduced in 1911 to help meet the costs, but this did not cover dependants, the long-term sick, or those needing specialist services. The system was also undermined by massive unemployment and many people exhausted their entitlement to assistance.

The development of services for children were greatly hindered during the first part of the twentieth century by two major national disasters. The first was the Great War of 1914-18, which was followed by a period of economic depression, mass unemployment and poverty for many people. The second disaster was the Second World War of 1939-45 which again had enormous economic consequences; food rationing, for example, continued until the 1950s.

However, the creation of the Ministry of Health in 1919 gave the newly appointed Minister for Health the authority, finance and responsibility to build a new public health system for the twentieth century. This underlines the beginning of the move away from individual and local provision of care, towards the welfare state and the full provision of services by the government.

The intervention of the government, through the emergency medical services, during the Second World War (1939 to 1945) is often considered to be a major reason for the creation of the **National Health Service.** However, the **Beveridge Report** of 1942 had already set out the broad framework for the welfare state of post-war Britain and indeed socialist proposals for state-provided health and social care can be traced back to the early 1900s.

## The Beveridge Report (1942)

The Beveridge Report was concerned with five aspects related to health: want, disease, ignorance, squalor and idleness – and it covered the whole population. The report prompted a 'cradle to the grave' provision of care, to be funded by a compulsory insurance scheme. The scheme would involve a single, weekly contribution which would cover sickness, medical care, unemployment, widows, orphans, old-age, maternity, industrial injury and funeral benefits. It promised universal social security (benefits), without means tests, uniformly administered by a Ministry for Social Security. It was even considered radical by Beveridge himself. The scheme was based on the notion of a redistribution of income, i.e. that wealth should be shared more evenly throughout the population.

There were various objections to the report's original proposals and many revisions were made. It was not until Aneurin Bevan became the Minister for Health, under a new Labour government in 1945, that an agreement was reached. Bevan affirmed that the proposed National Health Service (NHS), would be 'free at the time of use', financed mainly by taxation and that the hospitals would be nationalised.

The National Health Service Act was passed in mid-1946 and came into effect on 5 July 1948.

## The National Health Service 1948 to 1979

The original structure of the National Health Service (NHS) had three main 'arms' to the service:

- the regional/district system of hospitals and specialist services
- primary care services – including medicine, dentistry, pharmacy and optometry
- community and public health services.

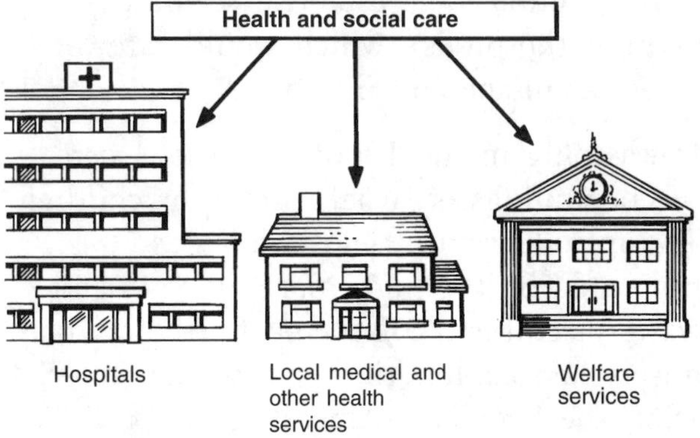


**Figure 5.1 The organisation of health and social care services under the National Health Service Act 1946**

The NHS provided a comprehensive health care system, with the potential to ensure a high standard of health care throughout the country. The bringing together of health and social care services under the Minister for Health meant that a more coherent, better planned and co-ordinated range of services could be developed. Health and social care policies were under-pinned by the principle of a free, comprehensive, universal and state-provided welfare system.

During the Second World War welfare officers had been appointed by the Minister of Health to deal with the problems of evacuation and, later, housing problems. Then by 1945, 70 local authorities had appointed social workers to help with the provision of social care. In addition to welfare and social workers, the Provisional Council for Mental Health was also appointing social workers to provide care for people with mental health problems. Following the introduction of the Children Act 1948 local authorities created separate children's departments and appointed child care officers.

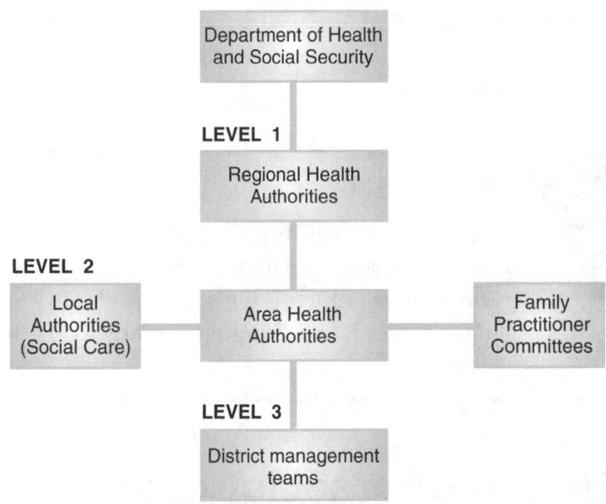


**Figure 5.2 The structure of the NHS 1974 to 1989**

During the 1960s, the demand rose for a family service in social care and in 1968 the Seebohm Report on personal social services was published. This resulted in the amalgamation of the children's departments and welfare services within local authorities. The subsequent Local Authorities Social Services Act 1970 required authorities to set up Social Services committees and set out a framework for social care provision. The 1960s, also highlighted problems in the structure of the NHS, with overlaps, duplication and lack of co-ordination of services. This eventually resulted in the reorganisation of the NHS, with three tiers of management being introduced at regional, area and district levels (see Figure 5.2).

> **Think it over**
>
> The numbers of doctors at consultant level in England and Wales roughly doubled between 1948 and 1973.

The 1970s saw a deterioration in industrial relations throughout the UK, including in the health care services. Disputes involved nurses, doctors and ancillary staff, with disruption to services contributing to long waiting lists, and occasional malpractice scandals. Again services were proved to be uncoordinated, duplicated or overlapping, with inequality in availability of services from area to area, and confusion regarding what constituted health care or social care in certain circumstances. In 1973 Parliament created the post of Health Service Commissioner to look at maladministration in the NHS. All this affected the public's support of the NHS

OVERTIME AT
RATES OF
WOULD YOU ACCEPT A CUT IN
JUNIOR DOCTORS DEMAND A FAIR DEAL


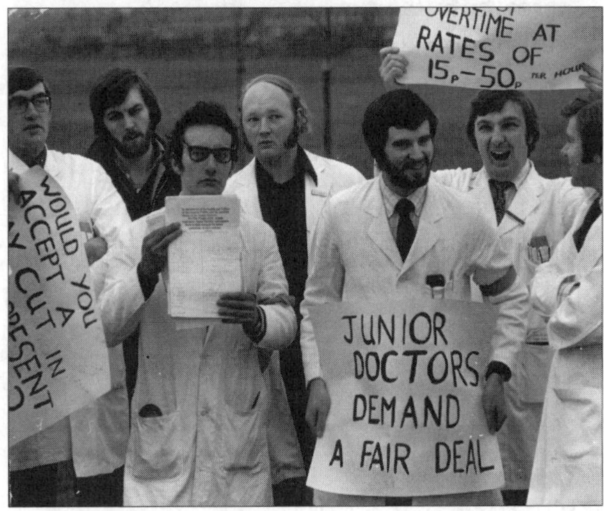

**NHS workers on strike**

and some people (those who could afford it) began to turn to the private sector for their health care.

**Think it over**

Find out what influenced the deterioration of industrial relationships between health care workers, the NHS management and the government in the 1970s.

## Health and social care since 1980

In May 1979 a Conservative government was elected to Parliament and this proved to be a watershed as far as the welfare services were concerned. Although support for care in the community, rather than in long-term hospitals, can be traced back to the 1960s, it wasn't until the mid-1970s that moves were made to promote and support this. The new government was keen to encourage community care for several reasons, and it was seen as a way of saving public money in health and social care. This meant that:

- people had to be transferred from long-term hospital care back into the community (this included the long-term sick or disabled, people with learning disabilities and people with non-acute mental health problems)
- there needed to be more involvement of the private and voluntary sector in the provision of care
- informal care by relatives, friends and neighbours had to be encouraged
- more efficient use of existing resources was required.

From 1979 to 1997 the Conservative government placed the emphasis on promoting self-reliance, the build-up of an **informal sector of care**, the promotion of an **independent sector**, eliminating waste and, even more vigorously, a reduction in public expenditure. The government began to create the notion of an **'internal market'** system for the delivery of care, especially in the health care sector. This meant that Health Authorities and, later, **GP fundholders**, held budgets and could 'buy' hospital treatment for their patients from any hospital that offered them 'the best deal'. The hospital was termed as the **provider** of services. It was thought by the supporters of the internal market idea that this would lead to better quality of care for patients (at no extra cost to the tax payer) and that competition between 'providers' meant greater efficiency. In addition, patients would be treated more like customers and have more say in their treatment. Opponents of the idea argued that certain individuals would be disadvantaged because their **'purchasers'** might not be in as powerful a position as others. Other opponents believed that the market would eventually lead to the privatisation of all services, which would result in certain types of care only being available to those who could afford to pay for them. (See Figure 5.3)

**Think it over**

What sort of health care might not be available to people on a low income and without access to other financial resources?

In May 1997 a Labour government was elected to Parliament with a policy for improving social welfare for all. The new government was keen to re-introduce the idea of co-operation between health and social care providers, while playing down

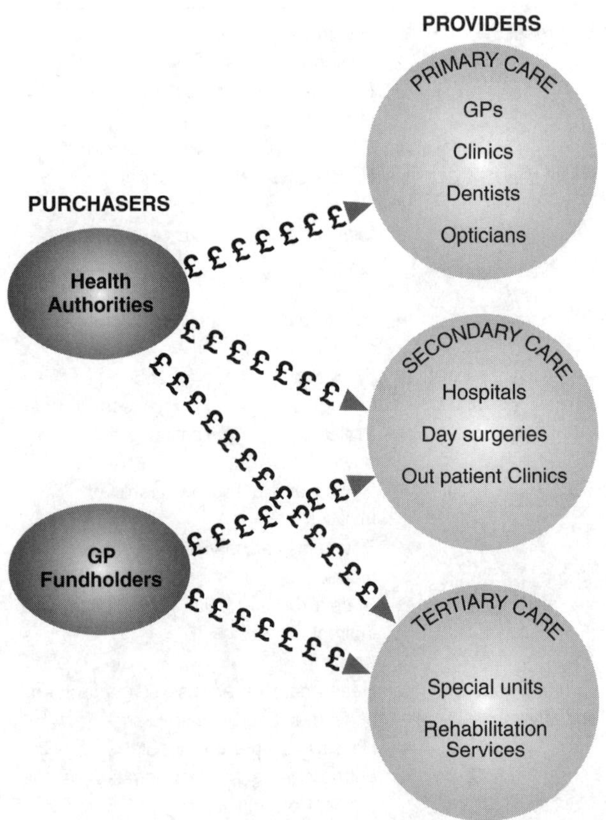


**Figure 5.3 Purchases and providers in the NHS (1990s)**

the issue of competition, abolishing the internal market and phasing out GP fundholding. However, the government still has a policy of continuing to reduce the direct provision of health and social care. In the health service this means that the long-term health care of people will be undertaken either in nursing homes, or in the person's own home. In social care it means that local authorities are reducing the number and range of services that they previously provided themselves (e.g. residential care, home care services, domestic assistance, meals-on-wheels) and are encouraging the development of private or voluntary organisations and agencies to provide these. It also promotes the role of 'informal' carers (i.e. people who are not paid for the care that they give, such as family, friends and neighbours). Additionally, the current government continues the trend towards promoting independence and personal responsibility. It sees the family unit as being 'at the heart of our society', with family members taking responsibility for each other. This combination of state-provided care and services provided by private, voluntary and informal sources is known as a **mixed economy** of care. (See Figure 5.4.)

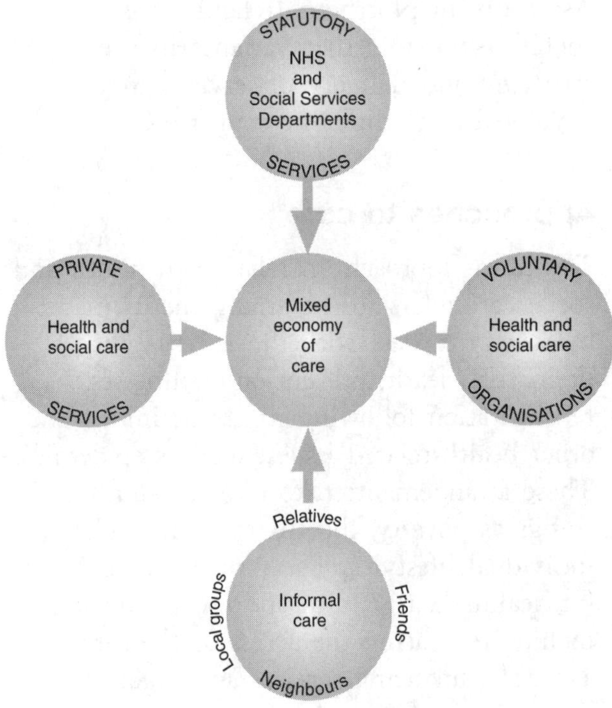


**Figure 5.4 Mixed economy of care**

Since 1997 the government have published three White Papers on the future of the NHS in England, Scotland and Wales. These are:

- *The New NHS: Modern and Dependable* (1998) (relating to England)
- *Designed to Care: Reviewing the NHS in Scotland* (1998)

- *Putting Patients First: The Future of the NHS in Wales* (1998)

All three of these papers uphold the fundamental principle of a National Health Service that is available to everyone, free of charge at the point of need, with services funded through general taxation. However, the responsibility for the NHS in Scotland has been devolved to the Scottish Parliament, in Wales to the Welsh Assembly and to the newly formed Assembly in Northern Ireland. It is therefore possible that variants in the structure and delivery of services may develop in the different countries.

## Approaches to care

The term 'approach' in relation to health and social care refers to the arrangements made by society to deal with illness, disability, premature death, prevention of illnesses, rehabilitation following illness or injury, and other health-related issues, such as epidemics. These arrangements take into account such things as poverty, the environment and individual lifestyles. The formal arrangements for dealing with health and social care will include regulating the access to the care available, financing services and organising the delivery of care. A number of health care systems have been developed throughout the industrial countries of the world. Field (1989) provides a useful overview of health care systems. Field identifies five main approaches, according to the way that services are allocated. These are:

- emergent
- pluralistic (USA)
- insurance/social security (France)
- National Health Service (UK)
- socialised (former Soviet Union).

(See Figure 5.5)

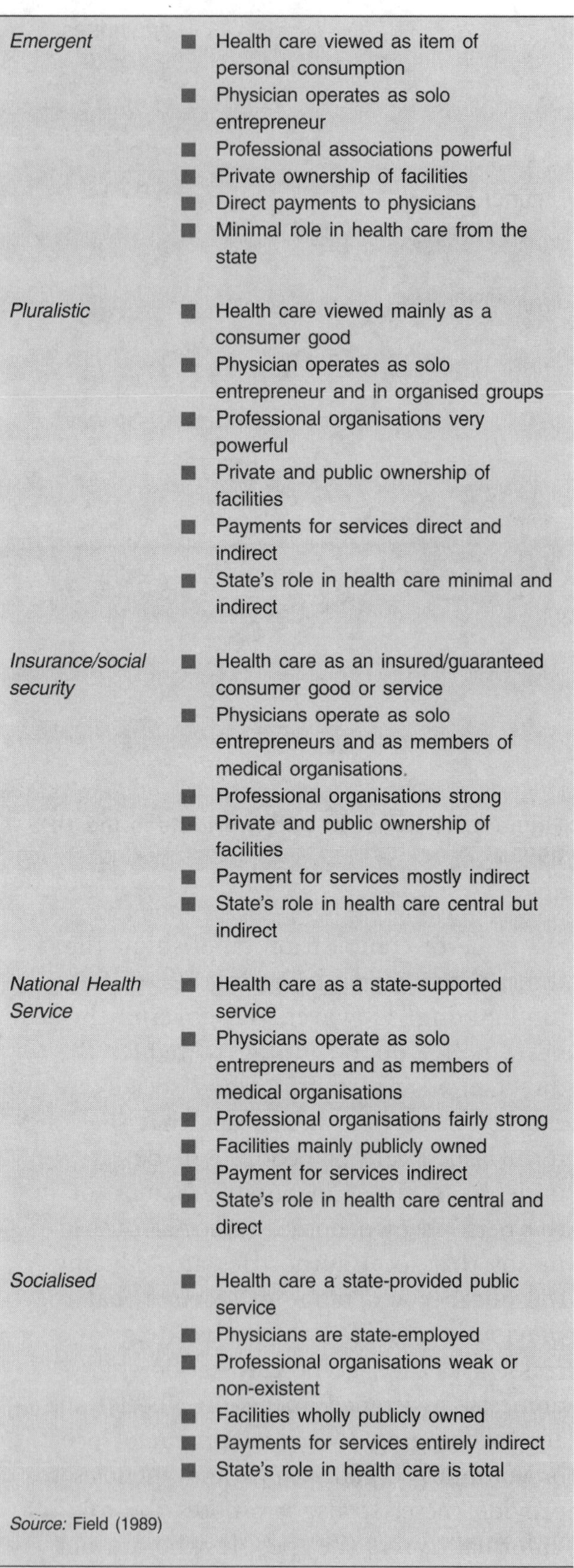

| Approach | Features |
|---|---|
| *Emergent* | ■ Health care viewed as item of personal consumption<br>■ Physician operates as solo entrepreneur<br>■ Professional associations powerful<br>■ Private ownership of facilities<br>■ Direct payments to physicians<br>■ Minimal role in health care from the state |
| *Pluralistic* | ■ Health care viewed mainly as a consumer good<br>■ Physician operates as solo entrepreneur and in organised groups<br>■ Professional organisations very powerful<br>■ Private and public ownership of facilities<br>■ Payments for services direct and indirect<br>■ State's role in health care minimal and indirect |
| *Insurance/social security* | ■ Health care as an insured/guaranteed consumer good or service<br>■ Physicians operate as solo entrepreneurs and as members of medical organisations.<br>■ Professional organisations strong<br>■ Private and public ownership of facilities<br>■ Payment for services mostly indirect<br>■ State's role in health care central but indirect |
| *National Health Service* | ■ Health care as a state-supported service<br>■ Physicians operate as solo entrepreneurs and as members of medical organisations<br>■ Professional organisations fairly strong<br>■ Facilities mainly publicly owned<br>■ Payment for services indirect<br>■ State's role in health care central and direct |
| *Socialised* | ■ Health care a state-provided public service<br>■ Physicians are state-employed<br>■ Professional organisations weak or non-existent<br>■ Facilities wholly publicly owned<br>■ Payments for services entirely indirect<br>■ State's role in health care is total |

*Source:* Field (1989)

**Figure 5.5 Types of health care approach**

It has been suggested that the health care policies of different countries are gradually moving closer together and so becoming increasingly similar. For example, the UK government is moving towards a pluralistic approach to care, while the US government is moving towards a more universal (or national) health scheme.

## Demographic influences on the provision of services

***Demography*** is the science of studying and measuring populations. The population of the UK was estimated to be 58.2 in mid-1993 and is relatively stable. The health of the population, and hence the health and social care needs, can be explored by using statistical information. Statistics are used as a basis to understand the major risks to health and for setting targets for general improvements in health. Population statistics are likely to become increasingly important as governments seek to reduce the health risks that face the population. Demographic changes in the population affect the need for health and social care services. For example, when there is an increase in the numbers of older people, more resources are required to meet their needs. Government policies therefore need to reflect actual and projected demographic changes. Recent government policies, such as care in the community and a mixed economy of care, have been responses aimed to cope with demographic changes. We will consider some demographic changes that are currently of concern to health and social care.

### The diminishing work force

The epidemic in the fourteenth century resulted in a diminishing number of people available for work compared with the number of people required for jobs. As described at the beginning of this chapter, this had a major influence on subsequent welfare policy. In recent years there has been considerable concern about the labour force of the future. It is predicted that there will be a shortage of appropriately skilled, educated staff. This has been an influence on the educational policies of recent governments.

A number of factors affect the population size, including birth rates, death rates, war and migration. (See Figure 5.6.) Until the nineteenth century births and deaths were in rough balance. As industrialisation and medical advances progressed, so there was a rapid increase in population and more people moved into the towns and cities. This resulted in the introduction of measures to improve sanitation and food hygiene. In the early part of the twentieth century, people began to limit the number of children they had and now the average number of births per woman is about 1.8 (below the replacement rate). There is also a decline of the number of people under the age of 16 (25 million in 1971, 20 million in 1991 and a predicted 18 million in 2011).

**Think it over**

Research has shown that higher earnings for women depress the birth rate, higher earnings for men raise it. Why do you think this might be?

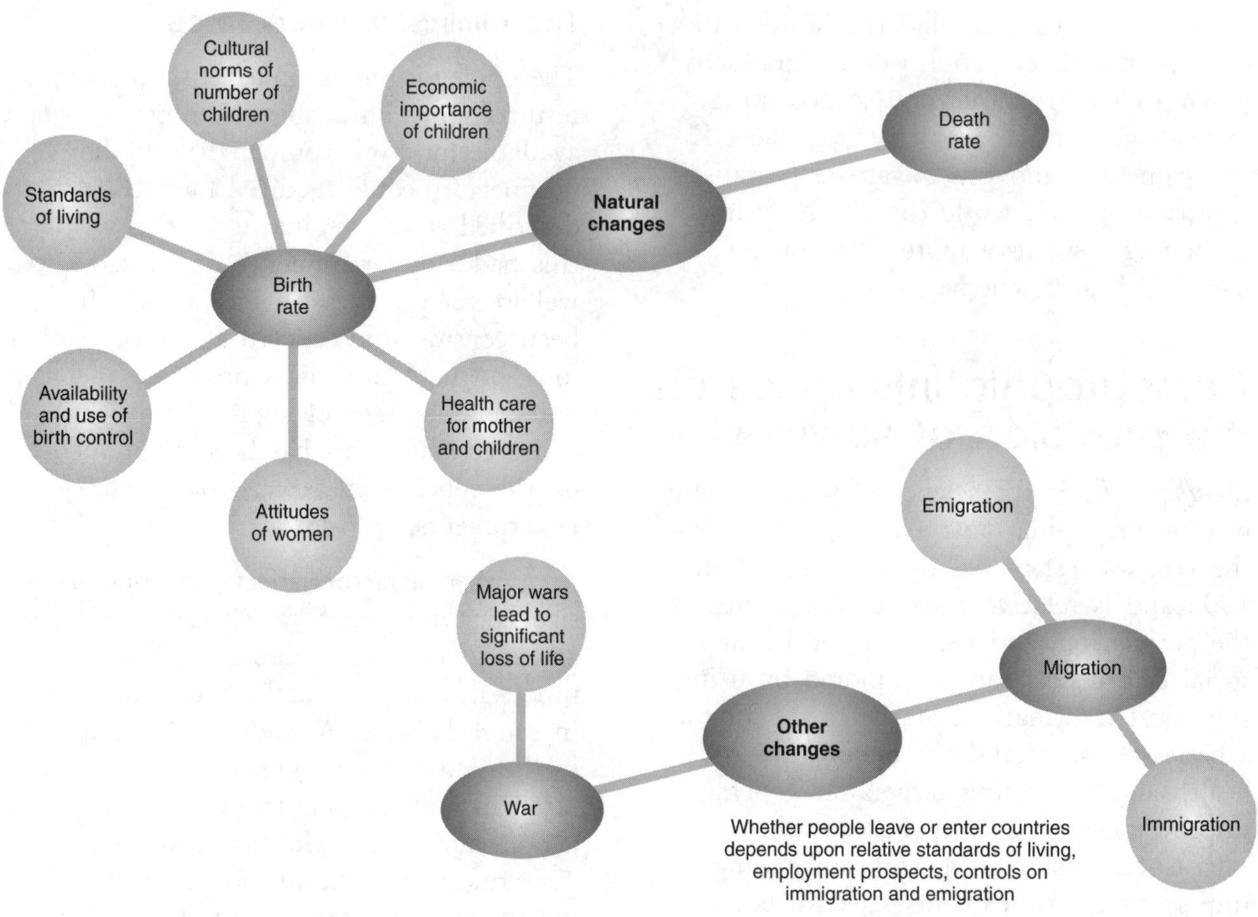


**Figure 5.6 Factors which influence population size**

## The ageing population

The average life expectancy has increased greatly in the twentieth century and is likely to continue in the foreseeable future. (See table below.)

| | 1911 | 1951 | 1991 | 2011 |
|---|---|---|---|---|
| Men | 50.4 | **66.1** | 73.1 | **77.4** |
| Women | 53.9 | **70.9** | 78.8 | **81.6** |

**Table 5.1 Increased life expectancy 1911–2011**

A fifth of the total of the population will be aged 65 and over by the year 2013 and one in 20 people will be aged over 80. (See Figure 5.7.)

For many people, their ability to remain independent will be determined by the level of help provided by relatives, friends and by voluntary services. However, as the population ages so do the people who would formerly have been carers. Also, as more women enter the work force, so there are fewer people available to be 'informal' carers.

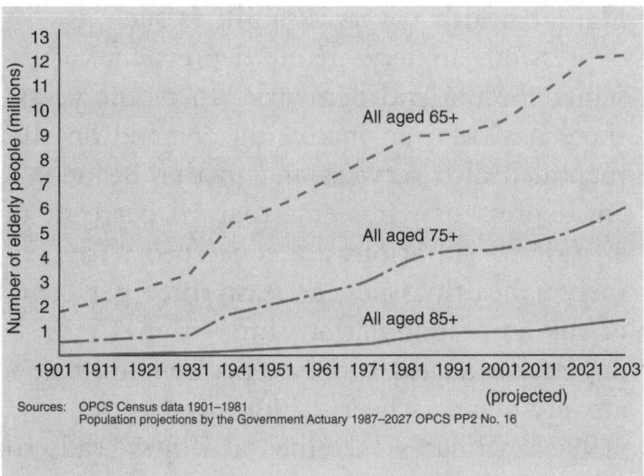


**Figure 5.7 The elderly population in Britain 1901 – 2031 (projected)**

The growing number of older people in itself is not a problem. However, the consequences of increased need for health and social care services could be problematic. Compared with other age groups, people aged over 75 are heavy users of health care services. For example, an ageing population means the number of people with dementia is growing at an alarming rate. Age is the most significant risk factor associated with dementia. Dementia currently affects more than 700,000 people in the UK. It is estimated that by 2040 there will be over 1.2 million people with the disease in the UK. The average cost of care for people with dementia ranges from £21,000 to £30,000 per year (1998 figures).

According to the International Labour Organisation's 1995 World Report, expenditure on pensions and health care for older people will soon be the largest single budget expense. The working population therefore faces an increasingly heavy burden of providing the resources necessary for the care of older people. In 1961 there were approximately six people of working age for every person over the age of 65. By 2011 there will be fewer than four people of working age to every person over 65. People are now encouraged to make provision for private pensions, rather than relying on a state pension for their total income in retirement.

## Incidence of disability, disease and mental illness

There has been a decline in the occurrence of many infectious diseases (such as measles, poliomyelitis and typhoid), although the level of others have risen again recently (e.g. tuberculosis, hepatitis and meningitis). The incidence of degenerative diseases (such as cancer, heart disease and strokes) has also risen; and it has been estimated that there are more than six million adults in the UK who have at least one form of disability, i.e. 15 per cent of the population.

> ? Heart disease, strokes and related illnesses currently cost the National Health Service an estimated £3.8 billion every year.

Modern lifestyles and environmental changes may have contributed to the increase in these degenerative diseases, and to other chronic diseases and dysfunctions. Lifestyle factors include smoking, alcohol abuse, poor diet, stress and lack of exercise. Other social, economic and environmental issues also affect people's health.

> **Think it over**
>
> - 120,000 lives are lost each year from smoking-related diseases
> - An estimated 40,000 deaths a year could be alcohol-related
> - 15 per cent of fatal road accidents are alcohol-related
>
> What do these figures suggest about lifestyle influences on life expectancy?

The Black Report, named after the chairperson responsible for it, was published in 1980. This report has led to wider acceptance that social and economic circumstances affect health. The report concluded that causes of ill-health include:

- physical environment – housing, working conditions, the general environment and air pollution
- social and economic factors – income, wealth and levels of employment
- behavioural factors and barriers to adopting healthier lifestyles
- access to appropriate and effective health and social services.

New approaches in public health seek to improve health by preventing disease. One key element is to convince people to choose a healthier lifestyle and there are various health campaigns that promote this. A healthier lifestyle would include:

- exercise – preferably a minimum of 20 minutes vigorous exercise a week
- healthy diet – low in saturated fat, high in fibre, vegetables and fruit
- avoiding obesity
- moderate drinking of alcohol
- avoidance of smoking
- avoidance of drug misuse
- avoidance of stress.

?

Almost 90 per cent of adults have one risk factor associated with heart disease and stroke according to the Department of Health.

Mental health covers disabilities such as depression, anxiety, manic depression, schizophrenia and dementia. In recent years there has been an increasing demand on the mental health services and in the use of antidepressants. It seems that 14 per cent of all GP consultations are concerned with mental health issues; at least three per cent of the adult population suffer from depressive illness and two per cent from anxiety states. The *Health of the Nation* (1992) estimates that mental illness leads to 14 per cent of certificated absence from work and 14 per cent of NHS in-patient health costs.

## Demographic influences on child health

Many of the wider demographic changes already mentioned have had an effect upon child health. Women are having fewer children, the birth rate has continued to decline overall, falling from 91 per thousand in 1961 to 59 per thousand in 1998. However, although there has been an overall decline, the rate among some age groups – women over 30, for example, has shown a slight increase.

| | 1961 | 1971 | 1981 | 1991 | 1997 | 1998 |
|---|---|---|---|---|---|---|
| Under 20 | 37 | 50 | 28 | 33 | 30 | 31 |
| 20 – 24 | 173 | 154 | 107 | 89 | 75 | 74 |
| 25 – 29 | 178 | 155 | 130 | 120 | 105 | 102 |
| 30 – 34 | 106 | 79 | 70 | 87 | 89 | 90 |
| 35 – 39 | 51 | 34 | 22 | 32 | 39 | 40 |
| 40 and over | 16 | 9 | 5 | 5 | 7 | 8 |
| All ages | 91 | 84 | 62 | 64 | 60 | 59 |

**Table 5.2 Fertility rates: by age of mother at childbirth**
Source: *Social Trends 2000,* Table 2.13

Family patterns have changed. There has been an increase in divorce rates and more couples are deciding to cohabit rather than marry. In 1998, 4 out of 10 births occurred outside of marriage. Births to teenage mothers in 1998 are four times higher than in 1974, and these are particularly likely to occur outside marriage. The average size of households has almost halved over the last century, with the number of one person households increasing over recent decades. The proportion of households where there is a lone parent with dependent children has trebled since 1961 but still only represents 7 per cent of all households.

### Try it out

In groups discuss differing definitions of the term 'lone parent'. How may this affect statistics?

Despite the increase in lone parent households the majority of dependent children do live in a family with two parents – 77 per cent in 1998. More women now choose to work outside the home and this has been reflected by increased provision of child care facilities – though many would say there are still not enough. The National Child Care Strategy aims to increase the provision of good quality and affordable child care.

The health of children has improved markedly over the last hundred years. There are many different measures of health, the infant mortality rate, or IMR (i.e. the number of babies that die before reaching one year old), being one that is frequently used. However the IMR for some regions in Britain is higher than others – the South East being the area with the lowest IMR and the West Midlands with the highest.

| | 1981 (%) | 1993 (%) | 1997 (%) |
|---|---|---|---|
| North East | 10.4 | 6.7 | 5.8 |
| North West | 11.3 | 6.5 | 6.8 |
| Yorkshire & Humber | 12.1 | 7.3 | 6.5 |
| East Midlands | 11.0 | 6.6 | 5.7 |
| West Midlands | 11.7 | 7.1 | 7.1 |
| East | 9.7 | 5.4 | 4.8 |
| London | 10.7 | 6.4 | 5.8 |
| South East | 10.3 | 5.3 | 5.0 |
| South West | 10.4 | 5.8 | 5.8 |

**Table 5.3 Infant mortality rate by region**

### Try it out

Look at the table above and answer the following questions.

- Have the areas with the highest and lowest IMR remained the same or changed?
- Which areas show the greatest change?
- What factors may explain these differences?

As well as regional variations there are also social class variations. A baby from a social class V household is twice as likely to die as a baby from a household in social class 1. In addition, the IMR tends to be higher among babies from ethnic minority group backgrounds.

| | 1981 | 1991 | 1996 | 1997 |
|---|---|---|---|---|
| **Inside marriage** | | | | |
| Professional | 7.8 | 5.0 | 3.6 | 4.4 |
| Managerial and technical | 8.2 | 5.3 | 4.4 | 4.0 |
| Skilled non-manual | 9.0 | 6.2 | 5.4 | 5.4 |
| Skilled manual | 10.5 | 6.3 | 5.8 | 5.3 |
| Semi-skilled | 12.7 | 7.2 | 5.9 | 6.4 |
| Unskilled | 15.7 | 8.4 | 7.8 | 6.8 |
| Other | 15.6 | 11.8 | 8.3 | 8.8 |
| **All inside marriage** | 10.4 | 6.3 | 5.4 | 5.2 |
| **Outside marriage** | | | | |
| Joint registration | 14.1 | 8.7 | 6.9 | 6.8 |
| Sole registration | 16.2 | 10.8 | 7.2 | 7.3 |
| **All outside marriage** | 15.0 | 9.3 | 7.0 | 6.9 |

**Table 5.4** Infant mortality by social class

Table 5.4 shows that while there is an overall fall in IMR it is actually increasing in some sections.

### Think it over

What lifestyle factors may affect the health of people in different social classes?

## Immunisation

It is generally agreed that improvements in health status have been due to a general rise in living standards, improved sanitation and immunisation. But as we have seen, these improvements have not been equally spread throughout the population. Although infectious diseases can still be a cause of death, some previously life-threatening diseases are now extremely rare, for example diptheria and polio.

| | 1981 | 1991-1992 | 1996-1997 |
|---|---|---|---|
| Diptheria | 82 | 94 | 96 |
| Tetanus | 82 | 94 | 96 |
| Whooping cough | 45 | 88 | 96 |
| Poliomyelitis | 82 | 94 | 94 |
| Measles, mumps, rubella | 52 | 90 | 92 |

**Table 5.5** Percentage of children immunised – United Kingdom

Table 5.5 shows that more than nine in ten children in the United Kingdom had been immunised by their second birthday against each of the diseases shown. The incidence of meningitis has increased, though it often occurs in 'outbreaks' and much publicity has been given to aid the early detection and treatment of the disease. An immunisation programme for babies and teenagers, the two age groups most at risk, is now underway, but it only protects against one form of the disease, meningitis C.

### Try it out

Find out what immunisation programme is offered to children. If you were a parent what factors would you consider when deciding whether or not to have your child immunised?

Measles is one of the diseases that almost everyone is aware of and some have experienced it themselves as children. It is now rarely fatal in this country and increased uptake of the MMR (measles, mumps, rubella) vaccine led to the notification of measles falling to its lowest level ever in 1997.

There are now a number of initiatives which seek to reduce the incidence of ill-health in later life by improving child health.

### Diet

Considerable information has been made available in newspapers, magazines and on television about healthy eating habits. However people do not always follow the healthy option, for a wide range of reasons. Health promotion programmes often rely upon people making appropriate choices. Heart and circulatory disease is a major cause of disease and premature death within our society, and it is well recognised that obesity is linked to these and a number of other diseases. Work by the National Children's Bureau (1987) suggests that there is an increase in obesity among children. Not only may this affect them physically, socially and emotionally as children, it will also have an impact on their health in later life. A survey undertaken by the Department of Health (reported 1989) among school children found that the main sources for dietary energy were bread, chips, milk, biscuits, meat products, cakes and puddings, whilst intake of certain vitamins and minerals was found to be below recommended levels.

Obesity is not the only dietary problem related to health. Comparisons with other countries have shown that poor diet will affect growth. So, although there may have been an increase in nutritional standards overall, there is evidence to suggest that there is a correlation between families with low incomes, where there is less expenditure on food, and poor growth in children.

### Exercise

The increase in television and multimedia entertainment, together with a greater tendency for children to be closely supervised, may play a part in the increase in child obesity. But it is also worth considering the role of education. There has been much debate recently about homework and its benefits, fuelled partly by the desire of government, school and parents to increase academic achievement. Although children do take part in sports within schools, they tend to play outside less and play less sport at school. The most common kind of exercise at school is competitive team games, which often come low on lists of sporting preferences (Sports Council 1985).

### Smoking

Despite many campaigns to encourage people to reduce smoking, there has been an increase in levels of smoking among young teenagers, particularly girls.

> **Think it over**
>
> What are the particular factors that may cause young teenagers, or even younger children, to begin smoking?

It is not only the rates of smoking among teenagers and children that affects child health. Children and babies in particular are more likely to suffer from respiratory infections and asthma if parents in the household smoke. In addition, it is well documented that smoking during pregnancy can cause lower birth weight. It is also known that babies with low birth weight are more likely to die in the first year of life. Asthma, which has become more widespread in recent years, is now the most common chronic disease of childhood in our society today, all age groups under 9 years showing an increase in the number of doctor-diagnosed cases of asthma in the period 1995 to 1997.

### Advances in medicine

The improved survival of very pre-term babies and greater life expectancy of children with certain degenerative conditions have contributed to an increase in the number of children with multiple disabilities. Children with disabilities are treated as children in need according to the Children Act, and many also have special educational needs as defined by the 1944 Education Act. In January 1999 there were almost 250,000 pupils with SEN statements in schools in England, showing a continued increase from previous years. Some of these children are educated in special schools and pupil referral units place others in mainstream schools.

Apart from the obvious emotional and practical problems that families with a child with disabilities may face, there is evidence to suggest (Parker 1997) that, regardless of social class, families with a disabled child were substantially worse off than other families. We have already seen the correlation between social class, income and health in our society today.

## Regional variations

As can be seen by the effect of the Industrial Revolution on public health, there are important variations in health and illness within industrial countries. For example, within the UK, variations can be seen in infant mortality rates; mortality rates are lower in England than in the rest of the UK. Scotland and Northern Ireland also have higher rates of coronary heart disease and diseases of the circulatory system. Within England itself there are also regional differences. In broad terms, there seems to be a north-south divide, with general health in the north being worse than in the south. However, there is evidence that the local environment is more significant than living in the north or south, with pockets of 'good' health and 'bad' being found in both.

Although one of the principles underpinning the NHS is to provide a universal health care service, it is still a local health service, with differing standards and level of provision, that has been developed around the country. For example, people with heart disease living in Huntingdon are three times more likely to receive surgery than those living in Great Yarmouth according to a Clinical Standards Advisory Group Report. Death rates from breast cancer are 23 per cent above the average in Hartlepool, but are 33 per cent below the national average in Darlington (Women and Home report, 1995). Also a report by the Audit Commission noted that survival rates for children with cancer are up to five times higher in specialist units than in general hospitals. Survival rates for premature babies are twice as high in special units, despite the fact that they deal with the most serious cases.

**Try it out**

Find out what the incidence of heart disease is in your area. Is it above or below the national average? What are the facilities for heart surgery in your area? (Your local Health Authority should be able to help you with this information.)

## Inequalities in health

Health inequalities are widening. The Black Report in 1980 identified strong, class-related differences in mortality rates, very marked differences in deaths from accidents, poisonings and violence, and respiratory disease. The government's Green Paper *Our Healthier Nation* 1997 emphasised that ill health is not spread evenly across our society:

- children in the bottom social class are five times more likely to die from an accident than those in the top social class
- more people die of lung cancer in the north of England than in the south
- in nearly every case, the highest incidence of illness is experienced by the poorest people.

The poorest people in our society are hit harder than the well-off by most major causes of illness and death. For example:

- premature deaths are more likely to occur in the lower classes: there are more than 17,000 extra early deaths each year among poor men under 65
- strokes in social class five occur more than three times more often than for social class one
- there is a fourfold higher rate of accidental death among the poorest compared to the richest
- mental health problems are at disproportionally higher levels among the poor
- infant mortality is higher in the lowest social classes.

Argyle (1987) states, 'The lower classes are affected by most illnesses more often, take days from work, and die sooner because of them (the illnesses). This is partly due to inequalities in the conditions of life – smaller homes, less heating, larger families, less food and so on'. Argyle goes on to argue that middle-class people make more use of preventative health services such as ante-natal clinics, vaccination programmes and cervical screening, than working-class people do.

Gordon and Forest (1995) produced an atlas for England based on the 1991 consensus data. It shows that most social variables like education, class and wealth, are not spread evenly across the country. Long-term sickness (including disability) is mapped in ratio to the number of health care professionals. A low ratio i.e. 9-34, suggests more care professionals in relation to need than a high ratio, such as 72-60. Some areas seem to be disadvantaged in comparison to others. (See Figure 5.8.)

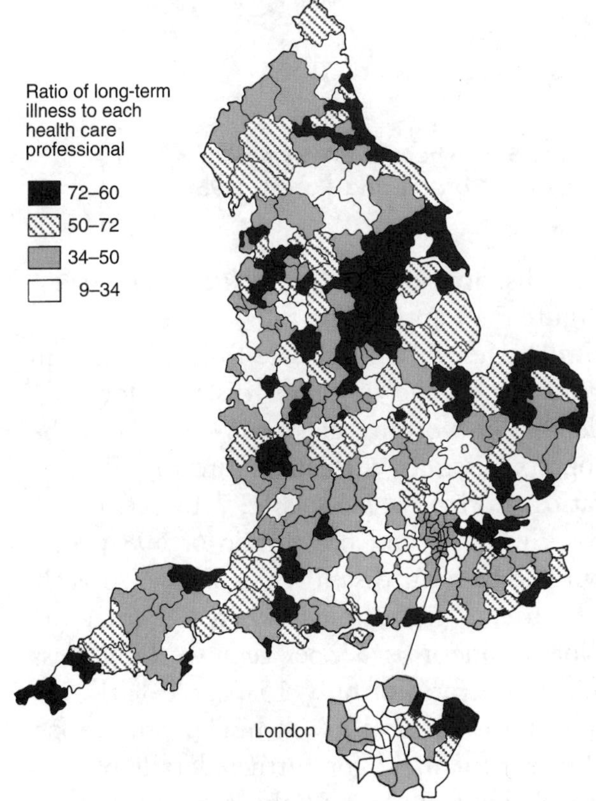


**Figure 5.8 Where to be sick in England: the ratio of long-term sickness to the number of health care professionals (Gordon and Forest, 1995)**

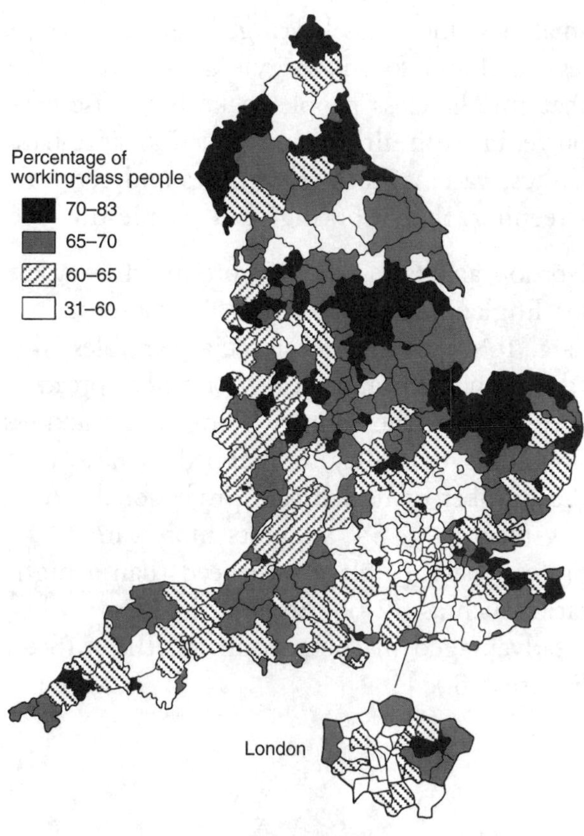


**Figure 5.9 Where the working class is in England (Gordon and Forest, 1995)**

The distribution of the working class (see Figure 5.9) appears to show some similarities with high care-to-need ratios in Figure 5.8. The top three districts for density of working class also come into the top six districts with high care-to-need ratios. Corby is listed as 82.7 per cent working class and has a ratio of 598 people with long-term disability or illness to each health care professional, whereas Barnet in North London is 51 per cent working class and has a ratio of only 15 people with long-term illness to each health professional. Please see Unit 4 for further details of health inequalities and the Acheson Report.

## 5.2 National and local provision of services

Many health and social care services are **statutory**: this means that they have been set up because Parliament has passed a law which requires these services to be provided. The two main providers of statutory services are the National Health Service (NHS) and social services departments. Although there are some differences in the way that these statutory services are organised in England, Wales, Scotland and Northern Ireland the provision of services is much the same.

Until recently the provision of health and social care services in England, Wales, Scotland and Northern Ireland was the responsibility of the central government's Secretary of State for Health. With the devolution of government this responsibility has also been devolved and is now delegated to the Welsh Assembly, the Scottish Parliament and the newly formed Northern Ireland Assembly.

### England

The Secretary of State for Health is responsible for the provision of both health and social care. In England health care is organised through the National Health Service (NHS) and administered by the NHS Executive and at a local level by Health Authorities. The provision of social care is administered by local authorities at local levels. (See Figure 5.10.)

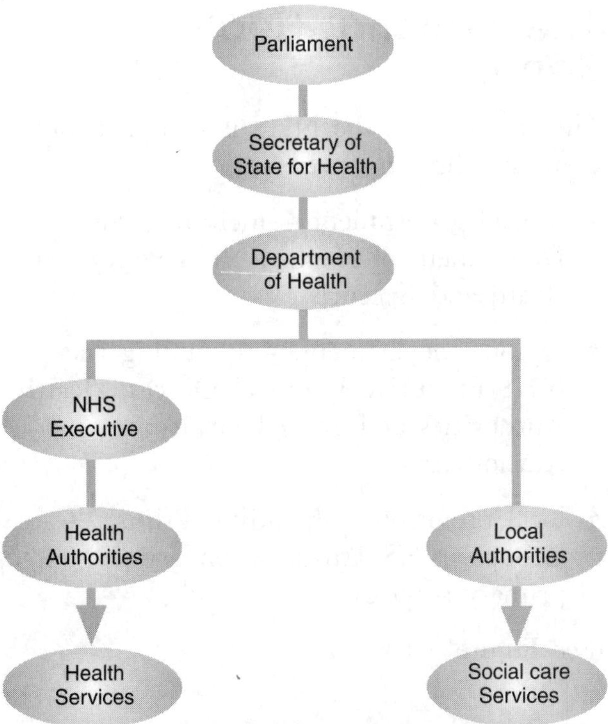


Figure 5.10 The structure of health and social care in England

## Wales

Services in Wales are organised in a similar way to England and the Secretary of State for Wales is accountable to the Welsh Assembly for health and social care services. Health Authorities and local authorities are responsible for services at a local levels. (See Figure 5.11.)

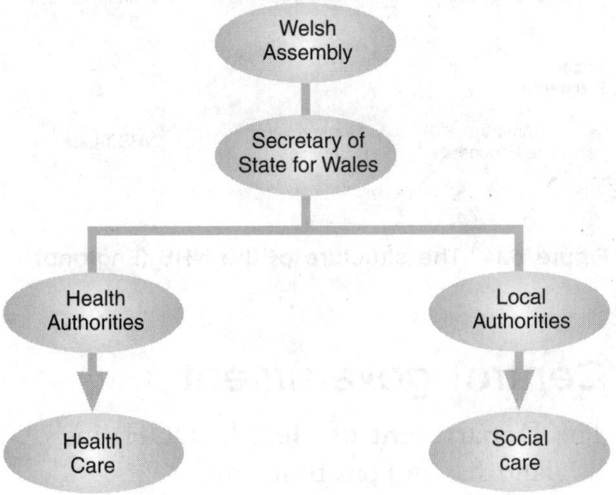


Figure 5.11 The structure of health and social care in Wales

## Scotland

The Secretary of State for Scotland is responsible to the Scottish Parliament for health and social care services in Scotland. The country's services are run by the Scottish Home and Health Department. Local Health Boards and local authorities administer the services at a local level. (See Figure 5.12.)

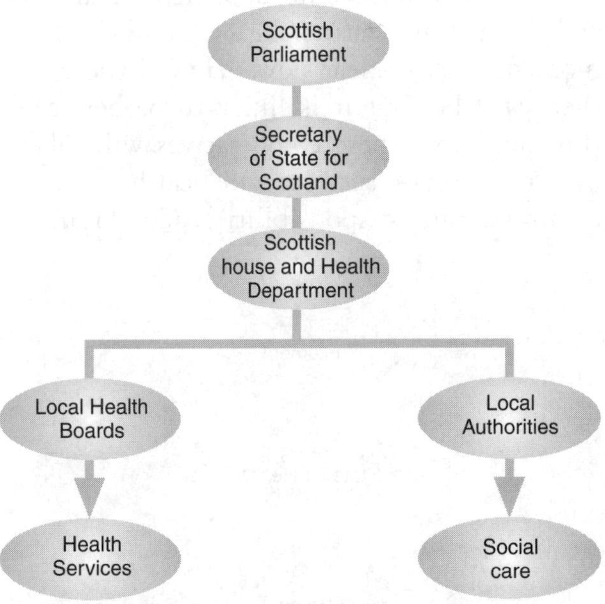


Figure 5.12 The structure of health and social care in Scotland

## Northern Ireland

In Northern Ireland health and social services are organised as a single agency. This is called a 'unified structure' and is outside political control. Once the new Northern Ireland Assembly is functioning, the minister of Health and Social Care for

Northern Ireland, and a newly formed Department of Health, Social Services and Public Safety will be the single, regional organisation responsible for policy, legislation, strategic planning and the management of health and social service. This is an example of an **integrated service.** Until the Assembly is operational, the Secretary of State for Health will retain overall responsibility.

Currently, four Health and Social Care Boards administer services at a local level in Northern Ireland. However, a recent government document has suggested that these may be replaced by new primary care co-operatives (and could be called 'Health and Social Care Partnerships'). At the moment it is unclear how many of these there will be, but it is likely to be between three and six. These co-operatives will take over most social services and health commissioning responsibilities. (See Figure 5.13.)

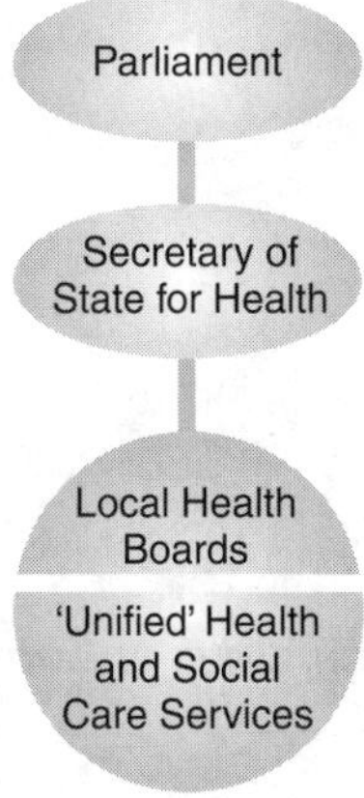


**Figure 5.13 The structure of health and social care in Northern Ireland (this structure will change when the Northern Ireland Assembly is operational)**

## The National Health Service

The structure of the NHS is complex, but there are three main tiers:

- central government – including the Department of Health, NHS Policy Board and Executive
- regional departments – including the NHS Executive Regional Offices, Health Authorities and Special Health Authorities
- local provision – including Primary Care Groups, NHS Trusts, secondary and primary services

(See Figure 5.14.)

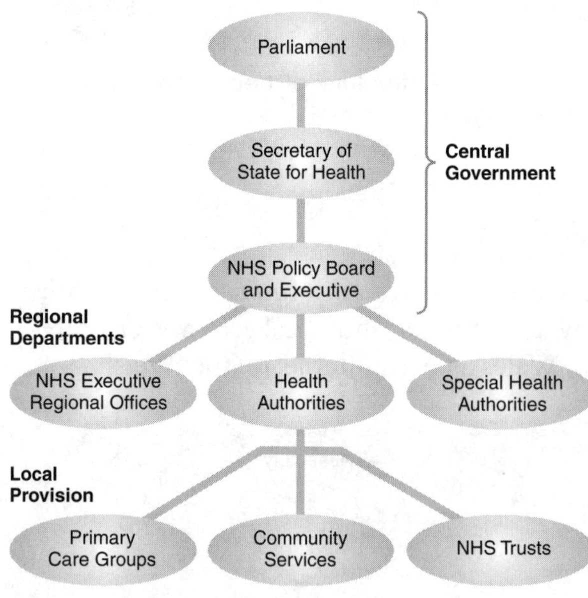


**Figure 5.14 The structure of the NHS (England)**

## Central government

The **Department of Health** (DOH) in England has responsibility for:

- making policies in relation to health and social care and for issuing guidelines

- monitoring the performance of health authorities and social services departments
- allocating resources for the provision of health and social care.

The Secretary of State is accountable for the financial resources spent on the Department of Health, the NHS, for the provision of social services and also has a general responsibility for promoting the health of all people. (The Welsh Assembly, the Scottish Home and Health Department and the Department of Health, Social Services and Public Safety in Northern Ireland have similar responsibilities to those of the DOH in England.)

### NHS Policy Board and Executive

The **NHS Policy Board** is responsible for the overall policy and strategic planning of the NHS and the **NHS Executive** has the responsibility of implementing the policies and strategies formulated by the Board. Both these departments were formed in 1989 in an attempt to separate policy-making from the management of the NHS.

### The General Social Care Council

In its White Paper *Modernising Social Services* the government set out its proposals to set up a **General Social Care Council** (GSCC). The Council's aims will be to:

- regulate the training of social workers
- set practical and ethical standards for staff
- register those working in the most sensitive areas e.g. social workers.

The Council will be an independent statutory body consisting of no more than 25 people. It is envisaged that most of these will be users of services and lay people. The Council will publish codes of conduct for staff groups and employers. It will be responsible for registering the whole of the workforce, although initially only social care workers will be registered. Heads of care homes are likely to be the next group of people to be registered. The Council will be able to de-register those who breach the codes of conduct. In addition, the Council will introduce a new national training strategy to improve training levels across all social care staff, through the National Training Organisation for social services.

### Department for Education

The central government department with the responsibility for education is the Department for Education and Employment. The overall aim of the department is, 'to give everyone the chance, through education, training and work, to realise their potential, and thus build an inclusive and fair society and a competitive economy'.

The education service is run by the Secretary of State for Education who is responsible for making education policy, approving the National Curriculum, the organisation and quality of teacher training, and educational standards. The Secretary of State for Education also has powers to close schools if standards are deemed unsatisfactory.

There are several other bodies concerned with education:

- Local education authorities
- Ofsted
- QCA.

Local education authorities are organised on a county or borough basis and are responsible for ensuring that there is adequate provision of education within the authority's area. Ofsted – the Office for Standards in

Education – is responsible for the inspection of schools and colleges. QCA – the Qualifications and Curriculum Authority – is responsible for overseeing and monitoring the standards and content of Key Stage curricula and public examinations (such as GCSE and A level).

## Regional departments

### Health Authorities

In April 1996 100 new **Health Authorities** (HAS) were formed. These were formed following the abolition of the Regional Health Authorities and by the amalgamation of the former District Health Authorities and Family Health Service Authorities. The boundaries for the new Health Authorities are approximately the same as the former District Health Authorities and have populations varying from 125,000 up to just over one million.

The Health Authorities are responsible for the provision of care for their resident population, and for making and administering arrangements with medical practitioners (GPs), dentists, pharmacists and opticians. They are also responsible for a whole range of acute, palliative, community and family health services, including mental health services. Health Authorities provide and secure the provision of health care services. They also administer the contracts that detail the services to be provided. These contracts may be filled by Trust Units within the NHS or by voluntary or private organisations. Consequently this gives the Health Authority the role of assessing the health needs of the local population and of deciding how those needs will best be met. The new Health Authorities also have the role of providing information about services, as well as developing and monitoring the quality of services. In addition they will manage the complaints system.

### Special Health Authorities

There are a number of health authorities outside the structure described above. They are called **Special Health Authorities** (SHAs) and they report directly to either the Department of Health in London or the NHS Executive. Special Health Authorities are providers of services and there are three types:

1 **Non-hospital SHAs; these provide a** service for the whole NHS which needs some co-ordination at national level. Examples are the NHS Supplies Authority and the Health Education Authority.

2 Hospital SHAs: specialist post-graduate teaching hospitals e.g. the National Heart and Chest Hospitals and the Royal Marsden Hospital.

3 Special Hospitals: i.e. those dealing with the care of seriously disturbed people e.g. Rampton.

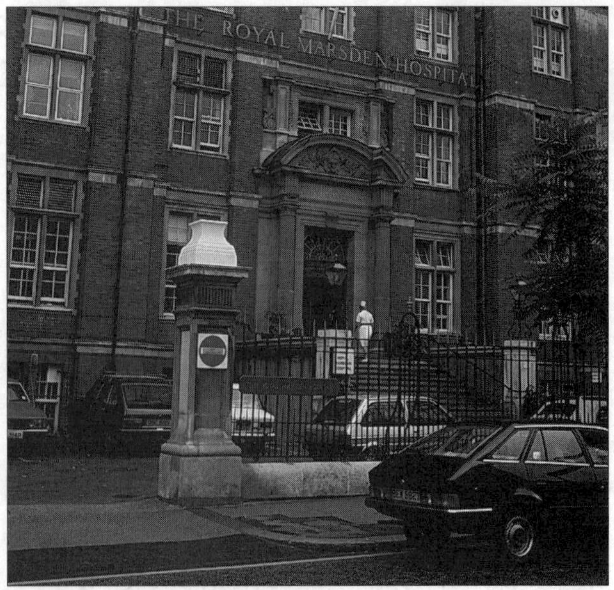


Royal Marsden Hospital

## Local provision

The local provision of health care can be seen as dividing into three main strands:

- primary care
- secondary and tertiary care
- community care and public health services.

**Primary care** means the first (or primary) contact with health services, for example GPs, practice nurses, dentists and opticians. GP practices often involve a group of GPs who may also have other health care professionals working with them, such as district nurses, community psychiatric nurses (and sometimes a social worker). These teams are called **primary care teams** (PCTs).

**Secondary care** focuses on hospital care, day surgeries and out-patient treatment. It is termed secondary care as a referral to these services is required following a recommendation from a primary service provider. The person being referred may require more intensive diagnosis, or more complicated treatment than can be provided through the primary health care services. **Tertiary care** relates to the more specialist services provided by some hospitals or rehabilitation units.

**Community services** comprise various nursing services (for example, district nurse, health visitor, community psychiatric nurses), therapy services (such as occupational therapy, physiotherapy, speech therapy, chiropody) and dental and optical services. **Public health services** are concerned with preventative work and health promotion e.g. vaccination and immunisation programmes.

### Primary Care Groups

In April 1999 **Primary Care Groups** were formed, replacing the former GP fund-holding arrangements. (The former GP fund-holding system meant that larger GP practices could hold budgets with which they could 'purchase' secondary care for their patients. This system was found to be unworkable and was very unpopular with the public.) In England Primary Care Groups (PCGs) are responsible for developing primary care (e.g. GP services, dentists and practice nurses) and community health services (e.g. district nurses, health visitors, domiciliary nurses, chiropodists, occupational and speech therapists).

Primary Care Groups are made up of GPs, community nurses and other professionals who work alongside them. Primary Care Groups cover populations of approximately one million people. Primary Care Boards consist of representatives from GPs, district nurses, the Health Authority, local authority and a member of the public; there will also be a PCG chief officer/manager.

The Boards have five key functions:

- contributing to the drawing up of Health Improvement Programmes (HIPs)
- promoting the health of the local population
- developing primary and community care services
- integrating primary and community care services
- contributing to the development and monitoring of the quality of services
- managing an allocated budget.

PCGs will operate on one of four levels, initially starting on level one or two and gradually progressing to levels three then four. (At level four they will become **Primary Care Trusts.**) These levels involve:

- *Level One:* acting in an advisory capacity only as a subcommittee of the Health Authority
- *Level Two:* holding a budget and responsible for commissioning services but still as a subcommittee of the Health Authority
- *Level Three:* as a 'free-standing body' responsible for purchasing all care for its patients
- *Level Four:* as Level Three but with added responsibilities for the provision of community services.

### Joint working and pooled budgets

Often when people have complex needs spanning both health and social care, there can be complications and delays in the delivery of services. Health and social services authorities are therefore beginning to plan services jointly. Joint working needs to be undertaken on three levels:

- at strategic levels when medium term plans are made for the development of services
- at the stage when services are commissioned
- at the service provision level so that the users of the service receive a coherent integrated service.

In order to achieve this, health and social services often have **pooled budgets**. Decisions regarding how these budgets should be used will be decided jointly.

In September 1998 the government announced their plans to remove legislative barriers to joint working between health and social services. It was envisaged that Primary Care Groups would hold 'pooled budgets' i.e. money to be used by the PCGs irrespective of whether it is a health or social service that is being provided. This would enable PCGs to commission services jointly and would lead to an **integrated** provision of health and social care.

In Wales, Local Health Groups (LHGs) bring together not only GPs and other health care professionals, but also social services departments and voluntary organisations. They may later hold a budget for the purchase of hospital and community health services, for prescribing medicines and for the funding of GP staff and premises, but initially only have an advisory role.

In Scotland, voluntary groups known as Local Health Care Co-operatives (LHCCs) have been formed, thus moving away from individual practices towards a more collective arrangement. The co-operatives hold a budget for primary and community health services, but are also responsible for purchasing secondary care (unlike the English PCGs).

As previously described, the arrangement for the commissioning and development of services in Northern Ireland are very different and are still to be confirmed. However it seems there is likely to be a system of 'Health and Social Care Partnerships'.

### NHS Trusts

**NHS trusts** are self-governing units within the NHS. At present there are two main kinds of trust: hospital trusts and community trusts. Hospital trusts can either be a single hospital or a group of hospitals and provide in-patient and out-patient services to local communities. Community trusts include many of the services that are found in the community such as district nurses, health visitors, bathing services, chiropody services, and a range of services provided in clinics, including services for children.

Trusts are run by boards of directors who manage all aspects of the unit within the policies and guidelines of the government and NHS Executive. Being a trust means these organisations are able to:

- determine their own management structures
- employ their own staff using their own terms and conditions of service
- acquire, own and sell their assets
- retain surpluses and borrow money.

Every trust must prepare a business plan each year, setting out proposals for service developments and capital investments. At the end of the year they prepare and publish annual reports and accounts.

**Think it over**

- In the first three months of 1999 English social services departments received 965,000 enquiries according to Department of Health data.
- 37 per cent of enquiries wanted information or advice only.
- 359,000 assessments were undertaken.
- 58 per cent of assessments were made on people aged 75 or over.

## Social services

### National level

In the 1998 White Paper *Modernising Social Services* the government set out its plans to develop a new General Social Care Council whose job it will be to raise the standards of social care staff, and to make sure that training levels are improved.

### Local level

The Secretary of State for Health is responsible for the provision of social care services. However, it is the **local authorities** that administer them. The powers and responsibilities of local authorities are defined by Parliament. Each local authority has a Social Services Committee which has the responsibility for developing the social care services within its area. It must also appoint a director of social services whose department administers the social care services. Social services departments are often organised into area offices from which the services for that area are operated (see Figure 5.15).

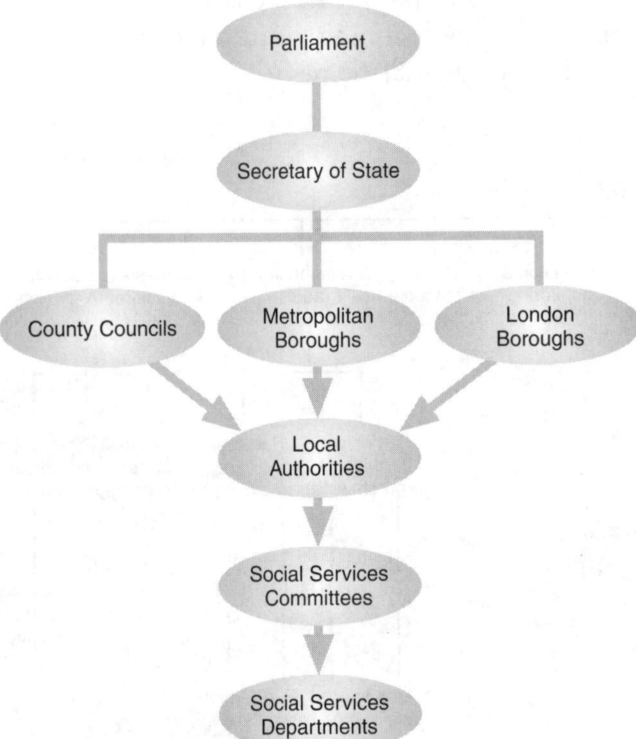


**Figure 5.15 The structure of social services**

Organisational structures within local authority social services departments have changed considerably in recent years. This has been necessary to enable them to carry out their new roles, as required by new legislation. For example, planning and development sections have become increasingly important now that the authorities are required to work more closely with their health service colleagues, as well as with the private and voluntary sectors. Also there is now a far greater emphasis on social services departments to act as 'purchasers' of care, rather than 'providing' care themselves. This change in function means that local authorities are moving away from owning and staffing residential, day care and home care services, into a role as assessors of need and purchasers of services. For example, today they are more likely to purchase residential care for individuals in private or non-profit making residential homes.

### Try it out

Find out from your local authority how many residential homes it owned and staffed ten years ago and how many it owns now. Also find out how many private residential homes are now registered with the authority compared to ten years ago.

In order to reflect this change of function, many social services departments have also re-organised their staffing structures to make a clear division between the purchasing and providing functions. In addition to this, social services are often divided in order to provide for specific client groups e.g. children and families, older people, and adults. The adults section is sometimes sub-divided into services for people with mental health problems, people with a learning disability, and people with a physical disability. (See Figure 5.16.)

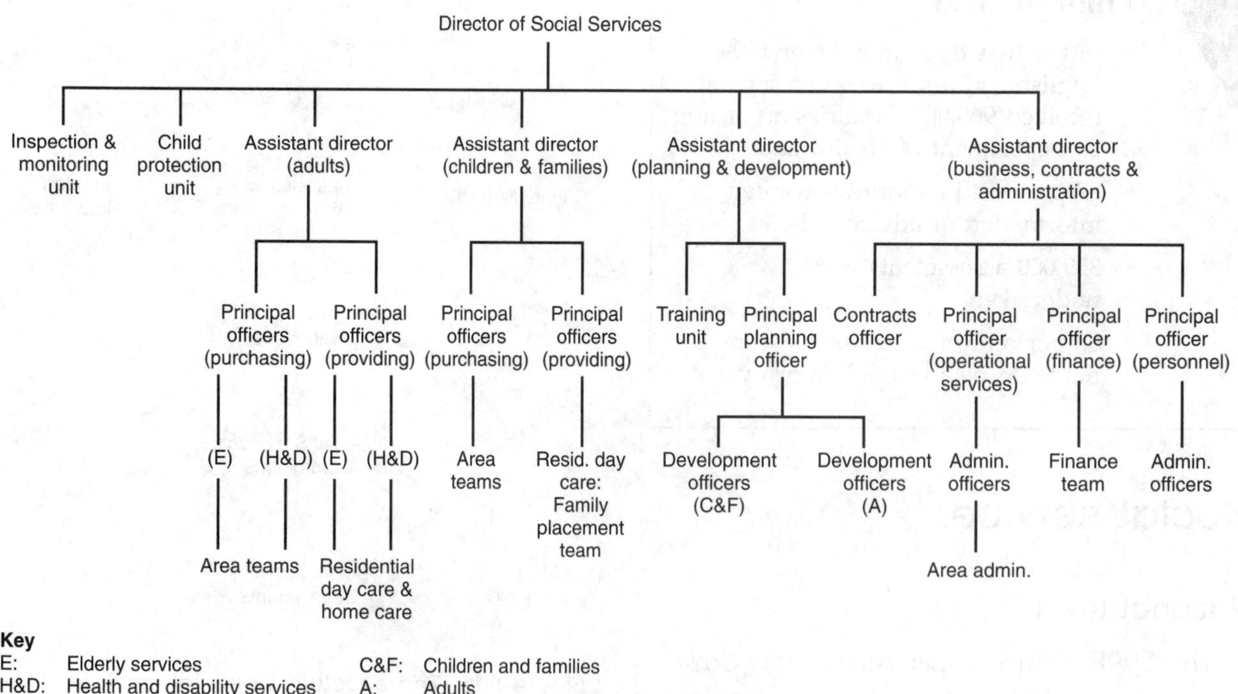


**Figure 5.16 An example of a social services department structure**

Some local authorities have undergone further major re-organisations in the past couple of years, bringing together children and families' services together with educational services; and 'community services' (i.e. the other social services functions) with housing and/or leisure services. (See Figure 5.17.)

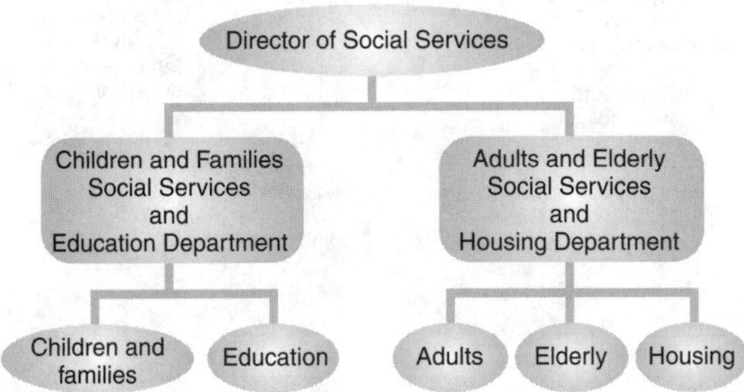


**Figure 5.17 Bringing social services together**

> **Try it out**
>
> Local authorities are required to publish their plans regarding the development of services. Obtain a copy of your local authority's 'Community Care Plan'. What services are provided by the authority and what services are being developed further?

# Early years services

There are three broad areas in the provision of services for early years:

- Health services
- Education
- Social services.

## Health services for children

There are a wide range of health services available to children and their families. These services are still provided without charge as successive governments have recognised the importance of early health care in preventing illness in later life. Health care for children begins long before they are born. There is also a growing awareness that care even before conception can sometimes improve the health of babies. The National Health Service provides three strands of services.

- **Primary care** – general practitioners, health visitors, district and practice nurses. These professionals are often based within GPs' surgeries and offer the first line of care for people. They are interested in prevention as well as treatment, so many surgeries now run well woman clinics and child health clinics. Access to other services is often through the primary care team. A GP may refer someone to a hospital consultant or a health visitor may refer a child for speech therapy.
- **Secondary care** – hospital services.
- **Community services** – school nurses and doctors, community dental services, etc. These services are offered to a local community regardless of the GP individuals may be registered with. A child in school will receive a medical in their second term and a sight and hearing test. This is offered to all children in the school.

The spidergrams which follow show some of these services and how they may be involved in child health care.

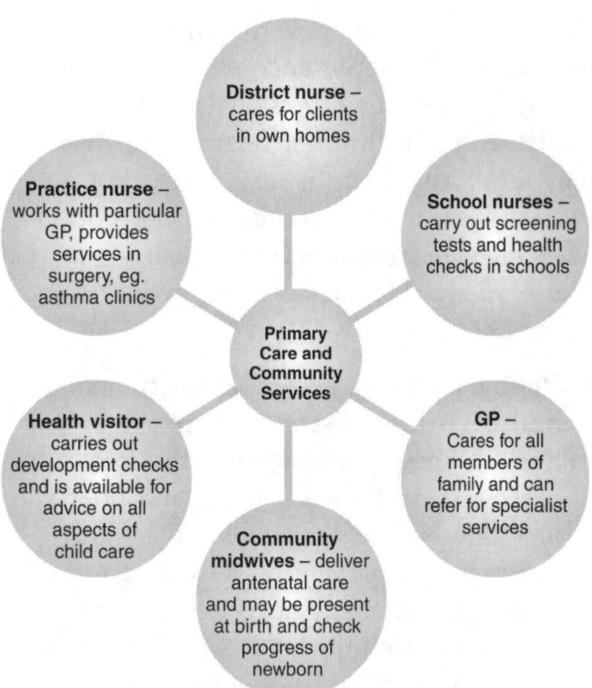


Figure 5.18 Examples of primary care services

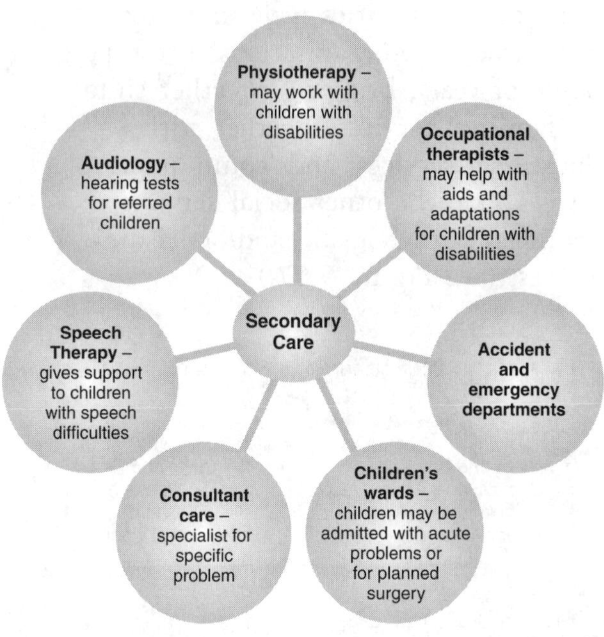


Figure 5.19 Examples of secondary care services for children

Newly formed primary care groups are now responsible for delivering and developing both primary care and community health services. They have control over resources, but have to account for the use of those resources in improving efficiency and quality of services. Primary care groups involve many different professionals and provide a range of services for a given locality. NHS trusts provide hospital services and have been responsible for some community health service provision through community NHS Trusts. It is envisaged that some of this will be done by the primary care groups, some of which may become primary care trusts, and will then be responsible for community services within their local area.

The focus of much health care in the early years is preventative, with regular developmental screening checks to ensure the early detection of any abnormalities. An example of developmental checks is given below.

| Age | Professional who carries out check |
|---|---|
| Birth | GP or paediatrician in hospital |
| 6 weeks | GP |
| 6–9 months | Health visitor or GP |
| 18–24 months | Health visitor |
| 3–3 $\frac{1}{2}$ years | GP or health visitor |

Table 5.6 Programme of developmental checks carried out by the health services

At each check the child will be measured to ensure that they are growing at the correct rate. This does vary from one child to another and percentile charts will show the acceptable range of normal. A physical

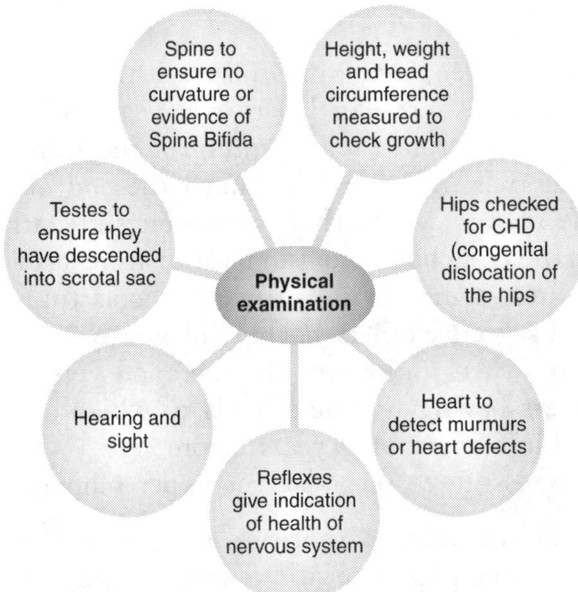


**Figure 5.20** Tests carried out during the physical examination of children

| Immunisation | Age |
|---|---|
| Diptheria, tetanus, pertussis (whooping cough) | 2, 3 and 4 months |
| Polio | 2, 3 and 4 months |
| Hib (meningitis) | 2, 3 and 4 months |
| MMR (measles, mumps, rubella) | 12 to 15 months |
| Diptheria, tetanus, polio and MMR booster | 3–5 years |
| Meningitis C | Babies and all children up to 18 |
| Tuberculosis | 10–14 years |
| Diptheria, tetanus, and polio booster | 15–19 years |

**Table 5.7** Immunisation programme

examination will be performed at birth, 6 weeks and three and a half years (and sometimes at the other checks as well), when the heart, hips, testes, spine and reflexes may also be checked. At each check the child's development is assessed to ensure that key developmental milestones are being reached.

Immunisation programmes are in place to reduce the incidence of certain infectious diseases (see above) and there are various screening programmes (see Table 5.8) for specific abnormalities, for example, screening for congenital dislocation of the hip. When problems are discovered, then the child will be referred to the appropriate specialist for treatment and care.

### Think it over

Jean has a three-year-old boy, Ryan, who has problems with his hearing and she is pregnant with her second child.

Figure 5.21 shows the professionals that Jean will come into contact with while she is pregnant and caring for her other child.

| Age | Condition | Referral to: |
|---|---|---|
| Birth | Congenital dislocation of hips | Consultant paediatrician |
| 11 days | Blood test for PKU (phenylketonuria) and growth hormone deficiency | Consultant paediatrician |
| 6–9 months | Hearing test (conducted by health visitor) | GP, then audiometrician. If hearing loss is found, then child may be referred on to paediatrician or ENT consultant and possible speech therapy. |

**Table 5.8** Specific screening tests

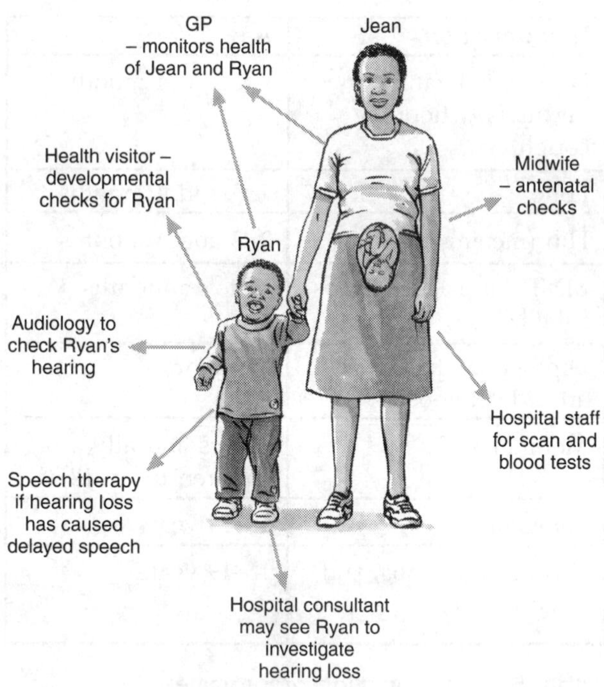


**Figure 5.21 Child health services**

Many services are concerned with prevention, early detection and health promotion. There has been considerable success in some areas, for example the incidence of some infectious diseases has been greatly reduced following immunisation programmes.

Throughout the health care services there has been growing recognition of the need to involve consumers in the planning and monitoring of services. Over recent years it has become increasingly apparent that the needs of children are very specific. The patients charter for children (Department of Health 1996) sought to protect the interests of children.

> **Try it out**
>
> Find out about the patients charter for children. What specific points does it raise? You could look it up on a government website.

## Education for children

All children, including those with disabilities, are entitled to receive education from the beginning of the term after their fifth birthday, until the end of the year in which they have their sixteenth birthday. School provision varies from area to area, some having primary schools (up to 11 years), others having infant (to 7 years) then junior (to 11 years) and yet others having middle schools to which children move at 9 years before progressing to secondary or upper schools.

Local education authorities, funded by the Department of Education, still control many schools, though the trend is for them to give a large proportion of their education budgets directly to schools. This local management of schools (LMS) enables the head teacher and governors of a school to decide how to spend the money. In addition to this, the Education Reform Act 1988 allowed schools to 'opt out' of local authority control and have grant-maintained status, by which they receive money directly from the government and not from the local authority, however this system is currently under review.

To ensure that all children follow a balanced and broad based curriculum it is

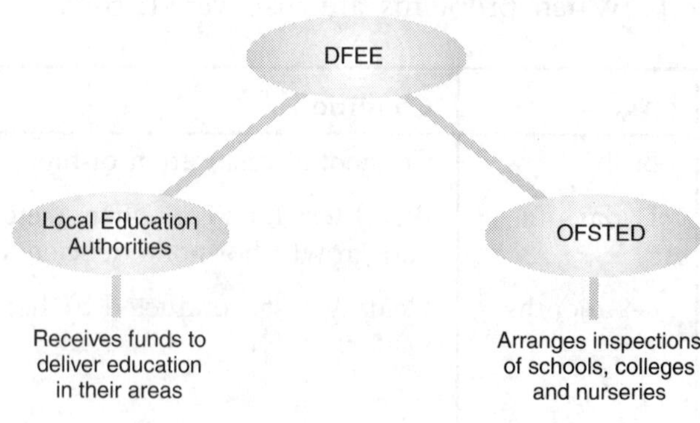


**Figure 5.22 Structure of education services**

required by law (Education Reform Act 1988) that all state schools follow the National Curriculum. The National Curriculum is divided into 'Key Stages' as follows.

| Key stage | Age | Test |
|---|---|---|
| 1 | 5–7 years | SATs at end of key stage |
| 2 | 7–11 years | SATs at end of key stage |
| 3 | 11–14 years | SATs at end of key stage |
| 4 | 14–16 years | GCSEs |

**Table 5.9 The National Curriculum Key Stages**

Parents are informed of their children's results in tests at the end of each Key Stage, and the performance of the school is made public through 'league tables'.

## Pre-school education

In addition to compulsory education from the age of five, many younger children attend nursery schools or classes. The provision of nursery education has been variable, but the government now fund education for all four-year-olds whether in state, private or voluntary establishments. Although many early years settings do not come under the direct control of LEAs, all establishments which receive funding are inspected for educational standards, by OFSTED.

These early years settings must demonstrate that they are following the Foundation Stage curriculum, for children aged three to five. The Foundation Stage is described as a series of stepping stones, ending in the 'Early Learning Goals', which are the goals most children are expected to achieve by the end of the reception year at school. The Foundation Stage curriculum is organised in six **areas of learning**:

- Personal, social and emotional development
- Communication, language and literacy
- Mathematical development
- Knowledge and understanding of the world
- Physical development
- Creative development.

As noted earlier, children with disabilities are entitled to education; for some this may be in a mainstream school, perhaps with support, for others the nature and extent of their problems may mean a more specialised environment is required.

### Try it out

Make a list under the following five headings of problems you can think of which might cause a child to have a special educational need: Physical, Psychological or Emotional, Sociocultural, Environmental, Political or Economic.

Following the Warnock Report in 1978, the Education Act 1981 made it a requirement that all children with special educational needs should be assessed to ascertain the best type of support that could be given. The assessment process should involve all those who have information about the child: parents, teachers, and health professionals and social workers. Assessments of this kind should take place regularly throughout the child's education as needs may change over time. Following the assessment a statement should be drawn up. This is a formal process of negotiation between the education authority and the parents and identifies the areas of need and the provision which will be made to meet those needs. What follows is a Statement of Special Educational Needs, which is a legal document. The Code of Practice introduced in 1994 gives guidelines on the procedures. Each school now has to appoint a Special Educational Needs Coordinator – SENCO – who takes an active role in the statementing and review of children with special needs. It is important to remember however that statements are only issued for a small number of children and there are many more who may have an IEP, Individual Education Plan, to help with one specific problem, for example ensuring that a child with a sight problem is able to sit near the front of the class.

## Social services for children

At a national level social services are responsible for the Benefits Agency and the Child Support Agency. There are many different types of benefit which can be claimed by children or which go towards supporting children, both contributory and

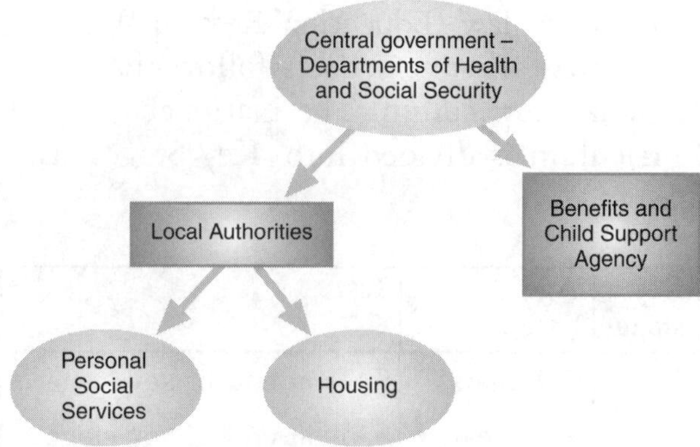


**Figure 5.23 Provision of social services for children**

non-contributory, some of which are illustrated in Table 5.10. Some people disagree with child benefit being a universal benefit, arguing that it is a waste of money as some people do not need it and there is therefore less money for those who do really need it. However, others argue that by paying benefit to everyone there is no shame in claiming it, and so families who do need the money actually get it, as often benefits go unclaimed.

Currently child benefit is paid to the mother (unless a specific request is made) and it remains a universal benefit, though

| Type of benefit | Examples | Conditions |
|---|---|---|
| Contributory benefits | Jobseekers allowance<br>State pensions<br>Statutory maternity pay | In order to claim the benefit people must have paid sufficient national insurance contributions |
| Non-contributory benefits usually | Income support<br>Family credit<br><br>Housing benefit | Claimants must meet given criteria, these benefits are means tested and people must show how much they are earning before a benefit is paid |
| Universal benefits | Child benefit | Given to everyone who fulfils criteria – regardless of income |
| Other benefits | Free prescriptions<br>Free school meals | People often qualify for these benefits by being in receipt of others |

**Table 5.10 Benefits that can be claimed for children and which go towards supporting children**

there are both advantages and disadvantages associated with the payment of universal benefits.

Growing numbers of women returning to work when children are below school age has led to an increased demand for child care. The National Child Care Strategy, a government-funded initiative, aims to ensure the provision of good quality, accessible and affordable child care for children up to the age of 14. A number of child care options exist, though the number of registered day nursery places available has shown a particularly large increase over recent years, rising from 32,000 in 1987 to 211,000 in 1998. In the same period the number of places with childminders has more than doubled from 153,000 to 388,000 while the number of places in play groups has fallen.

**Try it out**

Where are children cared for? List as many child care facilities as you can.

Social services departments have a duty to inspect and register all premises and persons who work with children under eight. This includes:

- Playgroups – may be voluntary or private and if registered for nursery grant for education of four-year-olds will be inspected by OFSTED. Playgroups usually offer sessional care.
- Creches – offer short-term care in shopping centres or sport centres or wherever there is demand.
- After school clubs – no set curriculum, they provide a safe environment for children whose parents may have to work beyond school hours. Often there is the opportunity for children to explore new hobbies or activities.
- Childminders – offer care usually in their own home often while parents are at work.
- Foster carers – care on a short or longer term basis for children who, for a variety of reasons, are not able to be cared for by their own parents.
- Nurseries – these may be attached to a school or privately or voluntarily run, a few being run by social services. Nurseries are required to follow the early years curriculum.

Working to guidelines in the Children Act, premises are inspected to ensure there is adequate space and toilet facilities, that food preparation is hygienic, that the environment is safe and that there are suitable and appropriate toys and play equipment. Guidelines for staff:child ratios are given and these vary depending upon the age of the children being looked after.

| Age of children | Required adult child ratio |
|---|---|
| 0–1 years | 1 adult to 3 children |
| 1–3 years | 1 adult to 4 children |
| 3–5 years | 1 adult to 8 children |

Table 5.11 Guidelines for staff:child ratios

Checks are also made on the people who work with children. In settings where more than three children are cared for Police screening is carried out to ensure that no one who has previous convictions for offences against children is allowed to work with children. It is essential that there is somebody with a recognised qualification in child care, though there may be unqualified helpers. Only when all the criteria have been fulfilled will a child care establishment be registered by social services. It is then inspected on a regular basis, usually each year, and the registration can be terminated, if standards fall. Similarly, childminders and foster carers are assessed and their homes inspected before they are registered by social services. In most areas some training is given, though the length of training courses may vary.

### Children in need

Social services departments, through local authorities, also have a duty towards children in need. The reason for such needs vary and can include children having no parent or guardian, being abandoned or the parent being unable to provide for them. Personal social services also help children who are considered to be at risk of abuse. A central register of such children is held by all local authority social services departments. This is called the child protection register. A case conference, at which decisions are made about the level of risk, is always held prior to a child's name being placed on the register and a plan is set out to protect the child. In 1998, 35,500 children in England and Wales were on child protection registers. Children with disabilities are also defined as being in need and local authorities have to keep a register of these children. As part of their work with children in need local authorities provide the following services:

- support, through social workers, counselling, home help, to enable children to stay with their families
- family centres, where parents may meet their children, or attend with children to receive support or specific guidance

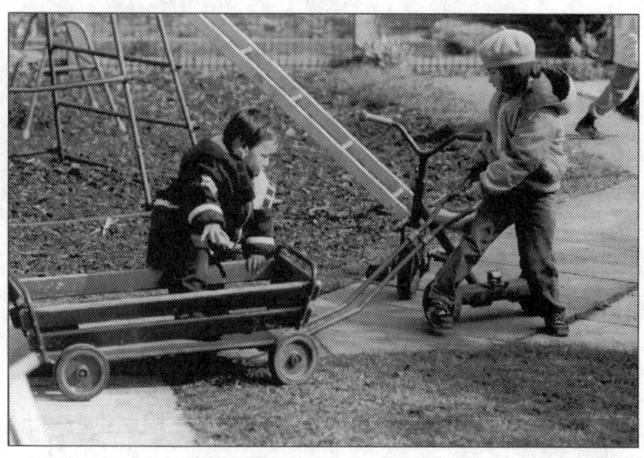

**Children with disabilities are defined as 'children in need'**

- day care, nurseries, childminders and out of school care.

### Working together

The vast range of services for early years provided by differing agencies has highlighted the need for liaison and integration of these services. In 1996 it became mandatory for local authorities to prepare and publish children's services plans. Social services produce plans, on behalf of local authorities, in consultation with health, education and other agencies. The plans were seen to be a tool to aid integration of services for children following a report by Utting (1991) on 'Children in Public Care'. The legal obligation for such plans relates particularly to children in need, however local authorities have been encouraged to consider plans in the context of services to all children in their locality.

#### Think it over

What may be the consequences if different agencies involved with families do not liaise or communicate effectively? Can you think of any examples from the media?

You may be able to remember particular cases where there have been tragic consequences. It is vital for the efficiency of services and therefore improved effectiveness that there is communication and liaison. It is also vital that people who have knowledge of local needs are involved in the planning of services. This is one of the aims behind the newly formed primary care groups, expressed in the NHS's White Paper 5, as . . . 'to better integrate primary and community health services and work more closely with social services on both planning and delivery. Services such as child health . . . where responsibilities have been split within the health service and where liaison with local authorities is often poor will particularly benefit.'

## Independent organisations

The work of the voluntary and private organisations in health and social care has always been of great importance. Some services to which people are statutorily entitled are provided by the independent sector, especially by voluntary organisations, although these services may have to be commissioned by the NHS or by the local authority. Services may be commissioned either by awarding grants to certain organisations, or by contracting with the organisations to provide the service. For example, some local authorities give grants to the local branches of Crossroads who provide a sitting service for sick or disabled people to allow their carer to have a break; while some Health Authorities may have a contract with a hospice to provide specialist palliative care services for people with an incurable terminal illness.

The **voluntary sector** has been established over a long period of time and is by far the largest provider of care within the **independent sector**, and in the past 30 years has seen a major growth. The range of activities of voluntary organisations is wide and may include self-help groups (such as Alcoholics Anonymous), pressure groups (such as Child Poverty Action Group), advisory groups (such as Release, which works with drug users), specific support groups (such as Arthritis Care), or umbrella organisations that help to co-ordinate a number of other agencies (such as the Organisation Development Unit, which acts as a development agency for black voluntary groups).

Many of the larger voluntary organisations are organised on national, regional and local levels. One such organisation is Age Concern. At a national level Age Concern England is responsible for developing policies and procedures in respect of the organisation, providing an information and advice service including publishing leaflets on all aspects of the welfare of older people and representing older people's needs to the public. At a regional level it co-ordinates services, monitors the quality of its services and provides support for local branches. Local branches are responsible for providing a range of services which may include day centre and luncheon club facilities, holidays and outings, counselling and befriending services, and help with practical activities such as gardening or decorating.

The private sector has also grown in recent years and is likely to continue to grow. However, it has always been susceptible to fluctuations in the economic state of the country and individuals.

The move away from a Welfare State to a **mixed economy** of health and social care will mean an increased role in care provision for the independent sector.

## 5.3 Informal carers

**Informal care** is a term used to describe the care given to someone who is ill or disabled by anyone other than a paid worker. The informal carer may be a family member, a friend or a neighbour; although informal care may also be provided by local groups, such as church groups or family support groups. The government's 1998 White Paper *Caring for People* acknowledged that 'the great bulk of community care is provided by friends, family and neighbours' and that 'carers need help and support if they are to continue to carry out their role'. In 1998 it was estimated that there was approximately 7 million carers in the UK, that is about one in eight adults giving informal care and one in six homes that have a carer. The General Household Survey of 1995 showed that 1.9 million provide more than 20 hours per week to a sick, disabled or elderly person.

The survey also showed that the majority of older people needing long-term care receive it from a family member, usually a spouse or an adult son or daughter. Carers play a vital role in looking after those who are sick, disabled, vulnerable or frail.

Informal carers have an invaluable role to play, providing all sorts of care, including:

- helping people get up from and return to bed
- helping them to get washed and dressed
- helping them to bathe or shower
- helping them with toileting
- preparing meals and refreshments
- monitoring and dispensing medicines
- providing transport for social and medical purposes
- providing leisure activities
- ensuring general safety and well-being.

### Needs of carers

Caring is a difficult task and is undertaken often at considerable personal cost – physical, emotional and financial. Caring for someone can be extremely tiring both emotionally and physically and carers undoubtedly experience higher than average levels of stress. Recent research has shown that in order to continue with this role, carers need help in various ways, including:

- time off from caring
- relief from isolation, and satisfaction with the help they receive from their family and others
- receipt of reliable and satisfactory services
- recognition of their role and contribution.

- 15 per cent of people aged 16 or over were carers in 1990.
- 60 per cent of adult carers are women; 40 per cent are men.
- 48 per cent of adult carers are caring for a parent or parent-in-law.
- 71 per cent of people receiving care are women.

(Taken from *Young Carers. The Facts* published by Reed Business

**Think it over**

Talk with a friend, family member or someone in a caring profession: why are there more women in a caring role than there are men?

## Case study: Yvonne

Yvonne is 47 years old and for the past three years has been looking after her 82-year-old mother, Yolanda, who has Alzheimer's disease, which is a form of dementia. Yvonne first noticed changes in her mother some years ago when she began to forget everyday things, couldn't find the right word to say what she wanted and kept repeating what she had just been talking about. Yolanda's short-term memory loss became far worse and her behaviour more erratic and aggressive as time went by. Three years ago Yolanda was found wandering the streets, unable to find her way home, which she insisted was in Poland. She had not lived in Poland since she was a teenager.

Since Yvonne, who is single, moved back to live with her mother (giving up a well-paid job and the company of her work colleagues), her mother's ability to hold any sort of sustained or rational conversation has deteriorated and it has not been possible to maintain any daily routines. She continually repeats what she has just said, asks the same question over and over again, and repeats the same actions over and over. She is unable to remember if she has eaten or not, does not recognise the house as being her home, or who her daughter is. It is very frustrating and frightening for her and for Yvonne, and both have become very isolated from friends and other family members. Yvonne feels that no-one is interested in her situation or understands how difficult things are for her. She says that it is like living with a stranger and feels her real mother 'died' three years ago.

***Questions***

1 List three things that might help Yvonne cope more easily with her caring role.

2 What things make it 'frustrating and frightening' for Yolanda?

3 Why does Yvonne say that she feels her 'real mother died three years ago'?

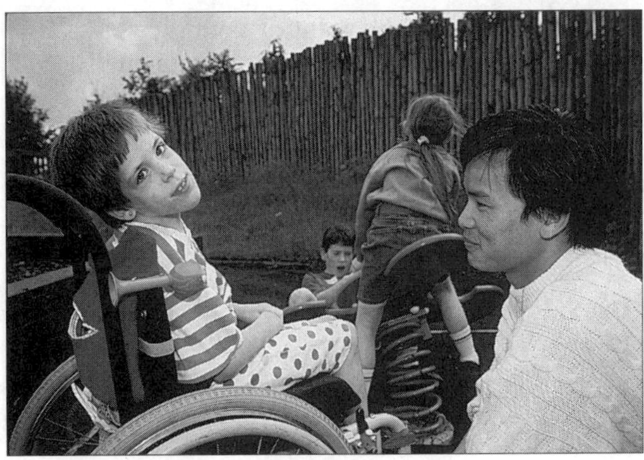

Informal carers play vital roles

The needs of individual carers will differ depending on their age, cultural background and whether they live in an inner city or rural area. For example, an older carer may also have health needs of his or her own; young carers may be juggling school and social activities with the caring role; a carer in a rural area may have less access to transport or the assistance of neighbours.

Carers need to know what help is available: what they can expect from health and social services. They also need to know how to access this help. Therefore it is essential to have clear information about the kind of support that is available.

Finances are often another issue for carers. Carers who give up paid work to care for someone may encounter financial difficulties that give rise to additional stresses; therefore some form of financial support may be needed. Many carers wish to combine part-time, or even full-time, work with their caring responsibilities. They need employment conditions that take account of their caring role and are flexible to help them in this.

> **Think it over**
>
> Do you know someone who is an informal carer? How does he or she help the person who is being cared for? Does the carer receive any support in carrying out this role?

## Young carers

**Young carers** are defined in the guidance issues by the Social Services Inspectorate in April 1995 as 'a child or young person (up to the age of 18) who is carrying out significant caring tasks and assuming a level of responsibility for another person, which would normally be undertaken by an adult'. The plight of young carers has been given a lot of media coverage in recent years. Research published by the Health Services Management Unit at Manchester University in March 1995 indicated that there are likely to be between 15,000 and 40,000 young carers nationally. However, accurate figures are difficult to obtain as many of those who are caring are 'hidden'. Most young carers are caring for a parent, commonly in a single parent family, but some may be taking care of a grandparent, brother or sister or other family member. Even when there are extended family members living near by, surveys by the Young Carers Research Group have shown that relatives will step in during a crisis, but do not offer day-to-day support. The range of caring responsibilities can include:

- domestic chores – cooking, cleaning, shopping
- personal care – washing, dressing, toileting their relative
- family responsibilities – caring for a brother or sister, managing the household budget
- medical care – administering medication, injections
- emotional support – for other family members.

Young carers are often isolated from their peers as they have little leisure time; but they are also in danger of losing out educationally, either because they miss time from school or are too tired to be able to participate fully. The family may also be on a low income and may be relying on state benefits. (People under 16 are not entitled to benefits in their own right.)

- 61 per cent of young carers are caring for their mothers.
- 30 per cent of young carers care for someone with a mental health problem.
- 61 per cent of young carers are female; 39 per cent are male.
- One in ten young carers is caring for more than one person.

(Taken from *Young Carers. The Facts* published by Reed Business Publishing/Young Carers Research Group, 1995)

## The needs of young carers

Young carers have very special needs and should be able to make informed choices about their situation. They need:

- someone to talk to who will listen and believe them
- recognition of their role as a carer
- information – about their relative's condition, about services and how to access them
- practical assistance and support.

## The Carers (Recognition and Services) Act 1995

This Act is a milestone for those who act as carers because it gives them a legal status for the first time. The Act places duties on local authorities to *assess* the ability of the carers to provide and to continue to provide for the person being cared for. They must assess the carers' needs separately from those of service users and have to take account of this assessment when making care arrangements for the service user. However, at present carers are not entitled to *receive* services in their own right independently from the user for whom they are caring. (There is a Bill, *The Carers and Disabled Children Bill*, going through Parliament at present that could remedy this.)

The Carers' National Association/ADSS survey, *In on the Act*, published in 1997, showed that 85 per cent of local authorities have already gone some way in meeting parts of the Act. However, due to increasing demand on services and financial constraints, the pace of the development of services for carers is slower than hoped.

The Act is concerned with:

- Adults (people aged 18 or over) who provide, or intend to provide, a *substantial* amount of care on a *regular* basis
- Children and young people (under 18) who provide, or intend to provide, a *substantial* amount of care on a *regular* basis. (This also includes brothers and sisters of disabled children.)
- Parents who provide, or intend to provide, a *substantial* amount of care on a *regular* basis for children with a disability.

Each local authority has to define what is meant by the terms *substantial* and *regular*. One definition could be *'Where the removal of the carer's support would mean that the cared for person's level of independence could not be maintained in the essential tasks of daily living; where the carer's health is likely to break down; or where the development of a child is likely to be impaired'*. It is possible that each local authority could have different definitions of these terms. This could lead to inequality of access to services across the country.

The Act states that:

- A carer is entitled, on request, to an assessment of need when a local authority carries out an assessment of the person cared for, in respect of Community Care Services or services for children.
- The results of the assessment should be taken into account when the local authority is making decisions about services to be provided to the user.

The Act places the responsibility on the carer to *ask* for an assessment. The local authority is under no obligation to automatically make an assessment of the carer's needs.

## Case study: Neil

Neil is eleven years old and lives with his mother who has epilepsy. He has a younger sister called Cathy. She is six years old. They have no contact with their father. When Neil's mother has a fit he cares for her and tries to ensure her safety. He also has to take care of Cathy at these times. Neil finds it very distressing when he sees his mother fitting. He gets very frightened and tearful. On one occasion his mother had to go to hospital and a neighbour looked after Neil and his sister. Neil is worried about what would happen to him and his sister if his mother had to go into hospital again. He knows very little about epilepsy and thinks that he might be responsible for causing his mother's fits sometimes, especially when he has been 'naughty'. Neil and his family have no help from anyone or any agency, other than their next door neighbour.

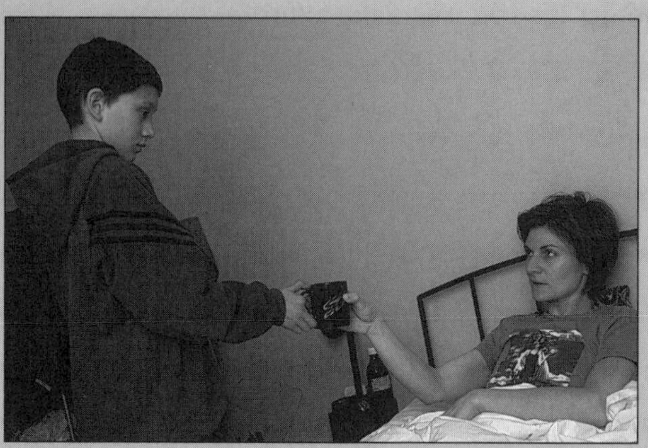

Young carers have very special needs and big responsibilities

***Question:***

What sort of help would Neil and his family benefit from? Where could he get this help?

The assessment might cover such things as:

- the carer's perception of the situation
- the tasks undertaken and consequent impact on the carer and the family
- the tasks the carer would like help with
- the carer's social contacts, family, employment and other commitments
- the carer's emotional, mental and physical health
- the carer's willingness and/or ability to continue to provide care.

In respect of young carers, local authorities should also consider:

- that the provision of community services should ensure that they do not carry inappropriate levels of caring responsibilities. It should not be assumed that young carers should take on similar levels of caring as adults
- how the young carer might be helping with both the care needs and parenting responsibilities, and ensure that they are not being exploited
- even if a young carer does not request an assessment, the local authority should still consider whether there is a need to assist or relieve the child. This can be done either through the provision of

community care services for the cared-for person, or through the provision of services to promote the welfare of the child

- where the development of the young carer is being impaired by their caring role, the local authority may consider whether they should exercise their existing duties towards children in need (see information on The Children Act)
- Social services departments should ensure that any young carers known to them have information on local arrangements for community care and that they are encouraged to discuss any concerns informally.

## Support for informal carers

Social service provision, such as home care, day care and respite care in a residential home, is provided specifically for the service user; however, these services do have the effect of lightening the practical load of the informal carer and of giving them a break from the caring role from time to time.

In addition to the practical support provided by social services, health services also have an important part to play in supporting carers. In response to a postal questionnaire sent out by the Carers' National Association in December 1997, 50 per cent of carers said they had received help from a district nurse, 28 per cent from a community nurse, 14 per cent from a community psychiatric nurse and 6 per cent from a night nurse. These services were highly valued by the people who received them.

The government has now set out a **National Strategy for Carers**, *Caring About Carers,* which aims to enhance the quality of life for all informal carers. The strategy emphasises that all organisations involved with caring must now not only focus on the person requiring care but also on the informal carers. To do this they state that means should be found to give carers:

- the freedom to have a life of their own
- time for themselves
- the opportunity to continue to work, if that is what they want to do
- control over their life and over the support they need in it
- better health and well-being
- integration into the community
- peace of mind.

The Strategy has three key elements:

- **information** for carers – providing the right information at the right time. The information must be accurate and given verbally as well as in writing
- **support** for carers in carrying out their caring responsibilities

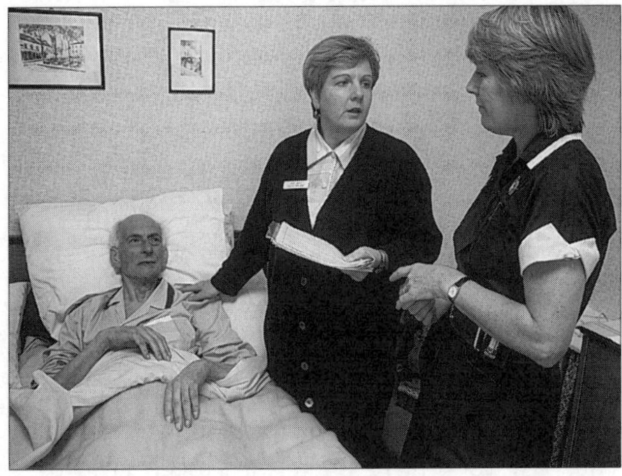

Hospices can provide respite care for someone who is seriously ill – and gives their usual carers a break

- **care** for the carers' own health and well-being.

Many health and local authorities are already beginning to make changes that recognise the need to support carers. These may include:

- recognising carers' needs in the work-force as part of their personnel policies (which supports their own employees who have a caring role)
- developing a strategy to support carers
- taking account of the views of carers as part of its consultation and planning processes.

In support of these aims the government has allocated £750 million for the three years 1999-2001 to promote the independence through prevention of illness, disability or disease, and through rehabilitation, for carers and the people that they care for. In addition to this they are making available a special grant to local authorities for the enhancement of services to allow carers to take a break from caring. Over the three years, the grant will total £140 million for England. The services that may be extended include domiciliary and sitting services that give the carer a short break, or longer breaks or holidays. It is up to each local authority to apply for the grant and then decide how it should be managed and spent. However, it is still unclear what will happen at the end of the three year period and whether the enhanced level of provision of services will be maintained or how they will be funded.

One of the problems facing carers is that in the past they have not always been able to rely on the quality of support that they have received. The King's Fund, as part of the National Strategy for Carers, has drafted standards for carer support services, which are aimed at services provided by statutory agencies and voluntary organisations. There are eight standards:

- information that is comprehensible, accurate and appropriate
- services accessible and responsive to individual needs
- to provide a break from care
- to work in partnership with the carer and person being supported
- to maintain the health and well-being of carers by offering training, health promotion and personal development opportunities
- to be flexible and give confidence
- offer emotional support and be sensitive to individual needs
- to have a voice which is accessible to all carers and is effective in bringing about change.

It is hoped that all organisations providing support to carers will adopt these standards.

### Voluntary organisations

There are many voluntary organisations that provide support for carers. One of these is **Crossroads**. This is a home-based respite service to relieve carers who are looking after dependent relatives or friends in their own homes. Services that can be provided include 'sitting services' or help with personal care. Carers can be of any age and the service is provided by paid and trained care attendants who are employed by Crossroads. There are over 235 schemes countrywide. In recognition of the particular needs of young carers, Crossroads has appointed an assistant director for young carers and is beginning to develop some projects aimed specifically at helping young carers.

The **Carers' National Association** (CNA) was established in 1988 to become the voice for all carers in the UK. The Association produces information for carers and professionals. In 1990 it also developed a Young Carers Project, funded by the Department of Health, to co-ordinate research, development and support work nationally. It now produces a newsletter for young carers. CNA has also been campaigning for practical measures which support working carers, such as statutory carers' leave and a right to flexible working. The government is now taking action to enable employees to take unpaid leave for family emergencies.

In 1991, Barnardos set up a project in the northwest of England to identify young carers and their needs and to raise awareness among organisations which provide care services. This began initially with three years funding from the Department of Health. Currently there are three projects working towards these aims and enabling young carers to get involved and help influence professionals.

## Helplines

Helplines are also being developed to help support carers. Some of these are well established, such as Mind, for people with mental health problems, while others are very new and may not yet be UK-wide, such as Healthline, which is a free confidential telephone service giving advice on all health-related issues to people in certain areas of London. A NHS Direct helpline for carers is also being developed. Other organisations that provide helplines include BACUP, for people whose lives are affected by cancer; SCOPE, for people affected by cerebral palsy or disability; Adfam National, for families and friends of drug users; and the Carers' National Association. However there are many others.

### Think it over

What other national organisations can you think of that give help, information or advice to carers? Which of these are aimed at people with specific problems and which are for all carers in general?

## Self-help groups

In addition to the national organisations, which often offer support to people with particular problems, local **self-help groups** may be developed. Self-help groups are set up by people who are, or have, experienced particular difficulties and members of the group use their own experiences, knowledge and skills to help one another. Self-help groups develop their own aims and objectives, depending on the specific interests and concerns of their members. These groups therefore develop in many varied ways, each with its own ideas and characteristics.

For example, in one area parents supporting bereaved children, where one parent has died, may get together to give one another support in this role and to give the children support by bringing them together with other bereaved children. As well as discussion groups, they may also organise social gatherings and outings. In another area, a self-help group might be developed by people who suffer from depression. The group may meet on a regular basis in order to give general emotional support to one another and may develop a system for providing immediate support at a time of crisis for its members. The group may also provide support for the families and carers of people who suffer from depression.

In another area a group may be started by the parents of children with disabilities. The group may aim to give general emotional and practical support to one another, but may also act as a negotiating body with local service providers regarding services in their area. They could even become a group that lobbies MPs regarding the rights of disabled children, or on the national provision of services.

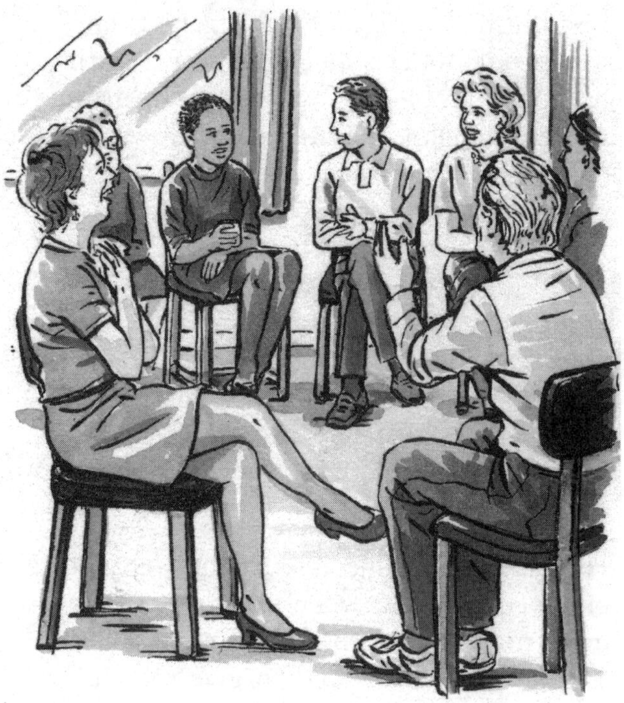

**Self-help groups can offer emotional and practical support to their members**

Some financial help is now available to carers who give up full-time work in order to look after someone. The Invalid Carers' Allowance (ICA) is a taxable benefit for carers who are looking after someone for at least 35 hours per week.

## 5.4 The funding of services

Health and social care may be resourced in a number of different ways, as shown in Figure 5.24 below.

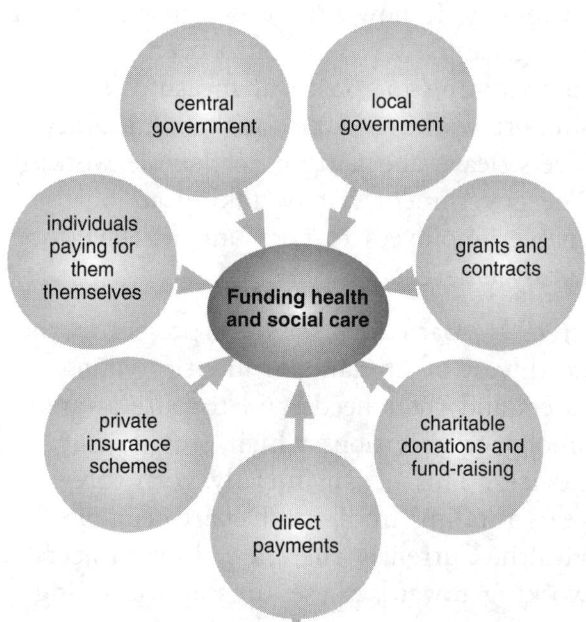


**Figure 5.24 Health and social care services may be funded in a variety of ways**

### Direct funding from central government

The NHS is funded by central government. Revenue is collected through national taxation – income tax, value added tax (VAT) and National Insurance contributions paid by individuals and organisations. The Treasury and the Department of Health have to decide how much money is to be spent on the NHS each year. The Department of Health then allocates money to the Health Authorities according to a formula based on size, age and health of their resident population. The Health Authorities can then purchase services to meet the needs of the population in their area.

In 1994 the estimated cost of the NHS in England was met as follows:

- 82 per cent from general taxation
- 12.7 per cent from national insurance contributions
- 3 per cent from various charges to patients
- 2.3 per cent from capital sales and other receipts.

The cost of welfare provision has continued to grow steadily over the years. The total cost of all welfare services (including education, housing and benefits) stood in excess of £131 billion in 1997, having risen from around £90 billion in 1973.

Expenditure on the NHS increased from £28.9 billion in 1993–4 to £36.5 billion in 1998-9 and is likely to rise to £46 billion in 2001–2.

Central government also gives monies to local authorities. The total amount that they give is determined by the Treasury and Department of Health, who then use a formula called the 'Standard Spending Assessment' (SSA), to determine how much each authority will receive and this is distributed through the revenue support grant. The formula takes into account such things as the number of old people living in the area, the percentage of rented accommodation, the number of single-parent families, the percentage of people from ethnic minority backgrounds, and the density of population.

Funding for social services has risen to £9.3 billion. Funding is broken down into three main areas:

- services for children – £2.1 billion
- residential care for older people – £3.2 billion
- domiciliary care for older people – £1.9 billion

*(Figures at December 1999.)*

Over the three years 1999 to 2002 the government will increase the funding available for social services by an annual average of 3.1 per cent above inflation. In addition to this, another £416 million has been allocated through special social services grants. There are four areas that these cover, three are aimed at promoting independence and the fourth is to enhance children's services.

There are also specific grants, totalling a further £194 million. These are:

- the training support grant – £42.5 million
- the AIDS support grant – £16 million
- the drug and alcohol misusers grant – £6.7 million
- the mental health grant – £129.4 million
- the secure accommodation grant – £14,000

*(Figures at December 1999.)*

From time to time central government will make special direct payments in order to fund special initiatives. For example, as part of the extra funding the government will be introducing a Social Services Modernisation Fund. The total for this over the three years 1999/00 to 2001/02 is £1347 million.

## Early years funding

In many ways the funding for services for the early years reflects the funding for more general services. The services for early years include statutory, voluntary and independently funded services.

> **Think it over**
>
> Think of some of the services for early years that you know about. How are they funded?

Figure 5.25 gives a broad outline of many of the services for early years.

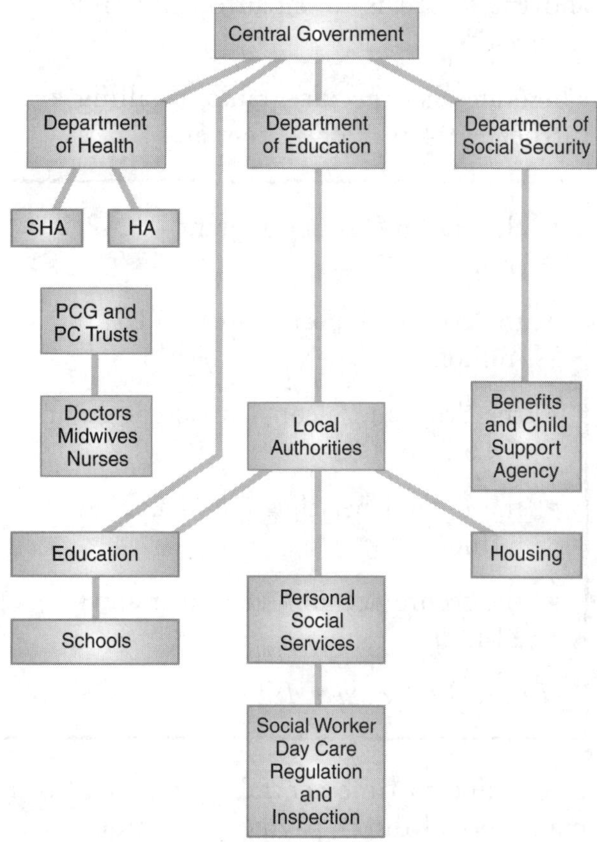


**Figure 5.25** Services for early years

### Statutory services

A large proportion of the health, education and social services for the early years are funded by the government. Recent years have seen many changes in the way the funding mechanisms operate and the level of autonomy that is given to local areas or departments in using the funding to provide services.

Central government expenditure on hospitals and community health services and family health services has more than doubled, rising from £21,771 million in 1988 to £45,346 million in 1998. In England the number of doctors on the family health services list has risen steadily to 26,855 in 1997, with the number of patients per doctor declining slightly from 1,902 in 1993 to 1,885 in 1997.

Primary care groups and the soon-to-be established primary care trusts will be responsible for the provision and development of primary health services and community health services.

Within education the majority of funding is still from central government. Table 5.12 opposite shows government expenditure on education over recent years.

Recent legislative changes have meant that schools can opt out from local authority control and access resources direct from central government. Schools that do not opt out still exercise more control over resources than previously as there is now a local management of schools initiative. This is generally regarded as being a positive change which has given local head teachers and governors more say in how resources are deployed, and they can therefore tailor provision to the needs of the local population. In addition to special school provision there were over 250,000 pupils in

| | 1988 | 1989 | 1990 | 1991 | 1992 | 1993 | 1994 | 1995 | 1996 | 1997 |
|---|---|---|---|---|---|---|---|---|---|---|
| Nursery & primary schools | 4,743 | 5,259 | 5,889 | 6,458 | 7,247 | 8,262 | 8,712 | 9,094 | 9,349 | 9,676 |
| Secondary schools | 5,991 | 6,437 | 6,832 | 7,147 | 7,787 | 8,347 | 8,615 | 8,875 | 8,987 | 9,253 |
| Special schools | 812 | 888 | 1,008 | 1,121 | 1,245 | 1,354 | 1,420 | 1,451 | 1,492 | 1,567 |

**Table 5.12 Government spending on education (£ in millions)**

schools in England in January 1999 who had a statement of special educational needs.

Personal social services provide a range of services for early years, both directly – for example social workers who work with families and children in need – and indirectly – for example in registering and inspecting nurseries and childcare facilities. In addition, families with dependent children are offered support by the social security system in the form of cash benefits. Child benefit was received by 7 million families in Britain in 1997-98. The growth in lone parent families means recipients on one-parent benefit has increased over the last decade from 469,000 in 1981-82 to over one million in 1997-98. Recent years have seen an increase in the provision of nursery places for children, though fewer are directly provided by local authorities.

| | 1987 | 1992 | 1997 | 1998 |
|---|---|---|---|---|
| Local authority provided | 29 | 24 | 20 | 19 |
| Registered | 32 | 96 | 180 | 211 |

**Table 5.13 Day nursery places for children (England & Wales) (in thousands)**

## Voluntary services

There are many voluntary services involved with early years provision. These may be very specific, for example the National Autistic Association, or more general, for example the NSPCC.

Although the aims of the organisations vary they usually share a common purpose in promoting awareness, raising funds and providing services for children and their families.

### Try it out

Working in groups produce a 'fact file' of the voluntary organisations which exist for children in your locality.

## Independent services

Recent years have seen considerable growth in private nurseries. These are run by individuals or companies, though they must be registered by social services. There are also a growing number of childminders, which reflects the trend of increasing numbers of women working away from home and the desire shown by an increasing number of parents for their children to begin education before statutory school age. The government has acknowledged this trend and education for four-year-olds is funded by the local authority, provided the establishment can show it is working towards the desirable outcomes of the early years curriculum.

## Local government

In addition to the money that local authorities receive from central government, they obtain funding from other sources which are raised locally. These include:

- local council taxes
- business rates
- charges for some services.

(See Figure 5.26.)

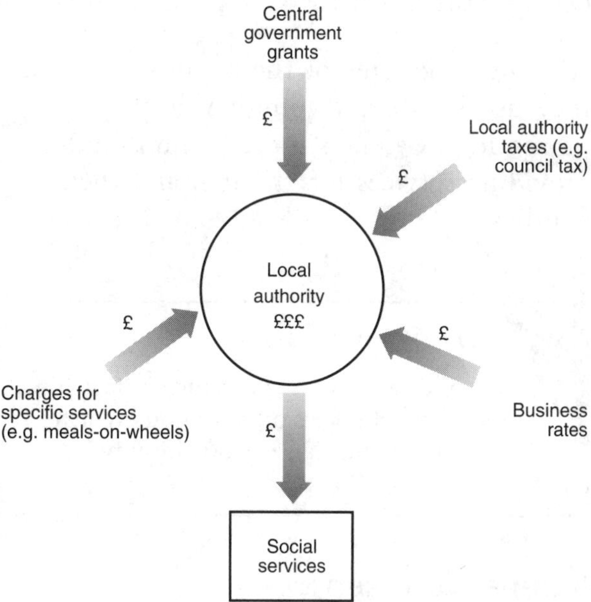


**Figure 5.26 Sources of funding for social services**

The local authority allocates money from all its sources to its various departments: housing, education, leisure, refuse collection, environmental health, etc. In many authorities the biggest expenditure is on education, with social services taking the next largest amount.

## Grants, contracts and other forms of fund-raising

Funding for voluntary organisations comes from five main sources:

- grants from central government, in order to carry out specific projects
- grants from local authorities, for the provision of specific services
- contracts from health authorities or social services departments
- charitable grants from organisations and businesses
- fund-raising through local events, donations and legacies.

(See Figure 5.27.)

Applications can be made to central government departments, usually by voluntary groups and organisations, for

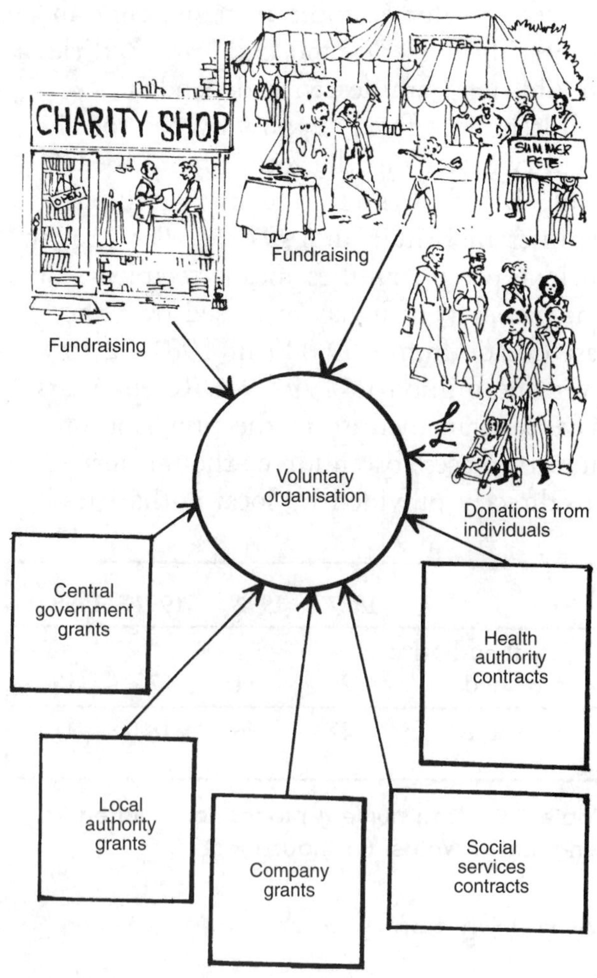


**Figure 5.27 Financing voluntary organisations**

grants towards various projects. Below are some examples of a few of the grants that are available from central government.

The Department of Health currently has three special grant programmes in operation. These are:

- *Health and personal social service – Section 64 grants*
  Mainly for setting up new initiatives in health and social care e.g. CRUSE Bereavement Care and Action Against Allergy
- *Opportunities for Volunteering Scheme*
  This aims to develop opportunities for unemployed people to undertake voluntary work and to expand voluntary work in health and social care services
- *Shared Training Grant programme*
  This aims to support services for people with learning difficulties e.g. Home Farm Trust.

The Department of Education also has three special programmes in operation:

- *Early Years Division – Section 64 grants*
  For voluntary organisations that help promote the government's policies for young children e.g. Kids Club Network
- *Adult and Community Learning Fund*
  To sustain and encourage new local schemes that help men and women gain access to education
- *National Voluntary Youth Organisation*
  To support planned programmes of informal and experimental education providing opportunities for young people which help them cope with the transition from childhood to adulthood.

Local authorities can also give grants, for example, they may give some funds to the local Age Concern group to provide day care facilities and luncheon clubs for older people in its area. A Health Authority may give a grant toward the setting up of a twenty-four hour home nursing service in order to provide a carer with respite at home.

Health and local authorities are beginning to reduce the amount of money available for grants and instead are increasingly 'contracting' services with the voluntary sector. A Health Authority may have a contract with a local hospice to provide palliative care for people with a terminal illness, such as cancer or AIDS. A local authority may contract with an organisation such as Crossroads to provide a sitting service for elderly and frail people in their area, so that their carer can go shopping or on a social outing. Although the contracting culture may provide more financial security for some voluntary organisations, others may not be able to survive. Many voluntary organisations only have short-term contracts with health and local authorities, making future planning very difficult and making workers in the organisation feel very insecure.

**Try it out**

Find out if there are any voluntary organisations in your area that are funded from contracts with the health or local authority.

Many private companies and organisations also give grants to voluntary agencies. These are often for specific projects, for example educational courses or building projects. They are rarely for the actual day-to-day running costs of the agency, i.e. staff salaries or for paying bills.

Often more than 50 per cent of a voluntary organisation's funds will come from fund-raising events. These may include:

sponsored events, discos, quiz evenings, summer and Christmas fairs; charity shops; donations from individuals and groups; or from legacies. Voluntary organisations rely on the general public; local communities, individuals and their own volunteer work force, to raise a high proportion of their funds in order to continue their services.

## Direct payments for services

In 1997 the Community Care (direct payment) Act 1996 came into force enabling local authorities to set up Direct Payment Schemes. These schemes enable disabled people aged 18 to 65 years to receive payments from the local authority which they then use to purchase their own care and to choose their own carers. This could result in the disabled person being the employer of the care giver. This places responsibilities as an employer on the disabled person but allows more flexibility in the way that care is received. The direct payment legislation is not mandatory and it seems that some local authorities have been reluctant to set up these schemes. However, the government plans to extend direct payment schemes to other groups, such as older people and people with learning difficulties.

The Carers and Disabled Children's Bill is currently being considered by Parliament. This could allow carers to receive vouchers to use when they want a break from caring and entitle them to receive direct payment, allowing them to decide what services to buy for their children. Disabled 16-17 year olds will also be able to demand direct payments. The Bill will also introduce a statutory duty on local authorities to provide services directly for the carer to meet their assessed needs.

**Think it over**

Do you know of anyone that might be able to receive direct payments? What sort of services do you think they would want to purchase?

## Free and paid-for services

This section will look at services which are free at the point of delivery and services which will require an assessment of the individual's ability to pay.

Services provided by the NHS are still largely free of charge. These include secondary health care, such as accident and emergency services, treatment for acute medical conditions (for example, following a stroke or the onset of an acute illness) and planned treatment (for example, eye surgery for the removal of cataracts or hip replacement surgery). However, other medical care, particularly primary health services, still require the user to make a payment towards the cost at the time that they require the service. These include payments for:

- drugs and appliances on prescription from a GP or dentist, or by hospital out-patient clinics
- the supply of dentures and spectacles
- dental treatment and eye tests
- the repair or replacement of appliances of any kind where this is necessary due to negligence
- the maintenance and incidental costs from persons receiving in-patient treatment but who leave the hospital during the day to work
- NHS hospital accommodation and services made available to private patients

- attending a person involved in a road traffic accident and in-patient and out-patient treatment resulting from a road traffic accident (the driver being charged)
- additional amenities e.g. a single hospital room, when this is not required for medical reasons.

Some people are exempt from these charges. These include people over the age of 65, pregnant women and women who have had a baby in the last twelve months, children under the age of 16 and young people under the age of 19 who are in full-time education. Other people who are on low incomes can also obtain help with these charges. Assistance with travel costs to hospital for treatment is also available to people on low incomes.

**Think it over**

What health care services are you and other members of your family entitled to receive 'free of charge'?

An increasing number of people now belong to private insurance schemes aimed to cover the cost of health and social care. People use the insurance to buy private health or social care when it is required. Private health care insurances have been available for many years, but increasingly people are taking out insurance that covers services previously received from the NHS. For example, there has been a marked increase in the number of people taking out dental insurance. Also, in the future it may be possible to take out insurance to pay for services that protect against residential or nursing home costs.

The National Assistance Act 1948 imposed a duty on local authorities to provide residential care for older people and people with disabilities. It empowered them to charge residents, according to their means, for residential care. Local authorities also have the power to make charges for other services that they provide, such as meals-on-wheels and home care services. Many authorities chose not to make a charge on home care services until very recently. The greater demand on services (as a result of the emphasis of people remaining in their own homes wherever possible), and the greater restrictions on public spending, has meant that many authorities have now begun to make charges for previously 'free' services. Local authorities often use a form of means-testing in order to decide what contribution the individual should make towards the cost of their care. Different authorities calculate this contribution in different ways and this has resulted in people feeling that inequalities exist across the country.

## Benefits

An individual's health and care problems may be linked to his or her social and financial situation. With the exception of Housing Benefit (which is dealt with by the local authority), financial matters are dealt with by the Department of Social Security (DSS) via the Benefits Agency. The DSS produces a number of leaflets which set out people's rights and entitlements to benefits.

Benefits can be universal and the same for everyone (such as child benefit), or they may be 'means-tested' (i.e. taking account of the individual's income and savings before the benefit is awarded). Some benefits are payable only if the person has made

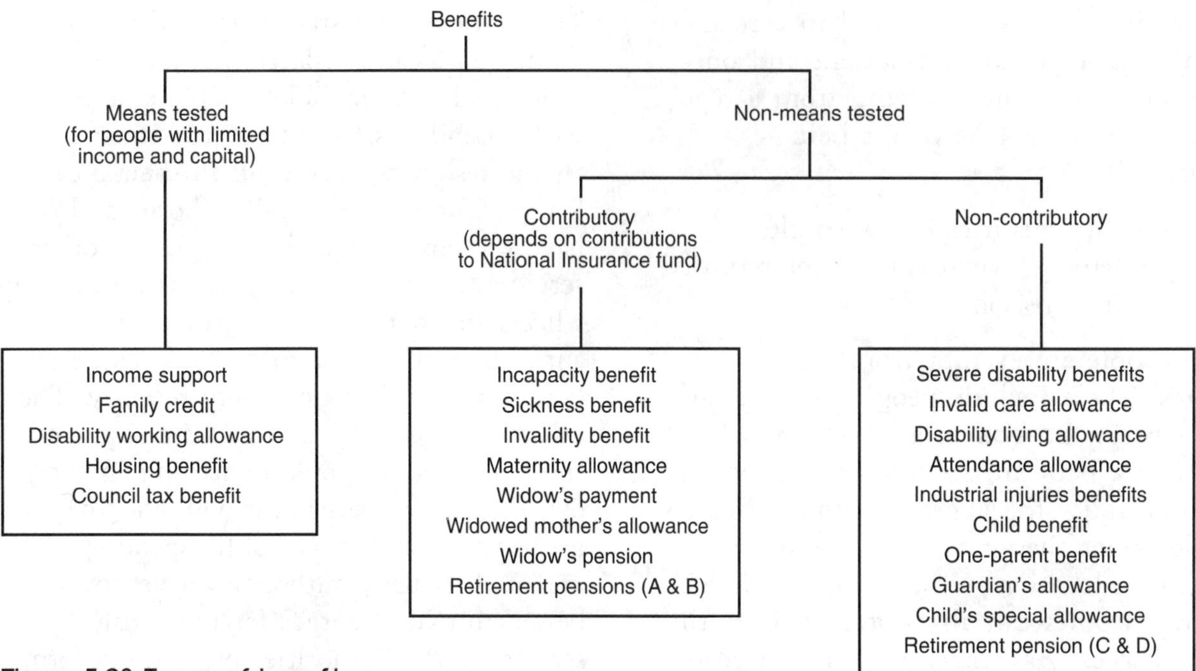


**Figure 5.28 Types of benefit**

contributions to the National Insurance scheme. These include incapacity benefit, sick pay, maternity payments and pensions. (See Figure 5.28.)

---

# 5.5 The effects of government policies on services

## Acts of parliament, White Papers and government circulars

Legislation prescribing the services is broadly divided between imposing **duties** (mandatory legislation) and those **empowering** government to do particular things (permissive legislation).

For example, the **Chronically Sick and Disabled Persons Act 1970** specifies that all or any of the following services for a person with a disability must be provided, or assistance given in obtaining them:

- practical assistance in the home
- radio, television, library or similar recreational facilities
- lectures, games, outings or other recreational facilities outside the home
- adaptations in the home to secure greater safety, comfort or convenience
- holidays
- provision of meals at home or elsewhere
- a telephone and any special equipment necessary to use it.

The Health Services and Public Health Act 1968 empowered local authorities to make arrangements for promoting the welfare of older people. DSS circular 19/71 lists the services that local authorities are empowered to provide, especially for older people. These are:

- meals and recreation in the home and elsewhere

- information on services available and arrangements to identify people in need of services
- transport and travel assistance to use special services
- visiting and advisory services and social work support
- practical assistance in the home, including adaptations to secure greater safety, comfort and convenience
- wardens for sheltered housing schemes.

Some permissive services that were previously provided by the social services department, such as help with domestic chores, have been withdrawn in recent years as restricted funding and more demand on other services has increased. Other services that were previously free of charge, such as home care assistance with personal care, now require the service user to make a payment towards the cost of the service.

From time to time the government publishes White Papers which set out reforms that it wishes to make to services. For example, in November 1998 it published the White Paper *Modernising Social Services: Promoting Independence, Improving Protection, Raising Standards*. This set out reforms to the way social services are provided and regulated. The White Paper proposed the following:

- a new independent inspection and monitoring service, made up of eight regional Commissions for Care, will inspect all types of care homes and will also have responsibilities for the inspection of care provided in people's own homes
- there will be better support for adults, with care being designed to allow people to remain in their own homes and live independently. To support this, a direct payment scheme will enable people to receive money, instead of services, to spend on their own choice of staff
- a special programme, called Quality Projects, will make sure children are properly protected against abuse, will raise standards in children's homes and give children in care better educational opportunities
- a new General Social Council will improve training levels for care staff.

The ways in which local authorities and the NHS are expected to carry out their duties are defined in government circulars. They are issued to all central government departments and can be mandatory or merely advisory. The circulars are used to instruct, give general policy guidelines and to explain new legislation.

**Try it out**

If you have access to the Internet, look up the latest information on the Department of Health's policies at www.doh.gov.uk/

Nettleton (1995) states, 'According to Lalonde (1976) any effective health policy must work at four levels: health care provision; lifestyle or behavioural factors; environmental pollution and biophysical factors; environmental pollution and biophysical factors.'

*The Health of the Nation (1992)* policy aims to change the way individuals behave in order to create a healthier nation. Healthier lifestyles are seen as the key to improving the health and well-being of the population. The second progress report on the *Health of the Nation* strategy, in July 1995, suggested that some aspects of health are improving. Death from heart disease in people under 65 years of age fell by 11 per cent in 1994, suicides fell by 6 per cent between 1993 and 1994, and a reduction in the incidence of gonorrhoea suggests that the 'safe sex' message may be taken seriously. On the other hand more teenagers are smoking, lung cancer among women may be rising, suicide in young men is increasing, and the number of obese men and women is rising.

Action to improve the safety of work and home environments and reduce risks from pollution are also built into the policy. Organisations work with the government to promote public safety and healthy lifestyles. The *Health of the Nation* strategy involves the National Health Service, local authorities, voluntary organisations, the media and employers all working to improve the health of the population.

**Health Improvement Programmes** (HIPs) are being developed by health and local authorities. These programmes set out to tackle health issues on a local basis and aim to combat and control diseases. It is proposed to do this through education and by improving services in hospitals and primary care.

### HIP targets

These might include:

- the reduction of death rates by cancer in the under 65s
- the reduction of death rates from heart disease and strokes
- the improvement of the health, social functioning and quality of life for people with serious mental illness
- improving the life expectancy and quality of life for people with respiratory disease
- helping to reduce the accident rate
- the reduction of young people's misuse of drugs and alcohol
- reducing the rate of conceptions amongst the under 16s
- reducing the effects of diabetes
- helping to reduce the number of suicides.

Practical work on improving health is also to be targeted on promoting cities, healthy schools, healthy hospitals, healthy workplaces, healthy homes and healthy environments. Legislation such as the Health and Safety at Work Act (1974) is designed to protect workers from hazards at work. Building regulations take health into account. There are regulations designed to protect the safety of drinking water, a range of regulations to provide road safety, and so on. Health promotion programmes are targeted at schools and in the workplace.

Regulation of pollution is widely accepted as a responsibility for central and local government. There is a growing concern about the effects of pollution. Environmental pollution is not an issue which can be left up to the individual. New policies and legislation are likely to

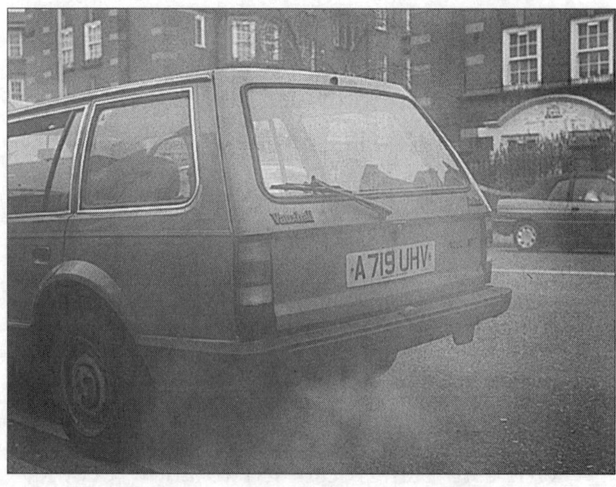


Environmental pollution concerns us all

## Landmarks in social care 1974–1999

**1974 Finer Report** – considered the need for a social security benefit for lone parents
**1974 Field-Fisher Report** – inquiry report on the care and supervision provided to Maria Colwell (who was neglected and abused); a key turning point in modern child protection
**1978 Warnock Report** – report on the commission of inquiry into the education of children and young people with learning difficulties or physical disabilities
**1978 Protection of Children Act**
**1979 Jay Report** – results of an inquiry into the health and social care of people with learning difficulties; care in the community recommended
**1980 Black Report** – inquiry into the relationships between social class, poverty, and health inequalities; buried for many years by the government
**1980 Child Care Act**
**1982 Barclay Report** – inquiry into the role and tasks of social workers, recommended a more community based approach
**1983 Mental Health Act**
**1983 Health and Social Services and Social Security Adjudications Act**
**1984 Health and Social Security Act**
**1986 Disabled Persons (Services, Consultation and Representation) Act**
**1988 Cleveland Report** – report of the inquiry into child abuse; recommended greater and more systematic awareness of the problem and improvements in the work of and collaboration between the agencies involved
**1988 Griffiths Report** – review of how non-health care policies and services operate abd how improvements could be made; forerunner to NHS and Community Care Act 1990
**1988 Wagner Report** – review of the role of residential care services provided by statutory, voluntary and private providers; recommended a major overhaul of training and quality standards, and closer involvement of social services departments
**1988 Social Security Act**
**1989 The Children Act**
**1990 NHS and Community Care Act**
**1992 Warner Report** – examined the selection and recruitment methods for staff working in childrens homes, recommended the licensing of care staff
**1992 The Health of the Nation** – White Paper which was intended to set out a strategy for improving health through self-help and developments in a wide range of health-related agencies
**1995 Carers (Recognition and Services) Act**
**1995 Children (Scotland) Act**
**1995 Disability Discrimination Act**
**1996 Burgner Report** – examined quality standards in residential care, recommended improvements in inspection and registration
**1996 Asylum, and Immigration Act**
**1996 Direct Payments Act**
**1997 House of Lords judgement** – on Gloucestershire Council decision to withhold services on resource grounds
**1997 People Like Us,** – Sir William Utting's review of standards for children in care
**1998 Modernising Social Services** – White paper
**1999 Crime and Disorder Act**
**1999 Health Bill,** – ushered in primary care groups
**1999 Quality Protects**
**1999 Welfare Reform and Pensions Bill**
**1999 With Respect to Old Age** – Report of Royal Commission on Long-Term Care for the Elderly
**1999 National Carers Strategy**

Figure 5.29 Reports, Acts, White and Green Papers that have impacted on social care 1974 to 1999

### Think it over

Can you think of any items over the past couple of years that have highlighted pollution? What were the concerns about?

be introduced in the future to combat air pollution.

Since 1974 there have been a number of Reports, Act of Parliament, White and Green Papers that have impacted on social care (see Figure 5.29). Since May 1997 the pace of measures that affect social services seems to have increased even further. (See Figure 5.30.)

## Government initiatives since May 1997

- Quality protects – response to Utting report On safeguarding children in care
- National Carers Strategy
- Review of Mental Health Act 1983
- Royal Commission on Long-Term Care for the Elderly
- Social Services White Paper – includes proposals On commissions for Care Standards, General Social Care Council and performance assessment framework
- Better Government for Older People programme
- National Service Frameworks
- National priorities Guidance
- Crime and Disorder Act 1998 – set up Youth Justice Board and Youth Offending Teams, and introduced curfews and parenting orders
- Welfare Reform Bill
- Comprehensive Spending Review
- Disability Rights Commission
- Sex Offenders Register
- Primary Care Groups
- Health Action Zones
- Education Action Zones
- Tackling Drugs to Build a Better Britain
- Family and Parenting Institute
- Sure Start programme
- Social Exclusion Unit
- National Childcare Strategy
- Training Organisations for the Personal Social Services
- Best Value proposals under Local Government Bill
- Acheson report on poverty and health
- Welfare to Work programmes for claimants
- New Deal for Communities regeneration programme
- Early Years Development Plans

Figure 5.30 Government-introduced measures that have impacted on social care since May 1997

In recent years, three of the most important Acts of Parliament have been the Mental Health Act, 1983; the Children Act 1989; and the NHS and Community Care Act, 1990.

## Mental Health Act, 1983

This Act deals with the rights of people who have a mental disorder, and the procedure that must be followed in order to provide them with appropriate care. It relates to a person's welfare when that person, due to a mental disorder, is not able to make decisions regarding his or her own welfare. Under the Act, local authorities must appoint **approved social workers** (ASWs), who have a duty to assess people for hospital admission. The approved social worker must interview the person in a suitable manner and make application for hospital admission, or guardianship, where appropriate. Other responsibilities of the approved social worker include a duty to:

- respond to a 'nearest relative's' request for assessment, and to inform the nearest relative in writing if no application is made for admission to hospital
- inform the nearest relative of application for admission to hospital, and to consult with him or her if the patient is to be admitted for treatment, or if guardianship is to be sought
- inform the nearest relative of his or her rights to make application for admission to hospital, and to discharge the patient.

The social services department also has the duty to arrange for a social worker (not necessarily an ASW) to provide reports to the hospital managers when a person is admitted, and to provide social circumstances reports for the mental health tribunals.

The definition of the term 'mental disorder' is central to the functioning of the Act. Section 12 of the Act refers to four specific forms of mental disorder:

- mental illness
- arrested or incomplete development of the mind
- psychopathic disorder
- 'any other disorder or disability of the mind'.

This definition means that people with learning difficulties may come within some sections of the Act. However, sexual deviancy and dependency on drugs or alcohol do not constitute a mental disorder and don't come within the scope of the Act.

Local authorities have the responsibility for providing approved social workers to assess the need for admission to hospital and, more recently, for supervising people returning to the community from psychiatric hospital care. However, it is the Health Authority which has the responsibility for developing services within the community for people with mental health problems. These services may include community psychiatric nurses (CPNs), who visit people in their own homes, giving them support on an individual basis, or in groups in clinics. Community service may also include out-patient or clinic consultations with a psychiatrist, short-term residential accommodation and resource centres.

The Government is in the process of implementing a **Mental Health Strategy** which aims to modernise mental health services, to make them 'safe, sound and supportive'. It hopes to improve mental health care and to build public confidence in the mental health services. A review of the Mental Health Act 1983 is part of the strategy.

A Green Paper proposing changes to the Mental Health Act was published in November 1999. The government has set out plans to impose compulsory treatment on people with a mental illness in their own homes or in hospital. The powers will apply differently for those who can make their own decisions about treatment, and those who are considered incapable of making a decision. The Green Paper also details changes in the way appeals against detention and compulsory treatment are governed. A new independent tribunal system will be responsible for deciding whether a patient should be made subject to a compulsory care and treatment order in the community, and for deciding how, where and when it should be implemented. The tribunal will be able to define the patient's place of residence and to force the patient to allow access to their home for treatment visits. In some cases police or paramedics will also be able to enter the patient's home forcibly and take them to hospital for compulsory treatment.

**Think it over**

Find out about the main points in the government's mental health strategy. Why do you think there could be some objections to plans to impose compulsory treatment on people with mental illness?

## The Children Act 1989

The Children Act came into force on 14 October 1991 after a long period of review and amendment. The main reasons why a review of the law was thought to be necessary were:

- the imbalance between relative powers of parents, local authorities and the courts
- the complex, confusing and disparate legislation concerning child welfare
- the powers and duties of local authorities were not always clear.

Aspects of public and private law were brought together in this comprehensive reform of child law. Private law affects children whose parents are separating or divorcing, for example; public law affects children who are in need of help from a local authority.

**Think it over**

How are children defined as being 'in need'?

The Children Act lays down a number of important principles that the court must follow in all cases involving children. Many of these relate specifically to children in need.

The Act defines a child being in need if:

a the child is unlikely to achieve or maintain, or to have the opportunity of achieving or maintaining, a reasonable standard of health or development without the provision of services

b the child's health or development is likely to be significantly impaired, or further impaired without services

c the child is disabled.

In relation to children in need the local authority must:

- identify the extent to which children are in need within their area

- provide day care, having regard to the different racial groups to which children in need belong within their area
- maintain a register of disabled children and provide services
- provide accommodation (residential or foster care)
- provide family services
- where children in need are living with their families provide, as appropriate, social, cultural and recreational activities, home help, facilities so that they can make use of these services, and assistance to enable the child and family to have a holiday
- where children in need are living away from home, take steps to enable them to live within their families, or to promote contact between children and their families if this is necessary to promote and safeguard their welfare.

There are various principles which underpin the provision of the Children Act.

### Paramountcy

The child's welfare must be the paramount consideration in any decision relating to the upbringing of a child. To make sure that the child's interests do take priority, a welfare checklist outlines the factors which must be taken into account when courts make decisions. These factors include:

- the child's own wishes
- the child's physical, emotional and educational needs
- the child's age, sex, background and other relevant considerations
- any harm which the child has suffered or might suffer in the future
- how able the child's parents (or other relevant people) are to meet his or her needs
- how the child might be affected by any change in circumstances
- the powers available to the court.

A principle of the Act is a presumption of no order. That means the court will only make an order when it is satisfied that to do so is positively better for the child than not doing so.

### Parental responsibility

The upbringing of children is primarily the responsibility of parents. This concept of parental responsibility replaces a notion of parental rights and places an emphasis on the duty and obligation towards children.

### Prevention

It is an assumption of the Act that in most circumstances the best place for children to be brought up and cared for is within their own family. Local authorities were given powers and duties to support children in need within the care of the family.

### Protection

Child protection is a priority and the Act made attempts to address the balance between unwarranted intervention into family life and the need to protect.

For a care order or supervision order to be made the court must be satisfied that the child concerned is suffering or is likely to suffer significant harm.

### Partnership

The local authority has a duty to consult all those concerned in the welfare of a child.

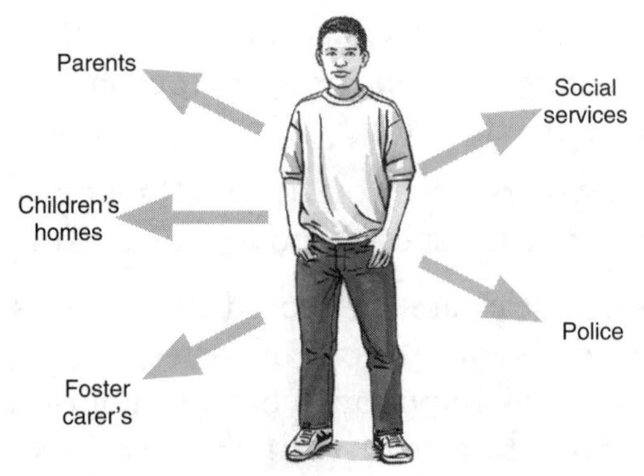


**Children can get lost in the middle of people responsible for them**

Services provided to families with children in need should be provided in partnership with:

- parents
- children and young people
- carers
- other local authority departments
- other agencies.

### Participation

The child, parents and other relevant agencies should all be involved in decision making, matters of welfare and provision of services. The Act represented a commitment to involving children in decision making.

### Planning

This is vital in both child care casework and the process of planning services.

### Permanency

As stated before, children are best looked after in their own family in most circumstances. All efforts of the local authority's preventative services should be directed towards assisting children to remain in the permanent care of their family. If substitute care is required, permanency and continuity should be provided.

In addition to those children who are in need the local authorities under the Children Act have some powers and duties towards ALL children. These include the registration of child care facilities.

## The NHS and Community Care Act, 1990

The NHS and Community Care Act incorporates the proposals set out in the Government White Paper *Working for Patients* (on reforming the NHS) and *Caring for People* (on care in the community).

There are six key objectives:

- to promote the development of home care, day care and short stays in residential units, to enable people to stay in their own homes for as long as possible
- to ensure that the needs of the carers are also taken into consideration by service providers
- to make full assessments of the needs of the individual and to promote good case management to ensure a high quality of care
- to encourage the development of the independent sector alongside good-quality public provision
- to clarify the responsibilities of both the social services and health authorities and to hold them accountable for their performance
- to secure better value for taxpayers' money by introducing a new funding structure for social and health care.

The Act is significant in that it incorporates important developments in the philosophy of community care and in the delivery of services called for in other legislation. The Act emphasises a care management approach, based on the assessment of individual need and the designing of tailor-made packages of care. It is important because it introduces a difference between the purchasing and providing of care. In addition to this, the Act encourages more involvement of private and voluntary sectors in the provision of services.

The Act places an obligation on health authorities to ensure that:

- health service staff contribute towards needs-led assessments
- appropriate health care is provided
- reviews of individual health care needs take place and service provisions are revised accordingly.

Local authorities are also required to:

- communicate assessments and decisions regarding service provision to the individual
- feed back information regarding changing community care needs into a planning system
- publish information to all users of services on the range of community services available.

## Ways that public opinion may affect government policy

It is tempting to think that government policy is directly designed to meet the wishes of the voting population. In practice, democracy does not work this way because:

- voters can only choose between a limited range of political parties, they cannot choose individual policies – only a general party package
- the voting public are very varied and there are many sub-groups with conflicting views on policy. It would be unusual for the majority of voters to have clearly expressed views on issues such as increasing taxation for spending on health or education
- many voters may vote for the 'image of a party' not for specific policy initiatives.

Political parties are influenced by opinions held by different sections of society. This influence is of importance because political parties hope to attract votes from various sections of society. It is quite possible that a party could ignore the opinions of a particular group (such as nurses) if the party is not concerned with obtaining their votes. Most governments are elected with around only one-third of the votes cast in a general election. Governments only have to get more votes per constituency than the other parties in order to win seats. Governments do not need to win the majority of votes given in the country.

### Pressure groups

Pressure groups may represent the self-interest of a professional group or they may act as voluntary organisations representing the needs of vulnerable groups in society. Some examples of voluntary groups and their aims – as stated in the *Voluntary Agencies Directory 2000* – are set out below:

- MIND – to raise awareness of mental health, and campaign for the rights of everyone experiencing mental distress.
- Macmillan Cancer Relief – works towards the day when everyone will have equal and ready access to the best information, treatment and cure for cancer.
- Shelter – to campaign for decent homes that everyone can afford. To provide advice and assistance to people in housing need.
- British Council of Disabled People – to serve as a national umbrella organisation

made up of national, regional and local groups and organisations run and controlled by disabled people. To unite the voice of disabled people in the UK.

These groups will also raise awareness, as well as campaigning for the interests of vulnerable groups.

### Publishing papers and leaflets

Some pressure groups seek to alter opinion directly through publicising themselves in newspaper adverts, **papers** and **leaflets**. Groups can 'raise awareness' and increase public interest in issues by their publication activities.

Papers and leaflets may influence politicians because politicians need to appear to be concerned with and working to promote 'good causes'. The effectiveness of using direct advertising to influence public opinion may depend on the popularity of a cause. A 'children in need' type of campaign is likely to attract public sympathy and political interest. A campaign for the needs of people with a very specific illness may attract less general concern and perhaps less political interest.

### Lobbying

Pressure groups can also attempt to influence government policy through **lobbying**. Lobbying involves trying to influence members of Parliament or civil servants directly. The name comes from the idea of catching the attention of important people as they walk through the lobby or entrance to a building. Although people still do try to 'catch attention' most lobbying is subtler than this. Michael Hunt (1997) argues that 'insider status' is a key issue in modern policy making. Policy-makers will often assume that experts in a given field should be consulted before policy is fixed. Civil servants and politicians will seek people who can advise them. If a voluntary group is respected, and perhaps even has royal sponsorship, then it might be an ideal group to consult about policy.

Hunt (1997) makes the point that many voluntary groups influence policy because they do *not* mount noisy campaigns or threaten direct action. Groups that do not organise political campaigns may be safer to consult and invite to committee meetings. Politicians and senior civil servants often represent a narrow social group. Hunt argues that many pressure groups seek to influence these people by holding out the offer of expertise together with the promise of not embarrassing them.

### Organised political campaigns

The opposite of being co-opted to work with policy-makers is to try and influence policy directly through organised political campaigns. Examples of this tactic might include union campaigns for status or campaigns aimed at increasing expenditure on the NHS. Organised campaigns can have an impact on government policy, but this may be mainly because they attract extensive support from the general public, or from sectors of voters who are perceived as significant for the electoral success of a party.

## Community Health Councils

**Community Health Councils** are bodies set up by the government to represent the interests of the public. They are independent from the management of the local Health Service and are the consumers' 'watchdog'. There is usually one Community Health Council (CHC) to each Health Authority, with the statutory function of representing the views of the community to the NHS. Each Council has representatives from the local authority, locally elected members and Health Authority members. The CHC has the legal right to inspect most health authority premises within the area and to make reports on their findings to the appropriate management board. CHCs will also continue to play an important role in helping patients to make complaints about any aspect of health services.

The main aims of the Community Health Council are:

- to form a representative view of the health needs of the population and the wishes of the public
- to monitor the operation of local health services and make relevant comparisons; to formulate a measure of local achievement, gaps and problem areas and quality of services
- to represent the public's interest and recommend improvements in order to influence the nature and quality of services
- to respond in a representative manner to consultation exercises, planning documents and proposals for change
- to inform and involve the public regarding the standard of local health services, the performances of the Health Authorities and activities of the CHC in order to facilitate an informed and participative community.
- to support individual users and voluntary groups in their dealings with the Health Authorities, especially regarding problem areas and complaints to help increase user input and the improvement of services.

(*Source:* Winchester and Central Hampshire Community Health Council – Annual Report, 1993/4.)

# 5.6 Access to services

Access to health and social care services can be achieved in one of four ways:

- through self-referral
- referral by a third party
- by recommendation of a professional
- by recall.

## Self referral

In order for people to refer themselves to a service, they must first know that it exists. People gain information about services that are available in various ways:

- from general publicity in the media e.g. television and newspapers
- from leaflets and posters in public places
- by word of mouth.

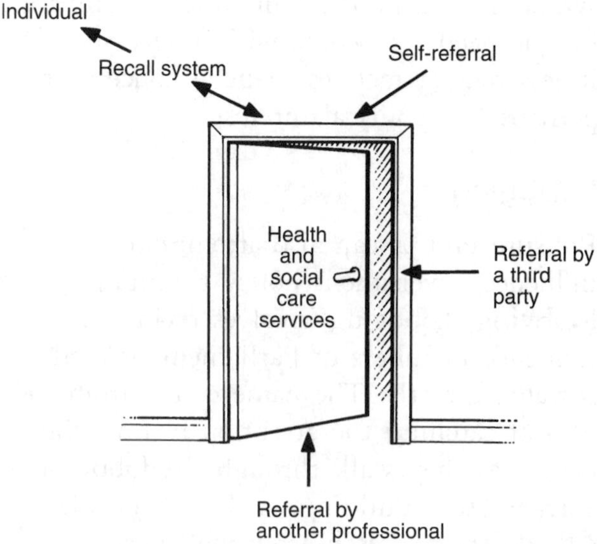


**Figure 5.31 Opening the door to health and social care services**

The health services to which people are able to refer themselves are the NHS primary care cervices – GPs, dentists, opticians – or for services for which they pay privately. People can refer themselves to social services departments, however they will be assessed as to whether they need any specific service before it is provided. People wishing to obtain social care through private or voluntary organisations can usually refer themselves.

## Referral by a third party

People may be referred to either the primary health care services or social services by a third party, often this will be a family member, friend or neighbour. In particular, referrals in respect of services for children are often made through a third party. Sometimes a person from one service will make a referral to another, for example a district nurse may refer someone to the social services department for additional help.

## Recommendation by a professional

Some services are only accessible through the recommendation of another professional. This applies particularly to the secondary health services, e.g. a GP will refer a patient to specialist hospital services. However, there are other services for which a referral by another professional is required e.g. a teacher will refer a child to the educational welfare officer or educational psychologist.

## Recall

For many services there may be a 'recall' system operating. For example, once a person has registered with a dentist or an optician, following the first visit a follow-up appointment may be sent out automatically after a certain period of time. Other services which often have a recall system are screening services, such as breast cancer screening programmes.

## Barriers to access and how access can be improved

### Attitudes to health

Nettleton (1995) quotes research from Stainton-Rogers, who identified different ways that people understand their health. For example, some people might see their body as a machine: this machine can break down or wear out; if the machine stops working properly it will need to be fixed. Another view is that the body is under attack from all the germs and dangers that exist in the world: health is a matter of fighting off all the attacks from outside. Some people see health as a matter of will-power: health depends on having the emotional strength to make the right choices. The research discovered that other people stressed the need for modern medicine, but were concerned that not everyone had an equal chance of getting the best treatment. Some people stressed the problems with modern medical treatments.

Whatever the theories, people seem to invent their own views of health. The way that people perceive health may influence them as to whether they use health services. For example, people who believe in *determinism* think that health is not something they can influence by choices in lifestyle. This is sometimes confirmed by their experience of life, for example they know people who did not smoke and yet died of cancer (and others who did smoke and lived to a healthy old age). They are less likely to believe in health education programmes and act on the information given. (See Argyle, 1997.)

Some people may not wish to acknowledge that they have a health problem, hoping that it will 'go away'. Emotionally they may feel unable to cope with the prospect of having a serious illness, what this would mean to them and their families. This state of 'denial' can last for a long time, even when other family members or friends have begun to notice that something has changed or is not quite right.

'I can't be ill. How would my family manage without my salary.....!

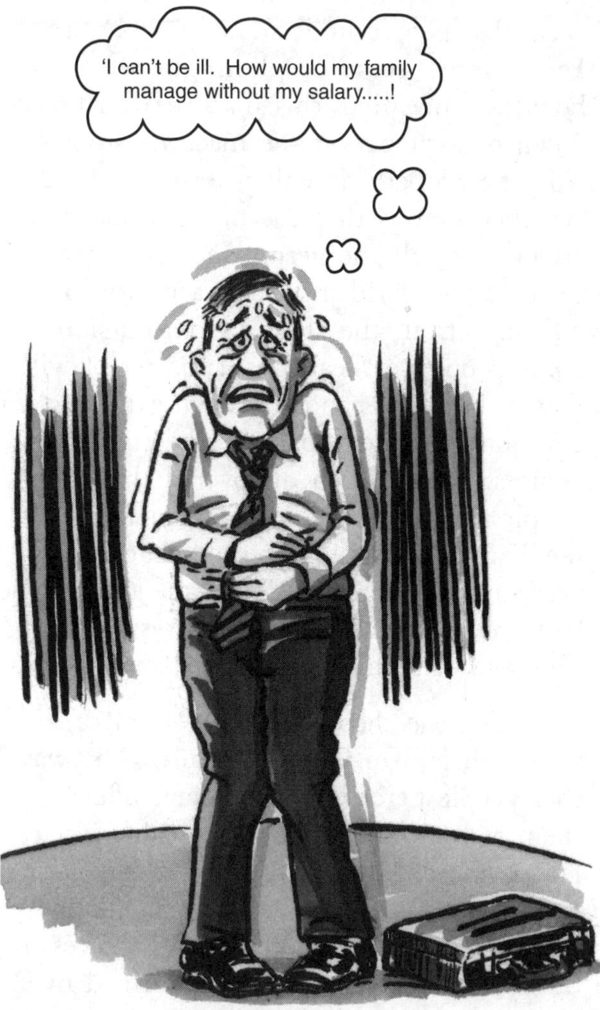

**Being in a state of denial can be a barrier to access**

The stigma that sometimes accompanies the accessing of services may also prevent people from applying for appropriate help and support. For example, there is still a stigma attached to having a mental health problem and people may not want to be seen as needing this type of help. Or where people are having difficulties in caring for children, either because of the child's behaviour, or due to lack of informal support, they might be afraid of the consequences of becoming involved with the social services department.

### Information regarding services

To enable people to take control of their own health and social care, and to be able to access services appropriately, it is essential that they can find information regarding the services that are available. This information should be in clear simple language which describes what that department can and cannot provide. Information systems should:

- ensure that information is straightforward and accurate
- ensure that everyone has access to the information in a form that is appropriate to them
- be regularly reviewed and up-dated.

Special account should be taken of those people who:

- have different cultures and languages
- have a sensory impairment
- have restricted mobility
- are isolated within their communities
- have difficulty with reading or writing
- are not motivated to seek or use help.

Information regarding services can be improved by:

- consulting users, their carers, community groups and those who provide services, about the content and style of the information
- building information networks on existing patterns of community life e.g. libraries and religious and community services
- using the expertise and experience of others to design the content and presentation of information
- giving better information to callers. The role of the people who are the first contact should be considered in relation to this.

Information for users, whose needs make them eligible for the service, should be brief and clear. It should say:

- for whom the service is intended
- what it does
- what its availability is
- what it costs
- how to apply for it.

## National Service Frameworks and Fair Access to Care Initiatives

The government believes that access to decent education, high quality health and social services, good local transport and affordable leisure services is important for the over-all health and well-being of people.

The consultation document *'A First Class Service: Quality in the NHS'* sets out the government's proposals for introducing a National Framework for Assessing Performance. This sets out six key areas for performance assessment:

- *health improvement* – to improve the general health of the population
- *effective delivery of health care* – effective, appropriate and timely care
- *efficiency* – the way in which resources are used achieves value for money
- *patient/carer experience* – the way in which patients and cares view the quality of treatment and care that they receive
- *health outcomes of care* – assessing the direct contribution of care to improvements in overall health
- *fair access* – to health services in relation to people's needs, irrespective of geography, socio-economic group, ethnicity, age or gender.

In respect of fair access for all, the government has set up ten health action zones as pilot schemes to encourage effective action. These pilot schemes provide a framework for the NHS, local authorities and other partners to work together in reducing health inequalities. The first wave of zones, introduced in 1998/99, received £4 million in additional resources.

Social Services inspectors will look at the fairness of provision in relation to need, the existence of clear eligibility criteria and the provision of accessible information about the provision of services. Indicators of performance might be the number of people over 65 helped to live at home, the day care provision for adults per head of population, spending on children in need to ensure they have fair access to educational opportunities, health care and social care, and/or the number of children looked after per 1,000 population.

(*Source*: Department of Health, *Modernising Social Services.*)

## Access to early years services

As we have seen there is a wide range of services for early years. Some of these need to be paid for by the service user, for example private nursery facilities, but many others are provided by statutory agencies, for example health services, and it would be easy to assume that these are equally accessible. In reality all kinds of barriers exist and these can be physical, psychological, financial and environmental.

### Physical barriers

Getting anywhere by public transport with two small children can be a challenge. It is often difficult to keep small children amused when attending a doctor's surgery or a hospital clinic and this can make listening to the professional very difficult. One answer would be to have the children cared for while Sally herself attends for antenatal care, but the cost and availability of care may make this difficult. The older child may attend a nursery school, however the younger child is unlikely to attend nursery unless a place had been offered in a nursery run by social services. If friends are in a similar position to herself, they are not likely to have the necessary resources, either physical or emotional, to care for additional children. Someone who can leave children with parents, partner, friends or in childcare and get in a car and drive to hospital may find it a lot easier to attend the hospital than Sally.

### Psychological barriers

Sally is probably spending a lot of time and energy each day ensuring that the basic needs of herself and her children are met. Financial and emotional constraints may make it difficult for Sally to socialise. The additional tiredness that may accompany pregnancy, perhaps fears for the future, perhaps loneliness, may all have an effect on her psychological well-being. If Sally feels 'low' it may be difficult for her to motivate herself to make certain choices, like attending for antenatal care. The social class difference between Sally and the health professionals she is likely to encounter may make Sally feel threatened. She may even be afraid the authorities will take away her children. The attitude of society in general may be critical of young women like Sally. These will all be disincentives in accessing services.

## Case study

Sally is 21 and has two young children aged 2 and $4^1/_2$. She lives in a two-bedroom flat in a tower block near the centre of a provincial market town. Sally is now pregnant. She spent most of her teenage years in the care of the local authority and became pregnant with her first child when she was just 16. Although Sally has no family she does have some support from friends, many of whom are in a similar position to herself.

### Try it out

Read the case study (left) and in small groups consider the barriers this mother would face when accessing services for herself and her children.

### Financial

Sally will be receiving various benefits, though her standard of living is still likely to be low. Certain choices are simply not available to her: private care or education for the children, private health care, or health insurance for herself, these choices would probably not be available to Sally. Even things like choosing a healthy diet can be difficult when income is limited. Some financial help may be available to purchase clothes and equipment for the new baby, but again the choice will be limited.

### Environmental barriers

Sally probably had little choice about where she lives. It may be some distance away from health care facilities or other amenities. For example, she is unlikely to have a garden where the children can play. She may live in an area with a high crime rate, and she prefers to stay indoors. If she lives in a tower block where the lifts are frequently vandalised she may find it difficult to get out with the children. All these factors can indirectly affect how prepared Sally is to access services.

The infant mortality rate, which is regarded as one of the indicators of child health, although showing great overall improvement, remains much higher in the lower social classes and in certain areas than others. Differential access to services does not explain this fully, but may be one of the many contributing factors.

**Try it out**

Look at a local service. Assess it for barriers under the four headings: physical, psychological, financial and environmental.

# Unit 5 Assessment

To obtain a pass in this unit you need to prepare a case study which shows an investigation into one local health, social care or early years organisation. Examples of these might include a health clinic, a residential home, a day centre (for elderly people, people with physical disabilities or people with learning disabilities) or a day nursery. The organisation may be set in the statutory, private or voluntary sector). You investigation can be based on a real or fictitious care setting.

Your investigation must include:

- the functions and purpose of the organisation
- information about how the local organisation provides services with reference to the function and purposes of the national framework, local demographic characteristics and government policies
- how individuals gain access to the services of the organisation, and barriers they may encounter
- ways in which one national and/or local organisation is funded
- recent changes in legislation that have affected the organisation.

## Obtaining an E grade

In order to obtain a grade E you must show that you can:

- explain clearly the functions and purpose of the organisation you have chosen
- explain clearly how clients gain access to the service and identify any barriers which they may face in accessing your chosen service
- explain accurately and clearly how the service is organised and funded at national level or regional and local level
- describe in detail the effects of any recent government reforms on your chosen organisation.

## Preparing your case study

In order to prepare your case study it may be helpful to get through the following steps:

- decide on the setting you wish to study
- think about what staff would be employed in this setting and who you might wish to interview
- think about the questions you may wish to ask them in order to obtain the information that you need
- interview the staff (if you are using a fictitious setting you will need to think about how this might have happened)
- analyse the information obtained through your interviews and observations.

You could then use the following headings in order to write up your case study:

- Purpose of the organisation and its functions
- Activities provided by the organisation
- Accessing the service
- Barriers to accessing the service
- Organisation of the service – national, regional and local levels
- Effects of recent government reforms.

## Obtaining a C grade

In order to obtain a C grade, in addition to the above you must also show that you can:

- analyse the impact of government policies on the way the organisation functions and is funded for the service it provided
- describe how your chosen organisation co-ordinates or interacts with at least one other service
- make realistic suggestions about how access to the service can be improved
- analyse the ways in which an aspect of the service has developed over a long period of time, as government policies have changed, and new legislation has been introduced.

Additional headings that you may wish to use could include:

- The impact of government policies on the function and funding of the organisation
- Interaction with other services
- Improvements to access
- Development of services.

## Obtaining an A grade

In order to obtain an A grade you must complete both of the parts above and in addition you must also show that you can:

- analyse the ways in which the public or clients have influenced the practices of the organisation
- evaluate the ways in which the organisation monitors changes in government policy and may alter the services it provides accordingly
- analyse how the work of the organisation relates to the work of other organisations at either local, regional, or national level, and how inter-agency co-ordination is managed.

Additional headings that you must wish to include:

- How the public/clients influence the organisation's practices
- Evaluation of the effect of government policies on the service
- Working with other organisations and how this is co-ordinated and managed.

# Case study: Wellborough Day Centre for Older People (run by Age Concern)

People interviewed:

- the manager of the day centre
- the activities co-ordinator
- a member of the care staff
- volunteer driver
- two clients.

*E grade*

- Purpose of the organisation and its functions
  - o To provide day care for people over the age of 65 years.
  - o To provide social activities that increase social contact, enhance mobility and mental functioning.
  - o To provide facilities to enhance personal care, self-esteem and confidence.
  - o Local demographic information shows that the number of older people in this area is 10 per

cent higher than the higher average.

- Activities provided by the organisation
  - o Leisure activities such as bingo, line dancing, short mat bowls, quizzes, discussion groups, exercise groups.
  - o Lunches; bathing service; hair dressing and barber services; chiropody services.

- Accessing the service
  - o Self-referral; referral by social services.
- Barriers to accessing the service
  - o Insufficient information, e.g. leaflets etc., in appropriate places such as libraries, GP surgeries or local authority offices.

- Organisation of the service – national, regional and local levels
  - o Age Concern England – concerned with the organisation's overall aims and objectives.
  - o Regional representatives – advise and assist local agencies.
  - o Local Age Concern organisation – develop services within national framework according to local needs.

- Effects of recent government reforms
  - o The NHS and Community Care Act (1990) resulted in many local authorities no longer directly providing luncheon clubs themselves and transferring this activity to local Age Concern day centres.

C grade

- The impact of government policies on the function and funding of the organisation
  - o Prior to the NHS and Community Care Act the Age Concern day centre's clients were mainly able-bodied people, now many of those attending the centre have mobility problems, or may be mentally frail.
  - o Local authorities has a three year contract with the centre and provides funding for the activities of the centre.

- Interaction with other services
  - o In addition to receiving funds from the local authority, the centre also receives many referrals from social workers based in the local authority social services department.
  - o The centre can also make referrals to the social services department if clients need more help at home.
  - o The centre therefore interacts with the local authority on various levels: at a management level in respect of agreeing the contract for services and funding, and on an individual client basis for receiving and making referrals.

- Improvements to access
  - o The centre could produce clearer, more user friendly leaflets about the services they offer. These could also be more readily available in places that older people might be able to see them, e.g. GP surgeries, libraries, supermarkets, local colleges or activity clubs aimed at retired people.

- Development of services
  - o Before the introduction of the NHS and Community Care Act the centre was used by able-bodied people for purely social purposes, where they could meet, talk and

perhaps have a light lunch. People attend now to have more specific needs met. Now the centre provides services and activities that help to meet these needs. The clientele and the activities have therefore changed over time.

A grade

- How the public/clients influence the organisation's practices
  - o Age Concern England has responded at a local level to the needs of the local population. People attending the centre are able to have a say in the activities that are provided at the centre, for example short-mat bowls. was introduced at the suggestion of one of the clients. Also many of the clients complained that they were unable to use, or felt unsafe using their bath at home. The centre therefore introduced an 'assisted bathing service' at the centre.
- Evaluation of the effect of government policies on the service
  - o As a result of many less able-bodied people using the centre, many of the previous more able-bodied people no longer meet the centre's criteria for admission; so although the centre provided more services for one group of people, it has had the effect of excluding another.
- Working with other organisations and how this is co-ordinated and managed
  - o The local social services department also has day centres for older people, however the people that attend these centres tend to be the very disabled, or even mentally frail, such as those with advanced dementia. There is some overlap between the two types of day centre, especially as the ability of someone attending the Age Concern centre begins to deteriorate. However it is over-come by a close liaison and effective referral system between the two organisations.
  - o Now that the centre has a contract with the local authority to provide specific services a representative of the centre now sits on the local authority's committee for planning older people's services and are representative of the local authority sits on the management committee of the centre.

## Sources of information

Useful sources of information may include:

- your local authority's community care plan
- *Social Trends* (regional and national) for demographic information
- local directories of independent health, social care and early years organisations
- local community health councils
- annual reports of organisations (including NHS trusts)
- newspapers and periodicals, which carry up-to-date information and comment on social policy
- books on social policy and services organisation
- government documents, such as white papers. Important ones are 'The New NHS: Modern Dependable, and Modernising Social Services

- the Department of Health website, which includes the latest information on policies – **www.doh.gov.uk/**
- websites of non-profit health, social care and early years organisations such as the National Children's Bureau (**www.ncb.org.uk**) and Disability Net (**www.disabilitynet.co.uk**)

## Self-test questions

**1** What were the main proposals of the 1942 Beveridge Report?

**2** What is meant by a 'mixed economy' of care?

**3** Name three of the main demographic effects that are influencing the provision of services today. What effects do they have?

**4** What are the main functions of Primary Care Groups (PCGs) in England?

**5** Under the 1995 Carers (Recognition and Services) Act, what should local authorities take into account when considering the needs of 'young carers'?

**6** What are the main sources of funding for:

**a** Health and social care services
**b** Local authorities
**c** Voluntary organisations.

**7** Why are health and local authorities developing Health Improvement Programmes (HIPs) and what areas of health might these be focused on?

## Self-test answers

**1** **a** A 'cradle to the grave' provision of care.
**b** A compulsory insurance scheme to fund the provision of services.
**c** That the insurance scheme would cover sickness, medical care, the unemployed, widows, orphans, old-age, maternity, industrial injury and funeral benefits.
**d** That there would be social security benefits that were not means-tested.

**2** This is an approach to health and social care which involves the public and independent sectors in the provision of care.

**3** **a** The aging population – increasing use of health and social care services.
**b** A diminishing work force – resulting in skills shortages and fewer people to finance welfare benefits schemes.
**c** Increase of degenerative diseases – increasing use of health and social care services.

**4** Primary Care Groups are responsible for developing primary care services (e.g. GP services, dentists' practices, nurses) and community services (e.g. district nurses, health visitors, domiciliary nurses, etc.) in their local area. PCGs cover populations of approximately 1000,000 people.

**5** Local authorities should ensure that:
- the provision of community services makes sure that young carers do not carry inappropriate levels of responsibility
- how young carers might be helped in both the care needs and parenting responsibilities, and ensure that the young carer is not being exploited
- whether a young carer needs assistance even if they have not asked for it
- if the young carers development is impaired, the local authority should

exercise their existing responsibility towards 'children in need'
- that young carers have information regarding the help that is available.

6 a Health and social care services:
- central government
- local government
- grants and contracts
- charitable donations and fund-raising
- direct payments
- private insurance schemes
- individuals paying for themselves.

b Local authorities
- grants from central government
- local council taxes
- business rates
- charges for services.

c Voluntary organisations
- grants from central government
- grants from local authorities
- contracts with health authorities and social services departments
- charitable grants
- fund-raising events
- donations from individuals
- legacies.

7 Health Improvement Programmes are schemes developed by health and local authorities that set out to tackle health issues on a local basis. HIP targets might include:

- reduction of death from cancer, heart disease and strokes
- improved quality of life for people with a mental illness and respiratory disease
- reduced accident rates and the number of suicides
- reduced conceptions amongst the under-16s
- reduce the effects of diabetes.

## References and recommended further reading

Baggott, R. (1994) *Health and health care in Britain* St Martin's Press

Carter, P. Heffs, A. and Smith, M.K. (eds) (1992) *Changing social work and welfare* Open University Press

Deakin, N. (1994) *The politics of welfare* Harvest Wheatsheaf

Department of Health (1991) *Care management and assessment, the manager's guide* HMSO

Field, M.G. (1989) *Success and crisis in the national health systems* Macmillan

Griffiths, K. (1988) *Community care: Agenda for action* HMSO

Leadbetter, P. (1990) *Partners in health: The NHS and the voluntary sector* National Association of Health Authorities and Trusts

Meredith, B. (1993) *The community care handbook: New systems explained* Age Concern

Ranade, V. (1994) *A future for the NHS? Health care in the 1990s* Longman

Whitefield, D. (1992) *The welfare state* Pluto Press

Wistow, G., et al (1993) *Social care in a mixed economy* Open University Press

## Fast Facts

**Approved social workers** A social worker especially appointed under the Mental Health Act 1983 to assess the need for admission to hospital.

**Beveridge Report** Published in 1942. The report set out the broad framework for the setting up of the Welfare State in the UK. The working party was chaired by William Beveridge.

**Care Management** A system for assessing and organising the provision of care for an individual.

**Carer** Anyone who is looking after someone who is ill or disabled.

**Caring for People** Government White Paper published in 1989 as a response to the Griffiths Report. It set out the proposals for care in the community, giving social service departments the lead responsibility.

**Carers (Recognition and Services) Act** An Act of Parliament, passed in 1995, which places duties on local authorities to assess the needs of the carers to provide and to continue to provide for the person being care for.

**Contract** A formal legal agreement to ensure the delivery of services.

**Community Care (direct payment) Act** An Act of Parliament, passed in 1996, which enables local authorities to set up direct payment schemes whereby disabled people, aged 18 to 65, can receive payments in order to buy in their own care.

**Community Health Councils** Government bodies set up to represent the interests of the public in respect of the quality of health care services.

**Demographic changes** Statistical changes that occur in the population and that can be used for planning services.

**Department of Health** A central government body which administers health and social care.

**Disabled Persons (Consultation and Representation) Act** An Act of Parliament, passed in 1986, which requires local authorities to provide information about services that are available. It also requires them to assess the needs of people requesting services.

**GP Fundholders** Groups of GPs who hold budgets and have the power to commission and purchase health care services.

**Griffiths Report** Published in 1988. The report set out the main principles for the provision of care in the community. The working party was chaired by Sir Roy Griffiths.

**Health Authorities** Purchasers of health care.

**Health Improvement Programmes** Programmes developed by health and local authorities in order to tackle health issues on a local basis which aim to combat and control diseases.

**Independent sector** Organisations providing health and social care other than statutory agencies.

**Informal care** Care provided by people and groups who are not paid for their services.

**Local authority social services departments** These departments are responsible for ensuring that people's social care needs are assessed and met.

**Marketplace economy** An approach to health and social care where the responsibility for purchasing and providing care is separate. It also puts providers in competition with one another in providing effective and efficient services.

**Mental Health Act** An Act of Parliament, passed in 1983, which sets out the framework for the provision of care for people with mental health problems.

**Mixed economy of care** An approach to health and social care which involves the public and independent sectors in the provision of care.

**National Health Service (NHS) and Community Care Act** An Act of Parliament, passed in 1990, which aims to allow vulnerable people to live as independently as possible, within their own homes or in a homely setting in the community.

**Need** A need is an essential requirement which must be met in order to ensure that the individual reaches a state of health and social well-being.

**Packages of care** A variety of integrated services that have been put together in order to meet an individual's assessed needs.

**Pooled budgets** Budgets held by health and social care agencies where decision regarding their use is made jointly.

**Poor Law** An Act of Parliament, passed in 1389, which fixed a legal maximum wage and made it illegal for labourers to leave the manor to which they belonged.

**Poor Law Act** An Act of Parliament, passed in 1601, which placed a duty on parishes to provide relief for their own poor and unemployed parishioners.

**Poor Law Amendment Act** An Act of Parliament, passed in 1834, which created a government body to supervise poor relief and elected Boards of Guardians to run each of the poor law unions and the infirmaries.

**Primary care** Health care provided in the community, often preventative in nature.

**Primary Care Groups** In England, groups of GPs and community nurses covering populations of about 100,000, with the responsibility for commissioning primary and secondary health care.

**Private Organisations** Agencies run on business lines, providing services for which a charge is made.

**Provider** An organisation that sells services to a purchaser.

**Purchaser** An organisation that buys in necessary services.

**Secondary care** Health care that is often curative in nature and is given in hospitals and clinics.

**Seebohm Report** Government report published in 1968 which resulted in the amalgamation of the children's department and the welfare departments within local authorities.

**Special Health Authorities** Special health services which operate at a national level, such as postgraduate and research hospitals, or which provide care for serviously disturbed offenders.

**Statutory organisations** Health and social care organisations providing care that must be given by law (statute). The National Health Service and local authority social services departments form the two main branches of the health and social care industry.

**Tertiary care** Health care often provided in specialist units and rehabilitative in nature.

**Trusts** Self-governing units within the NHS. They are run by boards of governors and are accountable directly to the NHS Management Executive.

**Voluntary organisations** Non-profit making organisation which provide services, usually free of charge.

**Welfare State** Where the state's role in health and social care is central and direct in the provision of services, with many facilities being publicly owned.

**Young carers** A child or young person (up to the age of 18) who is carrying out significant caring tasks and assuming a level of responsibility for another person, which would normally be undertaken by an adult.

# Research perspectives in health and social care

Unit 6

This unit is about developing your research skills. This means that you will need to find out about the research process and the skills needed to carry out research. You will also need to apply this knowledge in practice as you carry out a research project of your own.

The chapter is organised in five sections:

- The purpose of research in health and social care. This means looking at the uses that research is put to, and considering how your own work may be affected by research results and conclusions.
- Research methods used in health and social care. You will need to understand how research is carried out, and the differences between the variety of research methods that are available. Your understanding needs to be deep enough to enable you to choose and apply appropriate methods in your own research.
- Planning research, methods of analysis and validation of results. You need to understand the ways in which the information you collect can be analysed. This is crucial if useful conclusions are to be drawn from the research you do. You also need to be able to check the validity of your findings.
- Presenting research. The clear presentation of your findings is crucial. You will need to consider appropriate methods for presenting your research and suggest recommendations for developing research in the areas of your study.
- Ethical issues that must be considered when researching. Your research work must be carried out in an ethical fashion. You will need to be able to identify where ethical concerns may be a problem and deal with them appropriately.

The unit is entirely assessed through your portfolio of work; there is no test that you need to pass. Your portfolio must contain a report of a research project that you have designed and carried out. You can choose your own research topic, so long as it is relevant to a health, social care or early years setting.

Your research report must show your skills in research and your understanding of research methods used in health and social care. The report should include:

- a rationale for the research, and the research methods you have chosen
- a review of what is already known about the area you are researching
- an exploration of ethical issues that are relevant to your project

- a presentation of your findings which includes your conclusions, appropriate **data** and statistics, diagrams, charts and a bibliography.

## 6.1 The purpose of research in health and social care

Research can be described as the process of finding things out in an organised, systematic and thoughtful way. Information and knowledge are needed by practitioners in all fields, including health and social care. Research helps to ensure that the information and knowledge which underpins our work is as accurate and useful as possible.

Research is a widespread activity, carried out by governments, businesses, organisations and individuals all over the world. It could be a small-scale local research project, for example finding out if people would use a chocolate machine in an office, or a multi-million pound investigation involving a large team of professional researchers. Research of any type involves time and effort, so why do people make this investment in research and consider it to be so important?

The answer is that research produces information that is arrived at scientifically, and which is intended to be as accurate as possible. It aims to give us a true picture of the world. Of course, we already have a picture of the world that we have picked up through our socialisation and education; but how true a picture is it?

In our everyday lives we often hear assumptions made about social issues. They may be stated in the media, or crop up in conversations as 'common knowledge'. You may have heard statements like 'women don't really want a career' or 'people on state benefits are actually well off'. You may have given your own views on the subject in response. Without research, however, such discussions are just argument and opinion.

Several centuries ago it was 'common knowledge' that the earth was the centre of the universe, and that it was flat. European people were afraid to sail too far to the west for fear of falling off! This dramatically illustrates how incorrect assumptions about the world can affect people's behaviour, as well as their views. Eventually research showed that the earth was round and progress was made possible. Social research can address the social assumptions that we live with today, and allow progress to take place here too.

### Research in health and social care

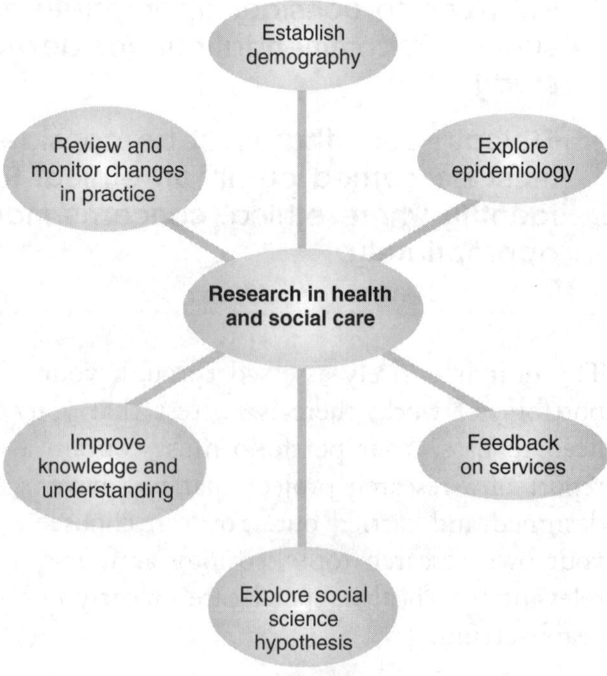


**Figure 6.1** Research in health and social care is carried out for a variety of reasons

Research in health and social care is carried out for a variety of purposes. It may be used to review existing knowledge, to describe a situation or a problem, or to provide explanations. Research is likely to have an influence on your career in health and social care, and on the organisations for which you work. It is important to understand how this may happen.

This chapter identifies six areas where research in health and social care may be directed. Research can be used to:

- plan service delivery by establishing the relevant **demography**
- explore patterns of disease (**epidemiology**)
- obtain feedback on services for quality assurance
- explore social science **hypotheses**
- extend and improve individual and collective knowledge, understanding and practice
- review and monitor changes in health and social care practice.

## Plan service delivery by establishing the relevant demography

Demography means the study of the personal characteristics of people within a group. These characteristics could include age, gender, height, income, disability, area of residence, or any other relevant feature. Information collected during research is known as **data**, and **demographic data** is collected to help plan service delivery.

For example, in order to plan for the provision of services for elderly people in a small town, demographic data about the ages, and geographical location, of people living in the town would be needed. The group of people who are the subjects of a research project are known as the research **population**, and the population for this research project would be people living in the town.

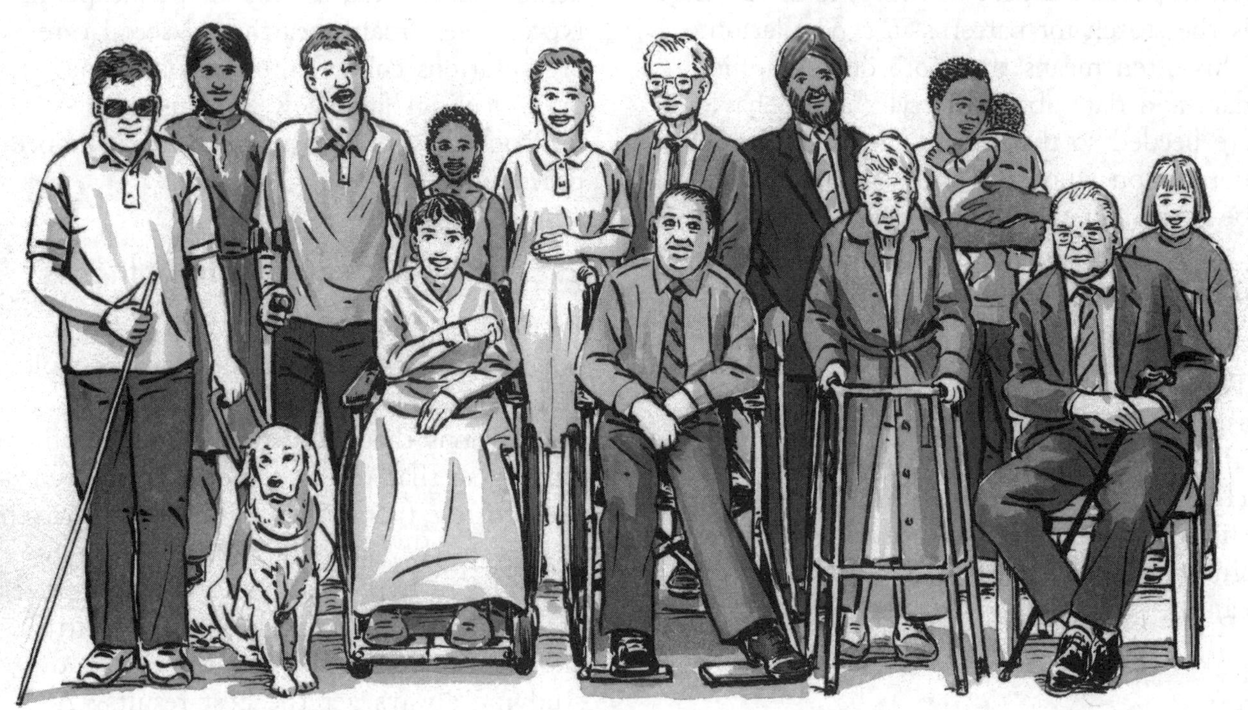

Demographic research is needed to help plan the delivery of local services

Demographic data has a big influence on the planning of service delivery. Decisions on the provisions of services are based on predictions about expected levels of need, and these predictions are in turn based largely on demographic data. For example, maternity services are provided to meet the needs of the expected number of new mothers in a population. Demographic data about age, gender, and maternity patterns helps to predict how many new mothers there are likely to be.

### Explore patterns of disease (epidemiology)

Research can also be used to collect data about the patterns of disease within a population. This information can be crucial for targeting a response to a disease. Treatments and preventative measures will only be effective if administered to the right people, and to the areas where they will be useful.

An important aspect of this type of research is the search for patterns in a population. This often means that both demographic data and data about lifestyles and behaviour are needed so those people in the population who are particularly at risk can be identified. Data about the personal characteristics and lifestyles of sufferers can help predict the numbers of sufferers likely in the future.

This research can also help to identify aspects of lifestyle that affect the spread of disease; for example, the transmission of HIV among intravenous drug users through the sharing of needles, and the links between cigarette smoking and lung cancer.

### Obtain feedback on services for quality assurance

Service providers need to know what users think about the services that they offer. The type of data collected may again be partly demographic and partly about people's opinions and views.

Providers may be interested in finding out the types of people who use their services. They may want to be sure that the service is helping those it is intended for, and that the number of clients properly represents the proportion of the population in need of the service. Demographic data would help answer these questions. For some services other types of demographic data, such as recovery rates, may be needed to help assess service quality.

Feedback in the form of clients' opinions may also be used for quality assurance. Opinion data is likely to be less straightforward to collect and interpret than demographic data, as this chapter explains. Nevertheless many health and social care organisations collect information about users' feelings and views and use this feedback to support their quality assurance procedures.

### Explore social science hypotheses

Research is also conducted by social scientists to test **hypotheses** about people and society. Hypotheses are ideas or propositions that are carefully framed and worded so that research methods can be used to test them. They are usually written as though they are a fact. Here are two examples of hypotheses: 'older people prefer being at home to attending a day centre' and 'students who spend the most time studying always get the best results'. A hypothesis may be a statement of a commonly held belief.

Scientists, including social scientists, carry out research to find out if a hypothesis holds when tested. They are not trying to prove that the hypothesis is true, they are looking for evidence that it may not be true. The idea that a proposition can never be proved, but *can* be disproved, comes from ideas about scientific method which are used in both the natural and social sciences. Physicists, chemists and other natural scientists work on the principle that a theory, or hypothesis, is never accepted as absolutely true, however many examples may seem to agree with it. If research reveals just one exception it shows that the theory doesn't always hold. A counter example forces scientists to revise the theory so that all cases are accounted for.

The same method can be applied to a hypothesis about social issues. For example, the hypothesis, 'older people prefer being at home to attending a day centre' would be disproved if research showed that there were some older people who preferred being at a day centre to being at home.

Research results may give indications of how hypotheses, and theories, should be revised and improved. In our fictitious example it may have been noticed that those older people who did prefer being at home often had family members living with them. This might suggest other lines of enquiry and the framing of new hypotheses. In this way the disproving of hypotheses can help us to develop better theories to explain it. This relationship between theory and research is an important aspect of scientific methods of enquiry.

### Extend and improve individual and collective knowledge, understanding and practice

Research has a crucial role to play in extending our collective knowledge and understanding. For example, research results linking smoking to ill health can help everyone to understand the risks that smokers face. The results obtained by professional researchers help to develop knowledge in the field that they are involved in, and so develop understanding of the world for humanity in general.

Individuals too can develop their knowledge, and improve their own professional practice, by finding things out. As a health and social care student you will be carrying out research of one sort or another throughout your studies. Research does not have to be carried out by large organisations and professional scientists to be useful. Small-scale research projects are not automatically less valuable than well-resourced professional studies. The thing that distinguishes good research from bad is how well other people can be convinced that the results are accurate and useful, and this means thinking carefully about what you are doing every step of the way.

### Review and monitor changes in health and social care practice

Research is often used to assess the effectiveness of changes to health and social care practice. Organisations and individuals involved in health and social care need to know that they are achieving what they set out to do. They need to check that the changes are working as intended. One of the roles of research is to discover how effective a change of practice has been, and whether further adjustments are necessary.

For example a local health centre may have developed a new equal opportunities policy, aimed at preventing discrimination effectively. The change will mean developing new ways of working to support the policy. This may include changes to the environment to ensure that physical access is available to all, and changes to administrative procedures and publicity materials so that all potential users are fully informed and made welcome. A research investigation into the effects of these practices can help to show whether aims are being met. The results may indicate that changes to the policy are necessary and suggest more effective approaches. They may indicate that working practices need to be altered to allow the policy to work.

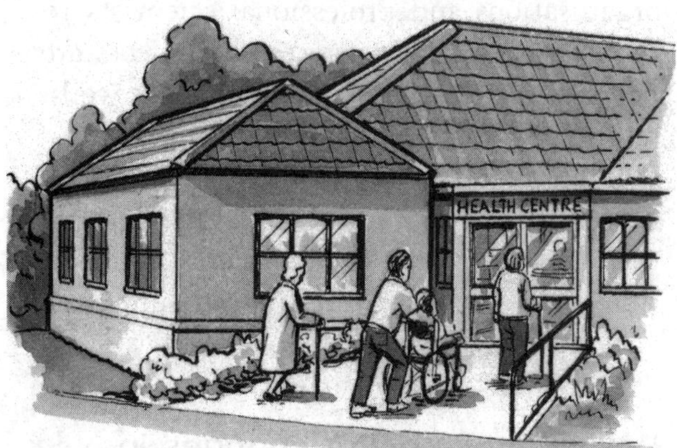


**Figure 6.2 Research can show that removing the barriers to access, so that wheelchair users can use the health centre, will improve the take-up of the service**

| **Try it out** | Think of at least 10 research questions or hypotheses. Decide into which of the six categories listed in Figure 6.1 each question would fit. Explain why you have chosen this category.<br>You could carry out this activity as a group. |
|---|---|

# 6.2 Research methods

## Quantitative and qualitative data

Data can take different forms. Some data is numerical, for example the number of people attending a day centre for older people. Other data may be more descriptive and personal, for example people's feelings about attending the day centre.

Data which is numerical and can be analysed using statistical methods is known as **quantitative data.** The number of single parent families in an area, or the number of people giving the same answer to a particular question, are examples of quantitative data. Quantitative results can be displayed using graphs, charts and tables.

Data which concerns attitudes, opinions and values often cannot be expressed in numerical form. It may include comments people have made about a subject; or accounts of their feelings about it, or reactions to it. This information is known as **qualitative data.** Qualitative data is expressed in words, not numbers, and

### Think it over

Suppose that you are planning to collect data from fellow students to find out how effective a recent anti-smoking poster campaign has been. Divide a sheet of paper into two columns, one headed 'Quantitative Data' and the other headed 'Qualitative Data'.

Try to think of examples of data that you might collect and write each one under the appropriate heading. An example of qualitative data might be people's feelings about smokers. An example of quantitative data might be whether a person smokes or not.

cannot be analysed and reported on using statistical methods.

It is important to understand that both quantitative and qualitative data can provide important and useful results. One is not better or more scientific than the other. The main issue is choosing the right type of data, and collection technique, for the questions you are interested in. Most really good research includes both types of data. This is the best way to provide background and balance in social investigations.

Whether you are looking for quantitative numerical data, or descriptive qualitative data, there are basically two ways of getting information. You can find out for yourself by carrying out an original research project, or you can look at work that has been done already by other people. Carrying out your own research project is called primary research, and data you gather in this way is known as **primary data**. Looking at the work of others is called secondary research, and data taken from the work of others is called **secondary data.** Methods of primary research that you can use are examined later in this section. We will look first at the issues involved in collecting secondary data.

## Secondary data and secondary research

### Why use secondary sources of data?

Collecting secondary data means looking at existing sources that contain information useful to your research. All researchers use secondary research methods to some extent, in fact some research is stimulated by the interesting results that others have published. Doing secondary research, or 'reading around' the research question, is important for any investigation and there are good reasons for looking at secondary sources at an early stage.

- You may pick up useful ideas and concepts about the subject you are interested in. You can relate your research question to existing theories and findings.
- You may get ideas for methods you could use for your own primary research. You may discover that others have already carried out basically the same research project that you are interested in! This last point shouldn't put you off. It can be very interesting to compare the results of your own carefully conducted research with other published results. It is often through repeating the work of others that new insights arise, and differences may point to interesting new areas of investigation.
- Secondary sources can provide data that it would be impossible to collect for yourself. For example, the government collects and publishes **official statistics** on a wide variety of topics. These include information on income, birth and death rates, and other features of the population at national and local level. Governments need these statistics, and have the resources to collect them. No research organisations can easily duplicate the endeavour needed to collect this data, and none would bother as the government's statistical department has an international reputation for the quality of its work.

| Health – England only | | | | | |
|---|---|---|---|---|---|
| | 1976–77 | 1986–87 | 1996–97 | 1997–98 | 1998–99 |
| **Health and Personal Social Services** | | | | | |
| Public Expenditure (£ million) National Health Services (NHS – net) | 5,032 | 15,173 | 32,997 | 34,664 | 36,611 |

| Consultant outpatient attendances | | | | | |
|---|---|---|---|---|---|
| New | 7,499 | 8,768 | 11,294 | 11,529 | N/A |
| Total | 32,396 | 37,728 | 40,873 | 41,635 | N/A |



**An example of official statistics published by the government.**

The places you look for secondary data will depend upon the subject you are interested in. Information of all sorts is published in books, government publications, newspapers, journals, on websites and in a variety of other places. Whatever you are researching it is likely that useful information exists somewhere. Research reports should always list secondary sources that have been consulted. If statistics and other material have been quoted or used to help the research work then it is particularly important that the source is stated clearly in the report. You should be suspicious of any anonymous or poorly attributed data since there is no way to gauge its accuracy.

## Doing secondary research

Doing secondary research around a hypothesis is a good way to begin your research development. There are many sources of secondary data and you need to begin by thinking about what sorts of information might be helpful and relevant to your research question. You may want statistical information about your population, and you may want to look at other studies that are related to your own. When you have some idea what you are looking for you then have the problem of finding it!

But this need not be so difficult as it may sound. Your thoughts about the research question might suggest where appropriate secondary data could be found. Tutors, library staff and other advisers should make it easier to identify and obtain useful secondary source materials.

Other problems crop up when you have found the material. All secondary sources need to be treated with some caution, and there are several points to bear in mind when using them.

- It is important that you understand the information you have found. Sometimes data appears in forms which are difficult to follow unless you are familiar with the field.

It's certainly weighty – but is it light on quality of research?

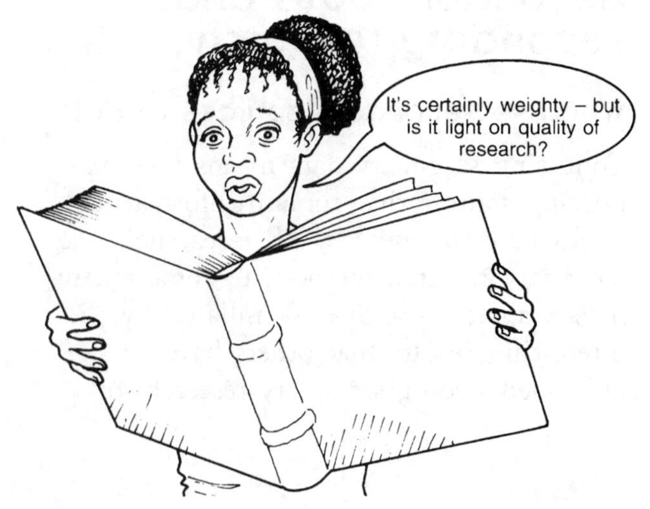

- You must assess how relevant the information is to your work. The people who collected and published the data will have had their own purposes in mind, and they are likely to differ from yours.
- There is the crucial question of the quality of other people's research work. Published data is by no means guaranteed to be accurate. Errors and distortions can result from careless or misguided research work. They can also occur because of deliberate bias. Unfortunately the quality of research behind secondary sources is often hard to judge.

## Sources of secondary data

### Official statistics

National and local government organisations produce a wide variety of official statistics. These bodies need facts and figures of all sorts to assist in planning and decision making.

The government carries out a **census** of the British population every ten years. The last one was in 1991. Every household in Britain is required to fill in a questionnaire, which asks questions about who lives in the house, their occupations and ages. There are also many other surveys and research projects which are carried out by, or on behalf of, government departments. These are not as comprehensive as the census, and usually concern specific topics such as transport or trade.

There are a variety of publications available which contain official statistics, all of which are available in local reference libraries. The census results are published in book form. They contain both national and regional information on a variety of topics. However, it is important to remember that some census results take several years to be published. The *Annual Abstract of Statistics* contain important government statistics. *Social Trends* is similar to the *Annual Abstract of Statistics* but may be more useful as it includes some discussion. It looks at changes over time, and is also published annually. *Regional Trends* is similar to *Social Trends* but contains information for particular regions. *Key Data* is an annual publication and covers important social and economic statistics. If you talk to the librarian you should easily be able to find these and other books containing official statistics in your local reference library.

Official statistics are usually straightforward and understandable. Most appear in the form of tables. You must make sure that you have read and understood the headings, and that you know what the figures represent.

Unfortunately the quality of all official statistics cannot be taken for granted. Although scrupulous care may be used in data collection and analysis, some official figures may not represent the true picture. For example, statistics on crime may seem straightforward to collect. Crimes known to the police are recorded, and totals for different types of crime can be presented as results. But figures can shift if the police decide to 'crack down' on particular areas. A sudden apparent increase in cases of fraud, for example, may be the result of increased police activity in fraud detection. Also, campaigns in the media can result in increased reporting of certain crimes by the public.

There are such a wide range of statistics available that you are likely to come across some data that is relevant to your work. One danger may be that you find a lot of interesting data and try to include too much of it in your final research report.

Remember to use secondary sources as a guide to carrying out your own research project. Quote secondary data only when it adds useful background to your work, or when it provides interesting comparisons with your own results.

### Think it over

Other official data may suffer from problems of distortion. Statistics on unemployment are also apparently easy to collect, but may not reflect the situation accurately.

Think about ways in which unemployment statistics may be affected by official policy and public behaviour.

### Books

Whatever area you are interested in there are probably books that can help you in libraries to which you have access. Books could include textbooks, reference books, or the published work of social researchers. Any of these may provide useful background, and introduce you to concepts and definitions relevant to your research. You may also find published results that you can compare with your own. If you make good use of library filing systems, and the advice of staff, you should find plenty of material.

But using books also has its pitfalls. The published research of social scientists is sometimes difficult to understand, and lengthy to read. It is often better to look at textbooks containing brief, condensed accounts of their work. Another problem is that data in textbooks and reference books may be out of date. Even recent works will have taken time to write and publish. Always try to check the age of any statistic quoted.

### Newspapers and magazines

Newspapers and magazines print research results of all types. In addition to quoting data produced by official sources, they sometimes print the results of their own 'polls'. Articles are likely to be easy to understand, but the big problem is with quality.

Newspapers tailor their content to suit the politics and expectations of their owners and readers, so information can easily be slanted in the direction the editor wishes. Statistics quoted may have been carefully chosen so as to project a particular point of view. The problem of bias makes it difficult to rely on information found in newspapers and magazines.

### Journals and professional publications

Journals and professional publications usually print much more reliable information than newspapers. Because they are aimed at people who are specialists in a particular field they report seriously on professional research results. The problem is that because they are aimed at specialists some articles may be written in technical language. Also, as with books, there is still no guarantee that the research reported has produced accurate results that are free from bias.

One way to judge the validity of information found in journals and other publications is to try to find out something about the author. If they are a supporter of a political party or pressure group you may look for the influence of this in their ideas and writings. It may be that the author has a particular philosophical approach which influences their work.

## Publications by other groups

Many groups and organisations produce information. Some are funded by government, like the Commission for Racial Equality (CRE). Some, such as Amnesty International or the RSPCA, are funded by donations from the public. Others, like the Trades Union Congress or the Confederation of British Industry, are paid for by members whose interests they represent. Political parties also sponsor and publish research. These organisations are usually happy to send you any data that they have if you write and ask for it.

The major drawback is that information from pressure groups may be heavily subject to bias, since the group is keen to get their message across. This is not likely to be a problem with officially sponsored organisations, but data produced by privately funded pressure groups should be treated with considerable caution.

## Using the internet for research

There is a vast amount of information available on the internet which you can access through any internet-connected computer. You may have tried searching the internet for information and found out how confusing it can be. Finding things can be made a lot easier if you know which web sites to visit for the information you need, so here are some useful links for sites to help you with secondary research.

### Centre for Applied Social Surveys – CASS

CASS is a web site run jointly by The National Centre for Social Research and the University of Southampton, with the University of Surrey. It provides short courses in survey methods and is developing a survey Question Bank for use by social scientists and social researchers in the academic world, government, market research and the independent and voluntary sectors. The internet address, or URL, of CASS is:

**http://www.natcen.ac.uk/cass/docs/fr_cass home.htm**

The Centre for Applied Social Surveys (CASS) Question Bank is a store of complete UK social survey questions, questionnaires and response forms. You can download tried and tested social survey materials and there is no cost for the service. The Question Bank's URL is:

**http://qb.soc.surrey.ac.uk/nav/fr_home3.h tm**

The CASS site has a lot of support and information for people involved in social research, many useful links to social research sites, and data available on line. This is a good site to look at for ideas and secondary data.

### Government Statistical Service

This is the web site of the Government Statistical Service (GSS) which produces and disseminates official UK statistics and data. Its URL is:

**http://www.statistics.gov.uk/**

The site describes itself as 'a Government Service, which aims to provide you with the information you need to access statistics, easily and quickly.'

One of the pages on this site is 'The UK in Figures: Official Statistics for the United Kingdom'. Information taken from Government Statistical Service publications and other sources is available here. The URL of this page is:

**http://www.statistics.gov.uk/stats/ukinfigs /ukinfig.htm**

### The Office for National Statistics

The Office for National Statistics (ONS) is a UK Government Agency that produces and disseminates social, health, economic, demographic, labour market and business statistics. Its internet address, or URL, is:

http://www.ons.gov.uk/

There are many types of statistics here as well as other useful information. For instance the Reference Information section of the site contains details of a health and social care research project titled 'Young teenagers and smoking in 1988'. The project looked at young people's attitudes to smoking and their awareness of anti-smoking promotions and campaigns. You can download the project report as a file in a format known as Adobe Acrobat. You may need to consult someone with IT expertise to find out how to download and read the report file.

| **Try it out** | Log on to the internet and have a look at the sites mentioned above. You may find some interesting background information to help your own research.<br><br>You could try using a search facility to look for information on other topics that you are interested in. Be careful to phrase your search carefully or you could find yourself swamped by a massive list of URLs to web sites that are of little or no use to you. Get advice from someone experienced in internet search techniques if you are unsure how to search the internet effectively. |
|---|---|

## Primary research methods

There are a variety of ways of doing primary research and each has strengths and weaknesses. This section examines several methods including:

- experiments
- self-completion questionnaires
- structured interviews
- in-depth interviews
- direct observation
- participant observation.

### Experiments

Experiments are often used by psychologists as a way of discovering how individuals behave. Scientists such as chemists and physicists use experiments as their main method of testing theories and hypotheses, and psychologists attempt to apply experimental techniques to the study of people. The principle of the experimental method is that the scientist has control of all the variables in the situation that is being studied. For example, a chemist can control variables like temperature, the amounts of each chemical, and the length of time allowed for them to react. By altering one variable and measuring the effect on another, the chemist can establish the experimental relationship between them and make predictions about the future behaviour of the same chemicals in similar circumstances.

However, applying the experimental method to the study of people is not so straightforward. The behaviour of a person is vastly more complex than that of a chemical substance. The range of variables that may influence a subject's behaviour is so large that it is difficult to list them, let

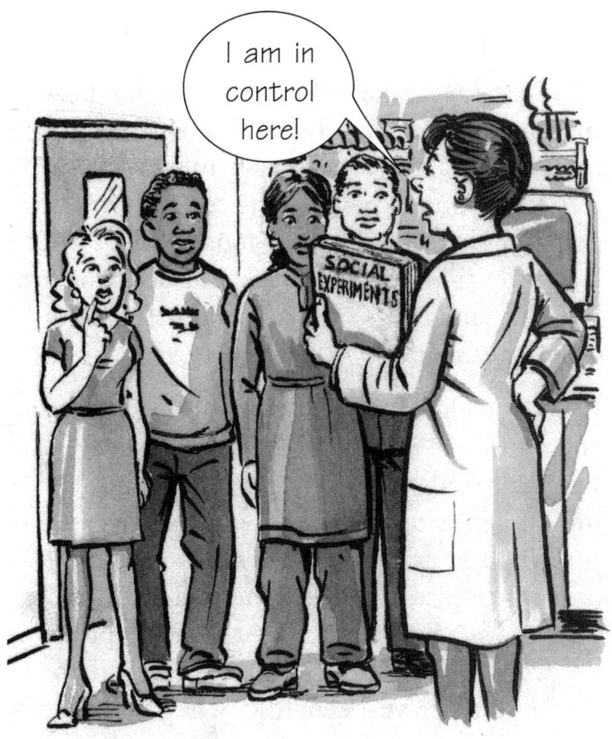


Applying the experimental method to the study of people is not always easy

alone control them. This becomes even more problematic when the behaviour of groups of people is being studied. One result of this difficulty is that experiments usually deal with a very narrow range of behaviour in very specific circumstances. Predictions about future behaviour need to take account of the complexity of real life where people's actions and behaviour are affected by ideas and influences that the experimenter cannot measure, and may not even be aware of.

Most social experimenters are sensibly cautious about the claims that they make for their research. Provided this scientific honesty is kept in mind, experiments can be a useful way of testing hypotheses about human characteristics and behaviour.

## Using experiments in a research project

Carrying out experiments in health and social care research can be difficult. Experiments are usually employed by scientists like biologists, or by psychologists who are interested in very specific aspects of people's abilities or behaviour. Some of the problems with applying the experimental method to the study of people are outlined above. Controlling, or even estimating, all the variables affecting human behaviour may be impossible. Researchers need to set up highly structured experimental situations so that outside influences are, as far as possible, identical for all the subjects tested.

Another difficulty is that experiments set out to measure things. This could be something like how far a person can jump, or how quickly they can press a button when ordered to do so. Taking

| Pros | Cons |
|---|---|
| Can be designed to test very specific theories and hypotheses | Range of enquiry limited to the specific aims of the experiment |
| The experimenter can control the circumstances in which the experiment takes place | Difficult for the experimenter to control all factors affecting the behaviour of subjects |
| Data collected is nearly always quantitative allowing statistical interpretation of the results | Artificial circumstances of the experimental situation may distort subjects' behaviour |
| It is possible for other researchers to duplicate the experiment and test the replicability of the results | 'Scientific' conduct of the experiment and statistical presentation of results may lend more credibility to the work than it deserves |

Table 6.1 Some pros and cons of experiments

measurements will mean having equipment available. Psychological and medical experiments often employ sophisticated equipment that has been specially designed and constructed for the research in question. This sort of specialised equipment is usually not available to the student researcher.

Even where everyday equipment is used, experimenters must be sure that they are able to carry out measurements accurately. For instance, you may decide to set up an experiment to find out how quickly and effectively the students on your course are able to apply a particular style of wound dressing. It is easy to time the efforts of each subject but it is much more difficult to judge the quality of their work. It would need someone with skill and experience to make accurate judgements.

Another thing to consider is safety. You are setting up a situation and are responsible for the outcomes. Apparently simple experiments can be hazardous to some subjects, and you may not be aware of personal circumstances that could make the experiment dangerous to a particular individual.

You also need to think about the ethics of the experiment you are planning. Researchers often need to keep subjects ignorant of the true purpose of the experiment because knowledge of this will affect how they behave. A researcher could tell subjects that they are researching one thing when they are really looking at another. In the past some classic psychological studies have relied on subjects being duped in this way. The ethical considerations may have been ignored, or taken to be less important than the advancement of human understanding. While professional researchers working in important areas may have some justification for their methods, it is generally not ethical to keep subjects in the dark about the true nature and aims of an experiment. If you feel that your experimental research will demand that subjects are fooled about your real intentions then you should abandon the method and carry out your research using other means.

If you do decide to carry out an experiment you must try to make the experience similar for all subjects. Carry out the method in a uniform way so that each subject has, as far as possible, a similar set of influences to all the others. Try to make sure that each subject has the same prior knowledge of what they will be asked to do. If some have been told what to expect well in advance their results may differ from those of subjects given less warning.

Finally, remember that there can be difficulties generalising the experimental results to other populations or situations. You have set up an artificial situation and the results may not apply outside that context. For example, our wound dressing skill experiment may have shown that one particular student excelled over all the rest, both in quality of the dressing and speed of execution. However, that person may, unknown to you, have a serious aversion to the sight of blood which prevents them using their skills effectively in a real emergency. What experiments show is how people have behaved on a particular occasion and under a particular set of circumstances. Going beyond this requires care and scientific honesty.

## Self-completion questionnaires

Self-completion questionnaires, as the name implies, are given to people for them to complete. It is up to the person, or

**respondent**, to read and interpret the questions for themselves. If it is a **postal questionnaire** then the respondent is left entirely to themselves; if not then the researcher may be present to help interpret the questions.

Questionnaires are used extensively in social research, and they can have several advantages:

- They give you the chance to collect information from a large **sample** of your population. It is fairly cheap to reproduce and distribute large numbers of questionnaires.
- There is less danger that the behaviour or appearance of an interviewer could affect the results. This problem occurs in all research which involves interaction between the researcher and the subjects. Distributing questionnaires is one way to avoid it.
- Respondents have time to consider their answers, and consult others if necessary. For example, if you stop somebody in the street and ask them how much their household spends on food per week they are likely to respond with 'don't know', or make a guess. To get an accurate answer it is probably better to give respondents time to think, and to ask other family members.
- Postal questionnaires may be the only practical way of contacting members of some populations. Postal questionnaires can be sent to people when physical distance makes interviewing impossible.
- Some busy people, such as doctors or other professionals, may be more willing to fill in a brief questionnaire than give up time for an interview.

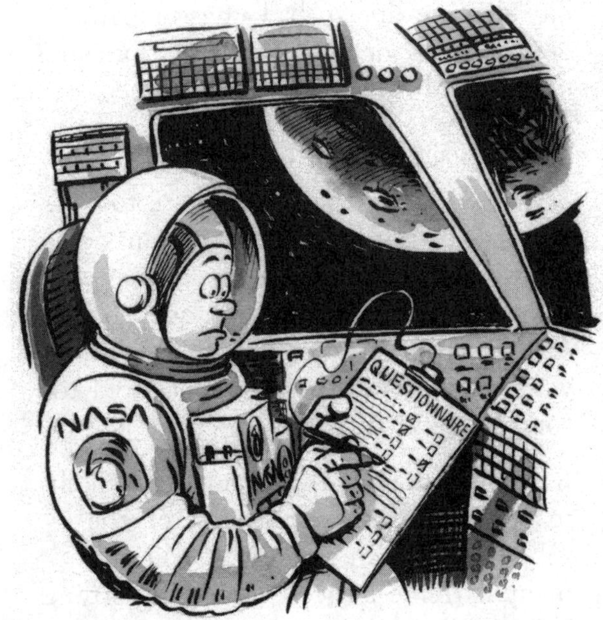

Postal questionnaires can reach people too far away to interview

Most questionnaires are designed to collect quantitative information. This means that results can be compared between respondents and analysed statistically. This can be seen as another advantage. Remember, however, that good looking statistics may mask sloppy research work. Well presented results are not necessarily good results.

When the information required is comparatively straightforward a questionnaire can be a very effective research instrument. However, there are problems associated with questionnaires that must be set against the advantages:

- Questionnaires often attract a very low **response rate.** Those who do respond cannot be taken as representative of the whole population, however carefully you selected your original sample. Statistical analysis of the data collected has little value in this situation. A poor response rate may be due to bad questionnaire design. Long or confusing questionnaires usually end up in the bin. Another possibility is that questions are asked which people are reluctant to answer, perhaps because the subjects are too personal or sensitive. The only answer to a low response rate is to make the subject and content of your questionnaire sufficiently interesting to members of your sample that they are motivated to complete and return them.

- Responses that you do receive are likely to be from those with a view on the subject. This can mean that you get many extreme answers indicating strong but divided opinions. In fact, opinion may be much more evenly spread within the population, but non-response by those who are not particularly interested will hide this.
- Questionnaires assume a certain level of literacy among respondents. This makes them inappropriate for surveying certain groups, for example small children. Even when this is not expected to be a problem, misunderstandings can and do occur. Without an interviewer present there is no check that the questions have been understood. Respondents cannot ask for clarification and may guess an answer, or throw the questionnaire away. Either way, the quality of the results will be reduced.
- The researcher has no control over who actually completes the questionnaire. It may be passed on to other members of the family or be filled in as a joke by a group of friends in the pub! Uncertainty over whose answers you actually receive can completely invalidate careful sampling work.

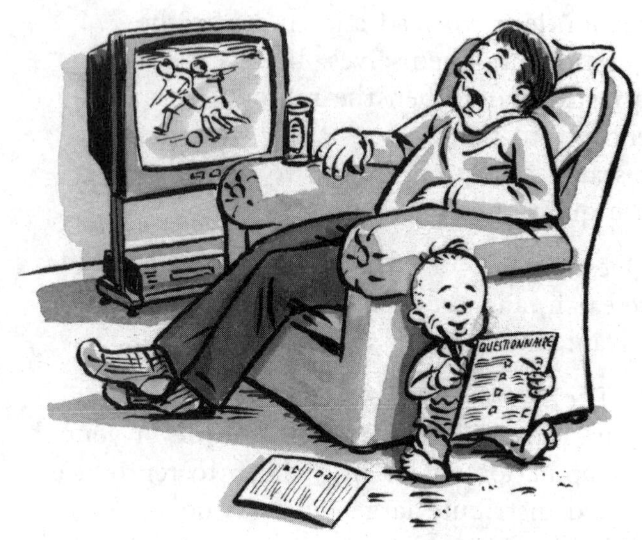


**You have no control over who completes a postal questionnaire**

- Sometimes researchers want to get people's spontaneous responses to a question. Respondents may give accurate answers to personal questions if they reply spontaneously; but if allowed time to think they can pick answers that support the image they wish to project. You cannot expect to receive spontaneous responses from questionnaires.
- Another limitation of questionnaires is that respondents can see all the questions at once. An interviewer can control the order in which questions are delivered, so that answers are not prejudiced by knowledge of questions still to come. For instance, in a postal questionnaire it is no use asking, 'Can you name the body set up by the government to promote good race relations?', if a later question asks, 'Do you think that the Commission for Racial Equality is effective in promoting good race relations?'.
- Interviewers can observe people's reactions to the questions as they are asked. This potentially useful information

| Pros | Cons |
|---|---|
| Data can be cheaply collected from a large number of respondents | Postal questionnaires often suffer from a poor response rate |
| No problem with the behaviour and appearance of the interviewer influencing results | Responses may be largely from people who have strong opinions on the subject |
| Respondents have time to consider answers and consult others if necessary | No check on whether respondents have really understood the questions |
| Postal methods may be the only way to contact some respondents | No control over who actually completes the questionnaire |
| May be more acceptable to some respondents than an interview | No opportunity to observe respondents' reactions to the questions |
| | Cannot expect to collect respondents' spontaneous answers |
| | No control over order in which questions are answered |
| | Respondents are limited to the questions and answer options presented and their authentic views may not be revealed |

Table 6.2 Some pros and cons of self-completion questionnaires

is not available with self-completion questionnaires.

## Using questionnaires in a research project

If you want to get information from a number of people quickly then a self-completion questionnaire may be a good way to go about it. Unfortunately self-completion questionnaires have a reputation for achieving poor response rates when postal methods are used. One answer to this is to make your questionnaire as interesting and relevant as possible to your subjects. Also, of course, it needs to be clear and simple enough not to put people off. Information technology resources can help you to produce a professional looking and easy to follow questionnaire. Subjects are much more likely to respond if your questionnaire has these qualities.

Postal questionnaires are simple to administer. You just send a copy of your questionnaire, together with a suitable covering letter, to each member of your sample and wait for the replies to come rolling in. In practice it may be necessary to include a stamped, addressed envelope to help encourage returns. This could be costly, but that is the price you pay for more accurate results!

If you are able to hand the questionnaires to your subjects, and collect them personally, your response rate should be much better. You may have thought of leaving a stack of questionnaires in a suitable place and providing a box for completed questionnaires to be placed in. This can be tempting if you want to get quick returns from people who use a particular facility. But beware because this method may give very distorted results. You are asking for a sample to select itself. Those who reply may do so because they have time or motivation. You will miss people in a hurry, and those who have moderate opinions on your research subject. People with strong opinions might fill in several forms so as to make their point. It is much better to take the trouble to use a simple sampling method and improve the quality of your results.

Questionnaires may be one of the research methods you use in your primary research project. It is useful if you are aware of the pitfalls and honest about possible sources of error when reporting on your results. Advice on designing questionnaires is given later in this chapter on page 456.

| **Try it out** | Self-completion questionnaires are a cheap and fairly easy way to collect data from a large number of people. Think about some of the research ideas you thought of in the activity on page 424. For each one, assess whether a self-completion questionnaire would be appropriate. List the pros and cons of using this research method in these specific areas of research. |
|---|---|

### Structured interviews

Interviews involve the researcher meeting with individual subjects and collecting data directly from them. It is up to the researcher to decide whether to make the interview a more or less formal meeting. An interview can follow an inflexible schedule, or it can be conducted in a more relaxed, less structured way. Interviews which follow a well defined and fairly rigid plan are known as **structured interviews.**

Interviews where the researcher allows the respondents to explore a question in their own way are called **unstructured** or **in-depth interviews.**

A main aim of structured interviews is to ensure that each interview is carried out in exactly the same way. Any factors that could bias a response are thus minimised, or at least are theoretically the same for all respondents. Uniformity in interviews is important if vital statistical comparisons are to be made between the responses of different subjects. Interviewers follow an **interview schedule** which dictates their input into the interview meeting. Interview schedules contains a list of questions, similar to a questionnaire. They also contain instructions for the interviewer to follow. Questions are read out to respondents and their answers recorded by the interviewer. To help maximise uniformity the schedule contains set comments to prompt a reply, or probe an area more deeply. Interviewers are not allowed to deviate from the questions and the **prompts** and **probes** are provided in the interview schedule.

In practice, the degree of uniformity described above is often very difficult to achieve. Nevertheless the structured interview is a useful and widely used research technique which has several advantages:

- The response rate obtained by structured interviewing is likely to be good. Provided that the sample chosen is small enough to handle and is easily accessible, the only difficulty is in pinning respondents down for an interview.
- Misunderstandings over the meaning of questions can easily be dealt with. Interviewers can repeat the question and add prompts allowed by the schedule.

- Interviews can be designed to follow up interesting lines of enquiry that a respondent's answers might suggest. The schedule can be structured so that certain responses result in an extra range of questions being asked.
- The pace of questioning is up to the interviewer, which allows him or her to draw subjects into giving quick answers. The result can be spontaneous responses which the subject has not had time to consider.
- Interviewers may pick up useful background data from observing a respondent's reactions to the questions. These observations can be recorded on the interview schedule if space is reserved for them.
- The responses can, of course be guaranteed to come from the respondents themselves. There is no danger of collusion with others if the subject is trapped in an interview.
- A main advantage of the structured interview technique is that quantitative data collected can be analysed statistically, and conclusions made about the population as a whole.

Many of the pitfalls of postal questionnaires are avoided because of the control an interviewer has over data collection. Uniformity of method attempts to offset any distortion that the presence of the interviewer creates. Structured interviewing attempts to be as 'scientific' as possible so that the results can be convincingly applied to the whole population.

However, structured interviews can also have disadvantages. Well-presented results can look convincing, particularly if charts and graphs are used to demonstrate a point. But structured interviewing can produce distorted data, and thus distorted results:

- A major problem is that sample size is often small. Interviewing is very time consuming. Contacting a representative sample may mean travelling, or waiting for respondents to turn up. Interviews that are really useful are likely to last for several minutes, and you need to add time to complete your notes. The lone researcher cannot hope to complete a large number of structured interviews and must select a sample small enough to be interviewed in the time available. But a very small sample is unlikely to be representative of the population as a whole. One way to overcome this problem is to set less ambitious aims for your investigation, and select a research topic which has a smaller population. For instance, if you are interested in attitudes to smoking then choose to research attitudes among local students, rather than attitudes among all young adults. This makes it much easier to select and interview a representative sample. The results may not be as far-reaching, but they are far more likely to be accurate.
- The interaction between respondent and interviewer is a source of distortion that can never be completely eliminated. An interview is a type of conversation. Even when verbal messages are standardised by an interview schedule the interviewer's appearance, accent and personal characteristics can affect what takes place. Non-verbal signals pass between the participants, and the respondent may be looking for cues that indicate what sort of answers the researcher wants. If they have negative perceptions of the interviewer, respondents may give deliberately provocative answers. If they wish to impress they may give answers that project a positive image of themselves. Distortions caused by interviewer-respondent interaction are difficult if not

| Pros | Cons |
|---|---|
| Very good response rates are possible | Time consuming interviews can mean that only a small unrepresentative sample is chosen |
| Interviewer is available to clarify questions and prevent misunderstandings | Interaction between respondent and interviewer can lead to distorted answers being given |
| Probes allow extra lines of enquiry to be followed up | Respondents are limited to the question and answer options presented, and their authentic views may not be revealed |
| Pace of questioning can induce spontaneous responses | Respondents need to be easily contactable |
| No uncertainty over who actually answers the questions | |
| Interviewers can observe and collect useful background data | |
| Uniformity of interview technique and content makes quantitative analysis of the data possible | |

**Table 6.3 Some pros and cons of structured interviews**

impossible to assess. But there is no doubt that they do occur. Studies have repeatedly shown that different interviewers often get different answers to the same questions. Awareness of this issue has led to attempts by researchers to reduce its effect. The formal nature of the structured interview is itself an attempt to minimise interviewer influence.

- Structured interviews rely on the honesty and good intentions of interviewing staff. Honesty can be checked, particularly if the data collected by one interviewer differs wildly from everyone else's. Deliberate influence, by gesture, tone of voice or deviations from the schedule, is much more difficult to detect.
- A structured interview is only as good as the questionnaire design and content allow. A poorly considered set of questions will not give useful data, however scrupulously the interviews are conducted and the results calculated.

## Using structured interviews in a research project

Structured interviews are one of the most commonly used research methods and the features that we have looked at help to explain why this is so.

When carrying out your own interviews you should try to stick to the principles that underlie the use of this research method. Structured interviewing stresses uniformity. It is essential that the effect of the interviewer on a respondent's answers is as small as possible. Even the stress interviewers put on words when reading out a question can exert an influence. Try reading out loud the question, 'Do you believe the government is doing a good job?' a few times, putting the stress on different parts of the question. Stressing the word *good* implies that there may be some doubt. Stressing the word *government* implies that they are being compared with something else. Interviewers should read out questions in as neutral a way as possible to reduce the possibility of biasing an answer.

- The questions asked must not be varied by the interviewer. If this is allowed it is even more likely that bias will occur. This is fine provided an interview goes smoothly, but in practice interviewers do not always have such an easy time. Problems with responses can take a variety of forms, but fortunately there are ways of dealing with them. You may get only a partial response, where the respondent does not give enough information for the response to be recorded. Or the response may be irrelevant to the question.
- Respondents could side-track the questioning process, perhaps by commenting on a previous question instead of answering the one just asked.
- Some responses are inaccurate, and obviously so. This may be an indication that the question has been misunderstood.
- Also you may get no response at all. Your question could be met with silence, perhaps because respondents are thinking it over, or because they do not know what to say.

Interviewers have the problem of dealing with response problems without biasing the results. The solution is to have a prepared list of statements, known as **prompts**, which can be used to tackle response problems. They can be printed on the interview schedule to ensure they are used similarly for each respondent. If interviewers vary the content and wording of these comments it defeats the object of using them.

'If you stand still does the pain go away or not?'

**IF RESPONDENT UNSURE, PROBE**: 'What happens to the pain on most occasions?'

**Figure 6.3 This question was used in the 1998 Health Survey for England. It was asked to people complaining of chest pains. It includes a specifically worded probe to be used in the event of a response problem**

Sometimes a non-verbal clue will help. If the problem is non-response it may be best to stay silent and allow a noticeable pause to develop. Respondents may pick up that it is their turn to speak and provide you with an answer. Another method is to use a nod, raised eyebrows, or similar non-verbal signal to indicate that you are waiting for a reply. Remember to standardise the non-verbal clues you intend to use, as haphazard use can introduce bias. If these tactics do not work you could ask if they would like you to repeat the question.

Partial responses may be solved by using silence or non-verbal cues. If there is no improvement verbal follow-ups could begin with 'I see' accompanied by a nod to indicate you want more. Or, more directly, 'Can you tell me more?'.

Responses which are irrelevant or inaccurate may be the result of a misunderstood question. This can be tricky since you need to avoid insulting or belittling respondents by highlighting their mistake. You could try saying, 'I'm sorry, I may not have asked that question very clearly,' and then repeat the question. Respondents may take care to listen closely as you have indicated that a problem of some kind has occurred, and the error has been transferred onto you. You could try stating the subject clearly before repeating the question. A statement like, 'This question is about . . .' can cover questions on many subjects. To minimise bias the subject of each question needs to be indicated on the schedule in case this statement has to be used.

### Think it over

Think about how you might deal with response problems during your interviews. Try to imagine the sorts of problems that could occur and what you could do or say to help.

Make a list of your ideas. You can decide which approaches to allow when you come to design your interview questionnaire.

When carrying out the interviews try to be friendly but professional. A standardised welcome and explanation of the purpose of the survey is needed, as are introductions to new parts of the interview. Remember that all the input of the interviewer needs to be scripted. Keep introductions brief and friendly, and be sure to stick to them with each respondent. Things go much more smoothly if the interviewer's input is clearly highlighted on the interview schedule, so use IT resources to make yours clear and well organised.

## In-depth interviews

Many aspects of opinion are difficult to explore through a fixed set of questions. People's attitudes, beliefs and opinions are a personal matter and formal quantitative techniques may not be the best way to bring out authentic views. Respondents often find it easier to make a safe, respectable response rather than think deeply about a sensitive issue on which their views are not so clear cut. Authentic opinion is more likely to emerge in a relaxed, less formal meeting.

Because questions in a structured interview schedule are fixed, the respondents have no room for manoeuvre. They may be forced into making choices, possibly between a set of equally inappropriate alternatives. Respondents may have other, strongly held, views that the questions fail to bring out and the interviewer never becomes aware of. The questionnaire and interview schedule define the territory to be explored, and define it in the researcher's terms. Answers may be obtained but are they important or relevant to the lives and outlook of the respondents themselves?

In-depth interviews, or unstructured interviews, are less fixed and formal than structured interviews. At the extreme, an in-depth interview can be more like a chat, with the interviewer supplying only the topic for conversation. The interviewer can provide guidance as things progress, to keep the topic in view. The aim of in-depth interviews is to encourage respondents to open up, and provide as much detail as possible.

In-depth interviews have big advantages when it comes to finding out what people really think. Subjects do not have to choose between alternative answers. They can introduce areas for discussion that are important to them, and they can give any information that they feel to be relevant. This means that the data is given according to the respondents' frame of reference and view of the world. Connections may be made that would never have occurred to the interviewer. Also there is likely to be a good deal of information collected since in-depth interviewers can last for a fairly long time, sometimes for several hours.

This open and flexible approach may be the best if not the only way to get information about people's real attitudes, values and opinions. In the informal atmosphere of the in-depth interview the respondents' inhibitions are reduced. They can be encouraged to talk about sensitive subjects and give views that they would not usually reveal to others. If interesting points arise that merit further investigation the interviewer has the freedom to steer the discussion towards them.

In-depth interviews provide rich information which is likely to represent respondents' views accurately. Of course, almost all the data collected is qualitative and the results cannot be analysed statistically. Comparing results between respondents is usually impossible since each will have given information in their own terms. Respondents may approach the same topic from a completely different viewpoint.

Different people will provide different items of data. Apart from this the sample size is likely to be very small because of the length of time needed to carry out and report on interviews. Even if comparisons between respondents can be made it is meaningless to try projecting the results onto the wider population. This is a characteristic of in-depth interviews, not a weakness of them. Researchers using the technique are aiming for depth and authenticity in difficult areas of enquiry, not for quantitative results.

The main issue that arises in in-depth interviewing is the level of skill required of the interviewer. Respondents must be put

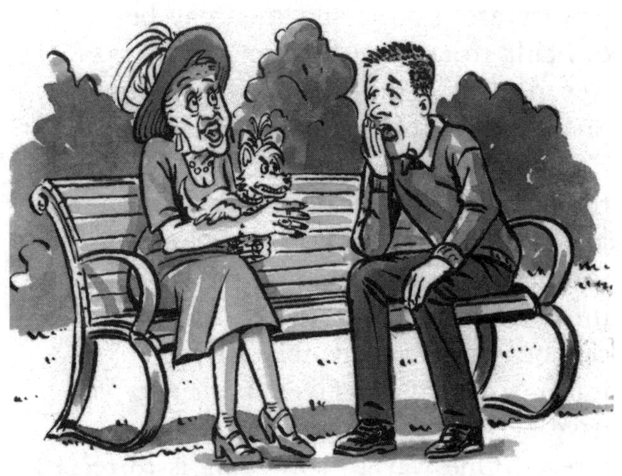

**In in-depth interviews, respondents must feel happy about talking openly to a stranger**

at ease and feel happy about talking openly to a stranger. Interviewers need to encourage their subject to speak while subtly keeping the conversation focused on the topic they are interested in. As well as this, interviewers must try to avoid imposing their own bias on the discussion. Egging on respondents to make out-of-character comments will not produce accurate results.

All the problems of interviewer influence that can occur in structured interviews apply also to in-depth interviews. In fact, the freedom and depth of interaction that occurs in in-depth situations make the problem even more serious. To some extent the length of the interview can help, since subjects have time to get used to the interviewer and begin to behave naturally. Apart from this it is the skill and integrity of the interviewer that is relied upon to make the interview useful.

In-depth interviews also pose practical problems. It is important that a suitable place is chosen for the interview. Time and privacy are needed and this may be difficult to arrange for some subjects. Recording the information is another problem. Taking notes is slow, and may inhibit the subject, reminding them that they are in an interview situation. Quickly jotted notes are likely to be at best a brief summary of the conversation, and later interpretation may lead to distortions. You cannot hope to remember all the information you receive, and things you have been too slow to write down are gone forever. One way to solve this is to record the interview on tape. Nothing verbal will be missed, but visual data about the subject's behaviour during the interview is not recorded. Some people are put off by the presence of a tape recorder and will not speak freely if you use one. Planting a hidden recorder is unethical practice, and you should resort to note-taking if a tape recorder puts subjects off.

### Using in-depth interviews in a research project

Carrying out in-depth research may seem to need less planning and preparation than methods which use questionnaires. There are, however, other demands placed on the researcher which it takes care and skill to deal with. In-depth interviews are about letting people 'open up'. This is how you expect to be able to collect accurate data from them. However, encouraging people to think and speak about deep personal feelings or events can lead to an interaction that you will need to handle with great care. Some respondents may find the interview a traumatic or even damaging experience. You need to prepare and carry out your research so as to avoid this happening, and to ensure that you are doing useful work towards your research question.

There may be advantages to using qualitative methods, perhaps before going on to design and use quantitative research approaches. You are likely to hear

| Pros | Cons |
|---|---|
| Subjects have the freedom to give an answer in their own terms | Interviewers must have very well developed communication skills |
| A large amount of information can be collected from each respondent | Each interview is time consuming so it is only possible to carry out a few |
| Answers can be very accurate representations of the subject's real opinions and feelings | Personal characteristics of the interviewer can affect answers given |
| Respondents have time to 'open up' on sensitive issues | Time and privacy are needed to carry out the interviews |
| Interviewers are free to explore any interesting areas that arise | Qualitative nature of data collected and small sample size limit the broader applicability of the results |
| Rich qualitative data can be gathered | |

Table 6.4 Some pros and cons of in-depth interviews

comments that you would never have expected, and you will have a much better understanding of the issues when your unstructured interviews are completed. You can use this knowledge and data to help create a questionnaire that is interesting to your respondents and covers the things that concern them. Qualitative research helps you to design better quantitative research instruments. Quantitative data can be included in your research report to give background and to help readers to assess how typical your subjects might be.

Next you need to decide who to interview, and how many interviews to carry out. You will probably want to allow at least an hour for each interview, perhaps much longer. How many will you be able to conduct in the time you have available? Each interview must be carried out somewhere which is private, quiet, where the respondent feels at ease, and where interruptions will not occur. One suitable place could be the respondent's own home, if you know them well enough to suggest it. Otherwise you may need to use a room in a suitable place. This may be a facility such as a day centre. Now you will have to consider whether you can get uninterrupted use of the room at times convenient to you and your subjects. All these issues will affect the number of interviews you can handle, and who you can use as subjects. If you intend to use in-depth techniques you should consider these implications at an early stage. You may need to reformulate your research question so that it concerns a population that you can easily contact and meet in private.

Another thing to plan is how you are going to record the data. A tape recorder is probably the best way, if your subjects are happy about it. Of course, it is unethical to record secretly. You must always warn respondents of your intentions, and most people will be happy for you to use this method. You might want to keep notes as well. You can record background data, such as a respondent's appearance and body language. Also you can note the time and content of important parts of the interview. This may speed things up later when you need to find them on the tape. Note taking can act as a barrier between you and your subject. But this may not be a bad thing since it reminds you both that you are having an interview, and may make it easier for you to keep the point in view.

The content of the interview will depend on your skills, the person you are interviewing, and the subject being discussed. An important issue that you need to think about in advance is the sensitivity of the research question for your respondents. Potentially traumatic subjects or events need handling with great care. You must pick respondents, and subjects, that minimise the likelihood of your interview causing someone serious upset. Areas like bereavement or the break-up of a relationship may become so upsetting that the interview becomes harmful to the respondent's psychological well-being. If you think that this is possible then it is unethical to continue your research along those lines.

Another ethical issue is the subject's right to confidentiality. In-depth methods collect a lot of data, and you will be reporting results from a very small sample of people. This might mean that respondents can be identified from your report if they are known to members of your target audience. You should simply avoid using subjects who may fall victim to this, and write your report carefully to prevent such identification.

In-depth research reports can help to remind us that social research really is about people. When writing your report try to include some quotes from your respondents that seem to sum up their views in their own words. It is rich original data of this sort that in-depth researchers are looking for.

## Reliability and validity

There is a marked contrast between the uniformity of the structured interview and the flexible openness of an in-depth interview. The differences between the two methods go further than interview style.

Structured interviews stress **reliability**. This means that repeats of the research using different samples should reliably produce the same results. Every aspect, from question design to interviewer style, is planned so as to maximise reliability. If the results of structured research seem not to be reliable then the research has failed on its own terms. Reliability can only be assessed if results are expressed statistically.

In-depth interviews stress validity. This means that the information collected comes very close to the subject's real views. It gives a valid picture of what they truly believe. In-depth interview data is not expected to have reliability. Subjects' responses are individual, and are not intended to be compared directly. Certainly they cannot be compared statistically since the data is qualitative.

Research which emphasises reliability may lose validity in the process. Questions that reliably receive a similar range of responses have to be carefully designed in order to achieve this. Questions which produce conflicting or erratic responses are pruned out so that reliability is ensured. This can result in questions that ask only about trite, safe subjects. More seriously it can result in real variations of opinion and attitude being ignored because they do not fit the researcher's notion of what he or she is trying to find out. Questions may reliably receive invalid responses.

Research which emphasises validity makes no attempt to be reliable. It is not expected that different respondents will give comparable data. Comparisons may be suggested but there is no list of allowed responses against which reliability can be assessed. The results do not help us to gauge the views of the wider population, and without wider applicability the research may be regarded as merely interesting.

In this discussion we have looked at two extreme positions in research methodology. In practice, many researchers pitch their work somewhere between them or try to use both methods. In-depth interviews may give you information that suggests a pattern of opinion worth exploring further. Structured interviews may be used to check how far that pattern of opinion extends into the wider population. Different research aims and methodologies should be seen as complementary, not in opposition to one another.

## Observation

Observation is another popular and useful research technique. There are two main variants: **direct observation,** where the researcher remains detached from the subjects, and **participant observation,** where the researcher joins in with the people being studied.

Observation means studying by looking. To be classed as research, rather then merely looking on, observations need to be structured. As with other research techniques, data collection has to be organised so that relevant and useful information is sought and recorded. Well-organised observation has several advantages as a research technique:

- You can observe what people actually do, not what they tell researchers that they do. People are studied in their own environment and should be expected to behave as they do naturally. Observation can detect 'taken for granted' behaviour that subjects are not aware of, and would thus not report if asked in an interview.
- Groups, and the interactions between their members, can be studied. Other research methods look at individuals, making group behaviour difficult to investigate.
- Observations can be done over time, allowing changes in groups or situations to be revealed.

### Direct observation

Direct observation can be regarded as similar to bird watching. Subjects are watched as they go about their normal lives and observations are recorded by the researcher.

Both qualitative and quantitative data can be collected through direct observation. For example, quantitative data about playground usage is probably best collected by this method. Observers can count arrivals and can group them in terms of sex, age, and other observable characteristics. Observers can also record qualitative data, such as how the children behave towards each other in the playground, and which seem to be friends.

Direct observation may be the only way to observe some groups, for example small children. It can be useful in any situation where your presence would be unobtrusive.

However, direct observation also has problems associated with it:

- One problem is that of recording the data. Making notes distracts the researcher from observation. It may be easy to miss something important, particularly when a fairly large group is being studied.
- Some methods of observation can raise ethical problems. Should researchers use secret techniques for collecting and recording data? This could be something fairly innocent, like fixing an electronic counter to a door to check how many people use it. However, it could include bugging phones, or using two-way mirrors to observe private behaviour.
- A more serious difficulty is interpreting what is observed. Direct observers are not 'inside', and they cannot see behaviour from the subject's point of view. For example, children may believe that they are playing a boisterous game, while the observer perceives a violent confrontation. Observers may project their own theories onto what they see, and fail to understand what is happening so far as the subjects are concerned.

It is because of the difficulties with interpretation that direct observation is a poor way to research opinions and values. Inferring beliefs from observed behaviour is likely to produce highly distorted results. Of course, observed behaviour may suggest lines of enquiry that can be followed up with other methods. For example, you may observe that staff at a day centre seem to spend less time talking to black clients. Further research using interview techniques could probe staff attitudes to race and discrimination.

## Observation sheet 3

**Observing an individual child for social development**

Name of candidate . . . . . . . . . . . . . . . . . . . . . . . . . . . . . . . . . . . . . . . . . . . . . . . . . .

Age/sex of child . . . . . . . . . . . . . . . . . . . . . . . . . . . . . . . . . . . . . . . . . . . . . . . . . . . .

Date . . . . . . . . . . . . . . . . . . . Time: From . . . . . . . . . . . . . . . To . . . . . . . . . . . . . .

Aim . . . . . . . . . . . . . . . . . . . . . . . . . . . . . . . . . . . . . . . . . . . . . . . . . . . . . . . . . . . .

Activity while observing

**Social development – interaction with peers**

Factors you might note

- Does the child seek out other children? . . . . . . . . . . . . . . . . . . . . . . . . . . . . . . . . . . . . .
- Does the child seek only certain children? . . . . . . . . . . . . . . . . . . . . . . . . . . . . . . . . . . .
- Does the child avoid some children? . . . . . . . . . . . . . . . . . . . . . . . . . . . . . . . . . . . . . . .
- Does the child take part in group activities with children of the same age? . . . . . . . . . . . .
- Is the child accepted by the other children in the group? . . . . . . . . . . . . . . . . . . . . . . . . .
- Does the child spend a lot of time watching other children? . . . . . . . . . . . . . . . . . . . . . . .
- Does the child share space, ideas and equipment? . . . . . . . . . . . . . . . . . . . . . . . . . . . . .
- Does the child want his/her own way most of the time? . . . . . . . . . . . . . . . . . . . . . . . . . .
- Does the child take a leadership role? . . . . . . . . . . . . . . . . . . . . . . . . . . . . . . . . . . . . . .
- Does the child take a follower's role? . . . . . . . . . . . . . . . . . . . . . . . . . . . . . . . . . . . . . .

**Candidate's signature** . . . . . . . . . . . . . . . . . . . **Supervisor's signature** . . . . . . . . . . . . . . . . . .

**Notes** . . . . . . . . . . . . . . . . . . . . . . . . . . . . . . . . . . . . . . . . . . . . . . . . . . . . . . . . . .

. . . . . . . . . . . . . . . . . . . . . . . . . . . . . . . . . . . . . . . . . . . . . . . . . . . . . . . . . . . . . .

. . . . . . . . . . . . . . . . . . . . . . . . . . . . . . . . . . . . . . . . . . . . . . . . . . . . . . . . . . . . . .

. . . . . . . . . . . . . . . . . . . . . . . . . . . . . . . . . . . . . . . . . . . . . . . . . . . . . . . . . . . . . .

Figure 6.4 An example of a child observation sheet

| Pros | Cons |
|---|---|
| Observers see what people actually do, not say that they do | Observers may miss important behaviour while note-taking |
| Subjects studied in their natural environment | Secretive observation leads to significant ethical problems |
| Can detect behaviour that subjects are unaware of | Inferences drawn from observed behaviour can lead to serious misinterpretations, so a poor way to look at values and beliefs |
| Can look at group behaviour and interactions between members | Lack of control over the sample observed limits broader applicability of results |
| May be the only suitable method with non-literate subjects, e.g. small children | |

Table 6.5 Some pros and cons of direct observation

## Using direct observation in a research project

Direct observation is a research method that is often used in combination with others. As we saw in the last section, observers can detect behaviour that participants are unaware of, but they are also capable of misinterpreting what they have seen. On its own, observation has major weaknesses if used for anything more complex than counting heads. If other methods are also used to confirm or illuminate the observations it can be a useful research tool.

You need to organise your observations to make them useful. As usual this begins with the research question and the population it concerns. Thinking about these things should help you to decide what behaviour you are going to be looking for. Observers are not trying to record everything that they see. They begin with a research plan that demands certain data and set out to collect only what they need. This means that you should think about what you are going to look for and devise ways of noting it easily. An observation checklist can be drawn up so that you can easily record incidents that fit your data needs.

You may decide to look at other things like body language, or how relaxed participants appear to be, if you think this data is relevant to the participants and the context of the interaction you are observing. The observation checklist can include anything that you feel is necessary. However, using a checklist in a live interaction might be very difficult if it is too complex. If you expect to be participating in most of the

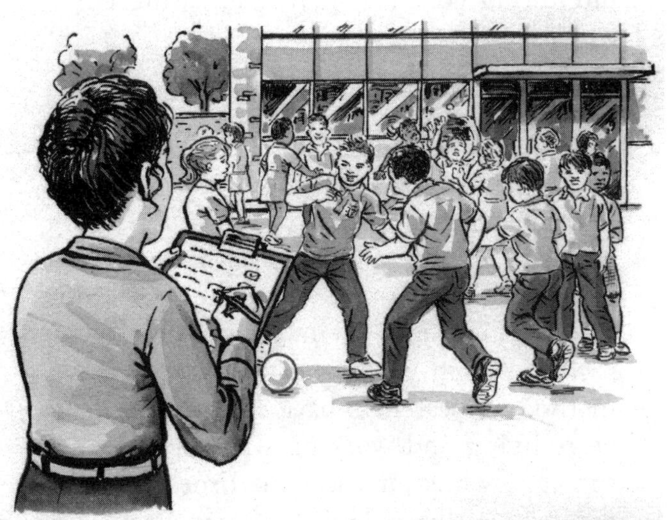

interaction it may be impractical to try to keep notes, even if they are merely ticks in a column when a particular behaviour is observed.

You could use a video recorder to tape the interaction, and play it back with your checklist in front of you. Now you will have plenty of time to note interesting observations in detail, and better still you can replay them if you are not sure what you saw. Remember that ethical standards demand that you must get your subject's permission before using video equipment. If anyone objects then you cannot use it. Also do not expect a video to pick up everything. You may not be able to film the whole group wherever you place the recorder, and you will have to rely on your own notes to record anything it misses.

When writing up your research report try to be honest about the quality of observational data. Do not assume that because you did not record seeing something it did not happen. Try to relate your observational results to data gathered by other means. For example, do your observations on levels of participation agree with the views expressed by the participants themselves? You may be able to draw interesting conclusions by comparing data in this way.

### Participant observation

Participant observation means that the researcher becomes part of the group being studied. There is probably no better way of really getting to understand the way groups work than to join them. Several classic social research projects have involved this method. Researchers have sometimes spent years living and working with their subjects, whilst at the same time recording data about them. This clearly requires dedicated professionalism, and a good deal of spare time. The commitment required puts participant observation beyond the scope of most researchers. Nevertheless there are several strengths to the technique.

The data provided by participant research is likely to be very valid. Researchers are living alongside the respondents and can see things from their point of view. There is little danger that serious misinterpretations will occur. Researchers can get to know their subjects so well that a valid picture of their values and opinions can be built up. Participant observation can produce excellent qualitative data.

Participant observation may also be the only way to study some groups. For example, people who are homeless and sleeping rough may only open up to someone who has become a familiar part of their world. Other groups, like gangs, may be so hostile to outsiders that participant observation is the only way to get close to them. This sort of social science is not for the faint hearted.

The main limitation of participant research is the time and commitment it demands. In addition to this, participant researchers need special skills if the study is to remain objective. It is all too easy to get sucked into the world you are now a part of. This can mean that things are only seen from the subjects' viewpoint. Researchers have to remain detached while being fully involved. Involvement can mean that only unusual events are noticed and recorded. Valuable background data may be unnoticed because it is now such a familiar part of everyday life for the researcher.

Where the researcher is so fully bound up in the life of his or her subjects it is certain that they are influenced by the researcher to some degree. The effects of this depend very much on the skills of the researcher, and how the research is being conducted. Some researchers reveal themselves to the group and seek acceptance as a harmless observer. This makes it much easier to take notes, and gives an excuse for the occasional probing interview. Others may try to pass themselves off as ordinary group members, and must thus scribble their notes in secret whenever they get a chance. This sort of secretive observation has its ethical difficulties. Is it right to record people's private lives in detail without their knowledge, particularly if you intend to publish the results?

Participant observation can lose quality because the researcher is not fully accepted by the group. A researcher may be kept on the fringes of the group's activities and never really find out what is going on. Observers may not be aware that this is happening and report what is observed as the whole picture.

### Using participant observation in a research project

The discussion of participant observation above mentioned the time and commitment needed to join a new group and develop an understanding of the members. This is certainly true if you have no connections at all with the subjects of your enquiry. However, you are already a member of many groups. You could include your family, your close friends, or your fellow students in a list of groups that you belong to.

It is possible to look at the behaviour or opinions of people you know and the data could be useful to you. But there are dangers in using family and friends as a data source. One problem is that of your own objectivity. Your existing relationships with the group members, as well as your role and status in the group, will affect your views of what you see and hear. This is a major problem for experienced social

| Pros | Cons |
|---|---|
| Can produce very valid and accurate qualitative data | Researcher needs time, commitment and high order social skills |
| May be the only method possible with closed or hostile groups | Researcher needs skills of objectivity and detachment |
| Little likelihood of serious misinterpretations of data | Researcher's influence on group behaviour almost inevitable |
| | Observers may be unknowingly ignorant of important aspects of group behaviour |
| | Secretive participant observation leads to serious ethical difficulties |

Table 6.6 Some pros and cons of participant observation

scientists working among complete strangers, so imagine how difficult it could be for you to remain objective among people you know well.

Another problem is that you could easily run into ethical difficulties. If you intend to try to shift from group member to observer you must tell the other members that you are doing so and ask their permission. If anyone objects you must abandon the method. Failure to do so is not only ethically wrong but could jeopardise your personal relationships. Confidentiality can be another problem, and you must be careful how you report your observations in order to make sure that it is preserved.

You may find that members of a group you belong to have no objections to your recording their views for a student research project. Your research must be organised and you need to be certain about what you are setting out to observe. You may want to instigate discussion on the ideas you are interested in so that you can collect the data you need. This also has the advantage of making it clear to the group when you are observing and when you are an ordinary member. It might make your relationships difficult if people are not sure whether you are 'on duty' or not. To record the data you could make notes and you could, with permission, tape the session. The data you are gathering will be qualitative. Good data may take the form of quotable passages which sum up a person's views in their own words.

Where you are working with subjects who are so close to you it is particularly important to make sure that they are happy with the way you have reported your findings. You should show your report to all the people concerned before you finalise it. If anyone objects then be prepared to make changes, or even abandon it altogether.

### Think it over

Go back to the research questions you listed for the activity on page 424. For each one, assess whether either interviews or observation would be appropriate methods of research. Once you have decided, list your reasons for your choice, giving the pros and cons of the method for each one.

## Research tools and techniques

This section looks at some of the techniques and resources used in health and social care research. It covers **sampling** methods, and questionnaire design.

### Sampling methods

Whatever research technique is used, researchers must decide who to collect information from. The term **population** is used to describe the total number of people that the research is interested in. For example if you are researching the attitudes of students towards smoking then your population would include all students.

Unless the population is particularly small, only vast projects like the government's census can survey all or most of their population. Therefore a smaller group, a **sample**, must be selected for questioning. Sampling methods have been developed to help make the sample as representative of the whole population as possible. This means that the proportions of people with different characteristics in the sample should reflect the proportions in the population as a whole. The sample should be a 'representative cross section' of the population being studied. This is particularly important to researchers seeking quantitative results, who want to apply their findings convincingly to the whole population.

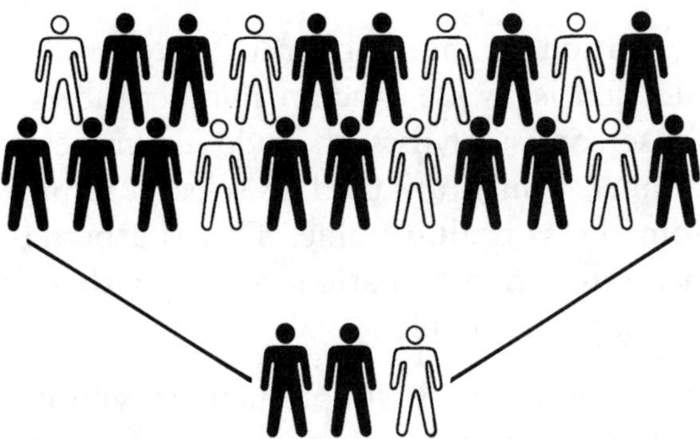

**Figure 6.5 The sample should be as representative of the whole population as possible**

Careful sampling is crucial if quantitative results are to claim broader applicability. Even if research is qualitative, subjects still need to be chosen. This is sampling of a sort, although being representative is seldom such an issue. All researchers should be able to explain how their sample was selected, and how representative it is likely to be.

How big should a sample be? To be representative it needs to contain a similar range of people to the population being studied. Very small samples run the risk of missing important groups. Social researchers want their sample to reflect the spread of things like age, gender, ethnic group and class background. The spread of such characteristics within a population is called **variance**. Some populations have much more **variability** than others. For instance, children in the same class at a primary school serving a local estate will have a lot in common. But variance among the passengers travelling on a bus is likely to be far greater. In practice, the size of samples usually depends on the researcher's resources. If you select as big a sample as you can manage then you have helped to make it representative and cover variance in the population.

> **Think it over**
>
> Think about the population concerned in a research project you are working on. What do you know about the variability in the population? You may know some things, such as age range within the population. Are there ways you can find out more?
>
> Variability in some areas may not affect your research whereas other areas are important. Are there personal characteristics that you know will probably affect the answers given by different members of the population? Can you list these characteristics? You need a sample big enough to cover important areas of variability in the population. How big a sample do you estimate that you would need to cover variability in your population?

## Random sampling

Even if samples are of a reasonable size it is possible for distortions to occur. If sample selection is left entirely to the choices of researchers then their own personal bias will be a problem. **Random sampling** methods are designed to eliminate the chance of personal bias influencing sample selection. Random sampling does not mean haphazard sampling. Rules of sample selection are strictly applied by professional researchers so that sampling errors can be calculated and stated mathematically. Of course, other factors such as interviewer bias, or poorly designed questionnaires, can influence and distort results in ways which are difficult to estimate. But if random sampling methods are used then at least errors due to sample selection can be precisely estimated.

Basically, random sampling means that a group is selected randomly from the whole population. All members of the population must have a measurable chance of being selected. Where all members of the population have the same chance of selection the method is known as simple random sampling. To begin random sampling the researcher needs to have a sampling frame. A **sampling frame** is a list containing the names of people from which a sample is to be drawn. It is important that the sampling frame provides complete coverage of the population. If the sampling frame is incomplete then some members of the population can never be selected, and the principle of randomness begins to break down.

A sample can be selected from the sampling frame in different ways. One method is known as **systematic sampling**. Names are picked at regular intervals from the sampling frame until the required size of sample is obtained. All members of the population must have a chance of selection and it is important that the size of the interval allows this to happen. For example, if the sampling frame has 1000 names, and you want to select a sample of 100, then you need to select every tenth name. This will give you a sample of the required size. The number of the first name picked also needs to be randomised.

There can be problems with the systematic sampling method. Sampling frames are usually acquired by researchers, seldom created by them from scratch. Most lists are not at all random in order. Many will be alphabetical, and some are grouped in other ways. In our example above, a list which is grouped in sets of ten would give a very biased sample. You could try to randomise the sampling frame before systematic sampling. However this is a long process, and introduces the problem of how to make the list truly random.

A solution to the problem of systematic selection is to use random number tables. These consist of lists of randomly chosen numbers which are used to select a sample from the sampling frame. This is a better method than systematic sampling although it takes a bit longer.

One problem with simple random sampling is that a biased sample may be chosen by chance. For example, suppose the population consists of 500 males and 500 females. It is quite possible, although extremely unlikely, for a random sample of 100 to be entirely composed of one sex, giving seriously biased results. A larger sample size does not guarantee balance, unless the whole population is selected. To overcome this **stratified random sampling** may be used.

### Stratified random sampling

Stratified random sampling is a way of making sure that important groups are represented in a sample. The sampling frame is split up into groups that need to be represented. Random methods are used to select a proportion of the sample from each group. In our example the sampling frame is split into two lists: one containing 500 males, and one containing 500 females. To get a sample of 100 subjects we randomly select 50 males and 50 females. Our sample is sure to reflect the gender balance in the population and has still been chosen randomly.

The method described above is an example of *proportionate stratified sampling*. The proportions of each group chosen for the sample were the same as their proportions in the population. If the population had consisted of 600 males and 400 females we would have chosen 60 males and 40 females to get our sample of 100.

Sometimes groups within the population may be small but are still important to the research. For example, a day centre may cater mainly for able-bodied people, but have a few disabled clients. Proportionate stratified sampling may allow only one or two disabled clients to be selected. The sample will thus fail to represent fully the views and needs of an important group. Disproportionate stratified sampling can be used to get over this problem. The researcher deliberately weights the proportions of different groups in the sample to include greater numbers of small but important groups.

Stratified random sampling is an improvement on simple random sampling but has some drawbacks. To stratify a sampling frame you need some prior knowledge of the groups within it. Unless the list contains extra information you may have to guess which groups people belong to. If you only have a list of names to go on, even guessing who is male or female can lead to mistakes. Apart from this, going through a sampling frame and identifying groups and proportions is a long process.

Another problem is that you could choose to stratify by characteristics which are not useful to your study. For example, you may stratify according to gender but not according to age. Later you could find that important differences of opinion occur between age groups. It is difficult to know how to stratify a population, even if it is possible to do so.

Both simple and stratified random sampling need a sampling frame. The problem is getting hold of a suitable list. Records kept for many purposes may be useful as sampling frames, but most are also confidential. Even if you do obtain a suitable list there is no guarantee that it is accurate and complete. Also it may be ordered in ways you are unaware of, making systematic sampling liable to bias. There are populations for which it is impossible to find or create a sampling frame. Then other sampling methods have to be used.

| Pros | Cons |
|---|---|
| Aims to ensure that results can be generalised to whole population | Researcher must be able to obtain a sampling frame |
| Sampling errors can be assessed and quantified mathematically | Simple random sampling may still give a biased sample |
| Stratification can ensure the inclusion of small but important groups | Implementing random sampling methods can be time consuming |
| Stratification can minimise the chance of selecting biased samples | Stratification requires you to have prior knowledge about the proportions of different types of people in the population |

**Table 6.7 Some pros and cons of random sampling methods**

## Quota sampling

Suppose you are interested in people's opinions about a new health education exhibition at a local hall. In this case, where members of the public come and go as they please, it is impossible to draw up a suitable sampling frame for your population. The best way to find a sample is to hang around the exhibition exit. You simply stop and question some of the people who come out. This sort of sampling has the advantage that the sample can always be ensured to be of the desired size. If there is a problem with no response from one person you simply ask another. The major problem is that the selection of the sample members is entirely at the interviewer's discretion. Interviewers may pick people who they like the look of. They are likely to avoid those who they perceive as looking demanding or threatening. One way of dealing with this is to introduce some controls on who the interviewer can choose.

**Quota sampling** is a type of stratified sampling, although it is not a random sampling method since the final selection of the sample is left to the interviewer. In quota sampling interviewers must pick a specified number of people from certain defined groups. For example, an interviewer might have to pick 50 men and 50 women for their sample. Quota sampling is much used for market research and **opinion polls**. Street interviews are the usual method, and interviewers have a quota of people in different categories to stop and question.

Quota sampling has several advantages:

- It is cheap and quick to do.
- There is no need to find a sampling frame and select a sample randomly from it.
- There is no problem with non response. If you need a particular quota of women with children you simply carry on until you have interviewed enough of them.
- Quota sampling gets quick results from a varied sample.

One problem with quota sampling is that it is not a random method. The final decision on who to talk to is left to the interviewer, and this introduces the problem of bias in selection. Even if interviewers must speak to a quota of people in a group their selection may still be biased. It may be easier to stop a parent with one child than one with four children to handle. Quotas of 'people over 65' are likely to under represent older members of the age group, particularly if interviewing is done in the street.

Most quota samples use gender, age and social class as the basis for setting quotas. Interviewers generally have no trouble identifying gender, and only a little more estimating age. However the identification of class by appearance is a risky business, likely to be heavily influenced by the interviewer's own perceptions and ideas.

Another problem is in drawing up the quotas for interview. Decisions can only be made if researchers have some prior knowledge of the population they are researching. This does not mean that a sampling frame is needed, but statistics indicating proportions of different groups in the population must be found.

Another important issue is where and when the sampling and interviewing takes place. If you interview in an upmarket shopping street it is likely that you will get a different type of sample than you would in a less prosperous area. If you interview on a midweek afternoon you are likely to miss working people. Unless you interview door-

| Pros | Cons |
|---|---|
| No need to obtain a sampling frame | Not a truly random sampling method |
| Refusals do not prevent the required sample size being achieved | Interviewer's choice will influence sample selection |
| Can be a quick method to implement | Quota setting requires prior knowledge of the proportions of groups in the population |
| May be the only way to sample views on an exhibition or event | Misses people who are difficult to bump into, e.g. people who are housebound or in hospital |

Table 6.8 Some pros and cons of quota sampling

to-door you will miss people who are housebound. In short, quota sampling misses people who are difficult to 'bump into'. Quota sampling is fine if you need simple approximate data from a section of the general public. It is less helpful if your population is more precisely defined.

## Sampling and observational research

The sampling methods we have looked at can be used to select subjects for self-completion questionnaires, for interviews or for experiments. If you decide to use observation as a research method you also have to make choices which result in sampling of a sort. Observation often deals with particular groups over time. Both group activities and group membership may vary at different times of the day, or week. There may be regular patterns to these changes that the observer is unaware of. For example, an observer who visits a nursery every day just after lunch will get a very biased view of the children's activity levels.

The timings of observations could be randomised to minimise distortions of this sort. Other types of observational study may be randomised in similar ways. The main point is that you should try to imagine what factors could introduce sampling bias into your observation, and attempt to deal with them.

The sampling method you choose will depend on who you are studying, and the resources available to you. Whatever method you pick try to think out your decision. Will your method give a biased result? Can you do anything to improve how representative and random your sample selection has been?

As a warning, consider the case of the disastrous poll carried out in 1936 by the American periodical *The Literary Digest.* The intention was to predict the result of the forthcoming presidential election between Landon and Roosevelt. A sample was chosen randomly from telephone directories and car registrations, and the result predicted an easy win for Landon. But Roosevelt won. The problem was that the sample was not representative of voters. Only the well-off had telephones and cars at that time. Poorer people were not asked and Roosevelt's popularity was seriously under-estimated. *The Literary Digest* claimed too much for their research. If you are aware of the problems that may have occurred due to your sampling method you can be more realistic about the accuracy of your own results.

### Think it over

You will need to select a sample from the population that you are researching. You need to think about the population and how you are going to make your sample as representative as possible.

- Think about the amount of variability in the population (see 'Think it over' on page 451).
- How random can you make your sampling? You will need a sampling frame to use random sampling methods, how could you obtain one or draw one up?
- What methods of sampling will you use? Will systematic random sampling be enough? Do you have enough information about your population to use stratified random sampling methods? Remember that careful sampling usually involves background research on the population and that this takes a lot of time and effort.
- Think about other sampling methods that may be suitable for your research. Would quota sampling be an appropriate technique to use?
- If you are thinking about doing observational research try to work out a schedule of observations that minimises bias. Can you observe at varying times to get as balanced a picture as possible?
- Think about the sort of errors that your chosen sampling method may give rise to. If you recognise and try to deal with these errors early on in your research you will add to the quality of your work.

## Designing questionnaires

This section is about how to write better questions and construct a questionnaire. It covers the following.

- **Open** and **closed questions**
- Measuring opinion
- Writing questions
- Question order
- Layout and presentation of self-completion questionnaires
- Designing a structured interview schedule.

*1 Open and closed questions*

Whether you intend using self-completion questionnaires or structured interviews you will need to create a questionnaire. The quality of your questionnaire largely depends on the questions it contains which need time and care which get to them right.

Question style is an important aspect of questionnaire design. There are two basic types of question: open and closed. Open (or open response) questions allow respondents to answer in their own words. Closed (or fixed response) questions ask respondents to choose from a set of alternative answers provided. Most surveys use both types of question.

**Open questions** can give very useful background data. Respondents do not have to choose between alternatives and can answer in their own terms. Open questions can be especially useful in a **pilot survey.** This is a small-scale trial of the survey proper which is intended to test the method and research tools to be used. Here open questions can indicate the sorts of things people regard as important to an issue, and help in the design of more relevant fixed response questions.

One problem with open questions can be that respondents' answers get rather lengthy.

In self-completion questionnaires answers can be limited by providing a restricted amount of space for them. The main limitation of open questions is that replies cannot be analysed statistically. Nevertheless they can be useful at the beginning of questionnaires as icebreakers, and they can be used to break up long strings of fixed response questions. Also they can be used to get people thinking about a topic, and establish a frame of reference before fixed response questions probe more specifically.

Fixed response questions restrict respondents to a choice between fixed alternatives. They can be used to collect data which is demographic or factual, such as gender, age group or religion. This data allows you to classify your respondents during the analysis stage and link, or correlate, their characteristics to their opinions. If quota sampling is used, demographic facts are vital to check that the respondent falls into a group you need to question. Responses to demographic questions can lead to a particular set of follow-up questions being asked. For instance *yes* answers to the factual question, 'Do you smoke cigarettes?' can lead to a set of questions specifically directed at smokers. This is usually known as **routing.**

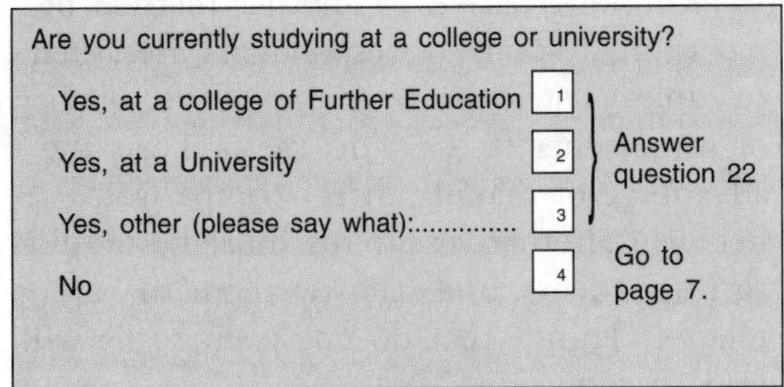
Are you currently studying at a college or university?

Yes, at a college of Further Education [1]
Yes, at a University [2]
Yes, other (please say what):.............. [3]
} Answer question 22

No [4] Go to page 7.

**Figure 6.6 This is an example of routing from the 1999 Survey of the Young People of Scotland. The options lead to further questions about studies after school jobs and training.**

Other fixed response questions seek data on opinions. There are different ways to design these questions, and the style of response required varies between them.

*2 Measuring opinion*

The most basic opinion question asks, 'Do you agree with . . .?', and allows respondents to choose between 'yes' and 'no'. Usually, however, it is better to allow more options so that strength of opinion can be indicated. Most opinion questions use some form of scaling or **ranking** method to allow differences between respondents to be measured more closely.

**Rating scales** are a way of measuring the strength of a person's opinion on an issue. A number of options, often five or seven, are offered for selection in answer to an opinion question. Options can be presented in a number of ways. They may be expressed verbally, say from 'strongly in favour' to 'strongly against', with tick boxes. Or it is possible to use a graphical scale with fixed points for respondents to indicate how strongly they are for or against.

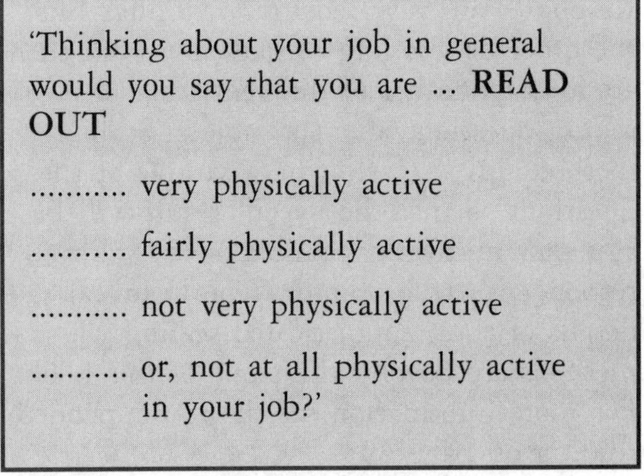
'Thinking about your job in general would you say that you are ... **READ OUT**

.......... very physically active

.......... fairly physically active

.......... not very physically active

.......... or, not at all physically active in your job?'

**Figure 6.7 This is an example of a rating scale from an interview schedule used in the 1998 Health Survey for England**

Please answer this question if you *currently* have a job or you are on a training scheme.
Otherwise, please go to question 38 on the next page.

| **Still thinking about this job (or training scheme), please tick a box to say whether you agree or disagree with each of the following.** | | Agree | Disagree |
|---|---|---|---|
| | I would leave this job (or scheme) if I could get a better job | ☐ 1 | ☐ 2 |
| | I will probably leave this job (or scheme) when I have got my qualification | ☐ 1 | ☐ 2 |
| | This is the kind of work I want to do in the future | ☐ 1 | ☐ 2 |
| | This is good experience and should help me to move on to something better | ☐ 1 | ☐ 2 |
| | This is the *only* job I have had since leaving school | ☐ 1 | ☐ 2 |
| | This job (or scheme) is teaching me useful skills | ☐ 1 | ☐ 2 |
| | The *main* reason I do this is for the money | ☐ 1 | ☐ 2 |

**Figure 6.8 This is an example of a sophisticated approach to scaling taken from the 1999 Survey of the Young People of Scotland**

The number of scale points offered can be odd or even. If an odd number is used, respondents can select a safe, middle of the road position. Respondents may cluster round this 'safe' option if it is available. An even number of options prevents respondents remaining neutral.

This form of rating scale is the most basic. Professional social researchers often use more sophisticated scaling methods, where responses from a group of questions are linked to give an overall view of opinion. Responses are very sensitive to things like the order or wording of questions, and there are a vast number of different ways of asking questions about a subject. Scaling methods involve selecting a sample of these questions so that the overall result will be as representative as possible of the respondent's true opinion. The technical details of these sophisticated scaling methods are beyond the scope of this book. For more information see the recommended reading on page 493.

### Grouped questions sets

You could use sets of questions to seek opinion on a topic from different angles. This prevents a small aspect of opinion from giving a distorted impression, which could happen if only one question was asked. For example, a respondent may say that he believes doctors to be very well qualified. He may nevertheless not believe in their ability to cure him. A grouped set of questions using a scaling method would reveal more accurately his lack of faith in doctors. You could try to design your questions so that different approaches are taken to the same subject. This allows a check of consistency of response, and helps to minimise the effects of badly constructed questions.

### Ranking order questions

Ranking alternatives is another method of recording responses. Respondents are asked to rank a list in order of preference, quality or some other factor. This method has the advantage of making direct comparisons between alternatives. Items must be familiar to respondents, and seen by them to be related. Things that do not seem to fit will lead to confusion.

Items can take a variety of forms. They could be statements, such as the different qualities associated with nurses. Here respondents could be asked to rank which qualities they thought most important, or items could be posts within the caring services, such as doctor or care assistant. Respondents could be asked to rank these in terms of the level of help they offer, or how hard working they seem to be. Ranking allows opinion on a linked group of items to be scaled, and is very useful when comparisons need to be made (Figure 6.9).

What features of this Day Care Centre do you like the best?

**(Please number the boxes 1 to 5 in order of preference)** (✓)

| | |
|---|---|
| Easy to get to | ☐ |
| Pleasant surroundings | ☐ |
| Friendly staff | ☐ |
| Meeting friends | ☐ |
| Good facilities | ☐ |

**Figure 6.9 An example of a ranking order question**

In this discussion we have looked at the styles of question that questionnaires can contain. The other important aspect of question design to be considered is the wording and content.

*3 Writing questions*

The quality of the questions is one of the most important aspects of survey design. All your careful planning is invalidated if the questions fail to collect the data intended. Unfortunately there are no strict rules to follow which will allows give good questions. There are, however, points to guide you which, together with your judgement, should make the job easier. Knowledge of your population, common sense and a pilot survey will all help you to write better questions.

One thing to decide is how many questions to include. Too many will exhaust the respondent, and the interviewer. Postal questionnaires are likely to suffer from a particularly poor response if they are too long or complicated. On the other hand too few questions will give very sketchy results. Try to strike a balance by thinking about your respondents. How long would they be prepared to spend on your questionnaire? How long will it take to carry out an interview? Guesswork can give you an idea of the answers, and a pilot survey will help refine them.

Question length is also important. Long questions should be avoided as they are likely to bore, and confuse respondents. If you seem to be producing long questions, try to split them into a number of shorter ones. Long questions may occur because you want to set the scene for respondents. You could get around the problem by using a

## Think it over

Think about an area of attitude or opinion that you need to collect data about. It could be for any of the research projects you will carry out during your studies where you intend using a self-completion questionnaire or structured interviews.

Try to think of a range of questions which you could ask that approach the attitude from different angles. Examine the list and make sure that there are no repetitions or questions that go off the point. All the questions in the set need to complement each other. Your question set can use a scale to allow respondents to indicate the strength of their opinion on each question in the set. Pre-coded number values in the scale give numerical scores for strength of opinion on each question. Combining a respondent's scores for the whole question set gives a value for strength of opinion on the issue which can be compared with that of other respondents.

general introduction and them asking several shorter questions around this theme.

Question content is crucial to the survey process. Respondents must be able to give answers to the questions they are asked. Questions about things that respondents have no knowledge of, or no opinion on, will produce worthless results. It is also important that questions are about subjects that respondents are willing to discuss. Even answers to factual questions can be biased by choice of subject. For example, responses to 'How often do you clean your teeth?' are likely to be biased in the direction of respectability. Opinion questions are even more likely to be affected by a respondent's willingness to answer on a particular subject.

Questions need to offer options which cover the full range of possible answers. Fact questions must have an option for every possible member of the population. For instance, if you ask 'How do you travel to college?' your options need to cover all possible modes of transport. You should always add an option for 'Other ....', for those whose response you failed to predict.

Another aspect of option choices is exclusivity. This means that respondents belong exclusively in one category, and are not left confused about which box to tick. The question above may have a problem with exclusivity. What about people who use both bus and train to travel? The need to cover all possible options may lead to a long list being created. In interviews this can lead to respondents forgetting earlier items, and inaccurately picking one they can remember in order to save face. A solution to this is to have a card containing the options which is given to the respondent as the question is read out. This is known as a prompt card.

The wording of opinion questions needs to be looked at carefully if bias is to be minimised. Questions must be specific. If you ask 'How would you rate the service in this canteen?' some respondents may have difficulty in answering. They may think that some staff give good service whereas others do not. They may think service is good at lunch times, but poor during morning breaks. A more specific set of questions would get a more accurate, and fuller, response. Wording needs to avoid being vague. Questions like 'Do you use this canteen often?' leave the respondent to decide what often means. The frame of reference of the question must be spelled out in specific terms.

Your questions must not make presumptions about the respondent. For example, if you ask elderly people 'Do you find it easy to live on a state pension?' you are presuming that they have no other source of income. Answers could often be a guess about how easy others may find it. Some respondents may be offended. You can insert factual questions to identify people who fit a particular category, if you need to ask particular questions of them.

Wording needs to be easy for respondents to understand. This means that language should be kept simple and non-technical. Try to avoid using an uncommon word when one or two simple ones would do. For example: use 'end' instead of 'terminate', 'worker' instead of 'practitioner', 'say' instead of 'state', 'need' instead of 'require'. There is nearly always a simpler way of expressing something. Clarity can also be obscured by confusing use of double negatives. The question, 'Do you think that not having enough money never affects people's quality of life?' is fairly difficult to understand. It is easy to reword it so that the double negative does not appear.

Wording also needs to be unambiguous. All respondents must understand the question in the same way. For example the question, 'Is work important to you?' is very ambiguous. Does it mean important in financial terms, or is it asking about personal attachment to a job? Is it about paid work, or about work in a more general sense? The same word can mean different things to different people.

Questions must not lead respondents into giving a particular answer. If you ask, 'You don't think that the health service is improving, do you?' you are obviously leading the reply. Questions can also lead in more subtle ways. If you ask, 'Do you think that social workers should get involved in people's private lives?' you are suggesting that they are being nosy rather than developing caring and supportive involvement. Leading questions can be difficult to spot. Try to examine the wording for signs that a loading, or value, is implied. Ask others how neutral the question sounds.

An important issue in question wording is that respondents should not find questions embarrassing or threatening. This can apply to factual as well as opinion questions. For instance, questions on income may seem threatening, and some respondents may find information about age or disability hard to give.

Opinion questions may be perceived as threatening if they touch on sensitive subjects. One problem is predicting which areas respondents are likely to find sensitive. Once again, a pilot survey with open questions will help. Sometimes threat can be reduced by careful wording, or by projecting the opinion onto someone else. For example, asking retired people, 'Do you feel less fulfilled now than when you were working?' is fairly threatening. You could change the question to, 'Some people find that they feel less fulfilled during retirement than when they were working. What do you think could cause this feeling among them?'. A follow-up question can ask whether respondents feel themselves to be a part of that group, and is now less likely to offend.

An important influence on how people respond to sensitive subjects is the way they are presented in the questionnaire or interview schedule. This brings us on to the issues of question order, layout and presentation.

### Think it over

Look at the questions that you have written for a questionnaire you are designing. Use the following checklist to assess the quality of your questions.

- Are there too many, putting respondents off, or too few to get the data you want?
- Will your subjects know the answer?
- Will they be willing to give the answer?
- Are any questions long and confusing?
- Do any questions make presumptions about respondents?
- Is each question specific enough to avoid ambiguity?
- Have you used wording that all respondents will understand?
- Are there any leading questions?
- Are any questions threatening or embarrassing?
- Do the options available cover all possible answers?
- Are the options offered mutually exclusive? (i.e. Could someone need to choose more than one option?)
- Do some questions need a prompt card?

Use this checklist before finalising your questions, and revise any that fall below standard. *Remember that your research will only be as good as the questions you ask allow it to be.*

*4 Question order*

The way you order and present your questions can influence the responses you receive. There are no strict rules on question order, but there are guidelines to help improve the quality of responses in different situations.

Respondents in interview situations must be put at ease early on. This means that opening with a sensitive opinion question is usually a bad idea. Opening with a battery of demographic factual questions can also put respondents in a less co-operative frame of mind. It is generally better to put these items lower down in the schedule. You could start with an open question which introduces the survey topic in a broad, non-threatening way. This should stimulate respondents' interest in the questions that follow, and prepare them for the sort of answers that may be expected of them.

If quota sampling is being used it is important to collect some demographic data fairly early on. Everyone's time will be wasted if interviews are conducted with people who do not fit the quotas. Usually only a few details are needed to establish whether a person fits a category needed for interview. These can often be found by a combination of observation and a couple of brief introductory questions. It is always a good idea to explain to respondents why you need to ask demographic questions, whenever they appear. This will make your enquiry seem less intrusive, and may help to get more accurate answers.

The order of the bulk of the questions is very much up to the researcher. One common device is to begin with general questions on a topic, then gradually narrow down the field of enquiry. This is intended to focus respondents down onto a topic by taking them from the general to the specific. It is sometimes known as the **funnel method**. The idea is that respondents are prepared for the specific questions when they arrive because they have been gradually orientated towards them. They may thus be more prepared to divulge sensitive information, or consider threatening topics. Also, respondents' answers to later questions may be more accurate because they have had time to think out their opinions.

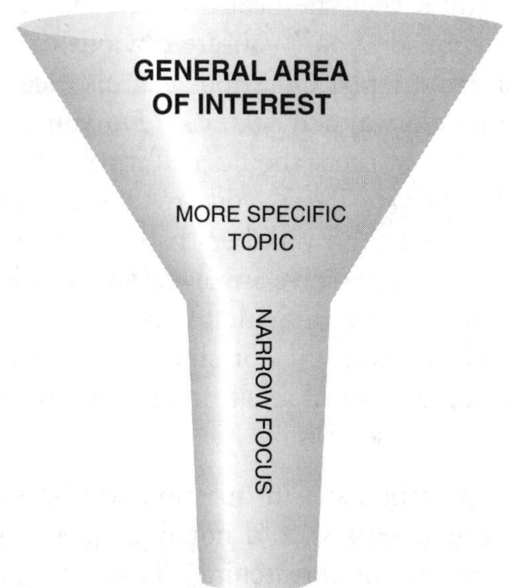


**Figure 6.10 The funnel method can bring your questioning to a focus**

There is another reason for putting general questions before more specific ones. Answers given to specific questions can bias answers to general questions which follow. People may have strong views of a particular aspect of a subject. If reminded of these by a specific question they may distort or exaggerate their response to questions about the subject as a whole.

Another point concerning question order is that perfectly good questions can become leading questions if they are badly placed. For instance, suppose you asked a string of questions designed to measure people's views on violence against children. If you followed these with the question, 'Do you think that police and social workers should be given more powers to deal with violence against children?' It is likely that some respondents will bias their answer because of feelings aroused by the preceding questions.

The way to eliminate sources of bias due to question order is by carefully reading through your questionnaire or interview schedule. A solution tried by some researchers is to randomise the question order for different respondents. However, this is time consuming and complicated to do. Also it does not attempt to eliminate bias. A randomised question order ensures that bias occurs with some, unidentified, members of the sample.

| **Try it out** | When designing your own questionnaire try to put questions in an order which minimises the problems mentioned above. Look at the questions you intend asking and order them with the following points in mind:<br>• Begin with easy questions that help set the context of the research.<br>• Do not begin with a battery of demographic questions, sprinkle them around the questionnaire.<br>• Avoid a question order which may lead respondents' answers<br>• Use the funnel method to focus on specific issues.<br>When you are satisfied with the order of your questions, show the whole questionnaire to other people and get their opinions on the content and order of your questions. Be prepared to make changes if this brings problems to light. |
|---|---|

*5 Layout and presentation of self-completion questionnaires*

Layout and presentation are particularly important with postal questionnaires. If they are cluttered or confused they will probably end up in the bin. Respondents must find questionnaires clear and easy to follow. They should also find them friendly. Introductions and directions that sound too scientific and formal can put people off.

You should always introduce your survey with an explanation of what the research is about and why you are asking them to respond by questionnaire. Failure to 'sell' your questionnaire at this stage may mean that a respondent never completes it. Keep the introduction short and simple, but try to convince respondents that the questionnaire is worth filling in and returning.

Questions should be clearly separated so that respondents have no difficulty making their way through them. Keep the layout neat and uncluttered to prevent confusion. Respondents must decide where their response to a particular question should be recorded. A clear layout should make it obvious which responses link with which questions.

Make sure that it is also clear how responses to particular questions are to be recorded on the questionnaire. If you use rating scales or ranking techniques you will have to explain how you want respondents to indicate their answers. Keep these explanations simple and brief, but make sure that they give clear and adequate instructions.

When planning the layout of questions and answers in your questionnaire you should remember that the respondent is not the only person you need to consider. If everything goes according to plan you will be receiving a large number of completed questionnaires, and will need to collate the data from them. Collating involves putting answers from different respondents together to build a picture of the overall response. If you lay the answers out clearly it can make this task much easier. It is made very much easier by the use of a computer, and this will help you towards the Information Technology Key Skills Unit. However you collate responses it is far easier and quicker if your pre-code the answers.

**Pre-coding** means assigning a number or letter to the possible responses for each question. For example you may code gender as simply M or F. Responses to a rating scale question could be coded 1 to 5, or however many are needed to cover all available answers. If pre-coding is not done the reply must be coded when the completed questionnaires are gone through, which is a much longer process.

**Some Scottish students sit English exams like GCSEs.**

Please tick *one* box to show how many *GCSEs* you have:

| | |
|---|---|
| None | 1 |
| 1 or more GCSE(s), *all* at grades D and below | 2 |
| 1–2 GCSEs at grades A–C | 3 |
| 3–4 GCSEs at grades A–C | 4 |
| 5 or more GCSEs at grades A–C | 5 |

**Figure 6.11 This is an example of a pre-coded question taken from the 1999 Survey of Young People of Scotland. Pre-coded questions are much easier to collate for data analysis**

The overall presentation of your questionnaire should be as professional as possible. People perceive professional looking documents to be more important than those which look amateurish. They are more likely to take your survey seriously if the questionnaire looks impressive. Your response rate is likely to be higher, which makes the research far more useful. The best way to produce a professional-looking questionnaire is again by using Information Technology.

One final point on postal questionnaire design is to remember to add a thank you at the end. Respondents need to feel motivated to return the completed form and a final word may help. You can use the opportunity to remind them why the

**Try it out**

You will have several opportunities to use self-completion questionnaires for carrying out research during your studies. The quality of your layout can be checked against the following list of recommendations:

- Include a brief, friendly introduction explaining the purpose of the research.
- Use a neat, uncluttered layout.
- Give clear instructions on how questions are to be answered.
- Make routing instructions easy to understand.
- Control the length of answers to open questions by limiting the space provided.
- Pre-code answer options to aid data analysis.
- Use IT resources to produce a professional looking survey document.
- Always add a thank you at the end, and perhaps a statement encouraging return of the questionnaire.

Check that any self completion questionnaire you create follows these guidelines. Poor questionnaires may well not get returned.

research is important and further increase the likelihood of getting a return. For example, if the survey is about services for the disabled you could end with 'Thank you for taking the time to fill out this questionnaire. Your answers will greatly help our research into services for disabled people'.

*6 Designing a structured interview schedule*
Structured interview schedules do not need such care in presentation as questionnaires, but layout is important if things are to go smoothly. A professional approach can again improve the quality of responses. Professionalism is likely to be judged on how smoothly the interview is conducted, and a well-organised schedule can help with this.

Interviewers must be able to keep track of the interview process. This may be straightforward when questions simply follow one after the other. But often interviews branch into different areas, depending on the responses given to certain questions. If you ask 'Do you smoke cigarettes?' you may have prepared a separate set of supplementary questions to ask smokers and non-smokers. Interview schedules can turn into complicated documents. It may be best to put questions belonging to a particular branch together on a separate sheet of paper. This way you can quickly flip to them, and return to the main run of questions when you have finished. Remember to include guidance notes, even if they are to yourself! It is all to easy to forget where to return to when a branch of questions has been completed.

As with self-completion questionnaires, make sure that answers are clearly linked to questions and pre-coded. Try to make the schedule as easy to use as possible. Do not forget to allow sufficient space for recording answers to open questions. You could also leave space for your own comments to collect qualitative background data. It is best to use Information Technology resources to design and create your interview schedule. A printed schedule is much easier to follow. You can use effects like *italic* and **bold** to separate clearly interviewer instructions from things to be read out to respondents. This will make the document much clearer and easier to use.

... **READ OUT** ...

*'Have you ever had an electrical recording of your heart (ECG) performed?':*

☐ 1 Yes

☐ 2 No

**If Yes**

**PROBE** *'Where did you have it?'* **CODE ALL THAT APPLY**

☐ 1 Hospital (in-patient)

☐ 2 Hospital (out-patient)

☐ 3 GP surgery

☐ 4 (Other)

**If No**
**Go to Question 14**

**Figure 6.12 This is a question from a structured interview schedule used in the 1998 Health Survey for England. The interviewer's instructions are in bold capitals and easy to follow. The coding and routing instructions are also clear.**

Prompt cards may be used to make respondents aware of the possible answers to a question. The interviewer can read out the options, prompting a respondent to choose one. Sometimes, however, it is useful to write prompts on a card which is handed to the respondent for them to pick an option.

Prompt cards have been discussed in connection with questions having many options, where respondents may have difficulty remembering the list if it was read out. They are also useful where information is sensitive or threatening. For example, questions on income may seem threatening, particularly if asked in a street interview. Respondents can be given a prompt card with income groups listed on it and coded. They only have to answer with a code number which the interviewer notes down. This can seem far less intimidating than saying an income level out loud. Prompt cards are also useful for ranking type questions. Here respondents need to consider comparisons, and putting all the options in front of them will help you get more accurate results.

**Try it out**

When designing a structured interview schedule you should keep the following recommendations in mind:

- Make routing easy to follow so that interviews go smoothly and you do not get lost.
- Leave sufficient room to record answers to open questions.
- Pre-code answer options in fixed response questions.
- Allow space for your own observations and comments.
- Provide yourself with prompts that you may need.
- Create prompt cards where necessary.
- Use bold or italic highlights to separate clearly questions from interviewer instructions.
- Use IT resources to create a smart, easy-to-use questionnaire.

Try to design a structured interview schedule that meets all these points. Remember that you are going to have to use it in the field. A well-designed document will make the interviews and data analysis far easier to do.

# 6.3 Planning research, methods of analysis and validation

## The research process

All research projects, whether small or large scale, should follow the same basic process. Research begins with a question or hypothesis. The overall aims of the research stem from the issues raised by the chosen question. This should lead to the identification of links between the research and existing findings and theories, and thus to opportunities for secondary research.

The identification of the population concerned and the type of data to be obtained from them should follow from an examination of the research question. The research methods decided upon will be linked to this and should be justified with reference to the question, population and data required.

The next stage involves the design and creation of research instruments, such as questionnaires or structured interview schedules. Many research projects will use more than one research method to gather the data needed. A representative sample needs to be chosen from the research population using an appropriate sampling method.

The data collection now begins and the members of the sample are contacted and data gathered. The data collected must be collated and organised so that it is in a form that can be analysed.

The data analysis stage comes next. This usually involves statistical analysis although other methods may be used, particularly if qualitative data is involved. Conclusions are then drawn from the analysis, which need to be related back to the research question.

The research can now be evaluated. Problems that have occurred during the project are taken into account, and limitations of the research results can be assessed.

The last stage is the report itself. This should contain the conclusions that the researcher has drawn from the data collected. The style of the conclusions will depend on the purpose of the research project. They may include recommendations for action, or an assessment of whether the hypothesis has been disproved or not. Suggestions for further study should also be made.

Good researchers are as open as possible about their work, and the questionnaire, interview schedule or observational checklist will allow others to judge for themselves the quality of the methods used. The research instruments devised and used are usually attached to the research report as appendices.

## Research questions and research structure

All research begins with an area of interest. This may be discrimination, health and lifestyle, clients' feelings about the care they receive, or any other area relevant to health and social care. From this area of interest specific questions emerge. Questions may be about situations people are in, such as

| | |
|---|---|
| **Planning** | 1 Identify the research area and narrow it to a research question or hypothesis to be studied.<br>2 Review prior research in the area.<br>3 Identify the population the research concerns, and the type of data needed from them.<br>4 Decide upon appropriate research methods to gather the data. |
| **Collecting research data** | 1 Design suitable research instruments to gather the data, and plan how to implement them.<br>2 Select a representative sample from the population to collect data from.<br>3 Contact the sample and gather the data.<br>4 Summarise and organise the data in preparation for analysis. |
| **Analysis and interpretation of data** | 1 Relate the data to the research question and the research aims.<br>2 Draw conclusions from the data analysis.<br>3 Evaluate the research, assessing problems in execution and the limitations of the results.<br>4 Offer suggestions for further study in the light of the results. |

Figure 6.13 Stages in the research progress

'What percentage of households live on low incomes?', or 'What is the ratio of male to female students on the Health and Social Care course you are following?'. They may be about their behaviour, such as 'How many people watch football on television?' or 'What percentage of students on your course smoke cigarettes?'. Questions may be about their beliefs and opinions, such as 'Do people think that the National Health Service is improving?' or 'Do young people believe that sex before marriage is morally wrong?'. The type of question you are interested in, and the people it applies to, will have a considerable influence on the planning and conduct of your research.

The research question will set the boundaries, or parameters, within which the work will take place. This means that you are able to define and clarify the area of study you are involved with. When you are clear about what you are looking at, it becomes possible to seek out work by other people that is relevant to your question. You can relate your research to existing findings and theories. This is important if you are to show that your research is serious and well prepared.

Research questions also set the parameters of hypotheses that researchers develop for testing. Most research questions can potentially yield many different hypotheses, and there are methods to help you uncover them which we will look at, below. However it is arrived at the hypothesis must address the research question at hand.

For example, suppose that you are interested in clients' experiences of health and social care provision, and particularly in the question of how older people feel about the care they receive. Within this question there are many possible areas of enquiry and further focusing down is needed before practical research can begin. You may come up with a number of possible hypotheses during this process. For instance, the hypothesis 'most older people attending the local day-care centre are satisfied with the care they receive there', might be one possibility. However, the hypothesis 'most older people using public transport are satisfied with the service they receive' would be rejected. It is not about health and social care services, and falls outside the parameters of the research question.

The research question may also suggest how you go about doing the research, and the type of information you need to collect. The first stage is to review prior research and do a thorough analysis of the secondary sources of information available to you. After that, a range of primary research methods are available and the question you are addressing is likely to indicate which are suitable and which are not. For example, long drawn-out interviews are not usually appropriate when studying young children.

Your research question may suggest likely sources of data to you. If you are interested in the number of disabled students attending a local college then the college's own records could be a good data source. If you are interested in the opinions of disabled people about the college then you need to get data directly from them. Most good research draws data from different sources so that background and context is provided for the results.

The research question itself is thus responsible for much of the structure of the research that addresses it. It defines the area of study, indicates relationships with existing theories and findings, sets the parameters of hypotheses, and suggests research methods and data sources. It is important to remember that research is not about collecting as much data as possible without considering why it is needed or what use it will be put to. Above all, research is a planned process which keeps the research question always in view.

## Developing a research question

The research question is the starting point of the research process. At first the question may cover a broad area which is too big to be dealt with. The question 'What perceptions do disabled people have about the health and social care services that they receive?' is interesting and important, but it is also extremely wide. To be able to answer with confidence you would need to check on all the possible options, or sub-questions, that the question contains. There are many sorts of disability, and many types of service, that people need to use. Perceptions about one service may be different to perceptions about others. After a few moments thought the range of permutations and combinations can be seen to be vast. The question needs to be narrowed down to something workable for research purposes.

Exploring the range of possibilities in a question is easier if you structure your approach to it. You can begin to 'unpack' the question by thinking about the range covered by each part of it. In our example you could begin by considering the range of disabilities that could be included, listing them on paper. Next you could think about the range of services that are available and list these also. Now the two lists could be related to each other. Looking at each entry in the list of disabilities in turn you could try to imagine which services may be particularly likely to link with it. For instance, you may have listed wheelchair users on the one hand and homecare services on the other. It is possible that some wheelchair users get help around the home from homecare services and you could indicate a link there. You should end up with many links between the two lists.

Now you need to make some decisions about which links to develop. It is probably best to choose links that are clear cut, or that you already know something about. You should also think about the ease with which you will be able to get data. The subject you pick will imply a particular population for your work, and the accessibility of the population is important whatever research method you eventually use. Bearing this in mind it should now be possible to make a list of the possible questions that could be written around the links you have made.

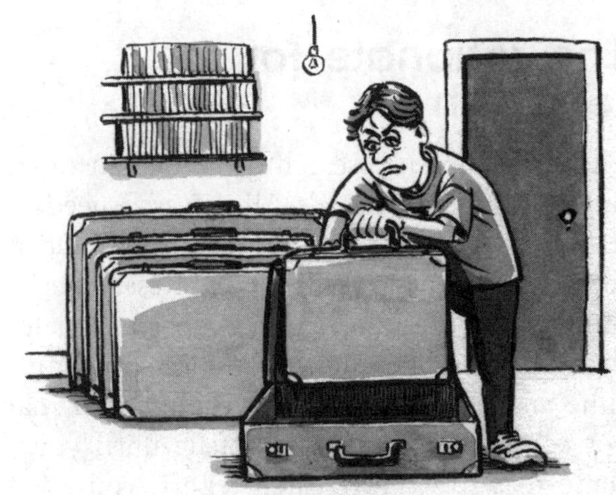

**'Unpacking' a research question takes time but is well worth the effort**

Each potential research question in the list can now be checked in detail by repeating the methods we have discussed. Further 'unpacking' may show that the subject is still too broad, or that the population is still too large, to be easily sampled. Eventually, a list of workable questions should emerge from which you can pick a specific research question to work on.

How far you take the unpacking process will depend on how wide you want your research project to be. In principle you could carry on unpacking until you have questions which cover a minute area of interest. You should stop when common sense indicates that you have a question that is within your scope. Further unpacking will now lead to lists of areas about which you need to gather data when carrying out your research.

Often the research question will be stated as an *hypothesis*, a statement which can be disproved or supported by the research results. There should be clear indications of the population concerned, and of course they need to be people that you can easily contact.

## The rationale for the research

The final chosen research question can now be considered in detail. All research needs to have a rationale: that is, a purpose and a set of reasons for taking place. Researchers must check that they have a clear rationale for their research question before spending time and effort on it. Even though you may not compose a detailed rationale until you come to write the research report, you should be sufficiently aware of the issues to confirm to yourself that it is worth proceeding.

One thing to consider is the original purpose of the research. Has the unpacking process drifted away from the reason why research was decided upon in the first place? You need to be able to state what it is that the research is now going to try to find out. Associated with this is the importance of the research to your own goals. Why is it useful for you to research this particular question? You should think about these points seriously before embarking on the considerable effort that research can involve. If you are not certain that the research question will serve the purpose then this is a good time to abandon it.

You should also think about who the audience for your research will be. Part of the rationale for the research should be an awareness of who is likely to be interested in the results. If you are not sure who the target audience is then the purpose of the research is not yet sufficiently clear. Another aspect of your rationale is the links that may exist between your research and other existing findings. The research question may have arisen through looking at other people's research, or you may have discovered them later through secondary research. If you know that the question has links with other work then this too establishes the purpose and context of your research.

Finally you should think about how widely your results are likely to apply. How far do you think the results of your research could be generalised to other situations and contexts? This may be a difficult question to answer precisely, but you should be able to suggest some possibilities. For instance, you might think that the results of your local enquiries could be relevant to the experiences of people in similar circumstances who live in other parts of the country.

A clear statement of the rationale for the research covering all these points should show precisely why the work is taking place, and demonstrate the value of carrying it out. You can then proceed without doubts that you might be wasting your efforts on pointless work.

| Try it out | |
|---|---|
| | You need to be able to describe the rationale for any research you undertake during your Health and Social Care studies. Research without a rationale is usually wasted effort.<br>Choose an area of your studies where you intend to do research and have a research question in mind. Think about the factors involved in the research rationale and check your ideas about each one. You need to think about:<br>• what the research question is trying to find out<br>• the relevance of the work to you, and your learning goals<br>• the intended target audience<br>• links with previous research<br>• the extent to which the results could be generalised.<br>Try to write a rationale for the research question which covers these points. If you are not sure that you have answers to each issue yet, think how you might work towards them.<br>You must have clear ideas about the rationale before you begin your research planning. All your research reports need to contain a description of the rationale covering each of the above points. |

# Analysing data

This section is about dealing with research data to produce conclusions, and ways of presenting your findings. It covers:

- analysing qualitative data
- analysing quantitative data
- statistical analysis
- making comparisons
- drawing valid conclusions.

When you have finished all your interviews, or collected in all your questionnaires, it is time to begin dealing with the data you have collected. You may have gathered data that is quantitative or qualitative, using any of the research methods we have discussed. Whatever form your data takes it needs to be processed before you can analyse what it might mean. You may have gained some initial impressions about your research results as you collected data, particularly if you used in-depth research methods. To find out if your impressions are supported by the data you need to organise it.

## Analysing qualitative data

Data that you intend to use towards your research needs to be relevant to the research question. With quantitative data collection methods you can make sure that this is the only data collected. Your questionnaire should aim to collect no more information than you need. However, with qualitative data methods the researcher has less control over the data coming in. This is particularly true of in-depth interview methods where respondents may have ranged into areas which are of great interest, but have nothing to do with your research question.

Interviews are frequently taped, and professional researchers may have them transcribed into print so that they are easier to examine and analyse. You will probably have to compromise and listen carefully through the tape yourself, pausing it and noting down passages that seem most useful to you. Your interview notes should help you with this, especially if you noted the time or tape counter number when interesting things came up.

You should not need to make a verbatim transcript but you must make sufficient notes to perform further analysis upon them. Also you should record verbatim any responses that could be quoted in your research report. It is wise to take down several quotes for each respondent, possibly covering different aspects of the issue. This will give you some choice later when you are more sure of what you need to use to illuminate your conclusions.

Further analysis of qualitative data from in-depth interviews requires imagination, and sensitivity to the meanings your respondents were expressing. You should try to sum up respondents' comments and opinions in a way that conveys accurately what they really think. Quotes used should clarify and establish your description of a respondent's views. At the same time you must relate these views to the research question, and to comments made by other respondents. You can use quotes to illustrate points of agreement, or otherwise.

Your analysis may seem to be more like reporting, but if you keep referring back to the relevance of the data to the research question a meaningful picture should emerge. You may find patterns which suggest further study. For instance, your subjects might have expressed similar views on a health and social care service that they all use. The conclusions that you draw will inevitably be difficult to generalise, but you should be able to claim that you have given a very accurate picture of your respondents' views.

Qualitative data may also have come from **semi-structured interviews**, or open questions in a structured interview or self-completion questionnaire. Here, responses are more controlled since the space for a response is limited and context is set by the surrounding questions. Subjects may still roam away from the point though, and you need to assess all qualitative data in terms of its relevance to the research question.

Short pieces of qualitative data using these more controlled methods should be easy to deal with. Semi-structured questionnaires may allow about around one side of a sheet of paper for each answer. Respondents may be aware of this and keep to the point. Also the interviewer controls what is noted down. It is usually good practice to try to record comments verbatim, that is word for word, since judgements about data should not be made in the heat of an interview. In practice you may find it hard to keep up with your subject and end up making decisions about what to jot down. This means that some, hopefully unneeded, data will be pruned out.

With fairly brief answers you can read through them and strike out any information that is irrelevant to the question. This leaves you with short pieces of useful qualitative data. You can use a similar approach to editing open questions in questionnaires, and here again short answers should minimise irrelevant data. Often open questions are seeking reasons for opinion expressed in a previous fixed response question so answers should be fairly specific and relevant.

With data from semi-structured interviews and open questions you can take a structured approach to data analysis. Here, you may expect respondents' answers to cover broadly similar points. If the questions asked were direct enough you should find that a range of possible answers emerges for a particular question. You can code the answers in order to get a much clearer view of the patterns in your subjects' responses.

Coding the results of open questions means drawing up a **coding frame** for the question. A coding frame is simply a list of all possible answers, with each one given a code. The difficulty is that each respondent's answer has to be read and judged to decide which code to apply. This process can introduce errors. Respondents will have expressed themselves in different ways, and you must use your judgement as to whether one answer means the same as another. The range of answers in your coding frame may not cover all the responses that you get. You need either to extend the range of the coding frame, i.e. add extra answers, or try to fit an answer into an existing slot.

In practice it is unlikely that all answers can be neatly pigeon-holed, and there is a practical limit to the length a coding frame can be allowed. A certain amount of approximation is likely to occur. The important thing is not to claim scientific accuracy for data that has been coded in this way. So long as you are honest about potential errors the procedure is perfectly valid. The results of your analysis can be examined statistically, and displayed on graphs or charts, using the methods outlined later in this chapter.

## Analysing quantitative data

The analysis of quantitative data may initially seem to be more of an arithmetic process than a creative one. You will be expecting this sort of data to demonstrate patterns or relationships numerically, and this means beginning to count and total the answers you have received. It is possible to do this using pen and paper, and until quite recently this was the only way. However, nowadays most researchers will use a computer to help with data analysis. You are expected to use information technology in your studies and research is a good opportunity to do so.

Whether you use IT or paper, the process of analysis begins with looking at each questionnaire form and listing the answers given for each question. You can summarise each respondent's answers into a list of codes. Hopefully, you will have been wise enough to pre-code the possible responses to each question and will find it easy to list the data in each questionnaire. If not you will need to code each answer as you go. Any open questions will need a coding frame so that you can assess and code respondents' answers.

As an example of *summarising responses* we will look at a fictitious questionnaire containing ten fixed response questions. Questions 1 and 2 are demographic questions. Question 1 asked for gender, coded 1 or 2. Question 2 asked for age, recorded in age bands coded 1, 2 and 3. Questions 3 to 10 had five coded fixed responses each, with an extra code for 'don't know'. Thus answers to these will be recorded as a code number from 1 to 6. The table below shows how the answers from three respondents have been summed up as rows of codes.

The same principles are used in computer-based analysis, and this method makes it much easier to quantify totals and relationships.

| Question number | 1 | 2 | 3 | 4 | 5 | 6 | 7 | 8 | 9 | 10 |
|---|---|---|---|---|---|---|---|---|---|---|
| Respondent 1 | 1 | 2 | 1 | 4 | 3 | 4 | 5 | 6 | 1 | 2 |
| Respondent 2 | 2 | 3 | 3 | 5 | 6 | 3 | 1 | 2 | 1 | 4 |
| Respondent 3 | 1 | 2 | 4 | 2 | 4 | 1 | 6 | 5 | 2 | 4 |

Table 6.9 An example of a table of coded results

When all the data has been taken from the questionnaires you can start to examine it. A good starting point is to look at the total responses for questions which are demographic or factual. How many men and women responded? What are the proportions of respondents in different age groups? These figures give a profile of the people who responded. They allow you to check whether your respondents were a representative sample of the population. Remember that even if your original sample was representative of the whole population, the people who actually responded from that sample may not be. Of course, if quota sampling was used you should already know the proportions of different people among your respondents.

The other set of totals you need are those for opinion questions. These will reveal how many people gave particular answers for each question. You can record numbers of people giving each answer and build up a picture of the way opinion differs within your sample. These totals, along with demographic totals, can be presented as tables. They can also be presented in graphical form as graphs or charts.

Although these totals are useful, the point of social research is usually to identify links between items of data. Your research question may indicate a need to do this. For example, suppose your hypothesis is 'Female students are more aware of the risks of smoking than male students'. To test the hypothesis you will need to link answers indicating awareness of the risks of smoking with the gender of respondents. The term used for linking responses in this way is **correlation.** In this example we are looking for a possible correlation between gender and smoking awareness. There are sophisticated statistical methods that can be used to give precise mathematical measures of correlation and significance. These methods are likely to be beyond your scope, but you can perform simple statistical analysis on your data to help you understand it better.

## Statistical analysis

When you have totalled the responses received you can begin a more detailed examination of your results. A good starting point for a closer examination of data is to draw up a **frequency distribution** diagram for the answers to each question. This is a graph which shows how often each answer has been reported. As an example, suppose we had asked the question 'Do you think that the caring services do a good job?'. We have allowed respondents to select an answer from a nine-point scale ranging from 'Agree strongly to 'Strongly disagree'. Our scale is coded from 1 = Strongly Agree to 9 = Strongly Disagree. We have received 50 answers from our sample and the results are as follows:

| Response | Number of answers |
|---|---|
| 1 Strongly agree | 2 |
| 2 | 4 |
| 3 | 6 |
| 4 | 9 |
| 5 Neutral | 10 |
| 6 | 8 |
| 7 | 6 |
| 8 | 4 |
| 9 Strongly Disagree | 1 |
| (Total responses = 50) | |

A table showing responses to the question 'Do you think that the caring services do a good job?'

A frequency distribution diagram for these responses would look like Figure 6.14.

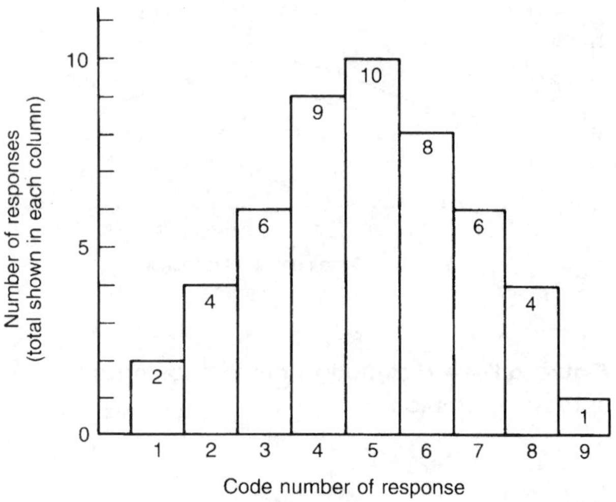


Figure 6.14 A frequency distribution diagram for responses to the question 'Do you think that the caring services do a good job?'

The data gives a roughly curved shape with a peak near the middle value, which indicates a neutral opinion on the question.

The number of answers tapers off towards each end of the diagram, indicating that extreme views are far less widely held. The shape of the diagram in our example is a familiar one in statistics. For many types of data a frequency distribution diagram will resemble a bell-shaped curve. It is so common that the shape is referred to as a **normal distribution curve**. A typical normal distribution curve is shown in Figure 6.15.

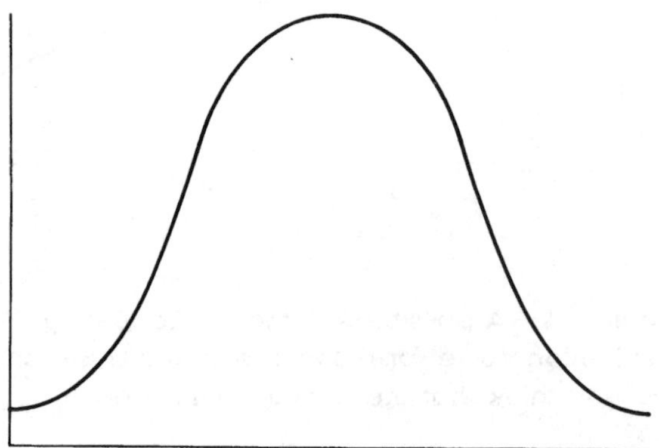

Figure 6.15 A normal distribution curve

All kinds of data give approximations to a normal distribution when plotted as a frequency distribution. Things like shoe sizes, income, or opinion, tend to follow the basic pattern. Most cases fall near the middle, and the numbers tail off towards the extremes. So common is the shape that researchers are alerted when a distribution fails to approximate to the normal curve.

The normal distribution curve has some very useful mathematical characteristics which can make data analysis easy and precise. These mathematical techniques are really a way of expressing quantitatively the messages that lie within the shape of the distribution curve for a particular set of data.

For instance, look again at the fictitious distribution of opinions on the caring services. The data could have been very different and we might have found that the distribution curve looked more like that in Figure 6.16.

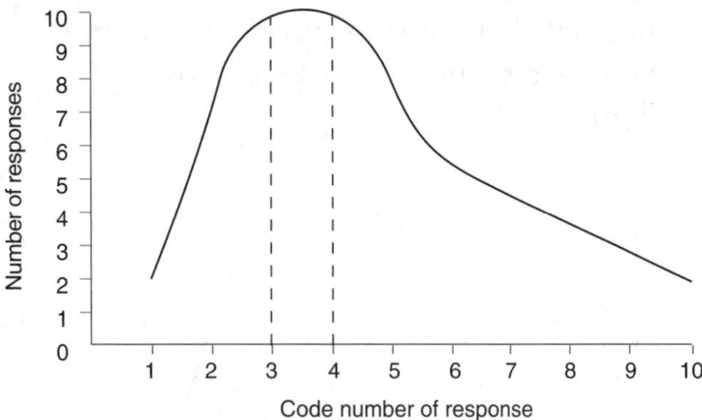


**Figure 6.16 A possible alternative frequency distribution curve for responses to the question 'Do you think that the caring services do a good job?'**

In Figure 6.16 the peak is over to the left of the neutral position. This indicates that opinion is clustered towards the 'satisfied' end of our response scale, which may be seen as an important finding. Other statistical measures can help us to clarify these implications.

- *The mean value*

One commonly used statistic is the **mean** value. The mean is simply the average of a set of data. To calculate the mean add together the values of all items in a set of data then divide the total by the number of items. The mean gives the point around which the data is clustered and can be marked on your frequency distribution diagram. In our example, the numbers 1 to 9 indicate the strength of respondents' opinions. Our first distribution curve (Figure 6.15) showed responses seeming to cluster around the neutral central position. The mean of this data is 4.94, which is very close to the neutral value of 5, and confirms our interpretation of the distribution curve.

In our second example (Figure 6.16), however, the curve was skewed over to the left-hand side. Calculation of the mean here would confirm our understanding of this distortion. Now the mean is likely to be somewhere between 3 and 4, indicating that people are inclined to agree that the caring services are indeed doing a good job. You have statistically identified the levels of satisfaction within your population.

- *Standard deviation*

However, the mean value is not always so useful. Look at the distribution curve in Figure 6.17.

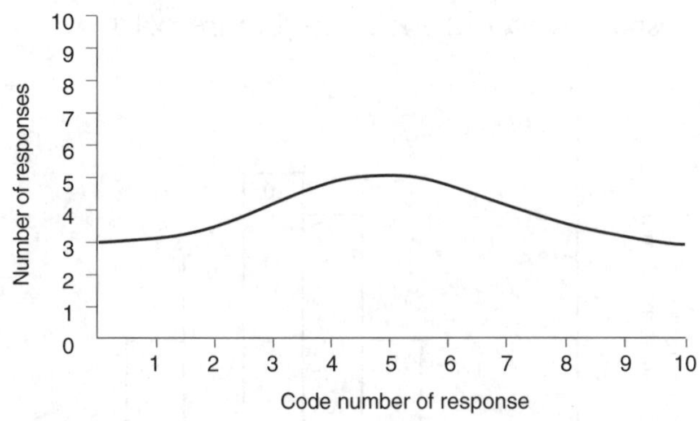


**Figure 6.17 A distribution curve showing a spread of opinion**

Here the curve is much flatter, which indicates that opinion is much more evenly spread across the range of possible views. It is easy to see that there is much less agreement in the sample on the question at issue. However, the mean value of the data could still be around 5, indicating neutral feelings. The mean only shows part of the picture. The shape of the distribution curve shows how people have deviated from the mean value. It gives a graphic view of the *variability*, or spread, of the results. You can see visually how much people's responses seem to have deviated from the mean. To get even more precision into your analysis you can use statistical methods to measure and quantify this deviation.

If data is normally distributed, or at least approximately so, variability can be shown by calculating the **standard deviation** of the data. Standard deviation is a way of showing how much the data varies from the mean. The size of the standard deviation indicates how spread out opinion on an issue really is.

To calculate standard deviation you need to measure the distance between each response and the mean value. Some data is higher than the mean and so gives a positive number. Other data is below the mean and so has a negative one. If you add all the deviations together the result should be zero, since this is how the mean is defined. To get positive numbers to work on, the deviations from the mean are squared, and these squares are then added together. This total is known, logically, as the sum of the squares. You are trying to find the average deviation from the mean so you now need to divide the sum of the squares by the number of data items. This gives the mean of the squares, also known as the variance. The standard deviation is the square root of the variance.

The calculations are not particularly difficult and can be made even easier if a computer is used. The point of finding the standard deviation is that you can now exploit some of the useful properties of the normal distribution curve. Fixed proportions of the curve fall within standard deviations from the mean. For example, 68.27 per cent of all responses fall within one standard deviation either side of the mean. Figure 6.18 shows the proportions of the curve that lie within standard deviations from the mean.

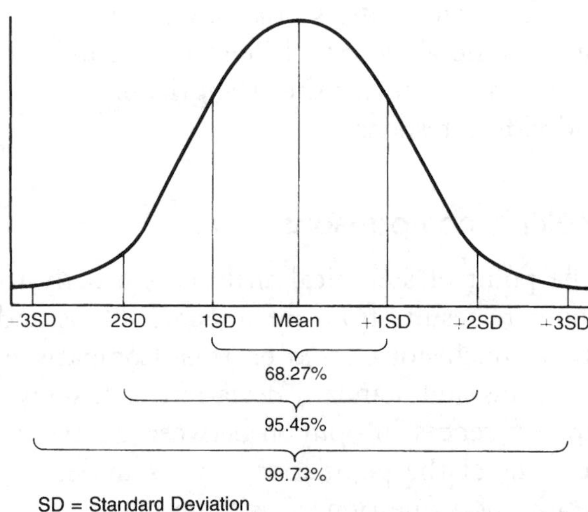


**Figure 6.18 Percentage proportions of a normal curve between standard deviations**

Standard deviation is often used to express probabilities associated with the data. You could say that there is a 68.27 per cent chance that an answer will lie within one standard deviation of the mean. To put it another way, you can say that there is a 68 per cent probability that an answer lies within one standard deviation from the mean, and a 99 per cent probability that it lies within three. Expressing your results in this way gives a statistical probability that future results will have a particular value. You have quantified your predictions based on statistical analysis of your data.

- *Median and mode*

Calculations of mean and standard deviation may not be necessary, or possible, for all your data. Other useful calculations are the median and the mode. If you have asked people to state their religion then the responses are not a measure of quantity or degree. Here it is more useful to take the **mode**, which is the most frequently occurring response.

Another statistic which is sometimes used is the **median**. This is the value which divides respondents so that an equal number lie above and below it. The median takes no account of the strengths of individual responses.

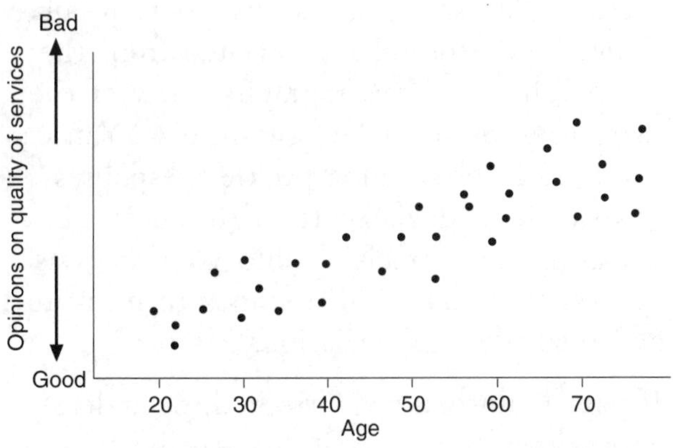


**Figure 6.19 A scattergram of age against opinion of the quality of health and social care services**

## Making comparisons

The point of statistical analysis is usually to compare results from different questions and draw conclusions based on this. Comparison of means and standard deviations can show up differences in opinion between different sections of the population. For example, results of a question on income may indicate that females have lower values for mean and standard deviation than males. This shows that on average women's pay was found to be lower than men's. It also implies that variability is higher among men, i.e. that women's income is more tightly clustered around the mean whereas men's income is more spread out across different income levels.

Another way of analysing data is to look for relationships between two variables. Suppose you are interested in the relationship between age and opinions on the quality of the health and caring services. If you plot a graph of age against opinion you could get results like those in Figure 6.19.

Each dot represents the age and opinion of an individual respondent. The graph is known as a **scattergram**. Here there seems to be a clear trend for opinions to become lower as age increases. A line of best fit would make the relationship more specific.

The relationship between the two variables is called correlation. If correlation was perfect all the points would lie on a straight line. There are mathematical techniques for finding the line of best fit exactly, and for expressing the degree of correlation shown by the data. These lie outside the scope of this book but more information can be found in the recommended reading at the end of the chapter. Often a correlation is fairly easy to spot. If, however, your scattergram shows a random pattern of dots it implies that there is no relationship between the variables you have chosen to plot.

You may want to compare different combinations of statistics in this way to check how groups in the population differ. Ideally you should have predicted which comparisons are relevant to the subject of your research. If you are researching with a hypothesis in mind then comparisons need to be related to it.

- *Sources of error*

Beware, however, because statistical analysis of your results can lead to errors and distortions. It is always possible that you have carried out the calculations incorrectly, although if you use a computer this risk is reduced. A more likely source of error is the way the statistics have been used.

One problem is misreading correlations between items of data. Correlations are often easy to identify, but difficult to explain or account for. You may find that a correlation seems to exist between two variables and wrongly assume that one is the cause of the other. There could be a third factor which is the cause of both effects. For example, there is a correlation between the number of leaves on oak trees and the amount of clothing people wear. This is not because oak leaves themselves bring about the wearing of light clothing, but because oaks bear their leaves during summer when the weather is warmer.

Another source of error when using statistics is **extrapolation**. This means extending your results beyond the range of your data, and attempting to predict what values a variable would have in extreme circumstances. The dangers of this can be shown by the scattergram in Figure 6.20.

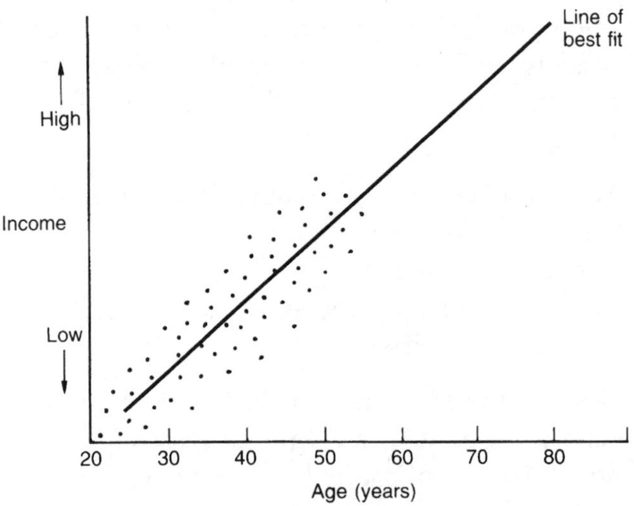


**Figure 6.20 A scattergram of age against income showing the dangers of extrapolation**

In Figure 6.20 the relationship between age and income has been plotted for people between the ages of 25 and 60. If the line of best fit is extended beyond the range of the data, it seems that most people are on a very high income indeed by the time they reach 80 years of age. In fact, we know that this is not the case, and income usually drops off sharply after retirement. Extrapolation is a very hazardous process. You should check your ideas carefully against other data, and in the light of common sense.

## Drawing valid conclusions

Analysis of your quantitative and qualitative data will help you to interpret what you have found out. The point of collecting and analysing data is to draw conclusions about the research question you began with. Now you need to consider the implications of your results for that question. It may be that all the results seem to agree and you feel fairly confident about declaring what your research has shown. More often, however, you will find that some results indicate one thing whereas other results indicate another.

Perhaps one section of your population seems to have different opinions to the rest, or people's feelings about different aspects of an issue are varied so that clear conclusions are hard to state. Do not feel that your results should always lead to definite conclusions. You must be prepared to conclude that the results do not allow you to give a clear answer to your research question, if this is what your data analysis indicates. The point is to make sure that the conclusions you do draw are supported by the data you have collected. The conclusion that further research is needed is a perfectly valid outcome.

The conclusions must also be clearly directed at the research question, and the purpose of the research. You may feel that your results allow you to draw conclusions about other things that lie outside the scope of your question. These findings can appear in your report, with suggestions that further research should be done. But remember that the main point of the report is to outline the relationship of your results to the research question, and the conclusions you are able to draw about it.

- *Sources of bias, inaccuracy and error*

Another point to consider is how confident you can be that your conclusions are accurate. Being honest about sources of error has been stressed in relation to all the aspects of the research process that we have looked at. Making valid claims for your data means being realistic about sources of error that may have occurred.

Errors can occur in the collection method. Was the method right for the population you are concerned with? Could you use it to collect the data that you wanted? If you used a postal questionnaire the number of responses you received is a good measure of the suitability of the method. A low response is a major source of error and should be indicated in your report. If structured interviews were used a likely source of error is interviewer-respondent interaction. These are very hard to estimate, but you should be able to remember how the interviews went. If respondents proved uncooperative, or you needed to use probes not written into the schedule, then it is likely that significant bias has occurred.

The collection tools themselves may have introduced errors. This may be shown by returned questionnaires that have obviously been misunderstood. Or your interviewing experiences may have revealed that certain questions simply do not work, needing many probes to get a relevant answer. Non-returned questionnaires can leave you guessing at the source of the problem. Was a questionnaire using the wrong approach, or were some of the questions too intrusive or confusing? Whatever the reason, non-returns represent a source of error in the results. Problems with interview schedules will be only too familiar to you by the time you have finished the field work.

Errors can also occur through the sampling process. There are ways of estimating errors when random sampling methods are used, although it is probably not worth calculating them for your research. For small samples such estimates are meaningless; and small samples are always prone to errors because they are not fully representative of the population. Representativeness can be checked by looking at the demographic balance among your respondents. Proportions of people within the sample should be available from your results, and can be compared with the profile a representative sample would have. Sometimes a sampling method is thrust upon you because no other is available. You need to consider how errors might have occurred through the method you ended up using.

Statistical analysis of your results can also lead to errors, as we have seen. It is possible that you have misinterpreted your results, or misused the statistical analysis tools that you have used.

Despite these points you do not need to report errors as a catalogue of disaster! All you need to do is briefly state the error factors that you are aware of, and estimate the possible effects of these factors on the conclusions you are able to draw. You need to state the confidence limits that surround

### Think it over

You need to think about the ways in which error or bias could have affected your research.

- How much did you know about your population when you began planning your research? Did you know enough to select a representative sample? Think about the limitations of the methods you used.
- How appropriate were the methods of data collection that you used? Think about the problems in data collection that you may have experienced. Do you think that they may have influenced the results?
- Were there response problems during your research? If you used self-completion questionnaires what was the response rate?
- In interviews were there many response errors, and perhaps more importantly did they seem to occur at the same point in the interview with different respondents? Did you need to deviate from the prepared set of prompts often, and what do you think the result of this might have been?
- Think about the accuracy of your data analysis. Did you use methods appropriate for the data? Are you sure that the conclusions you draw are backed up by the data you have collected?
- Think about these issues and note down your views on each point. Your list should indicate areas of uncertainty in your results but need not imply that they are unreliable. Try to sum up the overall effects of the sources of error and bias you have identified, and set them against the conclusions you draw. Can you make an estimate of the overall effects that errors and bias could have had on your conclusions?

your conclusions. In fact, few social researchers ever suggest that they are completely confident about the conclusions they have come to. They are aware of the many factors that can influence their results.

## 6.4 Presenting research

The research report is the culmination of all your hard work. It is therefore worth spending time to make the report as thorough and professional as possible or the care you took during planning, data collection and analysis will have been wasted. It is on the research report that the quality of your work will be judged by others. Use IT resources to produce your research report. Make sure that the language you use, and the style of the report are at an appropriate level for your target audience.

A research report generally follows a particular order.

A summary of the report structure we will look at below is as follows:

- title
- contents
- abstract
- introduction
- literature review
- objectives
- method
- results
- discussion
- conclusions
- recommendations
- bibliography
- appendices.

- **Title and contents**

The report is to some extent a catalogue of the research process. It begins with the *title* and a *list of the contents.*

- **Abstract**

Following this is an *abstract* of the report. An abstract is a very brief summing up of the research and its conclusions. You should aim for two to three paragraphs (less then 300 words). Try looking at the abstracts of other research reports to get some experience of how they should appear.

- **Introduction and literature review**

The *introduction* comes next. Here you can state your research question or hypothesis and the rationale for conducting research upon it. Following this you can review the literature surrounding the question. This will include the work you did during the secondary research phase of your project.

- **Objectives and method**

You can then deal with the *objectives* of your research project and your choice of *research method.* This means referring to the factors that influenced your decision to choose a particular research method, such as population characteristics and the nature of the research question. The sampling method you used can be briefly accounted for in the same way. You can outline how you implemented your data collection. This does not have to be a very full account of your experiences but should explain what procedures you followed, and what research tools you created and employed. Always attach a copy of your questionnaire to the report as an appendix. It will help readers to understand what you have done, and it is good scientific practice to be as open as possible about the tools used in research work.

Also include any comments you may have about possible sources of error that occurred in the data collection stage. This could form a brief 'how it went' section after your account of the procedures used.

- **Results**

Now you need to present the *results*. The way you do this depends on the research question and the data you wish to present. Qualitative data from in-depth interviews may be presented entirely in written form. You need to explain the threads that ran through the interview and relate them to the research question. You should attempt to sum up your respondents' views, and include quotes from them which illustrate the points that you are making. Provided that you keep to the point of the research question you have a lot of freedom in how you report this sort of data.

Quantitative data is usually easier to understand when presented in the form of charts and graphs. You should also show the data in a table to demonstrate how the charts or graphs are arrived at. Using IT methods you can quickly produce good looking graphics to display your results.

- **Discussion**

Of course, displaying your data is only part of the story. Your report must explain what

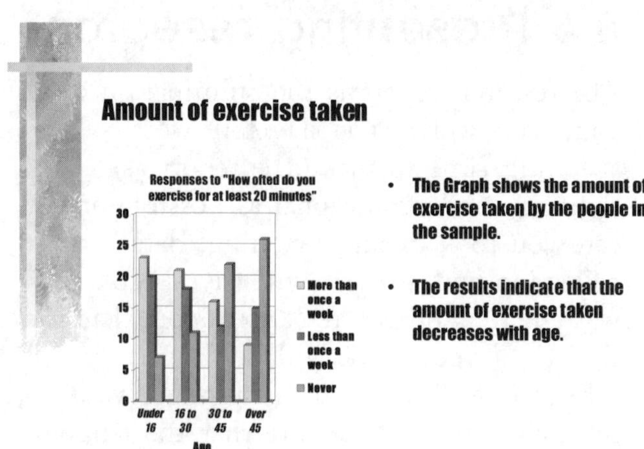


Figure 6.21 This graph is part of a PowerPoint presentation . . .

the data shows, and what conclusions you have come to in your examination of it. So now you need to *discuss the data* and show how you are led to your conclusions. You are summarising the thinking that led you to your research conclusions so it is important to be convincing. If you really believe that the data analysis has implied particular conclusions then you must explain why this is so. Use charts and graphs to help you make this point; remember that they are not an end in themselves.

- **Conclusions and recommendations**

A final summing up of your *conclusions* in relation to the research question should appear in this part of the report. You should also outline the *recommendations* that your conclusions lead you to make. These may concern a need for further research work that is indicated by your findings. There may be recommendations for practical action to deal with problems in the situation you have been looking at. Whatever form they take, your recommendations must be clearly linked to the conclusions your research has come to. Finally, consider how far your findings may be able to be generalised to other people and situations. Remember to be honest about the limitations of the methods you have used, and the errors that might limit the broader applicability of your results.

Your report should also include an account of the *ethical issues* that arose during your research. How you structure this is up to you. You could identify each issue in the part of your report which covers the stage where it occurred. Alternatively, you could have a section of the report devoted to ethical issues which discusses them in relation to the research project as a whole. However you deal with it, you must identify the issues and explain how you dealt with them.

- **Bibliography and references**

Finally, you should include a list of the references that you have consulted. You should use a standard referencing system throughout your report, such as the Harvard system. In the Harvard referencing system all sources that are mentioned in the report are listed at the end. The list is sorted alphabetically by the author's surname. When a source is referred to in the text of the report only the names of authors and the date of publication appear. For example the text of your report might say 'One of the disadvantages of postal questionnaires stated by Moser and Kalton (1971) is . . .'. Full details of the Moser and Kalton publication will appear in the list of references at the end of the report. The details normally include: author's surname and initials, date of publication, title, name of publisher. For the example given above the full details would be:

Moser, C.A. and Kalton, G. (1971) *Survey Methods in Social Investigation* Heinemann.

The appendix to your report can include a copy of your survey instrument, your covering letter if you used one, and any other research tools that you employed. The appendix can contain any documents that give background information about your research but which are not directly relevant to the main thrust of your report.

| **Try it out** | Investigate the IT resources that you will use to produce your report. Most software systems include a presentation package, for example Microsoft Powerpoint. Practise using the package to produce different displays such as charts and graphs. |
|---|---|

## Ethical issues

There are two main ethical issues involved in doing any research that involves collecting information from participants. The first is concerned with the effect of gender, race and culture on both researcher and participants. This may lead to a distortion of results, because these are influenced by the background and beliefs of the people involved. The second is the effect that being involved in research may have upon the participant. Causing harm or distress to participants is unacceptable and unethical.

All research is likely to encounter ethical problems of some sort. All researchers have their own opinions and outlook and it is impossible for these personal characteristics not to affect the research that they carry out. No social research is free from influence by the values of the researcher. The important thing is to be aware that ethical issues are likely to arise and to be honest in dealing with them.

## The effects of research on participants

Different methods of research raise their own ethical problems. As we have seen, ethical concerns are important and obvious in the application of observational methods. The use of two-way mirrors or hidden tape recorders by researchers is hard to justify. We would all wish to protect ourselves from becoming the victims of investigators using these sort of methods. However, ethical issues run through all social research and need to be considered seriously by researchers – whatever method of data collection they employ.

Social research deals with people, and there is considerable evidence to show that being the subject of research has an effect on individuals who are aware that this is happening. Some of these effects may be perceived as desirable by the subject. People may be flattered to be chosen as a sample member and feel that helping social researchers makes them special or important. If the research method involves a self-completion questionnaire or an interview it is possible to refuse to participate. Researchers are aware that non-participation by sample members will affect how representative the sample becomes. They will seek to persuade people to take part so that the scientific qualities of their research are maintained. The question is how far should researchers go with this persuasion to remain within the bounds of good ethical practice?

With self-completion questionnaires it is only possible to add a statement to the questionnaire form explaining the importance and relevance of the research in the hope that respondents will agree and go on to complete it. Adding statements which are threatening or intimidating is completely unethical, and could be regarded as unlawful!

Similar considerations apply to experiments and interview methods. Now the researcher is present to do the persuading, and this is one reason why interviews tend to get much better response rates than self-completion questionnaires. In fact, the ability of an interviewer to encourage participation is an important part of the selection process in professional research organisations. Again, however, the ethical issue is how far researchers should go to generate involvement. Lies or threats are unethical here too, and could be seen as threatening behaviour. People have a right to choose whether or not to become involved in a social research project and this right must be respected. Researchers can explain the importance of their work, and in fact should always explain truthfully what the research is

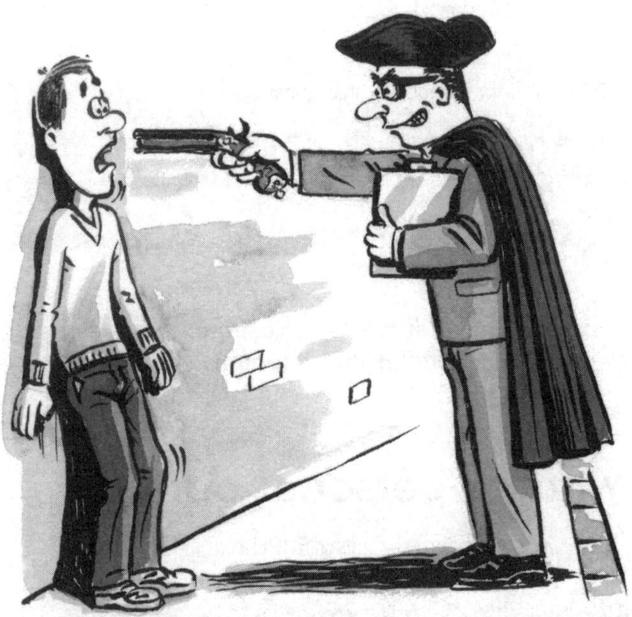

Persuading people to take part in research must keep within ethical boundaries

about. This may be enough to convince the slightly reluctant subject. Assurances about anonymity are also always necessary and may help a subject to agree.

If people still refuse, researchers need to be able to judge whether further discussion could be seen as unreasonable pressure. There is no simple guide to follow here, but perhaps putting yourself in the position of the reluctant respondent will help. Would you be happy to be on the receiving end of the persuasive techniques that you, as a researcher, intend to use? If the answer is 'no' then you should thank the person for their time and leave. A friendly, open and honest approach is the best way to find willing subjects, and data collected will be more accurate than that obtained through coercion.

Because observation can take place without subjects being aware of it, there is even more need to consider the ethics of the research. Much depends on the type of things being observed, and on the use to which the data will be put. If a researcher wants to collect data on the usage of a facility then counting heads may be the best way. Collecting this data may raise few ethical issues. But if the data being collected is more personal then subjects have a right to choose whether to participate or not. In practice it may be difficult or impossible to fully inform all subjects of your activities. In this case you may have to consider whether the research should carry on. If it seems that secretive observation will be the only way to deal with the research question, data and population that you are interested in then the research should be abandoned.

## Rights to confidentiality

Another ethical issue is the subject's right to confidentiality. Research reports should never identify the subjects personally, and should be written so that respondents cannot be identified. For example, if you are looking at a small group with easily identified members you must avoid giving clues about who gave what response to particular questions. If the group has only one male member then pointing to differences between the sexes clearly identifies how an individual responded and is unethical.

Researchers using participant observation have many ethical problems to face. It is likely to be a small group being studied, and the quantity of data gathered makes it hard to disguise who is being reported on. It is possible to be completely open about your intentions and seek the willing co-operation of your subjects. Although this may deal with the issue of a participant's rights to refuse to participate it still leaves open the question of confidentiality. Again, the research should be abandoned if it seems that confidentiality is impossible to preserve.

# 6.5 The Data Protection Act

The Data Protection Act (1998) is intended to safeguard people's rights when data about them is being collected and processed. You need to be aware of the principles of the Act since you will be collecting and processing data. The Act is particularly intended to address the ease with which information can be distributed with information technology, and if you are using IT resources to process data you need to be particularly careful.

The Act is implemented by the Data Protection Registrar's office and you can find out a lot more about how it works by visiting their web site.

The URL of the Data Protection Registrar's site is:

**http://www.dataprotection.gov.uk/commissioner.htm**

## Principles of data protection

Anyone processing personal data must comply with the eight enforceable principles of good practice. They say data must be:

1 fairly and lawfully processed
2 processed for limited purposes
3 adequate, relevant and not excessive
4 accurate
5 not kept longer than necessary
6 processed in accordance with the data subject's rights
7 secure
8 not transferred to countries without adequate data protection.

Thank you for completing this questionnaire

If you wish to receive a copy of the results of this research please tick this box ☐

**People who are subjects of research have a right to view the results of the research**

## What is personal data

The Act protects personal data. Personal data covers both facts and opinions about the individual. The Data Protection Act only covers the holding of personal data, that is data which relates to an identifiable living individual, the data subject, and which

- is being processed by computer or other automatic equipment
- or is recorded with the intention that it should be so processed
- or forms part of a relevant filing system or accessible record.

## Sensitive personal data

The Act introduces a new category of sensitive personal data. Sensitive personal data is any personal data whch includes information on

- racial or ethnic origin
- political opinions, religious or similar beliefs
- trade union membership
- physical or mental health

- sexual life
- the (alleged) commission of any offence, subsequent proceedings or sentence.

Sensitive personal data should normally only be processed if the data subjects have given their explicit consent to this processing.

## Information to be provided to the data subject

The 1998 Act imposes a new obligation to ensure fair processing by telling data subjects what is happening to their data. In simple terms, if we ask someone for data about themselves, we should tell them who will process the data, and for what purpose.

In practice you should not find that the Data Protection Act affects your research work too much if you follow the ethical principles of confidentiality that have been discussed in this chapter. If you try to ensure that the data you collect cannot be traced back to an individual respondent then you should avoid the problems that the Act is intended to deal with.

Subjects also have a right to view the results of the research and to comment of its outcomes. Self-completion questionnaires usually have a box to be ticked if respondents wish to see the results. The same consideration should be given to people agreeing to be interviewed. This can lead to difficulties if the research is carried out by street interview methods. Here the subjects are met in public and cannot be easily contacted to view the results. One simple solution is to offer subjects the opportunity to supply their address so that the results can be sent to them.

Research reports should include comments that respondents have made, and researchers need to allow time for these comments to arrive before completing their report. This is not only good ethical practice but could generate interesting and relevant observations on the quality of the results.

## The effects of gender, race and culture on research

A more subtle ethical problem concerns the way in which the researcher's own background can lead to presumptions and distortions in the analysis and reporting of data. All researchers carry with them their own cultural background and world view. They have attitudes and opinions just like everyone else. Social researchers need to be aware that this can lead to ethical difficulties. The danger is that researchers impose their own norms and values on the data they collect, and interpret the results in their own terms. This can distort the objectivity of the research and misrepresent the real meanings that lie behind their subjects' responses. Where there are significant differences between the culture of researcher and subject this may become an insurmountable difficulty. It is unethical to proceed with research in these circumstances. Imposing your own cultural values on the views of your subjects is arrogant, and leads to the production of irrelevant and unscientific results.

## Benefits of research

A final consideration in the ethics of research practice is the potential benefits of the research. This is sometimes set against the ethical issues outlined above, and used to justify continuation of the work when it may seem unethical to do so. There is a difficult moral problem here. Is it right to ignore the rights of the minority (the sample being looked at) if the majority will clearly benefit from the results?

Sometimes it is decided that society's need for information outweighs the rights of individuals. This is the case with the government's national census. This massive research project takes place every 10 years and legislation has been passed to compel people to respond. Other rights, such as confidentiality are, however, carefully preserved in the census reports.

Arguments about the benefits of research can be used to justify other, more contentious, research. For instance, secretive studies of deviant groups may claim that society's need to understand criminal behaviour allows researchers to disregard the rights of their subjects. Again this is a difficult moral area and judgements are not easily made. The general principle to be followed is that subjects' rights come first. Research which breaks this rule needs to have very exceptional reasons for doing so.

## Guidelines

Research organisations and professional bodies have published codes of conduct to guide their members in considering ethical issues. The British Psychological Society has produced 'Ethical Principles for Conducting Research with Human Participants'. These principles are intended to apply to all psychological researchers, from GCSE to postgraduate level. They cover areas such as participants' consent, researcher deception, confidentiality and the protection of participants from physical and psychological danger.

Another example is the 'Code of Conduct' produced by the Market Research Society. This code is intended to cover all market and social research. It is based on principles of willing co-operation of respondents, and their right to full confidentiality. It also covers the rights of children as research subjects.

These examples of published ethical guidelines are easily obtained and should be examined before any research project goes ahead. Details of how to obtain them are given in the suggestions for further reading at the end of this chapter.

| **Try it out** | Look up the 'Code of conduct' produced by the Market Research Society. Evaluate it from the point of view of researchers and participants in research. Is it clearly expressed and easy to understand? Write a brief summary with your own conclusions. |
|---|---|

# Unit 6 Assessment

For this unit you need to produce a report of a research project you have designed and carried out, and which is relevant to a health, social care or early years setting. Your report must show your skills in research and your understanding of research methods.

Your report must include:

- a rationale for the research, and the research methods you have chosen
- a review of what is already known in the area of your project
- an exploration of ethical issues that are relevant to your project
- a presentation of your findings and conclusions, including appropriate data and statistics, diagrams, charts and a bibliography.

## Ideas for achieving a grade E (a pass grade)

To achieve a grade E your work must show:

- an accurate description and application of an appropriate research methodology to a relevant issue in health, social care or early years
- a clear summary of what is already known in the area of your project
- an identification of the ethical issues that are relevant to your project
- the use of appropriate methods to present your findings.

To begin with you need to provide a suitable research question and a rationale for studying it. The rationale should show that your research is about an issue relevant to health, care or early years. You also need to provide a rationale for the research methods chosen; this shows that you have chosen an appropriate research methodology. You need to describe accurately how you have used the research methods in your work.

You must describe the results of your secondary research and reading around the topic of interest by providing a summary of what is known in the area. Remember to keep to information that is relevant to your area of interest. You must list the ethical issues that you have identified as relevant. At this level you need not go further than identifying the issues.

You must use appropriate methods to present your findings. This means using tables, charts, diagrams or text when they are suitable for the data being presented.

It is essential that you regularly review and monitor your research rationale, and that you provide evidence that you have done so. This means that you need to look back to the aims and purpose of your project as you carry it out, to make sure that you are not going off the track and losing sight of what you are trying to find out. The best way to do this is to carry out a regular review of your work and record the dates and results as a diary. You could note the work done so far and assess how it contributes to the aims of the project, and note down any issues that have arisen.

## Grade C

### Selecting a research methodology

For grade C your work will need to show that you have independently selected and applied an appropriate research methodology, and you will need to explain your decisions clearly. One way to provide evidence of these skills is to demonstrate that you have considered the advantages and disadvantages of using different research methods, including the ones chosen, in

| Research Question: *Do clients feel satisfied with the local meals-on-wheels service?* | | |
|---|---|---|
| **Method** | **Strengths** | **Weaknesses** |
| Questionnaire | Easy to produce and send out.<br><br>Can be answered in private. | Hard to get a list of client's addresses.<br><br>Clients may be reluctant or unable to complete and return them.<br><br>May not answer truthfully. |
| Structured interviews | No problem with uncompleted questionnaires.<br><br>Clients can be helped to understand questions and give the type of response required. | Time needed to carry out the interview.<br><br>Clients willing to be interviewed need to be found.<br><br>Difficult to select a representative sample unless demographic data about meals-on-wheels clients is known. |
| Observation | None | Will not provide useful data about people's opinions. |
| Unstructured interviews | Only a small sample needed.<br><br>Should allow real opinions and feelings to emerge.<br><br>Less need to worry about the selection of a representative sample. | Very time consuming, and intrusive for the client.<br><br>May provide data that is difficult to compare and analyse.<br><br>Results cannot be applied to the wider population of meals-on-wheels clients |

**Table 6.10 Strengths and weaknesses of different research methods as applied to a particular question**

order to study the question you are interested in. The tables of pros and cons for each research method that appear in this chapter could be used as a starting point.

You could draw up a table like the one below to show how the strengths and weaknesses of each method measure up when applied to your research question.

The table could be followed by a section which summarises the arguments for and against each method, and suggests which would be most effective. This would help to explain your decisions on research methodology.

## Reviewing research sources

For grade C you have to review the validity of your research resources and identify possible sources of error or bias in your own work that may have influenced your conclusions. This means that you have to go beyond summarising existing knowledge and look at the quality of your source material. The section on using secondary sources of data in this chapter should help you with this task. Try to categorise the data sources you use in terms of the headings given. Are they official statistics, or are they produced by independent researchers, or a pressure group? Look at the possible weaknesses of each source

| Stage | Methods used | Possible sources of error | Effect minimised by . . . |
|---|---|---|---|
| Primary data collection | Direct observation | a) Missing important behaviour<br>b) My presence influences subjects' behaviour | a) Attempting to watch a small number of subjects at once for manageable lengths of time |
| | | | b) Trying to stay in the background and remain |

**Table 6.11** An example of a 'Sources of error' checklist

and evaluate the ones you are using in the light of these points.

### Identifying sources of error

You also have to look at possible sources of error or bias in your own work. You could show evidence of this by drawing up a checklist of possible sources of error based on the stages of the research process that you have gone through. Look at Table 6.11 below as an example of how to do this.

Write the stages of your research process down the left column and your methods in the second one. Look at the sections in this chapter that deal with the method you are using and check the possible sources of error against your own work. In the third column list the sources of error that may have an effect at a particular stage, given the methods you have used. This shows that you are able to identify sources of error that could have occurred. In the fourth column write down the methods you have used to minimise the effects of each possible source or error.

Table 6.11 above shows an example of how part of a 'Sources or error checklist' could look.

You also need to evaluate the possible effect of errors on the overall research. You could provide evidence of this by a review of the effects your precautions seemed to have on the possible sources or error you have identified. Do you think your tactics worked? This summing up of the effects of possible sources of error should be related to your conclusions.

### Analyse the effects of ethical considerations

For grade C you need to go beyond an identification of ethical issues that are relevant to your project. Now you need to provide evidence that you have analysed the effects of these ethical considerations.

You should have thought about ethical issues as you designed and carried out your research. The list of issues that you have identified at each stage can be used as a starting point for collecting evidence here. Write down the ethical issues that you encountered as your research progressed and note how each was dealt with. Now consider how the action taken might have affected the outcomes of your research.

For example, suppose you are interested in people's behaviour in a care setting and are using observational methods. The most unbiased information could be obtained if the subjects were unaware that they were being observed. But it is unethical to collect data without the subjects' permission and awareness. This means that the subjects will know that they are being observed and therefore that their behaviour may be different from normal. You could note the possible effects of this ethical issue on the results of your observations.

### Presentation of findings

For a grade C your research report needs to present your research and findings accurately, clearly and coherently. The evidence of this is the overall quality of the report in terms of these factors. One way to make your report accurate, clear and coherent is to follow the advice in this chapter about designing and constructing a research report (see page 000). Make sure that you include information in each of the headings listed and that the logical process you followed is reported on appropriately.

## Grade A

### A comprehensive approach

For grade A you need to show evidence of taking a comprehensive approach to your research project. This applies to both the design of the research project and to the carrying out of the methods you have chosen. A comprehensive approach is one that includes everything needed, and leaves nothing out. To show evidence of this you need to ensure that you go about your research in a thorough way, following the principles of good practice.

You need to follow the procedures of the research process and demonstrate that at each stage you have worked carefully and thoughtfully, reviewing your progress and taking appropriate action to correct problems that arise. Most importantly, you need to provide evidence of having done this. A diary of the progress of your research project could help to demonstrate this work. You could review the contents of your diary when the project is completed, and write a commentary and evaluation of the research process you went through. This could help to show that your approach to the design and implementation of your research was thorough and comprehensive.

### Drawing conclusions

An important aspect of work at grade A is the quality of the conclusions drawn from the research. You need to draw conclusions that are realistic and valid, and you must be able to justify them with reference to your research work. This means that the conclusions you come to must follow from the results of your research and be tied to the research question. You must explain how the results suggest the conclusions you have come to, and show evidence that you are able to interpret the results.

Your conclusions should include recommendations for change. Your recommendations should be addressed to an appropriate individual or organisation and need to be based upon your research results.

You also need to suggest ways in which your research work might be improved. This means giving an honest appraisal of the limitations your research faced, and thinking about ways to do it better. Linked to this is the need to make recommendations for further research in your area of interest.

### Justify your choice of research method

For grade A you must justify your choice of the research methodology you used. This means that you need to explain how your research might have gone if different methods had been chosen, and how your findings might have been affected. Your evidence here should include an analysis of how other research methods could be brought to bear on the research question and how they might enhance or build on the methods you used.

## References and suggested further reading


Bell, J. (1993) *Doing your research project* Open University Press

Corston, R. (1992) *Research methods and statistics in the social sciences* Casdec Ltd

Dixon, B., Bouma, G., & Atkinson, G. (1987) *A handbook of social science research* Oxford University Press

Dooley. D. (1990) *Social research methods* Prentice-Hall

Dunsmuir, A., Williams, L. (1991) *How to do social research* Collins Educational

Hammersley, M (1993) *Social research. Philosophy, politics and practice.* Sage Pubs.

Hoinville, G., Jowell, R. et al (1978) *Survey research practice* Heinemann Educational

Jowell, R. et al (1994) *British social attitudes: The 11th report* Dartmouth Pubs.

Kidder, L. (1981) *Research methods in social relations* Holt, Rinehart and Winston

Langley. O. (1987) *Doing social research: A guide to coursework* Causeway Press

Moser, C.A., Kalton, G. (1971) *Survey methods in social investigation* Heinemann

North. P.J. (1980) *People in society* Longman

Oppenheim, A.N. (1992) *Questionnaire design, interviewing and attitude measurement* Pinter

Shipman. M. (1988) *The limitations of social research* Longman

Walker, R. (1985) *Applied qualitative research* Gower Publishing

'Ethical principles for conducting research with human participants' (British Psychological Society) in: Robson, C. (1994) *Real world research* Blackwell Publishers

Code of Conduct (for social and market research): The Market Research Society, 15 Northburgh Street, London EC1V OAH


## Relevant websites

**Centre for applied social surveys – CASS**
http://www.natcen.ac.uk/cass/docs/fr-casshome.htm

**CASS Question Bank**
http://qb.soc.survey.ac.uk/nav/fr-home3.htm

**Government Statistical Service – GSS**
http://www.statistics.gov.uk/

For information from GSS and others, http://www.statistics.gov.uk/stats/ukinfigs/ukinfig.htm

**The Office for National Statistics**
http://www.ons.gov.uk/

## Fast Facts

**Census** A vast social survey by the government every ten years. The census attempts to collect information from every British household.

**Closed question** A question which has a fixed set of answers pre-determined by the researcher to produce quantitative data.

**Coding frame** A list of the possible answers to open questions used to code responses.

**Correlation** Making links between separate groups of data. Correlation compares changes in one area to changes in another.

**Data** Information collected in the course of a research project.

**Demographic data** Data about respondents which is basically factual. Age and income group are examples of demographic data.

**Demography** The study of people in terms of their characteristics.

**Direct observation** A method of social research in which the behaviour of people and groups is watched. Direct observers do not become involved with the subjects.

**Epidemiology** The study of patterns of disease within a community or population.

**Extrapolation** Extending results beyond the range of the data to make predictions about other members of the population.

**Frequency distribution** A graphical method showing how often different answers occur. Frequency distributions often approximate to the normal distribution curve.

**Funnel method** A way of ordering questions in which general areas are covered first and more specific topics gradually introduced.

**Hypothesis** A statement which can be tested by research.

**In-depth interviewing** An interviewing method which has a loose structure. Respondents are encouraged to openly state their views.

**Interview schedule** A document used in structured interviewing to direct and control the process. A schedule contains the questions, and strict instructions for the interviewer to follow.

**Mean** The average value of a set of data.

**Median** The value that occurs in the middle of a ranked list of responses. Half the responses lie above the median, half below it.

**Mode** The mode is the most frequently recorded response in a set of data.

**Normal distribution curve** A bell-shaped curve which often results when frequency distributions are plotted. The mathematical properties of the normal distribution allow percentage probability statements to be made.

**Official statistics** Data collected by national and local government on a vast range of topics.

**Open question** A question which respondents answer in their own words. Open questions are often used to collect qualitative data.

**Opinion poll** A survey method intended to collect information on public opinion. Opinion polls often use street interviews and quota sampling techniques.

**Participant observation** A method of social investigation in which the researcher joins in with subjects and observes from the inside.

**Pilot survey** A test run of a survey which is carried out on a small sample. Pilot work is intended to help evaluate and refine methods.

**Population** The whole group that a survey or research project is concerned with. A population usually consists of people, although it can be other things such as households.

**Postal questionnaire** A research method where questionnaires are sent to respondents by post.

**Pre-coding** Giving a code to each available answer for a question. Pre-coding makes it easier to deal with the data during compilation of results.

**Primary data** Data that you have collected yourself. Primary research involves carrying out your own investigation to collect primary data.

**Probes** Comments designed to get further information from a respondent. Probes can help deal with response problems, and follow up lines of enquiry.

**Prompts** Statements made to respondents with possible answers to a question.

**Qualitative data** Data which cannot be expressed in numerical form. Qualitative data is descriptive, and is often about attitudes, opinions and values. Qualitative research methods seek this type of data.

**Quantitative data** Data which is expressed in numerical form. Quantitative research methods seek to collect this type of data.

**Questionnaire** A list of questions designed to collect primary data. Questionnaires are filled in by the respondents themselves, without an interviewer being present.

**Quota sampling** A method of sample selection where a population is stratified into types of people. Interviewers are given quotas of people to interview of each type.

**Random sampling** A method of choosing a sample which uses random methods to eliminate bias in selection.

**Ranking** A method of obtaining respondents' opinions of the differences between items in a group. Respondents rank the group in terms of the criteria set by the researcher.

**Rating scale** A method of recording answers to closed questions. Respondents indicate the strength of opinion by a scale point.

**Reliability** A property of research results. A result is reliable if it can be obtained again by the same research on another sample.

**Research** The process of finding things out in an organised and thoughtful way.

**Respondent** A person who provides data for a social investigation.

**Response rate** The proportion of sample members who return information. Postal questionnaires often have a poor response.

**Routing** Instructions included in self-completion questionnaires to indicate which question is to be answered next.

**Sample** A group chosen from the population on which research is conducted directly. Samples are intended to be representative of the population as a whole.

**Sampling frame** A list containing all members of a population from which a sample can be chosen.

**Scattergram** A graphical method of showing correlations between different sets of data.

**Secondary data** Data that has been collected by other people. Secondary research involves existing sources of information.

**Semi-structured interview** A method of data collection which uses a series of open questions. Semi-structured methods are less flexible than in-depth interviewing, but not as rigid as structured interviews.

**Standard deviation** A way of indicating the variability in a set of data. Fixed proportions of the normal curve lie within standard deviations of the mean.

**Stratified random sampling** A method of making a sample more representative. The population is grouped and a proportion of the sample picked from each group.

**Structured interviewing** A method of social research which uses tightly controlled interviews to collect data. Structured interviewing aims to minimise differences between each interview to help eliminate bias.

**Survey** An enquiry to collect primary data. Social surveys usually ask people questions.

**Systematic sampling** A method of choosing a random sample from a sampling frame. Names are picked at regular intervals from the list.

**Validity** A quality of research results. A result is valid if it accurately represents the view of a respondent.

**Variability** The degree of spread of a feature within a population.

**Variance** Within a research population the amount of spread of relevant characteristics.

# Index

The page numbers in brackets refer to Fast Facts